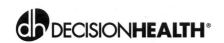

Plain English Descriptions for

ICD-10-CM

2016

2016 Plain English Descriptions for ICD-10-CM

Published by DecisionHealth
9737 Washingtonian Blvd., Ste. 2ØØ
Gaithersburg, MD 2Ø878-7364
www.codingbooks.com

Copyright © 2Ø15 DecisionHealth
All rights reserved

Please call 8ØØ.334.5724 for questions or technical support

Printed in the United States of America

ISBN: 978-1-58383-836-5

Item Number: MPB-PEDI10-16

Disclaimer

Acknowledgements

Tonya Nevin, *Vice President, Medical Practice Group*
Lori Becks, RHIA, *Clinical Technical Editor*
Lori Cipro, *Production Manager*
Juli Folk, *Books Manager*
Renee Dudash, *Senior Director of Operations*
Bethany Angleberger, *Desktop Publisher*
Bradley Clark, *Illustrator*

Contents

Introduction

The 2016 *Plain English Descriptions for ICD-10-CM* is a clinical diagnosis explanation for certain specially-selected and commonly used ICD-10-CM codes, written in plain English that is easily understood. Billing accuracy can be greatly increased when the user understands the medical relevance of the ICD-10-CM codes that are assigned for billing purposes, which can save both time and money.

Format

The *Plain English Descriptions for ICD-10-CM* is presented in a two column format using the same chapter and code category divisions used in the ICD-10-CM book. Page headers and individual page ends that identify chapter and code range provide a guide for quick reference. Three-digit categories with the official descriptions and appropriate rubric overview are presented first. Any fourth-, fifth-, or sixth-digit codes for which a clinical lay description at that particular code level is available are also presented, in chronological order, with their official descriptions in bold. Please note that code levels are not indented, nor is every available code within the ICD-10-CM system presented. Only those categories, subcategories, or codes for which additional, clinical lay information is being presented are listed in the book. Due to the size of the ICD-10-CM code system, it is not feasible to list every code with level indentations.

Where applicable, subcategories and subclassifications with their appropriate usage are identified under the rubric information. New and revised codes are notated with standard icon identifiers. A rationale pertaining to a code's incorporation or revision within the ICD-10-CM classification system is found in a separate text box under the clinical lay description. The *Plain English Descriptions for ICD-10-CM* also contains official coding guidelines, a listing of prefixes and suffixes found in general medical terminology, and anatomy charts.

The *Plain English Descriptions for ICD-10-CM* is not intended to be used for code selection. This reference book will be most useful if used in conjunction with an official ICD-10-CM book and a comprehensive medical dictionary. Using all of these resources in tandem will enable the coder to make the most accurate code selection.

ICD-10-CM Official Guidelines for Coding and Reporting

The Centers for Medicare and Medicaid Services (CMS) and the National Center for Health Statistics (NCHS), two departments within the U.S. Federal Government's Department of Health and Human Services (DHHS) provide the following guidelines for coding and reporting using the International Classification of Diseases, 10th Revision, Clinical Modification (ICD-10-CM). These guidelines should be used as a companion document to the official version of the ICD-10-CM as published on the NCHS website. The ICD-10-CM is a morbidity classification published by the United States for classifying diagnoses and reason for visits in all health care settings. The ICD-10-CM is based on the ICD-10, the statistical classification of disease published by the World Health Organization (WHO).

These guidelines have been approved by the four organizations that make up the Cooperating Parties for the ICD-10-CM: the American Hospital Association (AHA), the American Health Information Management Association (AHIMA), CMS, and NCHS.

These guidelines are a set of rules that have been developed to accompany and complement the official conventions and instructions provided within the ICD-10-CM itself. The instructions and conventions of the classification take precedence over guidelines. These guidelines are based on the coding and sequencing instructions in the Tabular List and Alphabetic Index of ICD-10-CM, but provide additional instruction. Adherence to these guidelines when assigning ICD-10-CM diagnosis codes is required under the Health Insurance Portability and Accountability Act (HIPAA). The diagnosis codes (Tabular List and Alphabetic Index) have been adopted under HIPAA for all healthcare settings. A joint effort between the healthcare provider and the coder is essential to achieve complete and accurate documentation, code assignment, and reporting of diagnoses and procedures. These guidelines have been developed to assist both the healthcare provider and the coder in identifying those diagnoses that are to be reported. The importance of consistent, complete documentation in the medical record cannot be overemphasized. Without such documentation accurate coding cannot be achieved. The entire record should be reviewed to determine the specific reason for the encounter and the conditions treated.

The term encounter is used for all settings, including hospital admissions. In the context of these guidelines, the term provider is used throughout the guidelines to mean any qualified health care practitioner who is legally accountable for establishing the patient's diagnosis. Only this set of guidelines, approved by the Cooperating Parties, is official.

The guidelines are organized into sections. Section I includes the structure and conventions of the classification and general guidelines that apply to the entire classification, and chapter-specific guidelines that correspond to the chapters as they are arranged in the classification. Section II includes guidelines for selection of principal diagnosis for non-outpatient settings. Section III includes guidelines for reporting additional diagnoses in non-outpatient settings. Section IV is for outpatient coding and reporting. It is necessary to review all sections of the guidelines to fully understand all of the rules and instructions needed to code properly.

Section I. Conventions, general coding guidelines and chapter specific guidelines

The conventions, general guidelines and chapter-specific guidelines are applicable to all health care settings unless otherwise indicated. The conventions and instructions of the classification take precedence over guidelines.

A. Conventions for the ICD-10-CM

The conventions for the ICD-10-CM are the general rules for use of the classification independent of the guidelines. These conventions are incorporated within the Alphabetic Index and Tabular List of the ICD-10-CM as instructional notes.

1. The Alphabetic Index and Tabular List

The ICD-10-CM is divided into the Index, an alphabetical list of terms and their corresponding code, and the Tabular List, a structured list of codes divided into chapters based on body system or condition. The Alphabetic Index consists of the following parts: the Index of Diseases and Injury, the Index of External Causes of Injury, the Table of Neoplasms and the Table of Drugs and Chemicals.

> *See Section I.C2. General guidelines*
>
> *See Section I.C.19. Adverse effects, poisoning, underdosing and toxic effects*

2. Format and Structure

The ICD-10-CM Tabular List contains categories, subcategories and codes. Characters for categories, subcategories and codes may be either a letter or a number. All categories are 3 characters. A three-character category that has no further subdivision is equivalent to a code. Subcategories are either 4 or 5 characters. Codes may be 3, 4, 5, 6, or 7 characters. That is, each level of subdivision after a category is a subcategory. The final level of subdivision is a code. Codes that have applicable 7th characters are still referred to as codes, not subcategories. A code that has an applicable 7th character is considered invalid without the 7th character. The ICD-10-CM uses an indented format for ease in reference.

3. Use of codes for reporting purposes

For reporting purposes only codes are permissible, not categories or subcategories, and any applicable 7th character is required.

4. Placeholder character

The ICD-10-CM utilizes a placeholder character "X". The "X" is used as a placeholder in certain codes to allow for future expansion. An example of this is at the poisoning, adverse effect and underdosing codes, categories T36-T50. Where a placeholder exists, the X must be used in order for the code to be considered a valid code.

5. 7th Characters

Certain ICD-10-CM categories have applicable 7th characters. The applicable 7th character is required for all codes within the category, or as the notes in the Tabular List instruct. The 7th character must always be the 7th character in the data field. If a code that requires a 7th character is not 6 characters, a placeholder X must be used to fill in the empty characters.

6. Abbreviations

a. Alphabetic Index abbreviations

NEC "Not elsewhere classifiable"

This abbreviation in the Alphabetic Index represents "other specified". When a specific code is not available for a condition, the Alphabetic Index directs the coder to the "other specified" code in the Tabular List.

NOS "Not otherwise specified"

This abbreviation is the equivalent of unspecified.

b Tabular List abbreviations

NEC "Not elsewhere classifiable"

This abbreviation in the Tabular List represents "other specified". When a specific code is not available for a condition the Tabular List includes an NEC entry under a code to identify the code as the "other specified" code.

NOS "Not otherwise specified"

This abbreviation is the equivalent of unspecified.

7. Punctuation

[ ] Brackets are used in the Tabular List to enclose synonyms, alternative wording or explanatory phrases. Brackets are used in the Alphabetic Index to identify manifestation codes.

( ) Parentheses are used in both the Alphabetic Index and Tabular List to enclose supplementary words that may be present or absent in the statement of a disease or procedure without affecting the code number to which it is assigned. The terms within the parentheses are referred to as nonessential modifiers. The nonessential modifiers in the Alphabetic Index to Diseases apply to subterms following a main term except when a nonessential modifier and a subentry are mutually exclusive, the subentry takes precedence. For example, in the ICD-10-CM Alphabetic Index under the main term Enteritis, "acute" is a nonessential modifier and "chronic" is a subentry. In this case, the nonessential modifier "acute" does not apply to the subentry "chronic".

: Colons are used in the Tabular List after an incomplete term which needs one or more of the modifiers following the colon to make it assignable to a given category.

8. Use of "and"

See Section I.A.14. Use of the term "And"

9. Other and Unspecified codes

a. "Other" codes

Codes titled "other" or "other specified" are for use when the information in the medical record provides detail for which a specific code does not exist. Alphabetic Index entries with NEC in the line designate "other" codes in the Tabular List. These Alphabetic Index entries represent specific disease entities for which no specific code exists so the term is included within an "other" code.

b. "Unspecified" codes

Codes titled "unspecified" are for use when the information in the medical record is insufficient to assign a more specific code. For those categories for which an unspecified code is not provided, the "other specified" code may represent both other and unspecified. *See Section I.B.18 Use of Signs/Symptom/Unspecified Codes.*

10. Includes Notes

This note appears immediately under a three-character code title to further define, or give examples of, the content of the category.

11. Inclusion terms

List of terms is included under some codes. These terms are the conditions for which that code is to be used. The terms may be synonyms of the code title, or, in the case of "other specified" codes, the terms are a list of the various conditions assigned to that code. The inclusion terms are not necessarily exhaustive. Additional terms found only in the Alphabetic Index may also be assigned to a code.

12. Excludes Notes

The ICD-10-CM has two types of excludes notes. Each type of note has a different definition for use but they are all similar in that they indicate that codes excluded from each other are independent of each other.

a. Excludes1

A type 1 Excludes note is a pure excludes note. It means "NOT CODED HERE!" An Excludes1 note indicates that the code excluded should never be used at the same time as the code above the Excludes1 note. An Excludes1 is used when two conditions cannot occur together, such as a congenital form versus an acquired form of the same condition.

b. Excludes2

A type 2 Excludes note represents "Not included here". An excludes2 note indicates that the condition excluded is not part of the condition represented by the code, but a patient may have both conditions at the same time. When an Excludes2 note appears under a code, it is acceptable to use both the code and the excluded code together, when appropriate.

13. Etiology/manifestation convention ("code first", "use additional code" and "in diseases classified elsewhere" notes)

Certain conditions have both an underlying etiology and multiple body system manifestations due to the underlying etiology. For such conditions, the ICD-10-CM has a coding convention that requires the underlying condition be sequenced first followed by the manifestation. Wherever such a combination exists, there is a "use additional code" note at the etiology code, and a "code first" note at the manifestation code. These instructional notes indicate the proper sequencing order of the codes, etiology followed by manifestation.

In most cases the manifestation codes will have in the code title, "in diseases classified elsewhere." Codes with this title are a component of the etiology/manifestation convention. The code title indicates that it is a manifestation code. "In diseases classified elsewhere" codes are never permitted to be used as first-listed or principal diagnosis codes. They must be used in conjunction with an underlying condition code and they must be listed following the underlying condition. See category F02, Dementia in other diseases classified elsewhere, for an example of this convention.

There are manifestation codes that do not have "in diseases classified elsewhere" in the title. For such codes, there is a "use additional code" note at the etiology code and a "code first" note at the manifestation code and the rules for sequencing apply.

In addition to the notes in the Tabular List, these conditions also have a specific Alphabetic Index entry structure. In the Alphabetic Index both conditions are listed together with the etiology code first followed by the manifestation codes in brackets. The code in brackets is always to be sequenced second.

An example of the etiology/manifestation convention is dementia in Parkinson's disease. In the Alphabetic Index, code G20 is listed first, followed by code F02.80 or F02.81 in brackets. Code G20 represents the underlying etiology, Parkinson's disease, and must be sequenced first, whereas codes F02.80 and F02.81 represent the manifestation of dementia in diseases classified elsewhere, with or without behavioral disturbance.

"Code first" and "Use additional code" notes are also used as sequencing rules in the classification for certain codes that are not part of an etiology/ manifestation combination.

See Section I.B.7. Multiple coding for a single condition.

14. "And"

The word "and" should be interpreted to mean either "and" or "or" when it appears in a title.

For example, cases of "tuberculosis of bones", "tuberculosis of joints" and "tuberculosis of bones and joints" are classified to subcategory A18.0, Tuberculosis of bones and joints.

15. "With"

The word "with" should be interpreted to mean "associated with" or "due to" when it appears in a code title, the Alphabetic Index, or an instructional note in the Tabular List.

The word "with" in the Alphabetic Index is sequenced immediately following the main term, not in alphabetical order.

16. "See" and "See Also"

The "see" instruction following a main term in the Alphabetic Index indicates that another term should be referenced. It is necessary to go to the main term referenced with the "see" note to locate the correct code.

A "see also" instruction following a main term in the Alphabetic Index instructs that there is another main term that may also be referenced that may provide additional Alphabetic Index entries that may be useful. It is not necessary to follow the "see also" note when the original main term provides the necessary code.

17. "Code also note"

A "code also" note instructs that two codes may be required to fully describe a condition, but this note does not provide sequencing direction.

18. Default codes

A code listed next to a main term in the ICD-10-CM Alphabetic Index is referred to as a default code. The default code represents that condition that is most commonly associated with the main term, or is the unspecified code for the condition. If a condition is documented in a medical record (for example, appendicitis) without any additional information, such as acute or chronic, the default code should be assigned.

B. General Coding Guidelines

1. Locating a code in the ICD-10-CM

To select a code in the classification that corresponds to a diagnosis or reason for visit documented in a medical record, first locate the term in the Alphabetic Index, and then verify the code in the Tabular List. Read and be guided by instructional notations that appear in both the Alphabetic Index and the Tabular List.

It is essential to use both the Alphabetic Index and Tabular List when locating and assigning a code. The Alphabetic Index does not always provide the full code. Selection of the full code, including laterality and any applicable 7th character can only be done in the Tabular List. A dash (-) at the end of an Alphabetic Index entry indicates that additional characters are required. Even if a dash is not included at the Alphabetic Index entry, it is necessary to refer to the Tabular List to verify that no 7th character is required.

2. Level of Detail in Coding

Diagnosis codes are to be used and reported at their highest number of characters available.

ICD-10-CM diagnosis codes are composed of codes with 3, 4, 5, 6 or 7 characters. Codes with three characters are included in ICD-10-CM as the heading of a category of codes that may be further subdivided by the use of fourth and/or fifth characters and/or sixth characters, which provide greater detail.

A three-character code is to be used only if it is not further subdivided. A code is invalid if it has not been coded to the full number of characters required for that code, including the 7th character, if applicable.

3. Code or codes from A00.0 through T88.9, Z00-Z99.8

The appropriate code or codes from A00.0 through T88.9, Z00-Z99.8 must be used to identify diagnoses, symptoms, conditions, problems, complaints or other reason(s) for the encounter/visit.

4. Signs and symptoms

Codes that describe symptoms and signs, as opposed to diagnoses, are acceptable for reporting purposes when a related definitive diagnosis has not been established (confirmed) by the provider. Chapter 18 of ICD-10-CM, Symptoms, Signs, and Abnormal Clinical and Laboratory Findings, Not Elsewhere Classified (codes R00.0 - R99) contains many, but not all codes for symptoms. *See Section I.B.18 Use of Signs/Symptom/Unspecified Codes.*

5. Conditions that are an integral part of a disease process

Signs and symptoms that are associated routinely with a disease process should not be assigned as additional codes, unless otherwise instructed by the classification.

6. Conditions that are not an integral part of a disease process

Additional signs and symptoms that may not be associated routinely with a disease process should be coded when present.

7. Multiple coding for a single condition

In addition to the etiology/manifestation convention that requires two codes to fully describe a single condition that affects multiple body systems, there are other single conditions that also require more than one code. "Use additional code" notes are found in the Tabular List at codes that are not part of an etiology/manifestation pair where a secondary code is useful to fully describe a condition. The sequencing rule is the same as the etiology/manifestation pair, "use additional code" indicates that a secondary code should be added.

For example, for bacterial infections that are not included in chapter 1, a secondary code from category B95, Streptococcus, Staphylococcus, and Enterococcus, as the cause of diseases classified elsewhere, or B96, Other bacterial agents as the cause of diseases classified elsewhere, may be required to identify the bacterial organism causing the infection. A "use additional code" note will normally be found at the infectious disease code, indicating a need for the organism code to be added as a secondary code.

"Code first" notes are also under certain codes that are not specifically manifestation codes but may be due to an underlying cause. When there is a "code first" note and an underlying condition is present, the underlying condition should be sequenced first.

"Code, if applicable, any causal condition first", notes indicate that this code may be assigned as a principal diagnosis when the causal condition is unknown or not applicable. If a causal condition is known, then the code for that condition should be sequenced as the principal or first-listed diagnosis.

Multiple codes may be needed for sequela, complication codes and obstetric codes to more fully describe a condition. See the specific guidelines for these conditions for further instruction.

8. Acute and Chronic Conditions

If the same condition is described as both acute (subacute) and chronic, and separate subentries exist in the Alphabetic Index at the same indentation level, code both and sequence the acute (subacute) code first.

9. Combination Code

A combination code is a single code used to classify:

Two diagnoses, or

A diagnosis with an associated secondary process (manifestation)

A diagnosis with an associated complication

Combination codes are identified by referring to subterm entries in the Alphabetic Index and by reading the inclusion and exclusion notes in the Tabular List.

Assign only the combination code when that code fully identifies the diagnostic conditions involved or when the Alphabetic Index so directs. Multiple coding should not be used when the classification provides a combination code that clearly identifies all of the elements documented in the diagnosis. When the combination code lacks necessary specificity in describing the manifestation or complication, an additional code should be used as a secondary code.

10. Sequela (Late Effects)

A sequela is the residual effect (condition produced) after the acute phase of an illness or injury has terminated. There is no time limit on when a sequela code can be used. The residual may be apparent early, such as in cerebral infarction, or it may occur months or years later, such as that due to a previous injury. Coding of sequela generally requires two codes sequenced in the following order: The condition or nature of the sequela is sequenced first. The sequela code is sequenced second.

An exception to the above guidelines are those instances where the code for the sequela is followed by a manifestation code identified in the Tabular List and title, or the sequela code has been expanded (at the fourth, fifth or sixth character levels) to include the manifestation(s). The code for the acute phase of an illness or injury that led to the sequela is never used with a code for the late effect.

See Section I.C.9. Sequelae of cerebrovascular disease

See Section I.C.15. Sequelae of complication of pregnancy, childbirth and the puerperium

See Section I.C.19. Application of 7th characters for Chapter 19

11. Impending or Threatened Condition

Code any condition described at the time of discharge as "impending" or "threatened" as follows:

- If it did occur, code as confirmed diagnosis.
- If it did not occur, reference the Alphabetic Index to determine if the condition has a subentry term for "impending" or "threatened" and also reference main term entries for "Impending" and for "Threatened."
- If the subterms are listed, assign the given code.

- If the subterms are not listed, code the existing underlying condition(s) and not the condition described as impending or threatened.

12. Reporting Same Diagnosis Code More than Once

Each unique ICD-10-CM diagnosis code may be reported only once for an encounter. This applies to bilateral conditions when there are no distinct codes identifying laterality or two different conditions classified to the same ICD-10-CM diagnosis code.

13. Laterality

Some ICD-10-CM codes indicate laterality, specifying whether the condition occurs on the left, right or is bilateral. If no bilateral code is provided and the condition is bilateral, assign separate codes for both the left and right side. If the side is not identified in the medical record, assign the code for the unspecified side.

14. Documentation for BMI, Non-pressure Ulcers and Pressure Ulcer Stages

For the Body Mass Index (BMI), depth of non-pressure chronic ulcers and pressure ulcer stage codes, code assignment may be based on medical record documentation from clinicians who are not the patient's provider (i.e., physician or other qualified healthcare practitioner legally accountable for establishing the patient's diagnosis), since this information is typically documented by other clinicians involved in the care of the patient (e.g., a dietitian often documents the BMI and nurses often documents the pressure ulcer stages). However, the associated diagnosis (such as overweight, obesity, or pressure ulcer) must be documented by the patient's provider. If there is conflicting medical record documentation, either from the same clinician or different clinicians, the patient's attending provider should be queried for clarification.

The BMI codes should only be reported as secondary diagnoses. As with all other secondary diagnosis codes, the BMI codes should only be assigned when they meet the definition of a reportable additional diagnosis (see Section III, Reporting Additional Diagnoses).

15. Syndromes

Follow the Alphabetic Index guidance when coding syndromes. In the absence of Alphabetic Index guidance, assign codes for the documented manifestations of the syndrome. Additional codes for manifestations that are not an integral part of the disease process may also be assigned when the condition does not have a unique code.

16. Documentation of Complications of Care

Code assignment is based on the provider's documentation of the relationship between the condition and the care or procedure. The guideline extends to any complications of care, regardless of the chapter the code is located in. It is important to note that not all conditions that occur during or following medical care or surgery are classified as complications. There must be a cause-and-effect relationship between the care provided and the condition, and an indication in the documentation that it is a complication. Query the provider for clarification, if the complication is not clearly documented.

17. Borderline Diagnosis

If the provider documents a "borderline" diagnosis at the time of discharge, the diagnosis is coded as confirmed, unless the classification provides a specific entry (e.g., borderline diabetes). If a borderline condition has a specific index entry in ICD-10-CM, it should be coded as such. Since borderline conditions are not uncertain diagnoses, no distinction is made between the care setting (inpatient versus outpatient). Whenever the documentation is unclear regarding a borderline condition, coders are encouraged to query for clarification.

18. Use of Sign/Symptom/Unspecified Codes

Sign/symptom and "unspecified" codes have acceptable, even necessary, uses. While specific diagnosis codes should be reported when they are supported by the available medical record documentation and clinical knowledge of the patient's health condition, there are instances when signs/symptoms or unspecified codes are the best choices for accurately reflecting the healthcare encounter. Each healthcare encounter should be coded to the level of certainty known for that encounter.

If a definitive diagnosis has not been established by the end of the encounter, it is appropriate to report codes for sign(s) and/or symptom(s) in lieu of a definitive diagnosis. When sufficient clinical information isn't known or available about a particular health condition to assign a more specific code, it is acceptable to report the appropriate "unspecified" code (e.g., a diagnosis of pneumonia has been determined, but not the specific type). Unspecified codes should be reported when they are the codes that most accurately reflects what is known about the patient's condition at the time of that particular encounter. It would be inappropriate to select a specific code that is not supported by the medical record documentation or conduct medically unnecessary diagnostic testing in order to determine a more specific code.

C. Chapter-Specific Coding Guidelines

In addition to general coding guidelines, there are guidelines for specific diagnoses and/or conditions in the classification. Unless otherwise indicated, these guidelines apply to all health care settings. Please refer to Section II for guidelines on the selection of principal diagnosis.

Chapter 1: Certain Infectious and Parasitic Diseases (A00-B99)

a. Human Immunodeficiency Virus (HIV) Infections

1) **Code only confirmed cases**

   Code only confirmed cases of HIV infection/illness. This is an exception to the hospital inpatient guideline Section II, H.

   In this context, "confirmation" does not require documentation of positive serology or culture for HIV; the provider's diagnostic statement that the patient is HIV positive, or has an HIV-related illness is sufficient.

2) **Selection and sequencing of HIV codes**

   (a) Patient admitted for HIV-related condition

   If a patient is admitted for an HIV-related condition, the principal diagnosis should be B20, Human immunodeficiency virus [HIV] disease followed by additional diagnosis codes for all reported HIV-related conditions.

(b) Patient with HIV disease admitted for unrelated condition

If a patient with HIV disease is admitted for an unrelated condition (such as a traumatic injury), the code for the unrelated condition (e.g., the nature of injury code) should be the principal diagnosis. Other diagnoses would be B20 followed by additional diagnosis codes for all reported HIV-related conditions.

(c) Whether the patient is newly diagnosed

Whether the patient is newly diagnosed or has had previous admissions/encounters for HIV conditions is irrelevant to the sequencing decision.

(d) Asymptomatic human immunodeficiency virus

Z21, Asymptomatic human immunodeficiency virus [HIV] infection status, is to be applied when the patient without any documentation of symptoms is listed as being "HIV positive," "known HIV," "HIV test positive," or similar terminology. Do not use this code if the term "AIDS" is used or if the patient is treated for any HIV-related illness or is described as having any condition(s) resulting from his/her HIV positive status; use B20 in these cases.

(e) Patients with inconclusive HIV serology

Patients with inconclusive HIV serology, but no definitive diagnosis or manifestations of the illness, may be assigned code R75, Inconclusive laboratory evidence of human immunodeficiency virus [HIV].

(f) Previously diagnosed HIV-related illness

Patients with any known prior diagnosis of an HIV-related illness should be coded to B20. Once a patient has developed an HIV-related illness, the patient should always be assigned code B20 on every subsequent admission/encounter. Patients previously diagnosed with any HIV illness (B20) should never be assigned to R75 or Z21, Asymptomatic human immunodeficiency virus [HIV] infection status.

(g) HIV Infection in Pregnancy, Childbirth and the Puerperium

During pregnancy, childbirth or the puerperium, a patient admitted (or presenting for a health care encounter) because of an HIV-related illness should receive a principal diagnosis code of O98.7-, Human immunodeficiency [HIV] disease complicating pregnancy, childbirth and the puerperium, followed by B20 and the code(s) for the HIV-related illness(es). Codes from Chapter 15 always take sequencing priority.

Patients with asymptomatic HIV infection status admitted (or presenting for a health care encounter) during pregnancy, childbirth, or the puerperium should receive codes of O98.7- and Z21.

(h) Encounters for testing for HIV

If a patient is being seen to determine his/her HIV status, use code Z11.4, Encounter for screening for human immunodeficiency virus [HIV]. Use additional codes for any associated high risk behavior.

If a patient with signs or symptoms is being seen for HIV testing, code the signs and symptoms. An additional counseling code Z71.7, Human immunodeficiency virus [HIV] counseling, may be used if counseling is provided during the encounter for the test.

When a patient returns to be informed of his/her HIV test results and the test result is negative, use code Z71.7, Human immunodeficiency virus [HIV] counseling.

If the results are positive, see previous guidelines and assign codes as appropriate.

b. Infectious agents as the cause of diseases classified to other chapters

Certain infections are classified in chapters other than Chapter 1 and no organism is identified as part of the infection code. In these instances, it is necessary to use an additional code from Chapter 1 to identify the organism. A code from category B95, Streptococcus, Staphylococcus, and Enterococcus as the cause of diseases classified to other chapters, B96, Other bacterial agents as the cause of diseases classified to other chapters, or B97, Viral agents as the cause of diseases classified to other chapters, is to be used as an additional code to identify the organism. An instructional note will be found at the infection code advising that an additional organism code is required.

c. Infections resistant to antibiotics

Many bacterial infections are resistant to current antibiotics. It is necessary to identify all infections documented as antibiotic resistant. Assign a code from category Z16, Resistance to antimicrobial drugs, following the infection code only if the infection code does not identify drug resistance.

d. Sepsis, Severe Sepsis, and Septic Shock

1) Coding of Sepsis and Severe Sepsis

(a) Sepsis

For a diagnosis of sepsis, assign the appropriate code for the underlying systemic infection. If the type of infection or causal organism is not further specified, assign code A41.9, Sepsis, unspecified organism.

A code from subcategory R65.2, Severe sepsis, should not be assigned unless severe sepsis or an associated acute organ dysfunction is documented.

(i)   Negative or inconclusive blood cultures and sepsis

Negative or inconclusive blood cultures do not preclude a diagnosis of sepsis in patients with clinical evidence of the condition, however, the provider should be queried.

(ii)   Urosepsis

The term urosepsis is a nonspecific term. It is not to be considered synonymous with sepsis. It has no default code in the Alphabetic Index. Should a provider use this term, he/she must be queried for clarification.

(iii)   Sepsis with organ dysfunction

If a patient has sepsis and associated acute organ dysfunction or multiple organ dysfunction (MOD), follow the instructions for coding severe sepsis.

(iv)   Acute organ dysfunction that is not clearly associated with the sepsis

If a patient has sepsis and an acute organ dysfunction, but the medical record documentation indicates that the acute organ dysfunction is related to a medical condition other than the sepsis, do not assign a code from subcategory R65.2, Severe sepsis. An acute organ dysfunction must be associated with the sepsis in order to assign the severe sepsis code. If the documentation is not clear as to whether an acute organ dysfunction is related to the sepsis or another medical condition, query the provider.

(b) Severe sepsis

The coding of severe sepsis requires a minimum of 2 codes: first a code for the underlying systemic infection, followed by a code from subcategory R65.2, Severe sepsis. If the causal organism is not documented, assign code A41.9, Sepsis, unspecified organism, for the infection. Additional code(s) for the associated acute organ dysfunction are also required.

Due to the complex nature of severe sepsis, some cases may require querying the provider prior to assignment of the codes.

2) Septic shock

Septic shock generally refers to circulatory failure associated with severe sepsis, and therefore, it represents a type of acute organ dysfunction.

For cases of septic shock, the code for the systemic infection should be sequenced first, followed by code R65.21, *Severe sepsis with septic shock* or code T81.12, *Postprocedural septic shock*. Any additional codes for the other acute organ dysfunctions should also be assigned. As noted in the sequencing instructions in the Tabular List, the code for septic shock cannot be assigned as a principal diagnosis

3) Sequencing of severe sepsis

If severe sepsis is present on admission, and meets the definition of principal diagnosis, the underlying systemic infection should be assigned as principal diagnosis followed by the appropriate code from subcategory R65.2 as required by the sequencing rules in the Tabular List. A code from subcategory R65.2 can never be assigned as a principal diagnosis.

When severe sepsis develops during an encounter (it was not present on admission) the underlying systemic infection and the appropriate code from subcategory R65.2 should be assigned as secondary diagnoses.

Severe sepsis may be present on admission but the diagnosis may not be confirmed until sometime after admission. If the documentation is not clear whether severe sepsis was present on admission, the provider should be queried.

4) Sepsis and severe sepsis with a localized infection

If the reason for admission is both sepsis or severe sepsis and a localized infection, such as pneumonia or cellulitis, a code(s) for the underlying systemic infection should be assigned first and the code for the localized infection should be assigned as a secondary diagnosis. If the patient has severe sepsis, a code from subcategory R65.2 should also be assigned as a secondary diagnosis. If the patient is admitted with a localized infection, such as pneumonia, and sepsis/severe sepsis doesn't develop until after admission, the localized infection should be assigned first, followed by the appropriate sepsis/severe sepsis codes.

5) Sepsis due to a postprocedural infection

(a) Documentation of causal relationship

As with all postprocedural complications, code assignment is based on the provider's documentation of the relationship between the infection and the procedure.

(b) Sepsis due to a postprocedural infection

For such cases, the postprocedural infection code, such as, T80.2, Infections following infusion, transfusion, and therapeutic injection, T81.4, Infection following a procedure, T88.0, Infection following immunization, or O86.0, Infection of obstetric surgical wound, should be coded first, followed by the code for the specific infection. If the patient has severe sepsis the appropriate code from subcategory R65.2 should also be assigned with the additional code(s) for any acute organ dysfunction.

(c) Postprocedural infection and postprocedural septic shock

In cases where a postprocedural infection has occurred and has resulted in severe sepsis and postprocedural septic shock, the code for the precipitating complication such as code T81.4, Infection following a procedure, or O86.0, Infection of obstetrical surgical wound should be coded first followed by code R65.21, Severe sepsis with septic shock and a code for the systemic infection.

6) Sepsis and severe sepsis associated with a noninfectious process (condition)

In some cases a noninfectious process (condition), such as trauma, may lead to an infection which can result in sepsis or severe sepsis. If sepsis or severe sepsis is documented as associated with a noninfectious condition, such as a burn or serious injury, and this condition meets the definition for principal diagnosis, the code for the noninfectious condition should be sequenced first, followed by the code for the resulting infection. If severe sepsis, is present a code from subcategory R65.2 should also be assigned with any associated organ dysfunction(s) codes. It is not necessary to assign a code from subcategory R65.1, Systemic inflammatory response syndrome (SIRS) of non-infectious origin, for these cases.

If the infection meets the definition of principal diagnosis it should be sequenced before the non-infectious condition. When both the associated non-infectious condition and the infection meet the definition of principal diagnosis either may be assigned as principal diagnosis.

Only one code from category R65, Symptoms and signs specifically associated with systemic inflammation and infection, should be assigned. Therefore, when a non-infectious condition leads to an infection resulting in severe sepsis, assign the appropriate code from subcategory R65.2, Severe sepsis. Do not additionally assign a code from subcategory R65.1, Systemic inflammatory response syndrome (SIRS) of non-infectious origin.

See Section I.C.18. SIRS due to non-infectious process

7) **Sepsis and septic shock complicating abortion, pregnancy, childbirth, and the puerperium**

See Section I.C.15. Sepsis and septic shock complicating abortion, pregnancy, childbirth and the puerperium

8) **Newborn sepsis**

See Section I.C.16.f. Bacterial sepsis of newborn

e. Methicillin Resistant *Staphylococcus aureus* (MRSA) Conditions

1) **Selection and sequencing of MRSA codes**

(a) *Combination codes for MRSA infection*

When a patient is diagnosed with an infection that is due to methicillin resistant *Staphylococcus aureus* (MRSA), and that infection has a combination code that includes the causal organism (e.g., sepsis, pneumonia) assign the appropriate combination code for the condition (e.g., code A41.02, Sepsis due to Methicillin resistant *Staphylococcus aureus* or code J15.212, Pneumonia due to Methicillin resistant *Staphylococcus aureus*). Do not assign code B95.62, Methicillin resistant *Staphylococcus aureus* infection as the cause of diseases classified elsewhere, as an additional code because the combination code includes the type of infection and the MRSA organism. Do not assign a code from subcategory Z16.11, Resistance to penicillins, as an additional diagnosis.

See Section C.1. for instructions on coding and sequencing of sepsis and severe sepsis.

(b) *Other codes for MRSA infection*

When there is documentation of a current infection (e.g., wound infection, stitch abscess, urinary tract infection) due to MRSA, and that infection does not have a combination code that includes the causal organism, assign the appropriate code to identify the condition along with code B95.62, Methicillin resistant *Staphylococcus aureus* infection as the cause of diseases classified elsewhere for the MRSA infection. Do not assign a code from subcategory Z16.11, Resistance to penicillins.

(c) *Methicillin susceptible *Staphylococcus aureus* (MSSA) and MRSA colonization*

The condition or state of being colonized or carrying MSSA or MRSA is called colonization or carriage, while an individual person is described as being colonized or being a carrier. Colonization means that MSSA or MSRA is present on or in the body without necessarily causing illness. A positive MRSA colonization test might be documented by the provider as "MRSA screen positive" or "MRSA nasal swab positive".

Assign code Z22.322, Carrier or suspected carrier of Methicillin resistant *Staphylococcus aureus*, for patients documented as having MRSA colonization. Assign code Z22.321, Carrier or suspected carrier of Methicillin susceptible *Staphylococcus aureus*, for patient documented as having MSSA colonization. Colonization is not necessarily indicative of a disease process or as the cause of a specific condition the patient may have unless documented as such by the provider.

(d) *MRSA colonization and infection*

If a patient is documented as having both MRSA colonization and infection during a hospital admission, code Z22.322, Carrier or suspected carrier of Methicillin resistant *Staphylococcus aureus*, and a code for the MRSA infection may both be assigned.

Chapter 2: Neoplasms (C00-D49)

General Guidelines

Chapter 2 of the ICD-10-CM contains the codes for most benign and all malignant neoplasms. Certain benign neoplasms, such as prostatic adenomas, may be found in the specific body system chapters. To properly code a neoplasm it is necessary to determine from the record if the neoplasm is benign, in-situ, malignant, or of uncertain histologic behavior. If malignant, any secondary (metastatic) sites should also be determined.

Primary malignant neoplasms overlapping site boundaries

A primary malignant neoplasm that overlaps two or more contiguous (next to each other) sites should be classified to the subcategory/code .8 ('overlapping lesion'), unless the combination is specifically indexed elsewhere. For multiple neoplasms of the same site that are not contiguous such as tumors in different quadrants of the same breast, codes for each site should be assigned.

Malignant neoplasm of ectopic tissue

Malignant neoplasms of ectopic tissue are to be coded to the site of origin mentioned, e.g., ectopic pancreatic malignant neoplasms involving the stomach are coded to pancreas, unspecified (C25.9).

The neoplasm table in the Alphabetic Index should be referenced first. However, if the histological term is documented, that term should be referenced first, rather than going immediately to the Neoplasm Table, in order to determine which column in the Neoplasm Table is appropriate. For example, if the documentation indicates "adenoma," refer to the term in the Alphabetic Index to review the entries under this term and the instructional note to "see also neoplasm, by site, benign." The table provides the proper code based on the type of neoplasm and the site. It is important to select the proper column in the table that corresponds to the type of neoplasm. The Tabular

List should then be referenced to verify that the correct code has been selected from the table and that a more specific site code does not exist.

See Section I.C.21. Factors influencing health status and contact with health services, Status, for information regarding Z15.0, codes for genetic susceptibility to cancer.

a. Treatment directed at the malignancy

If the treatment is directed at the malignancy, designate the malignancy as the principal diagnosis.

The only exception to this guideline is if a patient admission/encounter is solely for the administration of chemotherapy, immunotherapy or radiation therapy, assign the appropriate Z51.-- code as the first-listed or principal diagnosis, and the diagnosis or problem for which the service is being performed as a secondary diagnosis.

b. Treatment of secondary site

When a patient is admitted because of a primary neoplasm with metastasis and treatment is directed toward the secondary site only, the secondary neoplasm is designated as the principal diagnosis even though the primary malignancy is still present.

c. Coding and sequencing of complications

Coding and sequencing of complications associated with the malignancies or with the therapy thereof are subject to the following guidelines:

1) Anemia associated with malignancy

    When admission/encounter is for management of an anemia associated with the malignancy, and the treatment is only for anemia, the appropriate code for the malignancy is sequenced as the principal or first-listed diagnosis followed by the appropriate code for the anemia (such as code D63.0, Anemia in neoplastic disease).

2) Anemia associated with chemotherapy, immunotherapy and radiation therapy

    When the admission/encounter is for management of an anemia associated with an adverse effect of the administration of chemotherapy or immunotherapy and the only treatment is for the anemia, the anemia code is sequenced first followed by the appropriate codes for the neoplasm and the adverse effect (T45.1X5, Adverse effect of antineoplastic and immunosuppressive drugs).

    When the admission/encounter is for management of an anemia associated with an adverse effect of radiotherapy, the anemia code should be sequenced first, followed by the appropriate neoplasm code and code Y84.2, Radiological procedure and radiotherapy as the cause of abnormal reaction of the patient, or of later complication, without mention of misadventure at the time of the procedure.

3) Management of dehydration due to the malignancy

    When the admission/encounter is for management of dehydration due to the malignancy and only the dehydration is being treated (intravenous rehydration), the dehydration is sequenced first, followed by the code(s) for the malignancy.

4) Treatment of a complication resulting from a surgical procedure

    When the admission/encounter is for treatment of a complication resulting from a surgical procedure, designate the complication as the principal or first-listed diagnosis if treatment is directed at resolving the complication.

d. Primary malignancy previously excised

When a primary malignancy has been previously excised or eradicated from its site and there is no further treatment directed to that site and there is no evidence of any existing primary malignancy, a code from category Z85, Personal history of malignant neoplasm, should be used to indicate the former site of the malignancy. Any mention of extension, invasion, or metastasis to another site is coded as a secondary malignant neoplasm to that site. The secondary site may be the principal or first-listed with the Z85 code used as a secondary code.

e. Admissions/Encounters involving chemotherapy, immunotherapy and radiation therapy

1) Episode of care involves surgical removal of neoplasm

    When an episode of care involves the surgical removal of a neoplasm, primary or secondary site, followed by adjunct chemotherapy or radiation treatment during the same episode of care, the code for the neoplasm should be assigned as principal or first-listed diagnosis.

2) Patient admission/encounter solely for administration of chemotherapy, immunotherapy and radiation therapy

    If a patient admission/encounter is solely for the administration of chemotherapy, immunotherapy or radiation therapy assign code Z51.0, Encounter for antineoplastic radiation therapy, or Z51.11, Encounter for antineoplastic chemotherapy, or Z51.12, Encounter for antineoplastic immunotherapy as the first-listed or principal diagnosis. If a patient receives more than one of these therapies during the same admission more than one of these codes may be assigned, in any sequence.

    The malignancy for which the therapy is being administered should be assigned as a secondary diagnosis.

3) Patient admitted for radiation therapy, chemotherapy or immunotherapy and develops complications

    When a patient is admitted for the purpose of radiotherapy, immunotherapy or chemotherapy and develops complications such as uncontrolled nausea and vomiting or dehydration, the principal or first-listed diagnosis is Z51.0, Encounter for antineoplastic radiation therapy, or Z51.11, Encounter for antineoplastic chemotherapy, or Z51.12, Encounter for antineoplastic immunotherapy followed by any codes for the complications.

f. Admission/encounter to determine extent of malignancy

When the reason for admission/encounter is to determine the extent of the malignancy, or for a procedure such as paracentesis or thoracentesis, the primary malignancy or appropriate metastatic site is designated as the principal or first-listed diagnosis, even though chemotherapy or radiotherapy is administered.

g. Symptoms, signs, and abnormal findings listed in Chapter 18 associated with neoplasms

Symptoms, signs, and ill-defined conditions listed in Chapter 18 characteristic of, or associated with, an existing primary or secondary site malignancy cannot be used to replace the malignancy as principal or first-listed diagnosis, regardless of the number of admissions or encounters for treatment and care of the neoplasm.

See section I.C.21. Factors influencing health status and contact with health services, Encounter for prophylactic organ removal.

h. Admission/encounter for pain control/management

See Section I.C.6. for information on coding admission/encounter for pain control/management.

i. Malignancy in two or more noncontiguous sites

A patient may have more than one malignant tumor in the same organ. These tumors may represent different primaries or metastatic disease, depending on the site. Should the documentation be unclear, the provider should be queried as to the status of each tumor so that the correct codes can be assigned.

j. Disseminated malignant neoplasm, unspecified

Code C80.0, Disseminated malignant neoplasm, unspecified, is for use only in those cases where the patient has advanced metastatic disease and no known primary or secondary sites are specified. It should not be used in place of assigning codes for the primary site and all known secondary sites.

k. Malignant neoplasm without specification of site

Code C80.1, Malignant (primary) neoplasm, unspecified, equates to Cancer, unspecified. This code should only be used when no determination can be made as to the primary site of a malignancy. This code should rarely be used in the inpatient setting.

l. Sequencing of neoplasm codes

1) Encounter for treatment of primary malignancy

   If the reason for the encounter is for treatment of a primary malignancy, assign the malignancy as the principal/first listed diagnosis. The primary site is to be sequenced first, followed by any metastatic sites.

2) Encounter for treatment of secondary malignancy

   When an encounter is for a primary malignancy with metastasis and treatment is directed toward the metastatic (secondary) site(s) only, the metastatic site(s) is designated as the principal/first listed diagnosis. The primary malignancy is coded as an additional code.

3) Malignant neoplasm in a pregnant patient

   When a pregnant woman has a malignant neoplasm, a code from subcategory O9A.1-, *Malignant neoplasm complicating pregnancy, childbirth, and the puerperium*, should be sequenced first, followed by the appropriate code from Chapter 2 to indicate the type of neoplasm.

4) Encounter for complication associated with a neoplasm

   When an encounter is for management of a complication associated with a neoplasm, such as dehydration, and the treatment is only for the complication, the complication is coded first, followed by the appropriate code(s) for the neoplasm.

   The exception to this guideline is anemia. When the admission/encounter is for management of an anemia associated with the malignancy, and the treatment is only for anemia, the appropriate code for the malignancy is sequenced as the principal or first-listed diagnosis followed by code D63.0, Anemia in neoplastic disease.

5) Complication from surgical procedure for treatment of a neoplasm

   When an encounter is for treatment of a complication resulting from a surgical procedure performed for the treatment of the neoplasm, designate the complication as the principal/first listed diagnosis. See guideline regarding the coding of a current malignancy versus personal history to determine if the code for the neoplasm should also be assigned.

6) Pathologic fracture due to a neoplasm

   When an encounter is for a pathological fracture due to a neoplasm, if the focus of treatment is the fracture, a code from subcategory M84.5, *Pathological fracture in neoplastic disease*, should be sequenced first, followed by the code for the neoplasm.

   If the focus of treatment is the neoplasm with an associated pathological fracture, the neoplasm code should be sequenced first, followed by a code from M84.5 for the pathological fracture. The "code also" note at M84.5 provides this sequencing instruction.

m. Current malignancy versus personal history of malignancy

When a primary malignancy has been excised but further treatment, such as an additional surgery for the malignancy, radiation therapy or chemotherapy is directed to that site, the primary malignancy code should be used until treatment is completed.

When a primary malignancy has been previously excised or eradicated from its site, there is no further treatment (of the malignancy) directed to that site, and there is no evidence of any existing primary malignancy, a code from category Z85, Personal history of malignant neoplasm, should be used to indicate the former site of the malignancy.

See Section I.C.21. Factors influencing health status and contact with health services, History (of)

n. Leukemia, multiple myeloma, and malignant plasma cell neoplasms in remission versus personal history

The categories for leukemia, and category C90, Multiple myeloma and malignant plasma cell neoplasms, have codes indicating whether or not the leukemia has achieved remission. There are also codes Z85.6, *Personal history of leukemia*, and Z85.79, *Personal history of other malignant neoplasms of lymphoid, hematopoietic and related tissues.* If the documentation is unclear, as to whether the leukemia has achieved remission, the provider should be queried.

See Section I.C.21. *Factors influencing health status and contact with health services, History (of)*

o. Aftercare following surgery for neoplasm

See Section I.C.21. *Factors influencing health status and contact with health services, Aftercare*

p. Follow-up care for completed treatment of a malignancy

See Section I.C.21. *Factors influencing health status and contact with health services, Follow-up*

q. Prophylactic organ removal for prevention of malignancy

See Section I.C. 21, *Factors influencing health status and contact with health services, Prophylactic organ removal*

r. Malignant neoplasm associated with transplanted organ

A malignant neoplasm of a transplanted organ should be coded as a transplant complication. Assign first the appropriate code from category T86.-, *Complications of transplanted organs and tissue*, followed by code C80.2, *Malignant neoplasm associated with transplanted organ.* Use an additional code for the specific malignancy.

Chapter 3: Disease of the Blood and Blood-forming Organs and Certain Disorders Involving the Immune Mechanism (D50-D89)

Reserved for future guideline expansion.

Chapter 4: Endocrine, Nutritional, and Metabolic Diseases (E00-E90)

a. Diabetes mellitus

The diabetes mellitus codes are combination codes that include the type of diabetes mellitus, the body system affected, and the complications affecting that body system. As many codes within a particular category as are necessary to describe all of the complications of the disease may be used. They should be sequenced based on the reason for a particular encounter. Assign as many codes from categories E08 – E13 as needed to identify all of the associated conditions that the patient has.

1) Type of diabetes

The age of a patient is not the sole determining factor, though most type 1 diabetics develop the condition before reaching puberty. For this reason type 1 diabetes mellitus is also referred to as juvenile diabetes.

2) Type of diabetes mellitus not documented

If the type of diabetes mellitus is not documented in the medical record the default is E11.-, *Type 2 diabetes mellitus.*

3) Diabetes mellitus and the use of insulin

If the documentation in a medical record does not indicate the type of diabetes but does indicate that the patient uses insulin, code E11, *Type 2 diabetes mellitus*, should be assigned. Code Z79.4, *Long-term (current) use of insulin*, should also be assigned to indicate that the patient uses insulin. Code Z79.4 should not be assigned if insulin is given temporarily to bring a type 2 patient's blood sugar under control during an encounter.

4) Diabetes mellitus in pregnancy and gestational diabetes

See Section I.C.15. *Diabetes mellitus in pregnancy*

See Section I.C.15. *Gestational (pregnancy induced) diabetes*

5) Complications due to insulin pump malfunction

(a) Underdose of insulin due to insulin pump failure

An underdose of insulin due to an insulin pump failure should be assigned to a code from subcategory T85.6, *Mechanical complication of other specified internal and external prosthetic devices, implants and grafts*, that specifies the type of pump malfunction, as the principal or first listed code, followed by code T38.3x6-, *Underdosing of insulin and oral hypoglycemic [antidiabetic] drugs.* Additional codes for the type of diabetes mellitus and any associated complications due to the underdosing should also be assigned.

(b) Overdose of insulin due to insulin pump failure

The principal or first listed code for an encounter due to an insulin pump malfunction resulting in an overdose of insulin, should also be T85.6-, *Mechanical complication of other specified internal and external prosthetic devices, implants and grafts*, followed by code T38.3x1-, *Poisoning by insulin and oral hypoglycemic [antidiabetic] drugs, accidental (unintentional).*

6) Secondary Diabetes Mellitus

Codes under categories E08, Diabetes mellitus due to underlying condition, E09, Drug or chemical induced diabetes mellitus, and E13, Other specified diabetes mellitus, identify complications/manifestations associated with secondary diabetes mellitus. Secondary diabetes is always caused by another condition or event (e.g., cystic fibrosis, malignant neoplasm of pancreas, pancreatectomy, adverse effect of drug, or poisoning)

(a) Secondary diabetes mellitus and the use of insulin

For patients who routinely use insulin, code Z79.4, Long-term (current) use of insulin, should also be assigned. Code Z79.4 should not be assigned if insulin is given temporarily to bring a patient's blood sugar under control during an encounter.

(b) Assigning and sequencing secondary diabetes codes and its causes

The sequencing of the secondary diabetes codes in relationship to codes for the cause of the diabetes is based on the Tabular List instructions for categories E08, E09 and E13.

(i) Secondary diabetes mellitus due to pancreatectomy

For postpancreatectomy diabetes mellitus (lack of insulin due to the surgical removal of all or part of the pancreas), assign code E89.1, Postprocedural hypoinsulinemia. Assign a code from category E13 and a code from subcategory Z90.41-, Acquired absence of pancreas, as additional codes.

(ii) Secondary diabetes due to drugs

Secondary diabetes may be caused by an adverse effect of correctly administered medications, poisoning sequela of poisoning.

See Section I.C.19.e for *coding of adverse effects and poisoning*, and Section I.C.20 for *external cause code reporting*.

Chapter 5: Mental, Behavioral and Neurodevelopmental Disorders (F01 – F99)

a. Pain disorders related to psychological factors

Assign code F45.41, for pain that is exclusively related to psychological disorders. As indicated by the Excludes1 note under category G89, a code from category G89 should not be assigned with code F45.41.

Code F45.42, *Pain disorders with related psychological factors*, should be used with a code from category G89, *Pain, not elsewhere classified*, if there is documentation of a psychological component for a patient with acute or chronic pain.

See Section I.C.6. *Pain*

b. Mental and behavioral disorders due to psychoactive substance use

1) In Remission Selection of codes for "in remission" for categories F10-F19, Mental and behavioral disorders due to psychoactive substance use (categories F10-F19 with -.21) requires the provider's clinical judgment. The appropriate codes for "in remission" are assigned only on the basis of provider documentation (as defined in the *Official Guidelines for Coding and Reporting*).

2) Psychoactive Substance Use, Abuse And Dependence When the provider documentation refers to use, abuse and dependence of the same substance (e.g. alcohol, opioid, cannabis, etc.), only one code should be assigned to identify the pattern of use based on the following hierarchy:

   • If both use and abuse are documented, assign only the code for abuse

   • If both abuse and dependence are documented, assign only the code for dependence

   • If use, abuse and dependence are all documented, assign only the code for dependence

   • If both use and dependence are documented, assign only the code for dependence.

3) Psychoactive Substance Use

   As with all other diagnoses, the codes for psychoactive substance use (F10.9-, F11.9-, F12.9-, F13.9-, F14.9-, F15.9-, F16.9-) should only be assigned based on provider documentation and when they meet the definition of a reportable diagnosis (see Section III, Reporting Additional Diagnoses). The codes are to be used only when the psychoactive substance use is associated with a mental or behavioral disorder, and such a relationship is documented by the provider.

Chapter 6: Diseases of Nervous System (G00-G99)

a. Dominant/nondominant side

Codes from category G81, *Hemiplegia and hemiparesis*, and subcategories, G83.1, *Monoplegia of lower limb*, G83.2, *Monoplegia of upper limb*, and G83.3, *Monoplegia, unspecified*, identify whether the dominant or nondominant side is affected. Should the affected side be documented, but not specified as dominant or nondominant, and the classification system does not indicate a default, code selection is as follows:

• For ambidextrous patients, the default should be dominant.

• If the left side is affected, the default is non-dominant.

• If the right side is affected, the default is dominant.

b. Pain – Category G89

1) General coding information

   Codes in category G89, *Pain, not elsewhere classified*, may be used in conjunction with codes from other categories and chapters to provide more detail about acute or chronic pain and neoplasm-related pain, unless otherwise indicated below.

   If the pain is not specified as acute or chronic, post-thoracotomy, postprocedural, or neoplasm-related, do not assign codes from category G89.

   A code from category G89 should not be assigned if the underlying (definitive) diagnosis is known, unless the reason for the encounter is pain control/ management and not management of the underlying condition.

   When an admission or encounter is for a procedure aimed at treating the underlying condition (e.g., spinal fusion, kyphoplasty), a code for the underlying condition (e.g., vertebral fracture, spinal stenosis) should be assigned as the principal diagnosis. No code from category G89 should be assigned.

   (a) Category G89 Codes as Principal or First-Listed Diagnosis

   Category G89 codes are acceptable as principal diagnosis or the first-listed code:

   • When pain control or pain management is the reason for the admission/encounter (e.g., a patient with displaced intervertebral disc, nerve impingement and severe back pain presents for injection of steroid into the spinal canal). The underlying cause of the pain should be reported as an additional diagnosis, if known.

- When a patient is admitted for the insertion of a neurostimulator for pain control, assign the appropriate pain code as the principal or first-listed diagnosis. When an admission or encounter is for a procedure aimed at treating the underlying condition and a neurostimulator is inserted for pain control during the same admission/encounter, a code for the underlying condition should be assigned as the principal diagnosis and the appropriate pain code should be assigned as a secondary diagnosis.

(b) Use of Category G89 Codes in Conjunction with Site Specific Pain Codes

(i) Assigning Category G89 and Site-Specific Pain Codes

Codes from category G89 may be used in conjunction with codes that identify the site of pain (including codes from chapter 18) if the category G89 code provides additional information. For example, if the code describes the site of the pain, but does not fully describe whether the pain is acute or chronic, then both codes should be assigned.

(ii) Sequencing of Category G89 Codes with Site-Specific Pain Codes

The sequencing of category G89 codes with site-specific pain codes (including chapter 18 codes), is dependent on the circumstances of the encounter/admission as follows:

- If the encounter is for pain control or pain management, assign the code from category G89 followed by the code identifying the specific site of pain (e.g., encounter for pain management for acute neck pain from trauma is assigned code G89.11, *Acute pain due to trauma*, followed by code M54.2, *Cervicalgia*, to identify the site of pain).
- If the encounter is for any other reason except pain control or pain management, and a related definitive diagnosis has not been established (confirmed) by the provider, assign the code for the specific site of pain first, followed by the appropriate code from category G89.

2) Pain due to devices, implants and grafts

See Section I.C.19. *Pain due to medical devices.*

3) Postoperative Pain

The provider's documentation should be used to guide the coding of postoperative pain, as well as *Section III Reporting Additional Diagnoses* and *Section IV Diagnostic Coding and Reporting in the Outpatient Setting.*

The default for post-thoracotomy and other postoperative pain not specified as acute or chronic is the code for the acute form.

Routine or expected postoperative pain immediately after surgery should not be coded.

(a) Postoperative pain not associated with specific postoperative complication

Postoperative pain not associated with a specific postoperative complication is assigned to the appropriate postoperative pain code in category G89.

(b) Postoperative pain associated with specific postoperative complication

Postoperative pain associated with a specific postoperative complication (such as painful wire sutures) is assigned to the appropriate code(s) found in Chapter 19, Injury, poisoning, and certain other consequences of external causes. If appropriate, use additional code(s) from category G89 to identify acute or chronic pain (G89.18 or G89.28).

4) Chronic pain

Chronic pain is classified to subcategory G89.2. There is no time frame defining when pain becomes chronic pain. The provider's documentation should be used to guide use of these codes.

5) Neoplasm Related Pain

Code G89.3 is assigned to pain documented as being related, associated or due to cancer, primary or secondary malignancy, or tumor. This code is assigned regardless of whether the pain is acute or chronic.

This code may be assigned as the principal or first-listed code when the stated reason for the admission/encounter is documented as pain control/pain management. The underlying neoplasm should be reported as an additional diagnosis.

When the reason for the admission/encounter is management of the neoplasm and the pain associated with the neoplasm is also documented, code G89.3 may be assigned as an additional diagnosis. It is not necessary to assign an additional code for the site of the pain.

See Section I.C.2 for instructions on the sequencing of neoplasms for all other stated reasons for the admission/encounter (except for pain control/pain management).

6) Chronic pain syndrome

Central pain syndrome (G89.0) and chronic pain syndrome (G89.4) are different than the term "chronic pain," and therefore codes should only be used when the provider has specifically documented this condition.

See Section I.C.5. Pain disorders related to psychological factors

Chapter 7: Diseases of Eye and Adnexa (H00-IH59)

a. Glaucoma

1) Assigning Glaucoma Codes

Assign as many codes from category H40, Glaucoma, as needed to identify the type of glaucoma, the affected eye, and the glaucoma stage.

2) Bilateral glaucoma with same type and stage

When a patient has bilateral glaucoma and both eyes are documented as being the same type and stage, and there is a code for bilateral glaucoma, report only the code for the type of glaucoma, bilateral, with the seventh character for the stage.

When a patient has bilateral glaucoma and both eyes are documented as being the same type and stage, and the classification does not provide a code for bilateral glaucoma (i.e. subcategories H40.10, H40.11 and H40.20) report only one code for the type of glaucoma with the appropriate seventh character for the stage.

3) Bilateral glaucoma stage with different types or stages

When a patient has bilateral glaucoma and each eye is documented as having a different type or stage, and the classification distinguishes laterality, assign the appropriate code for each eye rather than the code for bilateral glaucoma

When a patient has bilateral glaucoma and each eye is documented as having a different type, and the classification does not distinguish laterality (i.e. subcategories H40.10, H40.11 and H40.20), assign one code for each type of glaucoma with the appropriate seventh character for the stage.

When a patient has bilateral glaucoma and each eye is documented as having the same type, but different stage, and the classification does not distinguish laterality (i.e. subcategories H40.10, H40.11 and H40.20), assign a code for the type of glaucoma for each eye with the seventh character for the specific glaucoma stage documented for each eye.

4) Patient admitted with glaucoma and stage evolves during the admission

If a patient is admitted with glaucoma and the stage progresses during the admission, assign the code for highest stage documented.

5) Indeterminate stage glaucoma

Assignment of the seventh character "4" for "indeterminate stage" should be based on the clinical documentation. The seventh character "4" is used for glaucomas whose stage cannot be clinically determined. This seventh character should not be confused with the seventh character "0", unspecified, which should be assigned when there is no documentation regarding the stage of the glaucoma.

Chapter 8: Diseases of Ear and Mastoid Process (H60-H59)

Reserved for future guideline expansion.

Chapter 9: Diseases of Circulatory System (I00-I99)

a. Hypertension.

1) Hypertension with Heart Disease

Heart conditions classified to I50.- or I51.4-I51.9, are assigned to, a code from category I11, *Hypertensive heart disease*, when a causal relationship is stated (due to hypertension) or implied (hypertensive). Use an additional code from category I50, *Heart failure*, to identify the type of heart failure in those patients with heart failure.

The same heart conditions (I50.-, I51.4-I51.9) with hypertension, but without a stated causal relationship, are coded separately. Sequence according to the circumstances of the admission/encounter.

2) Hypertensive Chronic Kidney Disease

Assign codes from category I12, Hypertensive chronic kidney disease, when both hypertension and a condition classifiable to category N18, Chronic kidney disease (CKD), are present. Unlike hypertension with heart disease, ICD-10-CM presumes a cause-and-effect relationship and classifies chronic kidney disease with hypertension as hypertensive chronic kidney disease.

The appropriate code from category N18 should be used as a secondary code with a code from category I12 to identify the stage of chronic kidney disease.

See Section I.C.14. *Chronic kidney disease*

If a patient has hypertensive chronic kidney disease and acute renal failure , an additional code for the acute renal failure is required.

3) Hypertensive Heart and Chronic Kidney Disease

Assign codes from combination category I13, *Hypertensive heart and chronic kidney disease*, when both hypertensive kidney disease and hypertensive heart disease are stated in the diagnosis. Assume a relationship between the hypertension and the chronic kidney disease, whether or not the condition is so designated. If heart failure is present, assign an additional code from category I50 to identify the type of heart failure.

The appropriate code from category N18, *Chronic kidney disease*, should be used as a secondary code with a code from category I13 to identify the stage of chronic kidney disease.

See Section I.C.14. *Chronic kidney disease*

The codes in category I13, *Hypertensive heart and chronic kidney disease*, are combination codes that include hypertension, heart disease and chronic kidney disease. The Includes note at I13 specifies that the conditions included at I11 and I12 are included together in I13. If a patient has hypertension, heart disease and chronic kidney disease then a code from I13 should be used, not individual codes for hypertension, heart disease and chronic kidney disease, or codes from I11 or I12.

For patients with both acute renal failure and chronic kidney disease an additional code for acute renal failure is required.

4) Hypertensive Cerebrovascular Disease

For hypertensive cerebrovascular disease, first assign the appropriate code from categories I60-I69, followed by the appropriate hypertension code.

5) Hypertensive Retinopathy

Subcategory H35.0, *Background retinopathy and retinal vascular changes*, should be used with a code from category I10 – I15, Hypertensive disease to include the systemic hypertension. The sequencing is based on the reason for the encounter.

6) Hypertension, Secondary

Secondary hypertension is due to an underlying condition. Two codes are required: one to identify the underlying etiology and one from category I15 to identify the hypertension. Sequencing of codes is determined by the reason for admission/encounter.

7) Hypertension, Transient

Assign code R03.0, *Elevated blood pressure reading without diagnosis of hypertension*, unless patient has an established diagnosis of hypertension. Assign code O13.-, *Gestational [pregnancy-induced] hypertension without significant proteinuria*, or O14.-, *Pre-eclampsia*, for transient hypertension of pregnancy.

8) Hypertension, Controlled

This diagnostic statement usually refers to an existing state of hypertension under control by therapy. Assign the appropriate code from categories I10-I15, Hypertensive diseases.

9) Hypertension, Uncontrolled

Uncontrolled hypertension may refer to untreated hypertension or hypertension not responding to current therapeutic regimen. In either case, assign the appropriate code from categories I10-I15, Hypertensive diseases.

b. Atherosclerotic coronary artery disease and angina

ICD-10-CM has combination codes for atherosclerotic heart disease with angina pectoris. The subcategories for these codes are I25.11, *Atherosclerotic heart disease of native coronary artery with angina pectoris* and I25.7, *Atherosclerosis of coronary artery bypass graft(s) and coronary artery of transplanted heart with angina pectoris*.

When using one of these combination codes it is not necessary to use an additional code for angina pectoris. A causal relationship can be assumed in a patient with both atherosclerosis and angina pectoris, unless the documentation indicates the angina is due to something other than the atherosclerosis.

If a patient with coronary artery disease is admitted due to an acute myocardial infarction (AMI), the AMI should be sequenced before the coronary artery disease.

See Section I.C.9. *Acute myocardial infarction (AMI)*

c. Intraoperative and Postprocedural cerebrovascular accident

Medical record documentation should clearly specify the cause- and-effect relationship between the medical intervention and the cerebrovascular accident in order to assign a code for intraoperative or postprocedural cerebrovascular accident. Proper code assignment depends on whether it was an infarction or hemorrhage and whether it occurred intraoperatively or postoperatively. If it was a cerebral hemorrhage, code assignment depends on the type of procedure performed.

d. Sequelae of Cerebrovascular Disease

1) Category I69, Sequelae of Cerebrovascular disease

Category I69 is used to indicate conditions classifiable to categories I60-I67 as the causes of late effects (neurologic deficits), themselves classified elsewhere. These "late effects" include neurologic deficits that persist after initial onset of conditions classifiable to categories I60-I67. The neurologic deficits caused by cerebrovascular disease may be present from the onset or may arise at any time after the onset of the condition classifiable to categories I60-I67.

Codes from category I69, *Sequelae of cerebrovascular disease*, that specify hemiplegia, hemiparesis and monoplegia identify whether the dominant or nondominant side is affected. Should the affected side be documented, but not specified as dominant or nondominant, and the classification system does not indicate a default, code selection is as follows:

- For ambidextrous patients, the default should be dominant.

- If the left side is affected, the default is non-dominant.

- If the right side is affected, the default is dominant.

2) Codes from category I69 with codes from I60-I67

Codes from category I69 may be assigned on a health care record with codes from I60-I67, if the patient has a current cerebrovascular disease and deficits from an old cerebrovascular disease.

3) Codes from category I69 and Personal history of transient ischemic attack (TIA) and cerebral infarction (Z86.73)

Codes from category I69 should not be assigned if the patient does not have neurologic deficits

See Section I.C.21.4. *History (of) for use of personal history codes*.

e. Acute myocardial infarction (AMI)

1) ST elevation myocardial infarction (STEMI) and non ST elevation myocardial infarction (NSTEMI)

The ICD-10-CM codes for acute myocardial infarction (AMI) identify the site, such as anterolateral wall or true posterior wall. Subcategories I21.0-I21.2 and code I21.3 are used for ST elevation myocardial infarction (STEMI). Code I21.4, *Non-ST elevation (NSTEMI) myocardial infarction*, is used for non ST elevation myocardial infarction (NSTEMI) and nontransmural MIs.

If NSTEMI evolves to STEMI, assign the STEMI code. If STEMI converts to NSTEMI due to thrombolytic therapy, it is still coded as STEMI.

For encounters occurring while the myocardial infarction is equal to, or less than, four weeks old, including transfers to another acute setting or a postacute setting, and the patient requires continued care for the myocardial infarction, codes from category I21 may continue to be reported. For encounters after the 4 week time frame and the patient is still receiving care related to the myocardial infarction, the appropriate aftercare code should be assigned, rather than a code from category I21. For old or healed myocardial infarctions not requiring further care, code I25.2, *Old myocardial infarction*, may be assigned

2) Acute myocardial infarction, unspecified

Code I21.3, *ST elevation (STEMI) myocardial infarction of unspecified site*, is the default for unspecified acute myocardial infarction. If only STEMI or transmural MI without the site is documented, assign code I21.3.

3) AMI documented as nontransmural or subendocardial but site provided

If an AMI is documented as nontransmural or subendocardial, but the site is provided, it is still coded as a subendocardial AMI.

See Section I.C.21.3 *for information on coding status post administration of tPA in a different facility within the last 24 hours.*

4) Subsequent acute myocardial infarction

A code from category I22, *Subsequent ST elevation (STEMI) and non ST elevation (NSTEMI) myocardial infarction*, is to be used when a patient who has suffered an AMI has a new AMI within the 4 week time frame of the initial AMI. A code from category I22 must be used in conjunction with a code from category I21. The sequencing of the I22 and I21 codes depends on the circumstances of the encounter.

Chapter 10: Diseases of Respiratory System (J00–J99)

a. Chronic Obstructive Pulmonary Disease [COPD] and Asthma

1) Acute exacerbation of chronic obstructive bronchitis and asthma

The codes in categories J44 and J45 distinguish between uncomplicated cases and those in acute exacerbation. An acute exacerbation is a worsening or a decompensation of a chronic condition. An acute exacerbation is not equivalent to an infection superimposed on a chronic condition, though an exacerbation may be triggered by an infection.

b. Acute Respiratory Failure

1) Acute respiratory failure as principal diagnosis

A code from subcategory J96.0, *Acute respiratory failure*, or code J96.2, *Acute and chronic respiratory failure*, may be assigned as a principal diagnosis when it is the condition established after study to be chiefly responsible for occasioning the admission to the hospital, and the selection is supported by the Alphabetic Index and Tabular List. However, chapter-specific coding guidelines (such as obstetrics, poisoning, HIV, newborn) that provide sequencing direction take precedence.

2) Acute respiratory failure as secondary diagnosis

Respiratory failure may be listed as a secondary diagnosis if it occurs after admission, or if it is present on admission, but does not meet the definition of principal diagnosis.

3) Sequencing of acute respiratory failure and another acute condition

When a patient is admitted with respiratory failure and another acute condition, (e.g., myocardial infarction, cerebrovascular accident, aspiration pneumonia), the principal diagnosis will not be the same in every situation. This applies whether the other acute condition is a respiratory or nonrespiratory condition. Selection of the principal diagnosis will be dependent on the circumstances of admission. If both the respiratory failure and the other acute condition are equally responsible for occasioning the admission to the hospital, and there are no chapter-specific sequencing rules, the guideline regarding two or more diagnoses that equally meet the definition for principal diagnosis (*Section II, C.*) may be applied in these situations.

If the documentation is not clear as to whether acute respiratory failure and another condition are equally responsible for occasioning the admission, query the provider for clarification.

c. Influenza due to certain identified influenza viruses

Code only confirmed cases of influenza due to certain identified influenza viruses (category J09), and due to other identified influenza virus (category J10). This is an exception to the hospital inpatient guideline Section II, H. (Uncertain Diagnosis).

In this context, "confirmation" does not require documentation of positive laboratory testing specific for avian or other novel influenza A or other identified influenza virus. However, coding should be based on the provider's diagnostic statement that the patient has avian influenza, or other novel influenza A, for category J09, or has another particular identified strain of influenza, such as H1N1 or H3N2, but not identified as novel or variant, for category J10.

If the provider records "suspected" or "possible" or "probable" avian influenza, or novel influenza, or other identified influenza, then the appropriate influenza code from category

J11, Influenza due to unidentified influenza virus, should be assigned. A code from category J09, Influenza due to certain identified influenza viruses, should not be assigned nor should a code from category J10, Influenza due to other identified influenza virus.

d. Ventilator associated Pneumonia

1) Documentation of Ventilator associated Pneumonia

As with all procedural or postprocedural complications, code assignment is based on the provider's documentation of the relationship between the condition and the procedure.

Code J95.851, *Ventilator associated pneumonia*, should be assigned only when the provider has documented ventilator associated pneumonia (VAP). An additional code to identify the organism (e.g., Pseudomonas aeruginosa, code B96.5) should also be assigned. Do not assign an additional code from categories J12-J18 to identify the type of pneumonia.

Code J95.851 should not be assigned for cases where the patient has pneumonia and is on a mechanical ventilator and the provider has not specifically stated that the pneumonia is ventilator-associated pneumonia. If the documentation is unclear as to whether the patient has a pneumonia that is a complication attributable to the mechanical ventilator, query the provider.

2) Ventilator associated Pneumonia Develops after Admission

A patient may be admitted with one type of pneumonia (e.g., code J13, *Pneumonia due to Streptococcus pneumonia*) and subsequently develop VAP. In this instance, the principal diagnosis would be the appropriate code from categories J12-J18 for the pneumonia diagnosed at the time of admission. Code J95.851, Ventilator associated pneumonia, would be assigned as an additional diagnosis when the provider has also documented the presence of ventilator associated pneumonia.

Chapter 11: Diseases of the Digestive System (K00-K94)

Reserved for future guideline expansion.

Chapter 12: Diseases of the Skin and Subcutaneous Tissue (L00-L99)

a. Pressure ulcer stage codes

1) Pressure ulcer stages

Codes from category L89, *Pressure ulcer*, are combination codes that identify the site of the pressure ulcer as well as the stage of the ulcer.

The ICD-10-CM classifies pressure ulcer stages based on severity, which is designated by stages 1-4, unspecified stage and unstageable.

Assign as many codes from category L89 as needed to identify all the pressure ulcers the patient has, if applicable.

2) Unstageable pressure ulcers

Assignment of the code for unstageable pressure ulcer (L89.--0) should be based on the clinical documentation. These codes are used for pressure ulcers whose stage cannot be clinically determined (e.g., the ulcer is covered by eschar or has been treated with a skin or muscle graft) and pressure ulcers that are documented as deep tissue injury but not documented as due to trauma. This code should not be confused with the codes for unspecified stage (L89.--9). When there is no documentation regarding the stage of the pressure ulcer, assign the appropriate code for unspecified stage (L89.--9).

3) Documented pressure ulcer stage

Assignment of the pressure ulcer stage code should be guided by clinical documentation of the stage or documentation of the terms found in the Alphabetic Index. For clinical terms describing the stage that are not found in the Alphabetic Index, and there is no documentation of the stage, the provider should be queried.

4) Patients admitted with pressure ulcers documented as healed

No code is assigned if the documentation states that the pressure ulcer is completely healed.

5) Patients admitted with pressure ulcers documented as healing

Pressure ulcers described as healing should be assigned the appropriate pressure ulcer stage code based on the documentation in the medical record. If the documentation does not provide information about the stage of the healing pressure ulcer, assign the appropriate code for unspecified stage.

If the documentation is unclear as to whether the patient has a current (new) pressure ulcer or if the patient is being treated for a healing pressure ulcer, query the provider.

6) Patient admitted with pressure ulcer evolving into another stage during the admission

If a patient is admitted with a pressure ulcer at one stage and it progresses to a higher stage, assign the code for the highest stage reported for that site.

Chapter 13: Diseases of the Musculoskeletal System and Connective Tissue (M00-M99)

a. Site and laterality

Most of the codes within Chapter 13 have site and laterality designations. The site represents either the bone, joint or the muscle involved. For some conditions where more than one bone, joint or muscle is usually involved, such as osteoarthritis, there is a "multiple sites" code available. For categories where no multiple site code is provided and more than one bone, joint or muscle is involved, multiple codes should be used to indicate the different sites involved.

1) **Bone versus joint**

    For certain conditions, the bone may be affected at the upper or lower end, (e.g., avascular necrosis of bone, M87, Osteoporosis, M80, M81). Though the portion of the bone affected may be at the joint, the site designation will be the bone, not the joint.

b. Acute traumatic versus chronic or recurrent musculoskeletal conditions

Many musculoskeletal conditions are a result of previous injury or trauma to a site, or are recurrent conditions. Bone, joint or muscle conditions that are the result of a healed injury are usually found in chapter 13. Recurrent bone, joint or muscle conditions are also usually found in chapter 13. Any current, acute injury should be coded to the appropriate injury code from chapter 19. Chronic or recurrent conditions should generally be coded with a code from chapter 13. If it is difficult to determine from the documentation in the record which code is best to describe a condition, query the provider.

c. Coding of Pathologic Fractures

7th character A is for use as long as the patient is receiving active treatment for the fracture. Examples of active treatment are: surgical treatment, emergency department encounter, evaluation and treatment by a new physician. 7th character, D is to be used for encounters after the patient has completed active treatment. The other 7th characters, listed under each subcategory in the Tabular List, are to be used for subsequent encounters for treatment of problems associated with the healing, such as malunions and nonunions, and sequelae.

Care for complications of surgical treatment for fracture repairs during the healing or recovery phase should be coded with the appropriate complication codes.

See Section I.C.19. *Coding of traumatic fractures*

d. Osteoporosis

Osteoporosis is a systemic condition, meaning that all bones of the musculoskeletal system are affected. Therefore, site is not a component of the codes under category M81, *Osteoporosis without current pathological fracture*. The site codes under category M80, *Osteoporosis with current pathological fracture*, identify the site of the fracture, not the osteoporosis.

1) **Osteoporosis without pathological fracture**

    Category M81, *Osteoporosis without current pathological fracture*, is for use for patients with osteoporosis who do not currently have a pathologic fracture due to the osteoporosis, even if they have had a fracture in the past. For patients with a history of osteoporosis fractures, status code Z87.31, *Personal history of osteoporosis fracture*, should follow the code from M81.

2) **Osteoporosis with current pathological fracture**

    Category M80, *Osteoporosis with current pathological fracture*, is for patients who have a current pathologic fracture at the time of an encounter. The codes under M80 identify the site of the fracture. A code from category M80, not a traumatic fracture code, should be used for any patient with known osteoporosis who suffers a fracture, even if the patient had a minor fall or

trauma, if that fall or trauma would not usually break a normal, healthy bone.

Chapter 14: Diseases of Genitourinary System (N00-N99)

a. Chronic kidney disease

1) **Stages of chronic kidney disease (CKD)**

    The ICD-10-CM classifies CKD based on severity. The severity of CKD is designated by stages I-V. Stage II, code N18.2, equates to mild CKD; stage III, code N18.3, equates to moderate CKD; and stage IV, code N18.4, equates to severe CKD. Code N18.6, *End stage renal disease (ESRD)*, is assigned when the provider has documented end-stage-renal disease (ESRD).

    If both a stage of CKD and ESRD are documented, assign code N18.6 only.

2) **Chronic kidney disease and kidney transplant status**

    Patients who have undergone kidney transplant may still have some form of chronic kidney disease (CKD) because the kidney transplant may not fully restore kidney function. Therefore, the presence of CKD alone does not constitute a transplant complication. Assign the appropriate N18 code for the patient's stage of CKD and code Z94.0, *Kidney transplant status*. If a transplant complication such as failure or rejection or other transplant complication is documented, see section I.C.19.g for information on coding complications of a kidney transplant. If the documentation is unclear as to whether the patient has a complication of the transplant, query the provider.

3) **Chronic kidney disease with other conditions**

    Patients with CKD may also suffer from other serious conditions, most commonly diabetes mellitus and hypertension. The sequencing of the CKD code in relationship to codes for other contributing conditions is based on the conventions in the Tabular List.

    See I.C.9. *Hypertensive chronic kidney disease*

    See I.C.19. *Chronic kidney disease and kidney transplant complications*

Chapter 15: Pregnancy, Childbirth, and the Puerperium (O00-O9A)

a. General Rules for Obstetric Cases

1) **Codes from chapter 15 and sequencing priority**

    Obstetric cases require codes from chapter 15, codes in the range O00-O9A, *Pregnancy, Childbirth, and the Puerperium*. Chapter 15 codes have sequencing priority over codes from other chapters. Additional codes from other chapters may be used in conjunction with chapter 15 codes to further specify conditions. Should the provider document that the pregnancy is incidental to the encounter, then code Z33.1, *Pregnant state, incidental*, should be used in place of any chapter 15 codes. It is the provider's responsibility to state that the condition being treated is not affecting the pregnancy.

2) **Chapter 15 codes used only on the maternal record**

Chapter 15 codes are to be used only on the maternal record, never on the record of the newborn.

3) **Final character for trimester**

The majority of codes in Chapter 15 have a final character indicating the trimester of pregnancy. The timeframes for the trimesters are indicated at the beginning of the chapter. If trimester is not a component of a code it is because the condition always occurs in a specific trimester, or the concept of trimester of pregnancy is not applicable. Certain codes have characters for only certain trimesters because the condition does not occur in all trimesters, but it may occur in more than just one.

Assignment of the final character for trimester should be based on the provider's documentation of the trimester (or number of weeks) for the current admission/encounter. This applies to the assignment of trimester for pre-existing conditions as well as those that develop during or are due to the pregnancy. The provider's documentation of the number of weeks may be used to assign the appropriate code identifying the trimester.

Whenever delivery occurs during the current admission, and there is an "in childbirth" option for the obstetric complication being coded, the "in childbirth" code should be assigned.

4) **Selection of trimester for inpatient admissions that encompass more than one trimesters**

In instances when a patient is admitted to a hospital for complications of pregnancy during one trimester and remains in the hospital into a subsequent trimester, the trimester character for the antepartum complication code should be assigned on the basis of the trimester when the complication developed, not the trimester of the discharge. If the condition developed prior to the current admission/encounter or represents a pre-existing condition, the trimester character for the trimester at the time of the admission/encounter should be assigned.

5) **Unspecified trimester**

Each category that includes codes for trimester has a code for "unspecified trimester." The "unspecified trimester" code should rarely be used, such as when the documentation in the record is insufficient to determine the trimester and it is not possible to obtain clarification.

6) **7th character for Fetus Identification**

Where applicable, a 7th character is to be assigned for certain categories (O31, O32, O33.3 - O33.6, O35, O36, O40, O41, O60.1, O60.2, O64, and O69) to identify the fetus for which the complication code applies.

Assign 7th character "0":

- For single gestations

- When the documentation in the record is insufficient to determine the fetus affected and it is not possible to obtain clarification.

- When it is not possible to clinically determine which fetus is affected.

b. Selection of OB Principal or First-listed Diagnosis

1) **Routine outpatient prenatal visits**

For routine outpatient prenatal visits when no complications are present, a code from category Z34, *Encounter for supervision of normal pregnancy*, should be used as the first-listed diagnosis. These codes should not be used in conjunction with chapter 15 codes.

2) **Prenatal outpatient visits for high-risk patients**

For routine prenatal outpatient visits for patients with high-risk pregnancies, a code from category O09, *Supervision of high-risk pregnancy*, should be used as the first-listed diagnosis. Secondary chapter 15 codes may be used in conjunction with these codes if appropriate.

3) **Episodes when no delivery occurs**

In episodes when no delivery occurs, the principal diagnosis should correspond to the principal complication of the pregnancy which necessitated the encounter. Should more than one complication exist, all of which are treated or monitored, any of the complications codes may be sequenced first.

4) **When a delivery occurs**

When a delivery occurs, the principal diagnosis should correspond to the main circumstances or complication of the delivery. In cases of cesarean delivery, the selection of the principal diagnosis should be the condition established after study that was responsible for the patient's admission. If the patient was admitted with a condition that resulted in the performance of a cesarean procedure, that condition should be selected as the principal diagnosis. If the reason for the admission/encounter was unrelated to the condition resulting in the cesarean delivery, the condition related to the reason for the admission/encounter should be selected as the principal diagnosis.

5) **Outcome of delivery**

A code from category Z37, *Outcome of delivery*, should be included on every maternal record when a delivery has occurred. These codes are not to be used on subsequent records or on the newborn record.

c. Pre-existing conditions versus conditions due to the pregnancy

Certain categories in Chapter 15 distinguish between conditions of the mother that existed prior to pregnancy (pre-existing) and those that are a direct result of pregnancy. When assigning codes from Chapter 15, it is important to assess if a condition was pre-existing prior to pregnancy or developed during or due to the pregnancy in order to assign the correct code.

Categories that do not distinguish between pre-existing and pregnancy-related conditions may be used for either. It is acceptable to use codes specifically for the puerperium with codes complicating pregnancy and childbirth if a condition arises postpartum during the delivery encounter.

d. Pre-existing hypertension in pregnancy

Category O10, *Pre-existing hypertension complicating pregnancy, childbirth and the puerperium*, includes codes for hypertensive heart and hypertensive chronic kidney disease. When assigning one of the O10 codes that includes hypertensive heart disease or hypertensive chronic kidney disease, it is necessary to add a secondary code from the appropriate hypertension category to specify the type of heart failure or chronic kidney disease.

See Section I.C.9. *Hypertension*

e. Fetal Conditions Affecting the Management of the Mother

1) Codes from categories O35 and O36

   Codes from categories O35, *Maternal care for known or suspected fetal abnormality and damage*, and O36, *Maternal care for other fetal problems*, are assigned only when the fetal condition is actually responsible for modifying the management of the mother, i.e., by requiring diagnostic studies, additional observation, special care, or termination of pregnancy. The fact that the fetal condition exists does not justify assigning a code from this series to the mother's record.

2) In utero surgery

   In cases when surgery is performed on the fetus, a diagnosis code from category O35, *Maternal care for known or suspected fetal abnormality and damage*, should be assigned identifying the fetal condition. Assign the appropriate procedure code for the procedure performed.

   No code from Chapter 16, the perinatal codes, should be used on the mother's record to identify fetal conditions. Surgery performed in utero on a fetus is still to be coded as an obstetric encounter.

f. HIV Infection in Pregnancy, Childbirth and the Puerperium

During pregnancy, childbirth or the puerperium, a patient admitted because of an HIV-related illness should receive a principal diagnosis from subcategory O98.7-, *Human immunodeficiency [HIV] disease complicating pregnancy, childbirth and the puerperium*, followed by the code(s) for the HIV-related illness(es).

Patients with asymptomatic HIV infection status admitted during pregnancy, childbirth, or the puerperium should receive codes of O98.7- and Z21, *Asymptomatic human immunodeficiency virus [HIV] infection status*.

g. Diabetes mellitus in pregnancy

Diabetes mellitus is a significant complicating factor in pregnancy. Pregnant women who are diabetic should be assigned a code from category O24, *Diabetes mellitus in*

pregnancy, childbirth, and the puerperium, first, followed by the appropriate diabetes code(s) (E08-E13) from Chapter 4.

h. Long term use of insulin

Code Z79.4, *Long-term (current) use of insulin*, should also be assigned if the diabetes mellitus is being treated with insulin.

i. Gestational (pregnancy induced) diabetes

Gestational (pregnancy induced) diabetes can occur during the second and third trimester of pregnancy in women who were not diabetic prior to pregnancy. Gestational diabetes can cause complications in the pregnancy similar to those of pre-existing diabetes mellitus. It also puts the woman at greater risk of developing diabetes after the pregnancy. Codes for gestational diabetes are in subcategory O24.4, *Gestational diabetes mellitus*. No other code from category O24, *Diabetes mellitus in pregnancy, childbirth, and the puerperium*, should be used with a code from O24.4

The codes under subcategory O24.4 include diet controlled and insulin controlled. If a patient with gestational diabetes is treated with both diet and insulin, only the code for insulin-controlled is required. Code Z79.4, *Long-term (current) use of insulin*, should not be assigned with codes from subcategory O24.4.

An abnormal glucose tolerance in pregnancy is assigned a code from subcategory O99.81, *Abnormal glucose complicating pregnancy, childbirth, and the puerperium*.

j. Sepsis and septic shock complicating abortion, pregnancy, childbirth and the puerperium

When assigning a chapter 15 code for sepsis complicating abortion, pregnancy, childbirth, and the puerperium, a code for the specific type of infection should be assigned as an additional diagnosis. If severe sepsis is present, a code from subcategory R65.2, Severe sepsis, and code(s) for associated organ dysfunction(s) should also be assigned as additional diagnoses.

k. Puerperal sepsis

Code O85, *Puerperal sepsis*, should be assigned with a secondary code to identify the causal organism (e.g., for a bacterial infection, assign a code from category B95-B96, *Bacterial infections in conditions classified elsewhere*). A code from category A40, *Streptococcal sepsis*, or A41, *Other sepsis*, should not be used for puerperal sepsis. If applicable, use additional codes to identify severe sepsis (R65.2-) and any associated acute organ dysfunction.

l. Alcohol and tobacco use during pregnancy, childbirth and the puerperium

1) Alcohol use during pregnancy, childbirth and the puerperium

   Codes under subcategory O99.31, *Alcohol use complicating pregnancy, childbirth, and the puerperium*, should be assigned for any pregnancy case when a mother uses alcohol during the pregnancy or postpartum. A secondary code from category F10, Alcohol related disorders, should also be assigned to identify manifestations of the alcohol use.

2) Tobacco use during pregnancy, childbirth and the puerperium

Codes under subcategory O99.33, *Smoking (tobacco) complicating pregnancy, childbirth, and the puerperium*, should be assigned for any pregnancy case when a mother uses any type of tobacco product during the pregnancy or postpartum. A secondary code from category F17, *Nicotine dependence*, should also be assigned to identify the type of nicotine dependence.

m.Poisoning, toxic effects, adverse effects and underdosing in a pregnant patient

A code from subcategory O9A.2, *Injury, poisoning and certain other consequences of external causes complicating pregnancy, childbirth, and the puerperium*, should be sequenced first, followed by the appropriate injury, poisoning, toxic effect, adverse effect or underdosing code, and then the additional code(s) that specifies the condition caused by the poisoning, toxic effect, adverse effect or underdosing.

See Section I.C.19. *Adverse effects, poisoning, underdosing and toxic effects.*

n. Normal Delivery, Code O80

1) Encounter for full term uncomplicated delivery

Code O80 should be assigned when a woman is admitted for a full-term normal delivery and delivers a single, healthy infant without any complications antepartum, during the delivery, or postpartum during the delivery episode. Code O80 is always a principal diagnosis. It is not to be used if any other code from chapter 15 is needed to describe a current complication of the antenatal, delivery, or perinatal period. Additional codes from other chapters may be used with code O80 if they are not related to or are in any way complicating the pregnancy.

2) Uncomplicated delivery with resolved antepartum complication

Code O80 may be used if the patient had a complication at some point during the pregnancy, but the complication is not present at the time of the admission for delivery.

3) Outcome of delivery for O80

Z37.0, *Single live birth*, is the only outcome of delivery code appropriate for use with O80.

o. The Peripartum and Postpartum Periods

1) Peripartum and Postpartum periods

The postpartum period begins immediately after delivery and continues for six weeks following delivery. The peripartum period is defined as the last month of pregnancy to five months postpartum.

2) Peripartum and postpartum complication

A postpartum complication is any complication occurring within the six-week period.

3) Pregnancy-related complications after 6 week period

Chapter 15 codes may also be used to describe pregnancy-related complications after the peripartum

or postpartum period if the provider documents that a condition is pregnancy related.

4) Admission for routine postpartum care following delivery outside hospital

When the mother delivers outside the hospital prior to admission and is admitted for routine postpartum care and no complications are noted, code Z39.0, *Encounter for care and examination of mother immediately after delivery*, should be assigned as the principal diagnosis.

5) Pregnancy associated cardiomyopathy

Pregnancy associated cardiomyopathy, code O90.3, is unique in that it may be diagnosed in the third trimester of pregnancy but may continue to progress months after delivery. For this reason, it is referred to as peripartum cardiomyopathy. Code O90.3 is only for use when the cardiomyopathy develops as a result of pregnancy in a woman who did not have pre-existing heart disease.

p. Code O94, Sequelae of complication of pregnancy, childbirth, and the puerperium

1) Code O94

Code O94, *Sequelae of complication of pregnancy, childbirth, and the puerperium*, is for use in those cases when an initial complication of a pregnancy develops a sequelae requiring care or treatment at a future date.

2) After the initial postpartum period

This code may be used at any time after the initial postpartum period.

3) Sequencing of Code O94

This code, like all sequela codes, is to be sequenced following the code describing the sequelae of the complication.

q. Termination of Pregnancy and Spontaneous abortions

1) Abortion with Liveborn Fetus

When an attempted termination of pregnancy results in a liveborn fetus, assign code Z33.2, *Encounter for elective termination of pregnancy* and a code from category Z37, Outcome of Delivery.

2) Retained Products of Conception following an abortion

Subsequent encounters for retained products of conception following a spontaneous abortion or elective termination of pregnancy are assigned the appropriate code from category O03, *Spontaneous abortion*, or code codes O07.4, *Failed attempted termination of pregnancy without complication* and Z33.2, *Encounter for elective termination of pregnancy*. This advice is appropriate even when the patient was discharged previously with a discharge diagnosis of complete abortion.

3) Complications leading to abortion

Codes from Chapter 15 may be used as additional codes to identify any documented complications of the pregnancy in conjunction with codes in categories in O07 and O08.

r. Abuse in a pregnant patient

For suspected or confirmed cases of abuse of a pregnant patient, a code(s) from subcategories O9A.3, *Physical abuse complicating pregnancy, childbirth, and the puerperium*, O9A.4, *Sexual abuse complicating pregnancy, childbirth, and the puerperium*, and O9A.5, *Psychological abuse complicating pregnancy, childbirth, and the puerperium*, should be sequenced first, followed by the appropriate codes (if applicable) to identify any associated current injury due to physical abuse, sexual abuse, and the perpetrator of abuse.

See Section I.C.19. *Adult and child abuse, neglect and other maltreatment.*

Chapter 16: Certain Conditions Originating in the Perinatal Period (P00-P96)

For coding and reporting purposes the perinatal period is defined as before birth through the 28th day following birth. The following guidelines are provided for reporting purposes.

a. General Perinatal Rules

1) Use of Chapter 16 Codes

   Codes in this chapter are *never* for use on the maternal record. Codes from Chapter 15, the obstetric chapter, are never permitted on the newborn record. Chapter 16 code may be used throughout the life of the patient if the condition is still present.

2) Principal Diagnosis for Birth Record

   When coding the birth episode in a newborn record, assign a code from category Z38, *Liveborn infants according to place of birth and type of delivery*, as the principal diagnosis. A code from category Z38 is assigned only once, to a newborn at the time of birth. If a newborn is transferred to another institution, a code from category Z38 should not be used at the receiving hospital.

   A code from category Z38 is used only on the newborn record, not on the mother's record.

3) Use of Codes from other Chapters with Codes from Chapter 16

   Codes from other chapters may be used with codes from chapter 16 if the codes from the other chapters provide more specific detail. Codes for signs and symptoms may be assigned when a definitive diagnosis has not been established. If the reason for the encounter is a perinatal condition, the code from chapter 16 should be sequenced first.

4) Use of Chapter 16 Codes after the Perinatal Period

   Should a condition originate in the perinatal period, and continue throughout the life of the patient, the perinatal code should continue to be used regardless of the patient's age.

5) Birth process or community acquired conditions

   If a newborn has a condition that may be either due to the birth process or community acquired and the documentation does not indicate which it is, the default is due to the birth process and the code

from Chapter 16 should be used. If the condition is community-acquired, a code from Chapter 16 should not be assigned.

6) Code all clinically significant conditions

   All clinically significant conditions noted on routine newborn examination should be coded. A condition is clinically significant if it requires:

   • clinical evaluation; or

   • therapeutic treatment; or

   • diagnostic procedures; or

   • extended length of hospital stay; or

   • increased nursing care and/or monitoring; or

   • has implications for future health care needs

   Note: The perinatal guidelines listed above are the same as the general coding guidelines for "additional diagnoses", except for the final point regarding implications for future health care needs. Codes should be assigned for conditions that have been specified by the provider as having implications for future health care needs.

b. Observation and Evaluation of Newborns for Suspected Conditions not Found

Reserved for future expansion.

c. Coding Additional Perinatal Diagnoses

1) Assigning codes for conditions that require treatment

   Assign codes for conditions that require treatment or further investigation, prolong the length of stay, or require resource utilization.

2) Codes for conditions specified as having implications for future health care needs

   Assign codes for conditions that have been specified by the provider as having implications for future health care needs.

   Note: This guideline should not be used for adult patients.

d. Prematurity and Fetal Growth Retardation

Providers utilize different criteria in determining prematurity. A code for prematurity should not be assigned unless it is documented. Assignment of codes in categories P05, *Disorders of newborn related to slow fetal growth and fetal malnutrition*, and P07, *Disorders of newborn related to short gestation and low birth weight, not elsewhere classified*, should be based on the recorded birth weight and estimated gestational age. Codes from category P05 should not be assigned with codes from category P07.

When both birth weight and gestational age are available, two codes from category P07 should be assigned, with the code for birth weight sequenced before the code for gestational age.

e. Low birth weight and immaturity status

Codes from category P07, *Disorders of newborn related to short gestation and low birth weight, not elsewhere classified*, are for use for a child or adult who was premature or had a low birth weight as a newborn and this is affecting the patient's current health status.

See Section I.C.21. *Factors influencing health status and contact with health services, Status*

f. Bacterial Sepsis of Newborn

Category P36, *Bacterial sepsis of newborn*, includes congenital sepsis. If a perinate is documented as having sepsis without documentation of congenital or community acquired, the default is congenital and a code from category P36 should be assigned. If the P36 code includes the causal organism, an additional code from category B95, *Streptococcus, Staphylococcus, and Enterococcus* as the cause of diseases classified elsewhere, or B96, *Other bacterial agents as the cause of diseases classified elsewhere*, should *not* be assigned. If the P36 code does not include the causal organism, assign an additional code from category B96. If applicable, use additional codes to identify severe sepsis (R65.2-) and any associated acute organ dysfunction.

g. Stillbirth

Code P95, *Stillbirth*, is only for use in institutions that maintain separate records for stillbirths. No other code should be used with P95. Code P95 should not be used on the mother's record.

Chapter 17: Congenital Malformations, Deformations, and Chromosomal Abnormalities (Q00-Q99)

Assign an appropriate code(s) from categories Q00-Q99, Congenital malformations, deformations, and chromosomal abnormalities when a malformation/deformation or chromosomal abnormality is documented. A malformation/deformation or chromosomal abnormality may be the principal/first listed diagnosis on a record or a secondary diagnosis.

When a malformation/deformation or chromosomal abnormality does not have a unique code assignment, assign additional code(s) for any manifestations that may be present.

When the code assignment specifically identifies the malformation/deformation or chromosomal abnormality, manifestations that are an inherent component of the anomaly should not be coded separately. Additional codes should be assigned for manifestations that are not an inherent component.

Codes from Chapter 17 may be used throughout the life of the patient. If a congenital malformation or deformity has been corrected, a personal history code should be used to identify the history of the malformation or deformity. Although present at birth, malformation/deformation or chromosomal abnormality may not be identified until later in life. Whenever the condition is diagnosed by the physician, it is appropriate to assign a code from codes Q00-Q99. For the birth admission, the appropriate code from category Z38, *Liveborn infants, according to place of birth and type of delivery*, should be sequenced as the principal diagnosis, followed by any congenital anomaly codes, Q00- Q99.

Chapter 18: Symptoms, Signs, and Abnormal Clinical and Laboratory Findings, Not Elsewhere Classified (R00-R99)

Chapter 18 includes symptoms, signs, abnormal results of clinical or other investigative procedures, and ill-defined conditions regarding which no diagnosis classifiable elsewhere is recorded. Signs and symptoms that point to a specific diagnosis have been assigned to a category in other chapters of the classification.

a. Use of symptom codes

Codes that describe symptoms and signs are acceptable for reporting purposes when a related definitive diagnosis has not been established (confirmed) by the provider.

b. Use of a symptom code with a definitive diagnosis code

Codes for signs and symptoms may be reported in addition to a related definitive diagnosis when the sign or symptom is not routinely associated with that diagnosis, such as the various signs and symptoms associated with complex syndromes. The definitive diagnosis code should be sequenced before the symptom code.

Signs or symptoms that are associated routinely with a disease process should not be assigned as additional codes, unless otherwise instructed by the classification.

c. Combination codes that include symptoms

ICD-10-CM contains a number of combination codes that identify both the definitive diagnosis and common symptoms of that diagnosis. When using one of these combination codes, an additional code should not be assigned for the symptom

d. Repeated falls

Code R29.6, *Repeated falls*, is for use for encounters when a patient has recently fallen and the reason for the fall is being investigated.

Code Z91.81, *History of falling*, is for use when a patient has fallen in the past and is at risk for future falls. When appropriate, both codes R29.6 and Z91.81 may be assigned together.

e. Coma scale

The coma scale codes (R40.2-) can be used in conjunction with traumatic brain injury codes, acute cerebrovascular disease or sequelae of cerebrovascular disease codes. These codes are primarily for use by trauma registries, but they may be used in any setting where this information is collected. The coma scale codes should be sequenced after the diagnosis code(s).

These codes, one from each subcategory, are needed to complete the scale. The 7th character indicates when the scale was recorded. The 7th character should match for all three codes.

At a minimum, report the initial score documented on presentation at your facility. This may be a score from the emergency medicine technician (EMT) or in the emergency department. If desired, a facility may choose to capture multiple coma scale scores.

Assign code R40.24, Glasgow coma scale, total score, when only the total score is documented in the medical record and not the individual score(s).

f. Functional quadriplegia

Functional quadriplegia (code R53.2) is the lack of ability to use one's limbs or to ambulate due to extreme debility. It is not associated with neurologic deficit or injury, and code R53.2 should not be used for cases of neurologic quadriplegia. It should only be assigned if functional quadriplegia is specifically documented in the medical record.

g. SIRS due to Non-Infectious Process

The systemic inflammatory response syndrome (SIRS) can develop as a result of certain non-infectious disease processes, such as trauma, malignant neoplasm, or pancreatitis. When SIRS is documented with a noninfectious condition, and no subsequent infection is documented, the code for the underlying condition, such as an injury, should be assigned, followed by code R65.10, *Systemic inflammatory response syndrome (SIRS) of non-infectious origin without acute organ dysfunction*, or code R65.11, *Systemic inflammatory response syndrome (SIRS) of non-infectious origin with acute organ dysfunction*. If an associated acute organ dysfunction is documented, the appropriate code(s) for the specific type of organ dysfunction(s) should be assigned in addition to code R65.11. If acute organ dysfunction is documented, but it cannot be determined if the acute organ dysfunction is associated with SIRS or due to another condition (e.g., directly due to the trauma), the provider should be queried.

h. Death NOS

Code R99, *Ill-defined and unknown cause of mortality*, is only for use in the very limited circumstance when a patient who has already died is brought into an emergency department or other healthcare facility and is pronounced dead upon arrival. It does not represent the discharge disposition of death.

Chapter 19: Injury, Poisoning, and Certain Other Consequences of External Causes (S00-T88)

a. Application of 7th Characters in Chapter 19

Most categories in chapter 19 have a 7th character requirement for each applicable code. Most categories in this chapter have three 7th character values (with the exception of fractures): A, initial encounter, D, subsequent encounter and S, sequela. Categories for traumatic fractures have additional 7th character values.

7th character "A", initial encounter is used while the patient is receiving active treatment for the condition. Examples of active treatment are: surgical treatment, emergency department encounter, and evaluation and treatment by a new physician.

7th character "D" subsequent encounter is used for encounters after the patient has received active treatment of the condition and is receiving routine care for the condition during the healing or recovery phase. Examples of subsequent care are: cast change or removal, removal of external or internal fixation device, medication adjustment, other aftercare and follow up visits following treatment of the injury or condition.

The aftercare Z codes should not be used for aftercare for conditions such as injuries or poisonings, where 7th characters are provided to identify subsequent care. For example, for aftercare of an injury, assign the acute injury code with the 7th character "D" (subsequent encounter).

7th character "S", sequela, is for use for complications or conditions that arise as a direct result of a condition, such as scar formation after a burn. The scars are sequelae of the burn. When using 7th character "S", it is necessary to use both the injury code that precipitated the sequela and the code for the sequela itself. The "S" is added only to the injury code, not the sequela code. The 7th character "S" identifies the injury responsible for the sequela. The specific type of sequela (e.g. scar) is sequenced first, followed by the injury code.

b. Coding of Injuries

When coding injuries, assign separate codes for each injury unless a combination code is provided, in which case the combination code is assigned. Code T07, *Unspecified multiple injuries* should not be assigned int the inpatient setting unless information for a more specific code is not available. Traumatic injury codes (S00-T14.9) are not to be used for normal, healing surgical wounds or to identify complications of surgical wounds

The code for the most serious injury, as determined by the provider and the focus of treatment, is sequenced first.

1) Superficial injuries

Superficial injuries such as abrasions or contusions are not coded when associated with more severe injuries of the same site.

2) Primary injury with damage to nerves/blood vessels

When a primary injury results in minor damage to peripheral nerves or blood vessels, the primary injury is sequenced first with additional code(s) for injuries to nerves and spinal cord (such as category S04), and/or injury to blood vessels (such as category S15). When the primary injury is to the blood vessels or nerves, that injury should be sequenced first.

c. Coding of Traumatic Fractures

The principles of multiple coding of injuries should be followed in coding fractures. Fractures of specified sites are coded individually by site in accordance with both the provisions within categories S02, S12, S22, S32, S42, S49, S52, S59, S62, S72, S79, S82, S89, S92 and the level of detail furnished by medical record content.

A fracture not indicated as open or closed should be coded to closed. A fracture not indicated whether displaced or not displaced should be coded to displaced.

More specific guidelines are as follows:

1) Initial vs. Subsequent Encounter for Fractures

Traumatic fractures are coded using the appropriate 7th character for initial encounter (A, B, C) while the patient is receiving active treatment for the fracture. Examples of active treatment are: surgical treatment, emergency department encounter, and evaluation and treatment by a new physician. The appropriate 7th character for initial encounter should also be assigned for a patient who delayed seeking treatment for the fracture or nonunion.

Fractures are coded using the appropriate 7th character for subsequent care for encounters after the patient has completed active treatment of the fracture and is receiving routine care for the fracture during the healing or recovery phase. Examples of fracture aftercare are: cast change or removal, removal of external or internal fixation device, medication adjustment, and follow up visits following fracture treatment.

Care for complications of surgical treatment for fracture repairs during the healing or recovery phase should be coded with the appropriate complication codes.

Care of complications of fractures, such as malunion and nonunion, should be reported with the appropriate 7th character for subsequent care with nonunion (K, M, N,) or subsequent care with malunion (P, Q, R).

A code from category M80, not a traumatic fracture code, should be used for any patient with known osteoporosis who suffers a fracture, even if the patient had a minor fall or trauma, if that fall or trauma would not usually break a normal, healthy bone.

See Section I.C.13. *Osteoporosis*

The aftercare Z codes should not be used for aftercare for traumatic fractures. For aftercare of a traumatic fracture, assign the acute fracture code with the appropriate 7th character.

2) Multiple fractures sequencing

Multiple fractures are sequenced in accordance with the severity of the fracture.

d. Coding of Burns and Corrosions

The ICD-10-CM makes a distinction between burns and corrosions. The burn codes are for thermal burns, except sunburns, that come from a heat source, such as a fire or hot appliance. The burn codes are also for burns resulting from electricity and radiation. Corrosions are burns due to chemicals. The guidelines are the same for burns and corrosions.

Current burns (T20-T25) are classified by depth, extent and by agent (X code). Burns are classified by depth as first degree (erythema), second degree (blistering), and third degree (full-thickness involvement). Burns of the eye and internal organs (T26-T28) are classified by site, but not by degree.

1) Sequencing of burn and related condition codes

Sequence first the code that reflects the highest degree of burn when more than one burn is present.

a. When the reason for the admission or encounter is for treatment of external multiple burns, sequence

first the code that reflects the burn of the highest degree.

b. When a patient has both internal and external burns, the circumstances of admission govern the selection of the principal diagnosis or first-listed diagnosis.

c. When a patient is admitted for burn injuries and other related conditions such as smoke inhalation and/or respiratory failure, the circumstances of admission govern the selection of the principal or first-listed diagnosis.

2) Burns of the same local site

Classify burns of the same local site (three-digit category level, T20-T28) but of different degrees to the subcategory identifying the highest degree recorded in the diagnosis.

3) Non-healing burns

Non-healing burns are coded as acute burns.

Necrosis of burned skin should be coded as a non-healed burn.

4) Infected Burn

For any documented infected burn site, use an additional code for the infection.

5) Assign separate codes for each burn site

When coding burns, assign separate codes for each burn site. Category T30, Burn and corrosion, body region unspecified is extremely vague and should rarely be used.

6) Burns and Corrosions Classified According to Extent of Body Surface Involved

Assign codes from category T31, *Burns classified according to extent of body surface involved*, or T32, *Corrosions classified according to extent of body surface involved*, when the site of the burn is not specified or when there is a need for additional data. It is advisable to use category T31 as additional coding when needed to provide data for evaluating burn mortality, such as that needed by burn units. It is also advisable to use category T31 as an additional code for reporting purposes when there is mention of a third-degree burn involving 20 percent or more of the body surface.

Categories T31 and T32 are based on the classic "rule of nines" in estimating body surface involved: head and neck are assigned nine percent, each arm nine percent, each leg 18 percent, the anterior trunk 18 percent, posterior trunk 18 percent, and genitalia one percent. Providers may change these percentage assignments where necessary to accommodate infants and children who have proportionately larger heads than adults, and patients who have large buttocks, thighs, or abdomen that involve burns.

7) Encounters for treatment of sequela of burns

Encounters for the treatment of the late effects of burns or corrosions (i.e., scars or joint contractures) should be coded with a burn or corrosion code with the 7th character "S" for sequela.

8) **Sequelae with a late effect code and current burn**

When appropriate, both a code for a current burn or corrosion with 7th character "A" or "D" and a burn or corrosion code with 7th character "S" may be assigned on the same record (when both a current burn and sequelae of an old burn exist). Burns and corrosions do not heal at the same rate and a current healing wound may still exist with sequela of a healed burn or corrosion.

9) **Use of an external cause code with burns and corrosions**

An external cause code should be used with burns and corrosions to identify the source and intent of the burn, as well as the place where it occurred.

e. Adverse Effects, Poisoning , Underdosing and Toxic Effects

Codes in categories T36-T65 are combination codes that include the substance that was taken as well as the intent. No additional external cause code is required for poisonings, toxic effects, adverse effects and underdosing codes.

1) **Do not code directly from the Table of Drugs**

Do not code directly from the Table of Drugs and Chemicals. Always refer back to the Tabular List.

2) **Use as many codes as necessary to describe**

Use as many codes as necessary to describe completely all drugs, medicinal or biological substances.

3) **If the same code would describe the causative agent**

If the same code would describe the causative agent for more than one adverse reaction, poisoning, toxic effect or underdosing, assign the code only once.

4) **If two or more drugs, medicinal or biological substances**

If two or more drugs, medicinal or biological substances are reported, code each individually unless a combination code is listed in the Table of Drugs and Chemicals.

5) The occurrence of drug toxicity is classified in ICD-10-CM as follows:

(a) Adverse Effect
When coding an adverse effect of a drug that has been correctly prescribed and properly administered, assign the appropriate code for the nature of the adverse effect followed by the appropriate code for the adverse effect of the drug (T36-T50). The code for the drug should have a 5th or 6th character "5" (for example T36.0X5-).

Examples of the nature of an adverse effect are tachycardia, delirium, gastrointestinal hemorrhaging, vomiting, hypokalemia, hepatitis, renal failure, or respiratory failure.

(b) Poisoning
When coding a poisoning or reaction to the improper use of a medication (e.g., overdose, wrong substance given or taken in error, wrong route of administration), first assign the appropriate code from categories T36-T50. The poisoning codes have an associated intent

as their 5th or 6th character (accidental, intentional self-harm, assault and undetermined. Use additional code(s) for all manifestations of poisonings.

If there is also a diagnosis of abuse or dependence of the substance, the abuse or dependence is assigned as an additional code.

Examples of poisoning include:

(i) Error was made in drug prescription

Errors made in drug prescription or in the administration of the drug by provider, nurse, patient, or other person.

(ii) Overdose of a drug intentionally taken

If an overdose of a drug was intentionally taken or administered and resulted in drug toxicity, it would be coded as a poisoning.

(iii) Nonprescribed drug taken with correctly prescribed and properly administered drug.

If a nonprescribed drug or medicinal agent was taken in combination with a correctly prescribed and properly administered drug, any drug toxicity or other reaction resulting from the interaction of the two drugs would be classified as a poisoning.

(iv) Interaction of drug(s) and alcohol

When a reaction results from the interaction of a drug(s) and alcohol, this would be classified as poisoning.

See Section I.C.4. *if poisoning is the result of insulin pump malfunctions.*

(c) Underdosing
Underdosing refers to taking less of a medication than is prescribed by a provider or a manufacturer's instruction. For underdosing, assign the code from categories T36-T50 (fifth or sixth character "6").

Codes for underdosing should never be assigned as principal or first-listed codes. If a patient has a relapse or exacerbation of the medical condition for which the drug is prescribed because of the reduction in dose, then the medical condition itself should be coded.

Noncompliance (Z91.12-, Z91.13-) or complication of care (Y63.6-Y63.9) codes are to be used with an underdosing code to indicate intent, if known.

(d) Toxic Effects
When a harmful substance is ingested or comes in contact with a person, this is classified as a toxic effect. The toxic effect codes are in categories T51-T65.

Toxic effect codes have an associated intent: accidental, intentional self-harm, assault and undetermined.

f. Adult and child abuse, neglect and other maltreatment

Sequence first the appropriate code from categories T74.- (Adult and child abuse, neglect and other maltreatment, confirmed) or T76.- (Adult and child abuse, neglect and other maltreatment, suspected) for abuse, neglect and other maltreatment, followed by any accompanying mental health or injury code(s).

If the documentation in the medical record states abuse or neglect it is coded as confirmed (T74.-). It is coded as suspected if it is documented as suspected (T76.-).

For cases of confirmed abuse or neglect an external cause code from the assault section (X92-Y08) should be added to identify the cause of any physical injuries. A perpetrator code (Y07) should be added when the perpetrator of the abuse is known. For suspected cases of abuse or neglect, do not report external cause or perpetrator code.

If a suspected case of abuse, neglect or mistreatment is ruled out during an encounter code Z04.71, *Encounter for examination and observation following alleged physical adult abuse, ruled out*, or code Z04.72, *Encounter for examination and observation following alleged child physical abuse, ruled out*, should be used, not a code from T76.

If a suspected case of alleged rape or sexual abuse is ruled out during an encounter code Z04.41, *Encounter for examination and observation following alleged physical adult abuse, ruled out*, or code Z04.42, *Encounter for examination and observation following alleged rape or sexual abuse, ruled out*, should be used, not a code from T76

See Section I.C.15. *Abuse in a pregnant patient.*

g. Complications of care

1) General Guidelines for complications of care

(a) Documentation of complications of care

See Section I.B.16. *for information on documentation of complications of care.*

2) Pain due to medical devices

Pain associated with devices, implants or grafts left in a surgical site (for example painful hip prosthesis) is assigned to the appropriate code(s) found in Chapter 19, Injury, poisoning, and certain other consequences of external causes. Specific codes for pain due to medical devices are found in the T code section of the ICD-10-CM. Use additional code(s) from category G89 to identify acute or chronic pain due to presence of the device, implant or graft (G89.18 or G89.28).

3) Transplant complications

(a) Transplant complications other than kidney

Codes under category T86, Complications of transplanted organs and tissues, are for use for both complications and rejection of transplanted organs. A transplant complication code is only assigned if the complication affects the function of the transplanted organ. Two codes are required to fully describe a transplant complication: the appropriate code from category T86 and a secondary code that identifies the complication.

Pre-existing conditions or conditions that develop after the transplant are not coded as complications unless they affect the function of the transplanted organs.

See I.C.21 *for transplant organ removal status*

See I.C.2. *for malignant neoplasm associated with transplanted organ*

(b) Kidney transplant complications

Patients who have undergone kidney transplant may still have some form of chronic kidney disease (CKD) because the kidney transplant may not fully restore kidney function. Code T86.1- should be assigned for documented complications of a kidney transplant, such as transplant failure or rejection or other transplant complication. Code T86.1- should not be assigned for post kidney transplant patients who have chronic kidney (CKD) unless a transplant complication such as transplant failure or rejection is documented. If the documentation is unclear as to whether the patient has a complication of the transplant, query the provider.

Conditions that affect the function of the transplanted kidney, other than CKD, should be assigned a code from subcategory T86.1, *Complications of transplanted organ, Kidney*, and a secondary code that identifies the complication.

For patients with CKD following a kidney transplant, but who do not have a complication such as failure or rejection, *see* Section I.C.14. *Chronic kidney disease and kidney transplant status.*

4) Complication codes that include the external cause

As with certain other T codes, some of the complications of care codes have the external cause included in the code. The code includes the nature of the complication as well as the type of procedure that caused the complication. No external cause code indicating the type of procedure is necessary for these codes.

5) Complications of care codes within the body system chapters

Intraoperative and postprocedural complication codes are found within the body system chapters with codes specific to the organs and structures of that body system. These codes should be sequenced first, followed by a code(s) for the specific complication, if applicable.

Chapter 20: External Causes of Morbidity (V00-Y99)

The external causes of morbidity codes should never be sequenced as the first-listed or principal diagnosis.

External cause codes are intended to provide data for injury research and evaluation of injury prevention strategies. These codes capture how the injury or health condition happened (cause), the intent (unintentional or accidental; or intentional, such as suicide or assault), the place where the event occurred and the activity of the patient at the time of the event, and the person's status (e.g., civilian, military).

There is no national requirement for mandatory ICD-10-CM external cause code reporting. Unless a provider is subject to a state-based external cause code reporting mandate or these codes are required by a particular payer, reporting of ICD-10-CM codes in Chapter 20, External Causes of Morbidity, is not required. In the absence of a mandatory reporting requirement, providers are encouraged to voluntarily report external cause codes, as they provide valuable data for injury research and evaluation of injury prevention strategies.

a. General External Cause Coding Guidelines

1) **Used with any code in the range of A00.0-T88.9, Z00-Z99**

   An external cause code may be used with any code in the range of A00.0-T88.9, Z00-Z99, classification that is a health condition due to an external cause. Though they are most applicable to injuries, they are also valid for use with such things as infections or diseases due to an external source, and other health conditions, such as a heart attack that occurs during strenuous physical activity.

2) **External cause code used for length of treatment**

   Assign the external cause code, with the appropriate 7th character (initial encounter, subsequent encounter or sequela) for each encounter for which the injury or condition is being treated.

3) **Use the full range of external cause codes**

   Use the full range of external cause codes to completely describe the cause, the intent, the place of occurrence, and if applicable, the activity of the patient at the time of the event, and the patient's status, for all injuries, and other health conditions due to an external cause.

4) **Assign as many external cause codes as necessary**

   Assign as many external cause codes as necessary to fully explain each cause. If only one external code can be recorded, assign the code most related to the principal diagnosis.

5) **The selection of the appropriate external cause code**

   The selection of the appropriate external cause code is guided by the Alphabetic Index of External Causes and by Inclusion and Exclusion notes in the Tabular List.

6) **External cause code can never be a principal diagnosis**

   An external cause code can never be a principal (first listed) diagnosis.

7) **Combination external cause codes**

   Certain of the external cause codes are combination codes that identify sequential events that result in an injury, such as a fall which results in striking against an object. The injury may be due to either event or both. The combination external cause code used should correspond to the sequence of events regardless of which caused the most serious injury.

8) **No external cause code needed in certain circumstances**

   No external cause code from Chapter 20 is needed if the external cause and intent are included in a code from another chapter (e.g. T36.0x1-- Poisoning by penicillins, accidental (unintentional)).

b. Place of Occurrence Guideline

Codes from category Y92, *Place of occurrence of the external cause*, are secondary codes for use after other external cause codes to identify the location of the patient at the time of injury or other condition.

A place of occurrence code is used only once, at the initial encounter for treatment. No 7th characters are used for Y92. Only one code from Y92 should be recorded on a medical record.

Do not use place of occurrence code Y92.9 if the place is not stated or is not applicable.

c. Activity Code

Assign a code from category Y93, Activity code, to describe the activity of the patient at the time the injury or other health condition occurred.

An activity code is used only once, at the initial encounter for treatment. Only one code from Y93 should be recorded on a medical record.

The activity codes are not applicable to poisonings, adverse effects, misadventures or sequela.

Do not assign Y93.9, *Unspecified activity*, if the activity is not stated.

A code from category Y93 is appropriate for use with external cause and intent codes if identifying the activity provides additional information about the event.

d. Place of Occurrence, Activity, and Status Codes Used with other External Cause Code

When applicable, place of occurrence, activity, and external cause status codes are sequenced after the main external cause code(s). Regardless of the number of external cause codes assigned, there should be only one place of occurrence code, one activity code, and one external cause status code assigned to an encounter.

e. If the Reporting Format Limits the Number of External Cause Codes

If the reporting format limits the number of external cause codes that can be used in reporting clinical data, report the code for the cause/intent most related to the principal diagnosis. If the format permits capture of additional external cause codes, the cause/intent, including medical misadventures, of the additional events should be reported rather than the codes for place, activity, or external status.

f. Multiple External Cause Coding Guidelines

More than one external cause code is required to fully describe the external cause of an illness or injury. The assignment of external cause codes should be sequenced in the following priority:

If two or more events cause separate injuries, an external cause code should be assigned for each cause. The first listed external cause code will be selected in the following order:

External cause codes for child and adult abuse take priority over all other external cause codes.

See Section I.C.19. *Child and Adult abuse guidelines*

External cause codes for terrorism events take priority over all other external cause codes except child and adult abuse

External cause codes for cataclysmic events take priority over all other external cause codes except child and adult abuse and terrorism.

External cause codes for transport accidents take priority over all other external cause codes except cataclysmic events, child and adult abuse and terrorism.

Activity and external cause status codes are assigned following all causal (intent) external cause codes.

The first-listed external cause code should correspond to the cause of the most serious diagnosis due to an assault, accident, or self-harm, following the order of hierarchy listed above.

g. Child and Adult Abuse Guideline

Adult and child abuse, neglect and maltreatment are classified as assault. Any of the assault codes may be used to indicate the external cause of any injury resulting from the confirmed abuse.

For confirmed cases of abuse, neglect and maltreatment, when the perpetrator is known, a code from Y07, Perpetrator of maltreatment and neglect, should accompany any other assault codes.

See Section I.C.19. *Adult and child abuse, neglect and other maltreatment*

h. Unknown or Undetermined Intent Guideline

If the intent (accident, self-harm, assault) of the cause of an injury or other condition is unknown or unspecified, code the intent as accidental intent. All transport accident categories assume accidental intent.

1) Use of undetermined intent

External cause codes for events of undetermined intent are only for use if the documentation in the record specifies that the intent cannot be determined

i. Sequelae (Late Effects) of External Cause Guidelines

1) Sequelae external cause codes

Sequela are reported using the external cause code with the 7th character "S" for sequela. These codes should be used with any report of a late effect or sequela resulting from a previous injury.

2) Sequela external cause code with a related current injury

A sequela external cause code should never be used with a related current nature of injury code.

3) Use of sequela external cause codes for subsequent visits

Use a late effect external cause code for subsequent visits when a late effect of the initial injury is being treated. Do not use a late effect external cause code for subsequent visits for follow-up care (e.g., to assess healing, to receive rehabilitative therapy) of the injury when no late effect of the injury has been documented.

j. Terrorism Guidelines

1) Cause of injury identified by the Federal Government (FBI) as terrorism

When the cause of an injury is identified by the Federal Government (FBI) as terrorism, the first-listed external cause code should be a code from category Y38, *Terrorism*. The definition of terrorism employed by the FBI is found at the inclusion note at the beginning of category Y38. Use additional code for place of occurrence (Y92.-). More than one Y38 code may be assigned if the injury is the result of more than one mechanism of terrorism.

2) Cause of an injury is suspected to be the result of terrorism

When the cause of an injury is suspected to be the result of terrorism a code from category Y38 should not be assigned. Suspected cases should be classified as assault.

3) Code Y38.9, *Terrorism, secondary effects*

Assign code Y38.9, *Terrorism, secondary effects*, for conditions occurring subsequent to the terrorist event. This code should not be assigned for conditions that are due to the initial terrorist act.

It is acceptable to assign code Y38.9 with another code from Y38 if there is an injury due to the initial terrorist event and an injury that is a subsequent result of the terrorist event.

k. External cause status

A code from category Y99, *External cause status*, should be assigned whenever any other external cause code is assigned for an encounter, including an Activity code, except for the events noted below. Assign a code from category Y99, *External cause status*, to indicate the work status of the person at the time the event occurred. The status code indicates whether the event occurred during military activity, whether a non-military person was at work, whether an individual including a student or volunteer was involved in a non-work activity at the time of the causal event.

A code from Y99, *External cause status*, should be assigned, when applicable, with other external cause codes, such as transport accidents and falls. The external cause status codes are not applicable to poisonings, adverse effects, misadventures or late effects.

Do not assign a code from category Y99 if no other external cause codes (cause, activity) are applicable for the encounter.

An external cause status code is used only once, at the initial encounter for treatment. Only one code from Y99 should be recorded on a medical record.

Do not assign code Y99.9, *Unspecified external cause status*, if the status is not stated.

Chapter 21: Factors Influencing Health Status and Contact with Health Services (Z00-Z99)

Note: The chapter specific guidelines provide additional information about the use of Z codes for specified encounters.

a. Use of Z codes in any healthcare setting

Z codes are for use in any healthcare setting. Z codes may be used as either a first listed (principal diagnosis code in the inpatient setting) or secondary code, depending on the circumstances of the encounter. Certain Z codes may only be used as first listed or principal diagnosis.

b Z Codes indicate a reason for an encounter

Z codes are not procedure codes. A corresponding procedure code must accompany a Z code to describe any procedure performed.

c. Categories of Z Codes

1)   Contact/Exposure

Category Z20 indicates contact with, and suspected exposure to, communicable diseases. These codes are for patients who do not show any sign or symptom of a disease but are suspected to have been exposed to it by close personal contact with an infected individual or are in an area where a disease is epidemic.

Category Z77, indicates contact with and suspected exposures hazardous to health.

Contact/exposure codes may be used as a first listed code to explain an encounter for testing, or, more commonly, as a secondary code to identify a potential risk.

2)   Inoculations and vaccinations

Code Z23 is for encounters for inoculations and vaccinations. It indicates that a patient is being seen to receive a prophylactic inoculation against a disease. Procedure codes are required to identify the actual administration of the injection and the type(s) of immunizations given. Code Z23 may be used as a secondary code if the inoculation is given as a routine part of preventive health care, such as a well-baby visit.

3)   Status

Status codes indicate that a patient is either a carrier of a disease or has the sequelae or residual of a past disease or condition. This includes such things as the presence of prosthetic or mechanical devices resulting from past treatment. A status code is informative, because the status may affect the course of treatment and its outcome. A status code is distinct from a history code. The history code indicates that the patient no longer has the condition.

A status code should not be used with a diagnosis code from one of the body system chapters, if the diagnosis code includes the information provided by the status code. For example, code Z94.1, *Heart transplant status*, should not be used with a code from subcategory T86.2, *Complications of heart transplant*. The status code does not provide additional information. The complication code indicates that the patient is a heart transplant patient.

For encounters for weaning from a mechanical ventilator, assign code J96.1, *Chronic respiratory failure*, followed by code Z99.11, *Dependence on respirator [ventilator] status*.

The status Z codes/categories are:

Z14 Genetic carrier

Genetic carrier status indicates that a person carries a gene, associated with a particular disease, which may be passed to offspring who may develop that disease. The person does not have the disease and is not at risk of developing the disease.

Z15 Genetic susceptibility to disease

Genetic susceptibility indicates that a person has a gene that increases the risk of that person developing the disease.

Codes from category Z15 should not be used as principal or first-listed codes. If the patient has the condition to which he/she is susceptible, and that condition is the reason for the encounter, the code for the current condition should be sequenced first. If the patient is being seen for follow-up after completed treatment for this condition, and the condition no longer exists, a follow-up code should be sequenced first, followed by the appropriate personal history and genetic susceptibility codes. If the purpose of the encounter is genetic counseling associated with procreative management, code Z31.5, *Encounter for genetic counseling*, should be assigned as the first-listed code, followed by a code from category Z15. Additional codes should be assigned for any applicable family or personal history.

Z16 Resistance to antimicrobial drugs

This code indicates that a patient has a condition that is resistant to antimicrobial drug treatment. Sequence the infection code first.

Z17 Estrogen receptor status

Z18 Retained foreign body fragments

Z21 Asymptomatic HIV infection status

This code indicates that a patient has tested positive for HIV but has manifested no signs or symptoms of the disease.

Z22 Carrier of infectious disease

Carrier status indicates that a person harbors the specific organisms of a disease without manifest symptoms and is capable of transmitting the infection.

Z28.3 Underimmunization status

Z33.1 Pregnant state, incidental

This code is a secondary code only for use when the pregnancy is in no way complicating the reason for visit. Otherwise, a code from the obstetric chapter is required.

Z66 Do not resuscitate

This code may be used when it is documented by the provider that a patient is on do not resuscitate status at any time during the stay

Z67 Blood type

Z68 Body mass index (BMI)

Z74.01 Bed confinement status

Z76.82 Awaiting organ transplant status

Z78 Other specified health status

Code Z78.1, *Physical restraint status*, may be used when it is documented by the provider that a patient has been put in restraints during the current encounter. Please note that this code should not be reported when it is documented by the provider that a patient is temporarily restrained during a procedure.

Z79 Long-term (current) drug therapy

Codes from this category indicate a patient's continuous use of a prescribed drug (including such things as aspirin therapy) for the long-term treatment of a condition or for prophylactic use. It is not for use for patients who have addictions to drugs. This subcategory is not for use of medications for detoxification or maintenance programs to prevent withdrawal symptoms in patients with drug dependence (e.g., methadone maintenance for opiate dependence). Assign the appropriate code for the drug dependence instead.

Assign a code from Z79 if the patient is receiving a medication for an extended period as a prophylactic measure (such as for the prevention of deep vein thrombosis) or as treatment of a chronic condition (such as arthritis) or a disease requiring a lengthy course of treatment (such as cancer). Do not assign a code from category Z79 for medication being administered for a brief period of time to treat an acute illness or injury (such as a course of antibiotics to treat acute bronchitis).

Z88 Allergy status to drugs, medicaments and biological substances

Except: Z88.9, *Allergy status to unspecified drugs, medicaments and biological substances status*

Z89 Acquired absence of limb

Z90 Acquired absence of organs, not elsewhere classified

Z91.0- Allergy status, other than to drugs and biological substances

Z92.82 Status post administration of tPA (rtPA) in a different facility within the last 24 hours prior to admission to a current facility

Assign code Z92.82, *Status post administration of tPA (rtPA) in a different facility within the last 24 hours prior to admission to current facility*, as a secondary diagnosis when a patient is received by transfer into a facility and documentation indicates they were administered tissue plasminogen activator (tPA) within the last 24 hours prior to admission to the current facility.

This guideline applies even if the patient is still receiving the tPA at the time they are received into the current facility.

The appropriate code for the condition for which the tPA was administered (such as cerebrovascular disease or myocardial infarction) should be assigned first.

Code Z92.82 is only applicable to the receiving facility record and not to the transferring facility record.

Z93 Artificial opening status

Z94 Transplanted organ and tissue status

Z95 Presence of cardiac and vascular implants and grafts

Z96 Presence of other functional implants

Z97 Presence of other devices

Z98 Other postprocedural states

Assign code Z98.85, *Transplanted organ removal status*, to indicate that a transplanted organ has been previously removed. This code should not be assigned for the encounter in which the transplanted organ is removed. The complication necessitating removal of the transplant organ should be assigned for that encounter.

See Section I.C19 *for information on the coding of organ transplant complications.*

Z99 Dependence on enabling machines and devices, not elsewhere classified

Note: Categories Z89-Z90 and Z93-Z99 are for use only if there are no complications or malfunctions of the organ or tissue replaced, the amputation site or the equipment on which the patient is dependent.

4) History (of)

There are two types of history Z codes, personal and family. Personal history codes explain a patient's past medical condition that no longer exists and is not receiving any treatment, but that has the potential for recurrence, and therefore may require continued monitoring.

Family history codes are for use when a patient has a family member(s) who has had a particular disease that causes the patient to be at higher risk of also contracting the disease.

Personal history codes may be used in conjunction with follow-up codes and family history codes may be used in conjunction with screening codes to explain the need for a test or procedure. History codes are also acceptable on any medical record regardless of the reason for visit. A history of an illness, even if no longer present, is important information that may alter the type of treatment ordered.

The history Z code categories are:

Z80 Family history of primary malignant neoplasm

Z81 Family history of mental and behavioral disorders

Z82 Family history of certain disabilities and chronic

diseases (leading to disablement)

Z83 Family history of other specific disorders

Z84 Family history of other conditions

Z85 Personal history of malignant neoplasm

Z86 Personal history of certain other diseases

Z87 Personal history of other diseases and conditions

Z91.4- Personal history of psychological trauma, not elsewhere classified

Z91.5 Personal history of self-harm

Z91.6- Personal history of other physical trauma

Z91.8- Other specified personal risk factors, not elsewhere classified

> Exception: Z91.83, *Wandering in diseases classified elsewhere*

Z92 Personal history of medical treatment

> Except: Z92.0, *Personal history of contraception*

> Except: Z92.82, *Status post administration of tPA (rtPA) in a different facility within the last 24 hours prior to admission to a current facility*

5) Screening

Screening is the testing for disease or disease precursors in seemingly well individuals so that early detection and treatment can be provided for those who test positive for the disease (e.g., screening mammogram).

The testing of a person to rule out or confirm a suspected diagnosis because the patient has some sign or symptom is a diagnostic examination, not a screening. In these cases, the sign or symptom is used to explain the reason for the test.

A screening code may be a first listed code if the reason for the visit is specifically the screening exam. It may also be used as an additional code if the screening is done during an office visit for other health problems. A screening code is not necessary if the screening is inherent to a routine examination, such as a pap smear done during a routine pelvic examination.

Should a condition be discovered during the screening then the code for the condition may be assigned as an additional diagnosis.

The Z code indicates that a screening exam is planned. A procedure code is required to confirm that the screening was performed.

The screening Z codes/categories:

Z11 Encounter for screening for infectious and parasitic diseases

Z12 Encounter for screening for malignant neoplasms

Z13 Encounter for screening for other diseases and disorders

> Except: Z13.9, *Encounter for screening, unspecified*

Z36 Encounter for antenatal screening for mother

6) Observation

There are two observation Z code categories. They are for use in very limited circumstances when a person is being observed for a suspected condition that is ruled out. The observation codes are not for use if an injury or illness or any signs or symptoms related to the suspected condition are present. In such cases the diagnosis/symptom code is used with the corresponding external cause code.

The observation codes are to be used as principal diagnosis only. Additional codes may be used in addition to the observation code but only if they are unrelated to the suspected condition being observed.

Codes from subcategory Z03.7 Encounter for suspected maternal and fetal conditions ruled out, may either be used as a first listed or as an additional code assignment depending on the case. They are for use in very limited circumstances on a maternal record when an encounter is for a suspected maternal or fetal condition that is ruled out during that encounter (for example, a maternal or fetal condition may be suspected due to an abnormal test result). These codes should not be used when the condition is confirmed. In those cases, the confirmed condition should be coded. In addition, these codes are not for use if an illness or any signs or symptoms related to the suspected condition or problem are present. In such cases the diagnosis/symptom code is used.

Additional codes may be used in addition to the code from subcategory Z03.7, but only if they are unrelated to the suspected condition being evaluated.

Codes from subcategory Z03.7 may not be used for encounters for antenatal screening of mother.

See Section I.C.21, *Screening.*

For encounters for suspected fetal condition that are inconclusive following testing and evaluation, assign the appropriate code from category O35, O36, O40 or O41.

The observation Z code categories:

Z03 Encounter for medical observation for suspected diseases and conditions ruled out

Z04 Encounter for examination and observation for other reasons

> Except: Z04.9, *Encounter for examination and observation for unspecified reason*

7. Aftercare

Aftercare visit codes cover situations when the initial treatment of a disease has been performed and the patient requires continued care during the healing or recovery phase, or for the long-term consequences of the disease. The aftercare Z code should not be used if treatment is directed at a current, acute disease. The diagnosis code is to be used in these cases.

Exceptions to this rule are codes Z51.0, *Encounter for antineoplastic radiation therapy*, and codes from subcategory Z51.1, *Encounter for antineoplastic chemotherapy and immunotherapy*. These codes are to be first listed, followed by the diagnosis code when a patient's encounter is solely to receive radiation therapy, chemotherapy, or immunotherapy for the treatment of a neoplasm. If the reason for the encounter is more than one type of antineoplastic therapy, code Z51.0 and a code from subcategory Z51.1 may be assigned together, in which case one of these codes would be reported as a secondary diagnosis.

The aftercare Z codes should also not be used for aftercare for injuries. For aftercare of an injury, assign the acute injury code with the appropriate 7th character (subsequent encounter).

The aftercare codes are generally first-listed to explain the specific reason for the encounter. An aftercare code may be used as an additional code when some type of aftercare is provided in addition to the reason for admission and no diagnosis code is applicable. An example of this would be the closure of a colostomy during an encounter for treatment of another condition.

Aftercare codes should be used in conjunction with any other aftercare codes or other diagnosis codes to provide better detail on the specifics of an aftercare encounter visit, unless otherwise directed by the classification. Should a patient receive multiple types of antineoplastic therapy during the same encounter, code Z51.0, *Encounter for antineoplastic radiation therapy*, and codes from subcategory Z51.1, *Encounter for antineoplastic chemotherapy and immunotherapy*, may be used together on a record. The sequencing of multiple aftercare codes depends on the circumstances of the encounter.

Certain aftercare Z code categories need a secondary diagnosis code to describe the resolving condition or sequelae. For others, the condition is included in the code title.

Additional Z code aftercare category terms include fitting and adjustment, and attention to artificial openings.

Status Z codes may be used with aftercare Z codes to indicate the nature of the aftercare. For example code Z95.1, *Presence of aortocoronary bypass graft*, may be used with code Z48.812, *Encounter for surgical aftercare following surgery on the circulatory system*, to indicate the surgery for which the aftercare is being performed. A status code should not be used when the aftercare code indicates the type of status, such as using Z43.0, *Encounter for attention to tracheostomy*, with Z93.0, *Tracheostomy status*.

The aftercare Z category/codes:

> *Z42 Encounter for plastic and reconstructive surgery following medical procedure or healed injury*
>
> *Z43 Encounter for attention to artificial openings*
>
> *Z44 Encounter for fitting and adjustment of external prosthetic device*
>
> *Z45 Encounter for adjustment and management of implanted device*
>
> *Z46 Encounter for fitting and adjustment of other devices*
>
> *Z47 Orthopedic aftercare*

> *Z48 Encounter for other postprocedural aftercare*
>
> *Z49 Encounter for care involving renal dialysis*
>
> *Z51 Encounter for other aftercare*

8) Follow-up

The follow-up codes are used to explain continuing surveillance following completed treatment of a disease, condition, or injury. They imply that the condition has been fully treated and no longer exists. They should not be confused with aftercare codes, or injury codes with 7th character for subsequent encounter, that explain ongoing care of a healing condition or its sequelae. Follow-up codes may be used in conjunction with history codes to provide the full picture of the healed condition and its treatment. The follow-up code is sequenced first, followed by the history code.

A follow up code may be used to explain multiple visits. Should a condition be found to have recurred on the follow-up visit, then the code for the condition should be assigned in place of the follow-up code.

The follow-up Z code categories:

> *Z08 Encounter for follow-up examination after completed treatment for malignant neoplasm*
>
> *Z09 Encounter for follow-up examination after completed treatment for conditions other than malignant neoplasm*
>
> *Z39 Encounter for maternal postpartum care and examination*

9) Donor

Codes in category Z52, *Donors of organs and tissues*, are used for living individuals who are donating blood or other body tissue. These codes are only for individuals donating for others, not for self donations. They are not used to identify cadaveric donations.

10) Counseling

Counseling Z codes are used when a patient or family member receives assistance in the aftermath of an illness or injury, or when support is required in coping with family or social problems. They are not used in conjunction with a diagnosis code when the counseling component of care is considered integral to standard treatment.

The counseling Z codes/categories:

> *Z30.0- Encounter for general counseling and advice on contraception*
>
> *Z31.5 Encounter for genetic counseling*
>
> *Z31.6- Encounter for general counseling and advice on procreation*
>
> *Z32.2 Encounter for childbirth instruction*
>
> *Z32.3 Encounter for childcare instruction*
>
> *Z69 Encounter for mental health services for victim and perpetrator of abuse*
>
> *Z70 Counseling related to sexual attitude, behavior and orientation*
>
> *Z71 Persons encountering health services for other counseling and medical advice, not elsewhere classified*
>
> *Z76.81 Expectant mother prebirth pediatrician visit*

11) Encounters for Obstetrical and Reproductive Services

See Section I.C.15. *Pregnancy, Childbirth, and the Puerperium, for further instruction on the use of these codes.*

Z codes for pregnancy are for use in those circumstances when none of the problems or complications included in the codes from the Obstetrics chapter exist (a routine prenatal visit or postpartum care). Codes in category Z34, *Encounter for supervision of normal pregnancy*, are always first listed and are not to be used with any other code from the OB chapter. Codes in category Z3A, *Weeks of gestation*, may be assigned to provide additional information about the pregnancy. The date of the admission should be used to determine weeks of gestation for inpatient admissions that encompass more than one gestational week.

The outcome of delivery, category Z37, should be included on all maternal delivery records. It is always a secondary code. Codes in category Z37 should not be used on the newborn record.

Z codes for family planning (contraceptive) or procreative management and counseling should be included on an obstetric record either during the pregnancy or the postpartum stage, if applicable.

Z codes/categories for obstetrical and reproductive services:

Z30 Encounter for contraceptive management

Z31 Encounter for procreative management

Z32.2 Encounter for childbirth instruction

Z32.3 Encounter for childcare instruction

Z33 Pregnant state

Z34 Encounter for supervision of normal pregnancy

Z36 Encounter for antenatal screening of mother

Z3A Weeks of gestation

Z37 Outcome of delivery

Z39 Encounter for maternal postpartum care and examination

Z76.81 Expectant mother prebirth pediatrician visit

12) Newborns and Infants

See Section I.C.16. *Newborn (Perinatal) Guidelines, for further instruction on the use of these codes.*

Newborn Z codes/categories:

Z76.1 Encounter for health supervision and care of foundling

Z00.1- Encounter for routine child health examination

Z38 Liveborn infants according to place of birth and type of delivery

13) Routine and administrative examinations

The Z codes allow for the description of encounters for routine examinations, such as, a general check-up, or, examinations for administrative purposes, such as, a pre-employment physical. The codes are not to be used if the examination is for diagnosis of a suspected condition or for treatment purposes. In such cases the diagnosis code is used. During a routine exam, should a diagnosis or condition be discovered, it should be

coded as an additional code. Pre-existing and chronic conditions and history codes may also be included as additional codes as long as the examination is for administrative purposes and not focused on any particular condition.

Some of the codes for routine health examinations distinguish between "with" and "without" abnormal findings. Code assignment depends on the information that is known at the time the encounter is being coded. For example, if no abnormal findings were found during the examination, but the encounter is being coded before test results are back, it is acceptable to assign the code for "without abnormal findings." When assigning a code for "with abnormal findings," additional code(s) should be assigned to identify the specific abnormal finding(s).

Pre-operative examination and pre-procedural laboratory examination Z codes are for use only in those situations when a patient is being cleared for a procedure or surgery and no treatment is given.

The Z codes/categories for routine and administrative examinations:

Z00 Encounter for general examination without complaint, suspected or reported diagnosis

Z01 Encounter for other special examination without complaint, suspected or reported diagnosis

Z02 Encounter for administrative examination

Except: Z02.9, *Encounter for administrative examinations, unspecified*

Z32.0- Encounter for pregnancy test

14) Miscellaneous Z codes

The miscellaneous Z codes capture a number of other health care encounters that do not fall into one of the other categories. Certain of these codes identify the reason for the encounter; others are for use as additional codes that provide useful information on circumstances that may affect a patient's care and treatment.

Prophylactic Organ Removal

For encounters specifically for prophylactic removal of an organ (such as prophylactic removal of breasts due to a genetic susceptibility to cancer or a family history of cancer), the principal or first listed code should be a code from category Z40, *Encounter for prophylactic surgery*, followed by the appropriate codes to identify the associated risk factor (such as genetic susceptibility or family history).

If the patient has a malignancy of one site and is having prophylactic removal at another site to prevent either a new primary malignancy or metastatic disease, a code for the malignancy should also be assigned in addition to a code from subcategory Z40.0, *Encounter for prophylactic surgery for risk factors related to malignant neoplasms*. A Z40.0 code should not be assigned if the patient is having organ removal for treatment of a malignancy, such as the removal of the testes for the treatment of prostate cancer.

Miscellaneous Z codes/categories:

Z28 Immunization not carried out

Except: Z28.3, *Underimmunization status*

Z40 Encounter for prophylactic surgery

Z41 Encounter for procedures for purposes other than remedying health state

Except: Z41.9, *Encounter for procedure for purposes other than remedying health state, unspecified*

Z53 Persons encountering health services for specific procedures and treatment, not carried out

Z55 Problems related to education and literacy

Z56 Problems related to employment and unemployment

Z57 Occupational exposure to risk factors

Z58 Problems related to physical environment

Z59 Problems related to housing and economic circumstances

Z60 Problems related to social environment

Z61 Problems related to negative life events in childhood

Except: Z61.81-, *Personal history of abuse in childhood*

Z62 Problems related to upbringing

Z63 Other problems related to primary support group, including family circumstances

Z64 Problems related to certain psychosocial circumstances

Z65 Problems related to other psychosocial circumstances

Z72 Problems related to lifestyle

Z73 Problems related to life management difficulty

Z74 Problems related to care provider dependency

Except: Z74.01, *Bed confinement status*

Z75 Problems related to medical facilities and other health care

Z76.0 Encounter for issue of repeat prescription

Z76.3 Healthy person accompanying sick person

Z76.4 Other boarder to healthcare facility

Z76.5 Malingerer [conscious simulation]

Z91.1- Patient's noncompliance with medical treatment and regimen

Z91.83 Wandering in diseases classified elsewhere

Z91.89 Other specified personal risk factors, not elsewhere classified

15) Nonspecific Z codes

Certain Z codes are so non-specific, or potentially redundant with other codes in the classification, that there can be little justification for their use in the inpatient setting. Their use in the outpatient setting should be limited to those instances when there is no further documentation to permit more precise coding. Otherwise, any sign or symptom or any other reason for visit that is captured in another code should be used.

Nonspecific Z codes/categories:

Z02.9 Encounter for administrative examinations, unspecified

Z04.9 Encounter for examination and observation for unspecified reason

Z13.9 Encounter for screening, unspecified

Z41.9 Encounter for procedure for purposes other than remedying health state, unspecified

Z52.9 Donor of unspecified organ or tissue

Z86.59 Personal history of other mental and behavioral disorders

Z88.9 Allergy status to unspecified drugs, medicaments and biological substances status

Z92.0 Personal history of contraception

16) Z Codes That May Only be Principal/First-Listed Diagnosis

The following Z codes/categories may only be reported as the principal/first-listed diagnosis, except when there are multiple encounters on the same day and the medical records for the encounters are combined:

Z00 Encounter for general examination without complaint, suspected or reported diagnosis

Z01 Encounter for other special examination without complaint, suspected or reported diagnosis

Z02 Encounter for administrative examination

Z03 Encounter for medical observation for suspected diseases and conditions ruled out

Z04 Encounter for examination and observation for other reasons

Z33.2 Encounter for elective termination of pregnancy

Z31.81 Encounter for male factor infertility in female patient

Z31.82 Encounter for Rh incompatibility status

Z31.83 Encounter for assisted reproductive fertility procedure cycle

Z31.84 Encounter for fertility preservation procedure

Z34 Encounter for supervision of normal pregnancy

Z39 Encounter for maternal postpartum care and examination

Z38 Liveborn infants according to place of birth and type of delivery

Z42 Encounter for plastic and reconstructive surgery following medical procedure or healed injury

Z51.0 Encounter for antineoplastic radiation therapy

Z51.1- Encounter for antineoplastic chemotherapy and immunotherapy

Z52 Donors of organs and tissues

Except: Z52.9, *Donor of unspecified organ or tissue*

Z76.1 Encounter for health supervision and care of foundling

Z76.2 Encounter for health supervision and care of other healthy infant and child

Z99.12 Encounter for respirator [ventilator] dependence during power failure

Section II. Selection of Principal Diagnosis

The circumstances of inpatient admission always govern the selection of principal diagnosis. The principal diagnosis is defined in the Uniform Hospital Discharge Data Set (UHDDS) as "that condition established after study to be chiefly responsible for occasioning the admission of the patient to the hospital for care."

The UHDDS definitions are used by hospitals to report inpatient data elements in a standardized manner. These data elements and their definitions can be found in the July 31, 1985, *Federal Register* (Vol. 50, No, 147), pp. 31038-40.

Since that time the application of the UHDDS definitions has been expanded to include all non-outpatient settings (acute care, short term, long term care and psychiatric hospitals; home health agencies; rehab facilities; nursing homes, etc).

In determining principal diagnosis the coding conventions in the ICD-10-CM, the Tabular List and Alphabetic Index take precedence over these official coding guidelines. (*See* Section I.A., *Conventions for the ICD-10-CM*).

The importance of consistent, complete documentation in the medical record cannot be overemphasized. Without such documentation the application of all coding guidelines is a difficult, if not impossible, task.

A. Codes for symptoms, signs, and ill-defined conditions

Codes for symptoms, signs, and ill-defined conditions from Chapter 18 are not to be used as principal diagnosis when a related definitive diagnosis has been established.

B. Two or more interrelated conditions, each potentially meeting the definition for principal diagnosis.

When there are two or more interrelated conditions (such as diseases in the same ICD-10-CM chapter or manifestations characteristically associated with a certain disease) potentially meeting the definition of principal diagnosis, either condition may be sequenced first, unless the circumstances of the admission, the therapy provided, the Tabular List, or the Alphabetic Index indicate otherwise.

C. Two or more diagnoses that equally meet the definition for principal diagnosis

In the unusual instance when two or more diagnoses equally meet the criteria for principal diagnosis as determined by the circumstances of admission, diagnostic workup and/or therapy provided, and the Alphabetic Index, Tabular List, or another coding guidelines does not provide sequencing direction, any one of the diagnoses may be sequenced first.

D. Two or more comparative or contrasting conditions.

In those rare instances when two or more contrasting or comparative diagnoses are documented as "either/or" (or similar terminology), they are coded as if the diagnoses were confirmed and the diagnoses are sequenced according to the circumstances of the admission. If no further determination can be made as to which diagnosis should be principal, either diagnosis may be sequenced first.

E. A symptom(s) followed by contrasting/comparative diagnoses

When a symptom(s) is followed by contrasting/comparative diagnoses, the symptom code is sequenced first. However, if the symptom code is integral to the conditions listed, no code for the symptom is reported. All the contrasting/comparative diagnoses should be coded as additional diagnoses.

F. Original treatment plan not carried out

Sequence as the principal diagnosis the condition, which after study occasioned the admission to the hospital, even though treatment may not have been carried out due to unforeseen circumstances.

G. Complications of surgery and other medical care

When the admission is for treatment of a complication resulting from surgery or other medical care, the complication code is sequenced as the principal diagnosis. If the complication is classified to the T80-T88 series and the code lacks the necessary specificity in describing the complication, an additional code for the specific complication should be assigned.

H. Uncertain Diagnosis

If the diagnosis documented at the time of discharge is qualified as "probable", "suspected", "likely", "questionable", "possible", or "still to be ruled out", or other similar terms indicating uncertainty, code the condition as if it existed or was established. The bases for these guidelines are the diagnostic workup, arrangements for further workup or observation, and initial therapeutic approach that correspond most closely with the established diagnosis.

Note: This guideline is applicable only to inpatient admissions to short-term, acute, long-term care and psychiatric hospitals.

I. Admission from Observation Unit

1. Admission Following Medical Observation

When a patient is admitted to an observation unit for a medical condition, which either worsens or does not improve, and is subsequently admitted as an inpatient of the same hospital for this same medical condition, the principal diagnosis would be the medical condition which led to the hospital admission.

2. Admission Following Post-Operative Observation

When a patient is admitted to an observation unit to monitor a condition (or complication) that develops following outpatient surgery, and then is subsequently admitted as an inpatient of the same hospital, hospitals should apply the Uniform Hospital Discharge Data Set (UHDDS) definition of principal diagnosis as "that condition established after study to be chiefly responsible for occasioning the admission of the patient to the hospital for care."

J. Admission from Outpatient Surgery

When a patient receives surgery in the hospital's outpatient surgery department and is subsequently admitted for continuing inpatient care at the same hospital, the following guidelines should be followed in selecting the principal diagnosis for the inpatient admission:

- If the reason for the inpatient admission is a complication, assign the complication as the principal diagnosis.

- If no complication, or other condition, is documented as the reason for the inpatient admission, assign the reason for the outpatient surgery as the principal diagnosis.
- If the reason for the inpatient admission is another condition unrelated to the surgery, assign the unrelated condition as the principal diagnosis.

K. Admissions/Encounters for Rehabilitation

When the purpose for the admission/encounter is rehabilitation, sequence first the code for the condition for which the service is being performed. For example, for an admission/encounter for rehabilitation for right-sided dominant hemiplegia following a cerebrovascular infarction, report code I69.351, *Hemiplegia and hemiparesis following cerebral infarction affecting right dominant side*, as the first-listed or principal diagnosis.

If the condition for which the rehabilitation service is no longer present, report the appropriate aftercare code as the first-listed or principal diagnosis. For example, if a patient with severe degenerative osteoarthritis of the hip, underwent hip replacement and the current encounter/admission is for rehabilitation, report code Z47.1, *Aftercare following joint replacement surgery*, as the first-listed or principal diagnosis.

See Section I.C.21.c.7, Factors influencing health states and contact with health services, Aftercare.

Section III. Reporting Additional Diagnoses

GENERAL RULES FOR OTHER (ADDITIONAL) DIAGNOSES

For reporting purposes the definition for "other diagnoses" is interpreted as additional conditions that affect patient care in terms of requiring:

- clinical evaluation; or
- therapeutic treatment; or
- diagnostic procedures; or
- extended length of hospital stay; or
- increased nursing care and/or monitoring.

The UHDDS item #11-b defines Other Diagnoses as "all conditions that coexist at the time of admission, that develop subsequently, or that affect the treatment received and/or the length of stay. Diagnoses that relate to an earlier episode which have no bearing on the current hospital stay are to be excluded." UHDDS definitions apply to inpatients in acute care, short-term, long term care and psychiatric hospital setting. The UHDDS definitions are used by acute care short-term hospitals to report inpatient data elements in a standardized manner. These data elements and their definitions can be found in the July 31, 1985, *Federal Register* (Vol. 50, No, 147), pp. 31038-40.

Since that time the application of the UHDDS definitions has been expanded to include all non-outpatient settings (acute care, short term, long term care and psychiatric hospitals; home health agencies; rehab facilities; nursing homes, etc).

The following guidelines are to be applied in designating "other diagnoses" when neither the Alphabetic Index nor the Tabular List in ICD-10-CM provide direction. The listing of the diagnoses in the patient record is the responsibility of the attending provider.

A. Previous conditions

If the provider has included a diagnosis in the final diagnostic statement, such as the discharge summary or the face sheet, it should ordinarily be coded. Some providers include in the diagnostic statement resolved conditions or diagnoses and status-post procedures from previous admission that have no bearing on the current stay. Such conditions are not to be reported and are coded only if required by hospital policy.

However, history codes (categories Z80-Z87) may be used as secondary codes if the historical condition or family history has an impact on current care or influences treatment.

B. Abnormal findings

Abnormal findings (laboratory, x-ray, pathologic, and other diagnostic results) are not coded and reported unless the provider indicates their clinical significance. If the findings are outside the normal range and the attending provider has ordered other tests to evaluate the condition or prescribed treatment, it is appropriate to ask the provider whether the abnormal finding should be added.

Please note: This differs from the coding practices in the outpatient setting for coding encounters for diagnostic tests that have been interpreted by a provider.

C. Uncertain Diagnosis

If the diagnosis documented at the time of discharge is qualified as "probable", "suspected", "likely", "questionable", "possible", or "still to be ruled out" or other similar terms indicating uncertainty, code the condition as if it existed or was established. The bases for these guidelines are the diagnostic workup, arrangements for further workup or observation, and initial therapeutic approach that correspond most closely with the established diagnosis.

Note: This guideline is applicable only to inpatient admissions to short-term, acute, long-term care and psychiatric hospitals.

Section IV. Diagnostic Coding and Reporting Guidelines for Outpatient Services

These coding guidelines for outpatient diagnoses have been approved for use by hospitals/providers in coding and reporting hospital-based outpatient services and provider-based office visits.

Information about the use of certain abbreviations, punctuation, symbols, and other conventions used in the ICD-10-CM Tabular List (code numbers and titles), can be found in Section IA of these guidelines, under "Conventions Used in the Tabular List." Section I.B. contains general guidelines that apply to the entire classification. Section I.C. contains chapter-specific guidelines that correspond to the chapters as they are arranged in the classification. Information about the correct sequence to use in finding a code is also described in Section I.

The terms encounter and visit are often used interchangeably in describing outpatient service contacts and, therefore, appear together in these guidelines without distinguishing one from the other.

Though the conventions and general guidelines apply to all settings, coding guidelines for outpatient and provider reporting of diagnoses will vary in a number of instances from those for inpatient diagnoses, recognizing that:

The Uniform Hospital Discharge Data Set (UHDDS) definition of principal diagnosis applies only to inpatients in acute, short-term, long-term care and psychiatric hospitals.

Coding guidelines for inconclusive diagnoses (probable, suspected, rule out, etc.) were developed for inpatient reporting and do not apply to outpatients.

A. Selection of first-listed condition

In the outpatient setting, the term first-listed diagnosis is used in lieu of principal diagnosis.

In determining the first-listed diagnosis the coding conventions of ICD-10-CM, as well as the general and disease specific guidelines take precedence over the outpatient guidelines.

Diagnoses often are not established at the time of the initial encounter/visit. It may take two or more visits before the diagnosis is confirmed.

The most critical rule involves beginning the search for the correct code assignment through the Alphabetic Index. Never begin searching initially in the Tabular List as this will lead to coding errors.

1. Outpatient Surgery

When a patient presents for outpatient surgery (same day surgery), code the reason for the surgery as the first-listed diagnosis (reason for the encounter), even if the surgery is not performed due to a contraindication.

2. Observation Stay

When a patient is admitted for observation for a medical condition, assign a code for the medical condition as the first-listed diagnosis.

When a patient presents for outpatient surgery and develops complications requiring admission to observation, code the reason for the surgery as the first reported diagnosis (reason for the encounter), followed by codes for the complications as secondary diagnoses.

B. Codes from A00.0 through T88.9, Z00-Z99

The appropriate code(s) from A00.0 through T88.9, Z00-Z99 must be used to identify diagnoses, symptoms, conditions, problems, complaints, or other reason(s) for the encounter/visit.

C. Accurate reporting of ICD-10-CM diagnosis codes

For accurate reporting of ICD-10-CM diagnosis codes, the documentation should describe the patient's condition, using terminology which includes specific diagnoses as well as symptoms, problems, or reasons for the encounter. There are ICD-10-CM codes to describe all of these.

D. Codes that describe symptoms and signs

Codes that describe symptoms and signs, as opposed to diagnoses, are acceptable for reporting purposes when a diagnosis has not been established (confirmed) by the provider. Chapter 18 of ICD-10-CM, Symptoms, Signs, and Abnormal Clinical and Laboratory Findings Not Elsewhere Classified (codes R00-R99) contain many, but not all codes for symptoms.

E. Encounters for circumstances other than a disease or injury

ICD-10-CM provides codes to deal with encounters for circumstances other than a disease or injury. The Factors Influencing Health Status and Contact with Health Services codes (Z00-99) is provided to deal with occasions when circumstances other than a disease or injury are recorded as diagnosis or problems.

See Section I.C.21. *Factors influencing health status and contact with health services*

F. Level of Detail in Coding

1. ICD-10-CM codes with 3, 4, 5, 6 or 7 characters

ICD-10-CM is composed of codes with 3, 4, 5, 6 or 7 characters. Codes with three characters are included in ICD-10-CM as the heading of a category of codes that may be further subdivided by the use of fourth, fifth, sixth or seventh characters which provide greater specificity.

2. Use of full number of characters required for a code

A three-character code is to be used only if it is not further subdivided. A code is invalid if it has not been coded to the full number of characters required for that code, including the 7th character, if applicable.

G. ICD-10-CM code for the diagnosis, condition, problem, or other reason for encounter/visit

List first the ICD-10-CM code for the diagnosis, condition, problem, or other reason for encounter/visit shown in the medical record to be chiefly responsible for the services provided. List additional codes that describe any coexisting conditions. In some cases the first-listed diagnosis may be a symptom when a diagnosis has not been established (confirmed) by the physician.

H. Uncertain diagnosis

Do not code diagnoses documented as "probable", "suspected," "questionable," "rule out," or "working diagnosis" or other similar terms indicating uncertainty. Rather, code the condition(s) to the highest degree of certainty for that encounter/visit, such as symptoms, signs, abnormal test results, or other reason for the visit.

Please note: This differs from the coding practices used by short-term, acute care, long-term care and psychiatric hospitals.

I. Chronic diseases

Chronic diseases treated on an ongoing basis may be coded and reported as many times as the patient receives treatment and care for the condition(s)

J. Code all documented conditions that coexist

Code all documented conditions that coexist at the time of the encounter/visit, and require or affect patient care treatment or management. Do not code conditions that were previously treated and no longer exist. However, history codes (categories Z80-Z87) may be used as secondary codes if the historical condition or family history has an impact on current care or influences treatment.

K. Patients receiving diagnostic services only

For patients receiving diagnostic services only during an encounter/visit, sequence first the diagnosis, condition, problem, or other reason for encounter/visit shown in the medical record to be chiefly responsible for the outpatient services provided during the encounter/visit. Codes for other diagnoses (e.g., chronic conditions) may be sequenced as additional diagnoses.

For encounters for routine laboratory/radiology testing in the absence of any signs, symptoms, or associated diagnosis, assign Z01.89, Encounter for other specified special examinations. If routine testing is performed during the same encounter as a test to evaluate a sign, symptom, or diagnosis, it is appropriate to assign both the Z code and the code describing the reason for the non-routine test.

For outpatient encounters for diagnostic tests that have been interpreted by a physician, and the final report is available at the time of coding, code any confirmed or definitive diagnosis(es) documented in the interpretation. Do not code related signs and symptoms as additional diagnoses.

Please note: This differs from the coding practice in the hospital inpatient setting regarding abnormal findings on test results.

L. Patients receiving therapeutic services only

For patients receiving therapeutic services only during an encounter/visit, sequence first the diagnosis, condition, problem, or other reason for encounter/visit shown in the medical record to be chiefly responsible for the outpatient services provided during the encounter/visit. Codes for other diagnoses (e.g., chronic conditions) may be sequenced as additional diagnoses.

The only exception to this rule is that when the primary reason for the admission/encounter is chemotherapy or radiation therapy, the appropriate Z code for the service is listed first, and the diagnosis or problem for which the service is being performed listed second.

M. Patients receiving preoperative evaluations only

For patients receiving preoperative evaluations only, sequence first a code from subcategory Z01.81, *Encounter for pre-procedural examinations*, to describe the pre-op consultations. Assign a code for the condition to describe the reason for the surgery as an additional diagnosis. Code also any findings related to the pre-op evaluation.

N. Ambulatory surgery

For ambulatory surgery, code the diagnosis for which the surgery was performed. If the postoperative diagnosis is known to be different from the preoperative diagnosis at the time the diagnosis is confirmed, select the postoperative diagnosis for coding, since it is the most definitive.

O. Routine outpatient prenatal visits

See Section I.C.15. *Routine outpatient prenatal visits*

P. Encounters for general medical examinations with abnormal findings

The subcategories for encounters for general medical examinations, Z00.0-, provide codes for with and without abnormal findings. Should a general medical examination result in an abnormal finding, the code for general medical examination with abnormal finding should be assigned as the first listed diagnosis. A secondary code for the abnormal finding should also be coded.

Q. Encounters for routine health screenings

See Section I.C.21. *Factors influencing health status and contact with health services, Screening*

Appendix I Present on Admission Reporting Guidelines

Introduction

These guidelines are to be used as a supplement to the *ICD-10-CM Official Guidelines for Coding and Reporting* to facilitate the assignment of the Present on Admission (POA) indicator for each diagnosis and external cause of injury code reported on claim forms (UB-04 and 837 Institutional).

These guidelines are not intended to replace any guidelines in the main body of the *ICD-10-CM Official Guidelines for Coding and Reporting*. The POA guidelines are not intended to provide guidance on when a condition should be coded, but rather, how to apply the POA indicator to the final set of diagnosis codes that have been assigned in accordance with Sections I, II, and III of the official coding guidelines. Subsequent to the assignment of the ICD-10-CM codes, the POA indicator should then be assigned to those conditions that have been coded.

As stated in the Introduction to the *ICD-10-CM Official Guidelines for Coding and Reporting*, a joint effort between the healthcare provider and the coder is essential to achieve complete and accurate documentation, code assignment, and reporting of diagnoses and procedures. The importance of consistent, complete documentation in the medical record cannot be overemphasized. Medical record documentation from any provider involved in the care and treatment of the patient may be used to support the determination of whether a condition was present on admission or not. In the context of the official coding guidelines, the term "provider" means a physician or any qualified healthcare practitioner who is legally accountable for establishing the patient's diagnosis.

These guidelines are not a substitute for the provider's clinical judgment as to the determination of whether a condition was/was not present on admission. The provider should be queried regarding issues related to the linking of signs/symptoms, timing of test results, and the timing of findings.

General Reporting Requirements

All claims involving inpatient admissions to general acute care hospitals or other facilities that are subject to a law or regulation mandating collection of present on admission information. Present on admission is defined as present at the time the order for inpatient admission occurs – conditions that develop during an outpatient encounter, including emergency department, observation, or outpatient surgery, are considered as present on admission.

POA indicator is assigned to principal and secondary diagnoses (as defined in Section II of the Official Guidelines for Coding and Reporting) and the external cause of injury codes.

Issues related to inconsistent, missing, conflicting or unclear documentation must still be resolved by the provider.

If a condition would not be coded and reported based on UHDDS definitions and current official coding guidelines, then the POA indicator would not be reported.

Reporting Options

Y – Yes; N – No; U – Unknown; W – Clinically undetermined
Unreported/Not used – (Exempt from POA reporting)

Reporting Definitions

Y = present at the time of inpatient admission

N = not present at the time of inpatient admission

U = documentation is insufficient to determine if condition is present on admission

W = provider is unable to clinically determine whether condition was present on admission or not

Timeframe for POA Identification and Documentation

There is no required timeframe as to when a provider (per the definition of "provider" used in these guidelines) must identify or document a condition to be present on admission. In some clinical situations, it may not be possible for a provider to make a definitive diagnosis (or a condition may not be recognized or reported by the patient) for a period of time after admission. In some cases it may be several days before the provider arrives at a definitive diagnosis. This does not mean that the condition was not present on admission. Determination of whether the condition was present on admission or not will be based on the applicable POA guideline as identified in this document, or on the provider's best clinical judgment.

If at the time of code assignment the documentation is unclear as to whether a condition was present on admission or not, it is appropriate to query the provider for clarification.

Assigning the POA Indicator

Condition is on the "Exempt from Reporting" list

Leave the "present on admission" field blank if the condition is on the list of ICD-10-CM codes for which this field is not applicable. This is the only circumstance in which the field may be left blank.

POA Explicitly Documented

Assign Y for any condition the provider explicitly documents as being present on admission. Assign N for any condition the provider explicitly documents as not present at the time of admission.

For further information on POA Guidelines and exempt categories and codes, visit the following web site: http://www. cdc.gov/nchs/data/icd10/Detailed%20List%20of%20Codes%20 Exempt%20from%20POA.pdf

Prefixes and Suffixes

Prefixes and suffixes are elements used in medical terminology that consist of one or more syllables placed before or after root words to show various kinds of relationships. Prefixes come before the root word and suffixes come after the root word. They are never used independently but function to modify the meaning. Many prefixes and suffixes are added to other words with a hyphen, but medical dictionary publishers are opting to drop the hyphen on many of the more commonly prefixed medical words.

Examples:

Prefixes
micro = small
peri = surrounding

Suffixes
algia = pain
an = pertaining to

The following are lists of prefixes and suffixes typically seen in medical terminology.

Prefixes

a(d)-	towards
a(n)-	without
ab-	from
ab(s)-	away from
ad-	towards
allo-	other, another
ambi-	both
amphi-	on both sides, around
ana-	up to, back, again, movement from
aniso-	different, unequal
ante-	before, forwards
anti-	against, opposite
ap-, apo-	from, back, again
bi(s)-	twice, double
bio-	life
brachy-	short
cata-	down
circum-	around
con-	together
contra-	against
cyte-	cell
de-	from, away from, down from
deca-	ten
di(s)-	two
dia-	through, complete
di(a)s	separation
diplo-	double
dolicho-	long
dur-	hard, firm
dys-	bad, abnormal
e-, ec-	out, from out of
ecto-	outside, external
ek-	out
em-	in
en-	into
endo-	into
ent-	within
epi-	on, up, against, high
eso-	will carry
eu-	well, abundant, prosperous
eury-	broad, wide
ex-, exo-	out, from out of
extra-	outside, beyond, in addition
haplo-	single
hapto-	bind to
hemi-	half
hept-	seven
hetero-	different
hex-	six
homo-	same
hyper-	above, excessive
hypo-	below, deficient
im-, in-	not
in-	into, to
infra-	below, underneath
inter-	among, between
intra-	within, inside, during
intro-	inward, during
iso-	equal, same
juxta-	adjacent to
kata-	down, down from
macro-	large
magno-	large
medi-	middle
mega-	large
megalo-	very large
meso-	middle
meta-	beyond, between
micro-	small
neo-	new
non-	not
ob-	before, against
octa-	eight
octo-	eight
oligo-	few
pachy-	thick
pan-	all
para-	beside, to the side of, wrong

pent-	five
per-	by, through, throughout
peri-	around, round-about
pleo-	more than usual
poly	many
post-	behind, after
pre-	before, in front, very
pros-	besides
prox-	besides
pseudo-	false, fake
quar(r)-	four
re, red-	back, again
retro-	backwards, behind
semi-	half
sex-	six
sept-	seven
sub-	under, beneath
super-	above, in addition, over
supra-	above, on the upper side
syn-	together, with
sys-	together, with
tetra-	four
thio-	sulfur
trans-	across, beyond
tri-	three
uni-	one
ultra-	beyond, besides, over

Suffixes

-ase	fermenter
-ate	do
-cide	killer
-c(o)ele	cavity, hollow
-ectomy	removal of, cut out
-form	shaped like

-ia	got
-iasis	full of
-ile	little version
-illa	little version
-illus	little version
-in	stuff
-ism	theory, characteristic of
-itis	inflammation
-ity	makes a noun of quality
-ium	thing
-ize	do
-logy	study of, reasoning about
-megaly	large
-noid	mind, spirit
-oid	resembling, image of
-ogen	precursor
-ol(e)	alcohol
-ole	little version
-oma	tumor (usually)
-osis	full of
-ostomy	"mouth-cut"
-pathy	disease of, suffering
-penia	lack
-pexy	fix in place
-plasty	re-shaping
-philia	affection for
-rhage	burst out
-rhea	discharge, flowing out
-rhexis	shredding
-pagus	Siamese twins
-sis	idea (makes a noun, typically abstract)
-thrix	hair
-tomy	cut
-ule	little version
-um	thing (makes a noun, typically abstract)

Anatomy

The Right Ear

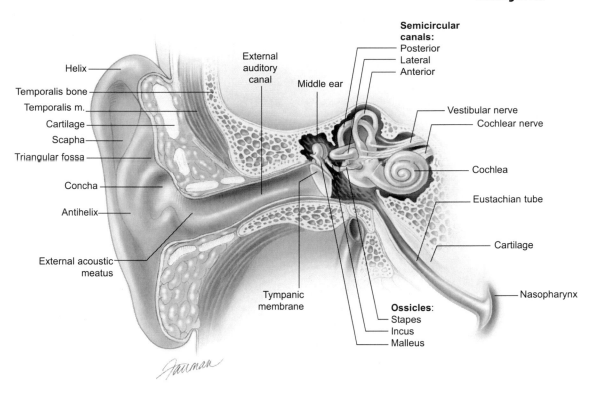

Helix

Temporalis bone

Temporalis m.

Cartilage

Scapha

Triangular fossa

Concha

Antihelix

External acoustic meatus

External auditory canal

Middle ear

Tympanic membrane

Semicircular canals:
Posterior
Lateral
Anterior

Vestibular nerve

Cochlear nerve

Cochlea

Eustachian tube

Cartilage

Nasopharynx

Ossicles:
Stapes
Incus
Malleus

The Right Eye
(Transverse Section)

Lateral rectus m.

Zonular fibers

Conjunctiva

Canal of Schlemm

Iris

Lens

Cornea

Pupil

Aqueous humor

Anterior chamber

Posterior chamber

Sclera

Ciliary body

Ora serrata

Medial rectus m.

Vitreous body

Hyaloid canal

Macula lutea

Optic disc

Retinal vessels

Optic nerve

Nerve sheath

Retina

Choroid

Male Figure
(Anterior View)

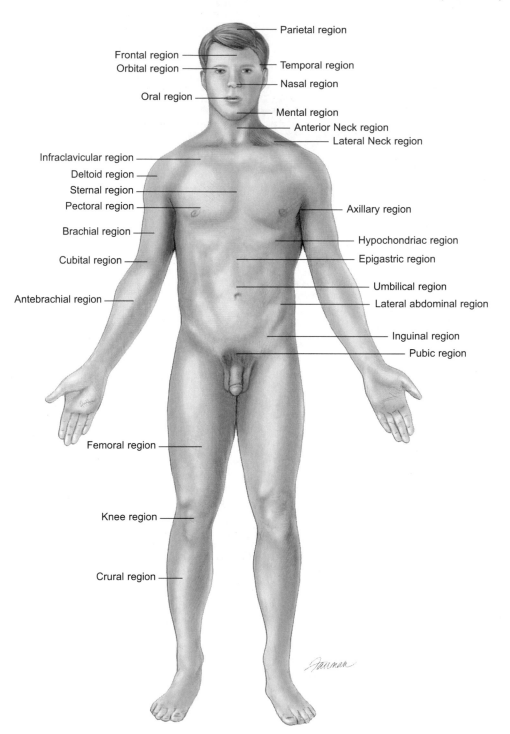

Parietal region

Frontal region

Orbital region

Temporal region

Nasal region

Oral region

Mental region

Anterior Neck region

Lateral Neck region

Infraclavicular region

Deltoid region

Sternal region

Pectoral region

Axillary region

Brachial region

Hypochondriac region

Cubital region

Epigastric region

Umbilical region

Antebrachial region

Lateral abdominal region

Inguinal region

Pubic region

Femoral region

Knee region

Crural region

Muscular System
(Anterior View)

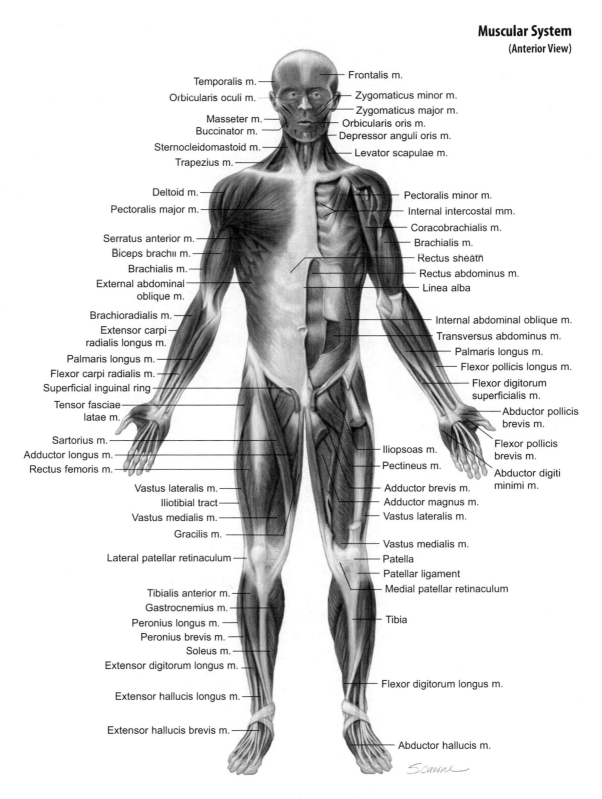

Temporalis m.
Orbicularis oculi m.
Masseter m.
Buccinator m.
Sternocleidomastoid m.
Trapezius m.

Frontalis m.
Zygomaticus minor m.
Zygomaticus major m.
Orbicularis oris m.
Depressor anguli oris m.
Levator scapulae m.

Deltoid m.
Pectoralis major m.

Pectoralis minor m.
Internal intercostal mm.
Coracobrachialis m.

Serratus anterior m.
Biceps brachii m.
Brachialis m.
External abdominal oblique m.

Brachialis m.
Rectus sheath
Rectus abdominus m.
Linea alba

Brachioradialis m.
Extensor carpi radialis longus m.
Palmaris longus m.
Flexor carpi radialis m.
Superficial inguinal ring
Tensor fasciae latae m.
Sartorius m.
Adductor longus m.
Rectus femoris m.

Internal abdominal oblique m.
Transversus abdominus m.
Palmaris longus m.
Flexor pollicis longus m.
Flexor digitorum superficialis m.
Abductor pollicis brevis m.
Flexor pollicis brevis m.
Abductor digiti minimi m.

Iliopsoas m.
Pectineus m.

Vastus lateralis m.
Iliotibial tract
Vastus medialis m.
Gracilis m.

Adductor brevis m.
Adductor magnus m.
Vastus lateralis m.

Lateral patellar retinaculum

Vastus medialis m.
Patella
Patellar ligament
Medial patellar retinaculum

Tibialis anterior m.
Gastrocnemius m.
Peronius longus m.
Peronius brevis m.
Soleus m.
Extensor digitorum longus m.

Tibia

Extensor hallucis longus m.

Flexor digitorum longus m.

Extensor hallucis brevis m.

Abductor hallucis m.

Scarline

© Fairman Studios, LLC, 2002. All Rights Reserved.

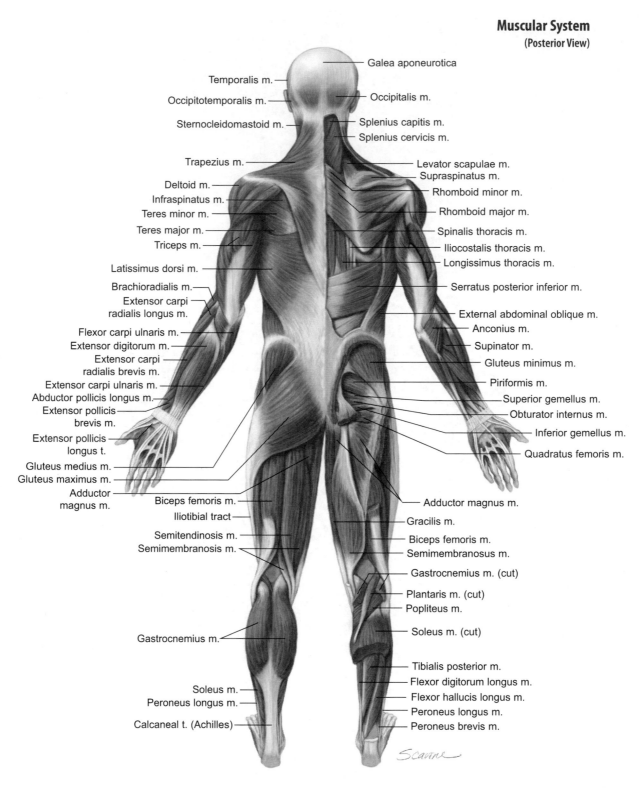

Muscular System
(Posterior View)

Galea aponeurotica

Temporalis m.

Occipitalis m.

Occipitotemporalis m.

Sternocleidomastoid m.

Splenius capitis m.

Splenius cervicis m.

Trapezius m.

Levator scapulae m.

Supraspinatus m.

Deltoid m.

Rhomboid minor m.

Infraspinatus m.

Rhomboid major m.

Teres minor m.

Spinalis thoracis m.

Teres major m.

Iliocostalis thoracis m.

Triceps m.

Longissimus thoracis m.

Latissimus dorsi m.

Serratus posterior inferior m.

Brachioradialis m.

Extensor carpi radialis longus m.

External abdominal oblique m.

Anconius m.

Flexor carpi ulnaris m.

Supinator m.

Extensor digitorum m.

Extensor carpi radialis brevis m.

Gluteus minimus m.

Extensor carpi ulnaris m.

Piriformis m.

Abductor pollicis longus m.

Superior gemellus m.

Extensor pollicis brevis m.

Obturator internus m.

Inferior gemellus m.

Extensor pollicis longus t.

Quadratus femoris m.

Gluteus medius m.

Gluteus maximus m.

Adductor magnus m.

Biceps femoris m.

Adductor magnus m.

Iliotibial tract

Gracilis m.

Semitendinosis m.

Biceps femoris m.

Semimembranosis m.

Semimembranosus m.

Gastrocnemius m. (cut)

Plantaris m. (cut)

Popliteus m.

Soleus m. (cut)

Gastrocnemius m.

Tibialis posterior m.

Flexor digitorum longus m.

Soleus m.

Flexor hallucis longus m.

Peroneus longus m.

Peroneus longus m.

Calcaneal t. (Achilles)

Peroneus brevis m.

Skeletal System
(Anterior View)

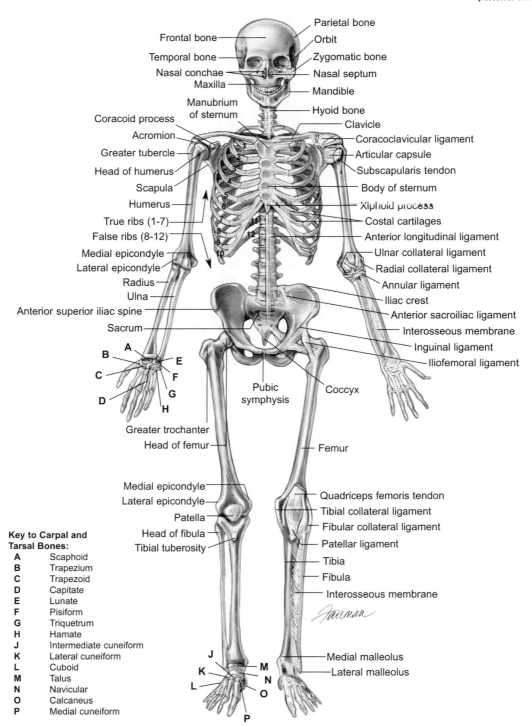

Frontal bone
Parietal bone
Orbit
Temporal bone
Zygomatic bone
Nasal conchae
Nasal septum
Maxilla
Mandible
Manubrium of sternum
Hyoid bone
Coracoid process
Clavicle
Acromion
Coracoclavicular ligament
Greater tubercle
Articular capsule
Head of humerus
Subscapularis tendon
Scapula
Body of sternum
Humerus
Xiphoid process
True ribs (1-7)
Costal cartilages
False ribs (8-12)
Anterior longitudinal ligament
Medial epicondyle
Ulnar collateral ligament
Lateral epicondyle
Radial collateral ligament
Radius
Annular ligament
Ulna
Iliac crest
Anterior superior iliac spine
Anterior sacroiliac ligament
Sacrum
Interosseous membrane
Inguinal ligament
Iliofemoral ligament
Pubic symphysis
Coccyx
Greater trochanter
Head of femur
Femur
Medial epicondyle
Quadriceps femoris tendon
Lateral epicondyle
Tibial collateral ligament
Patella
Fibular collateral ligament
Head of fibula
Patellar ligament
Tibial tuberosity
Tibia
Fibula
Interosseous membrane
Medial malleolus
Lateral malleolus

Key to Carpal and Tarsal Bones:

A	Scaphoid
B	Trapezium
C	Trapezoid
D	Capitate
E	Lunate
F	Pisiform
G	Triquetrum
H	Hamate
J	Intermediate cuneiform
K	Lateral cuneiform
L	Cuboid
M	Talus
N	Navicular
O	Calcaneus
P	Medial cuneiform

Skeletal System
(Posterior View)

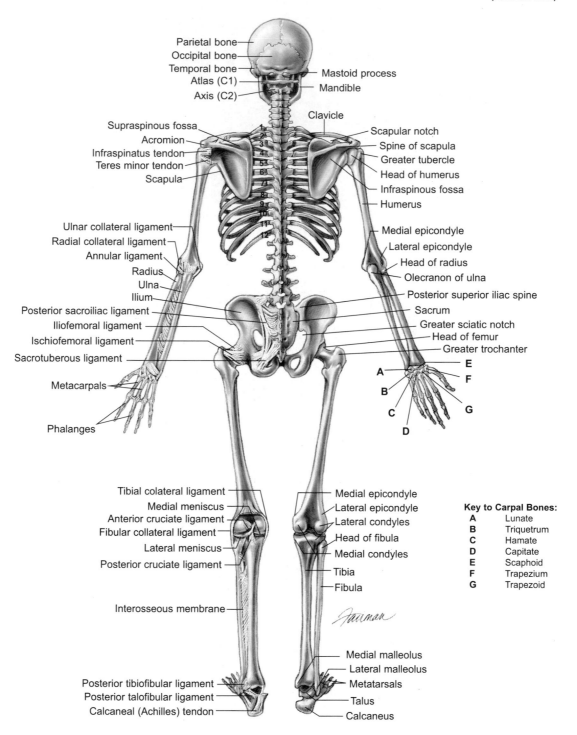

Parietal bone
Occipital bone
Temporal bone
Atlas (C1)
Axis (C2)

Mastoid process
Mandible

Clavicle

Supraspinous fossa
Acromion
Infraspinatus tendon
Teres minor tendon
Scapula

Scapular notch
Spine of scapula
Greater tubercle
Head of humerus
Infraspinous fossa
Humerus

Ulnar collateral ligament
Radial collateral ligament
Annular ligament
Radius
Ulna
Ilium
Posterior sacroiliac ligament
Iliofemoral ligament
Ischiofemoral ligament
Sacrotuberous ligament

Medial epicondyle
Lateral epicondyle
Head of radius
Olecranon of ulna
Posterior superior iliac spine
Sacrum
Greater sciatic notch
Head of femur
Greater trochanter

Metacarpals

E
F
G

A
B
C
D

Phalanges

Tibial colateral ligament
Medial meniscus
Anterior cruciate ligament
Fibular collateral ligament
Lateral meniscus
Posterior cruciate ligament

Medial epicondyle
Lateral epicondyle
Lateral condyles
Head of fibula
Medial condyles
Tibia
Fibula

Interosseous membrane

Key to Carpal Bones:

A	Lunate
B	Triquetrum
C	Hamate
D	Capitate
E	Scaphoid
F	Trapezium
G	Trapezoid

Posterior tibiofibular ligament
Posterior talofibular ligament
Calcaneal (Achilles) tendon

Medial malleolus
Lateral malleolus
Metatarsals
Talus
Calcaneus

Skeletal System
(Vertebral Column – Left Lateral View)

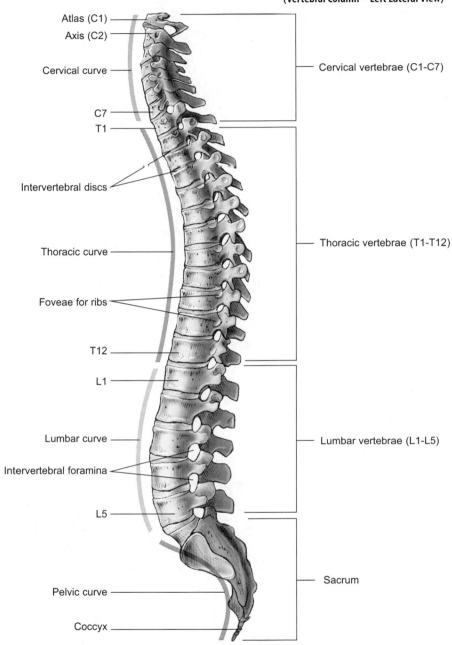

Atlas (C1)

Axis (C2)

Cervical curve

Cervical vertebrae (C1-C7)

C7

T1

Intervertebral discs

Thoracic curve

Thoracic vertebrae (T1-T12)

Foveae for ribs

T12

L1

Lumbar curve

Lumbar vertebrae (L1-L5)

Intervertebral foramina

L5

Sacrum

Pelvic curve

Coccyx

© Fairman Studios, LLC, 2002. All Rights Reserved.

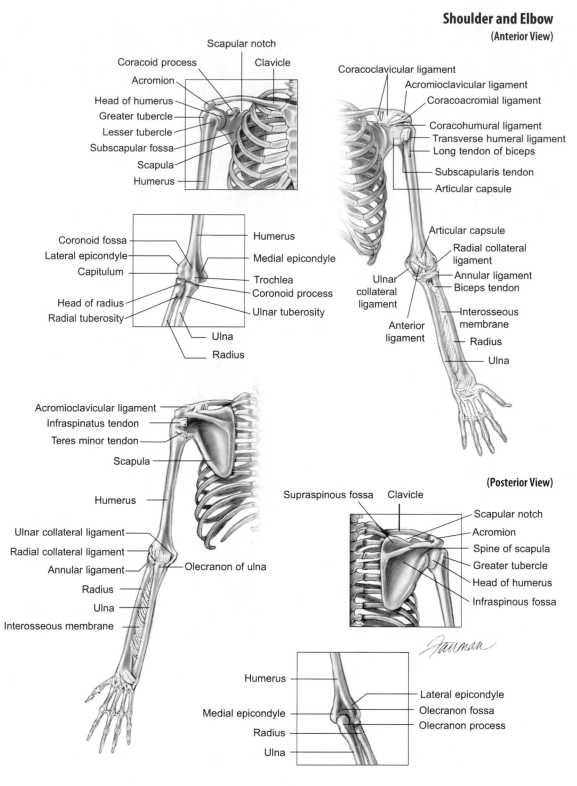

Shoulder and Elbow
(Anterior View)

Scapular notch
Coracoid process
Acromion
Head of humerus
Greater tubercle
Lesser tubercle
Subscapular fossa
Scapula
Humerus
Clavicle

Coracoclavicular ligament
Acromioclavicular ligament
Coracoacromial ligament
Coracohumural ligament
Transverse humeral ligament
Long tendon of biceps
Subscapularis tendon
Articular capsule

Coronoid fossa
Lateral epicondyle
Capitulum
Head of radius
Radial tuberosity
Humerus
Medial epicondyle
Trochlea
Coronoid process
Ulnar tuberosity
Ulna
Radius

Articular capsule
Radial collateral ligament
Annular ligament
Biceps tendon
Ulnar collateral ligament
Interosseous membrane
Anterior ligament
Radius
Ulna

Acromioclavicular ligament
Infraspinatus tendon
Teres minor tendon
Scapula
Humerus
Ulnar collateral ligament
Radial collateral ligament
Annular ligament
Olecranon of ulna
Radius
Ulna
Interosseous membrane

(Posterior View)

Supraspinous fossa
Clavicle
Scapular notch
Acromion
Spine of scapula
Greater tubercle
Head of humerus
Infraspinous fossa

Humerus
Medial epicondyle
Radius
Ulna
Lateral epicondyle
Olecranon fossa
Olecranon process

Musculoskeletal System – Hand and Wrist
(Dorsal and Palmar Views)

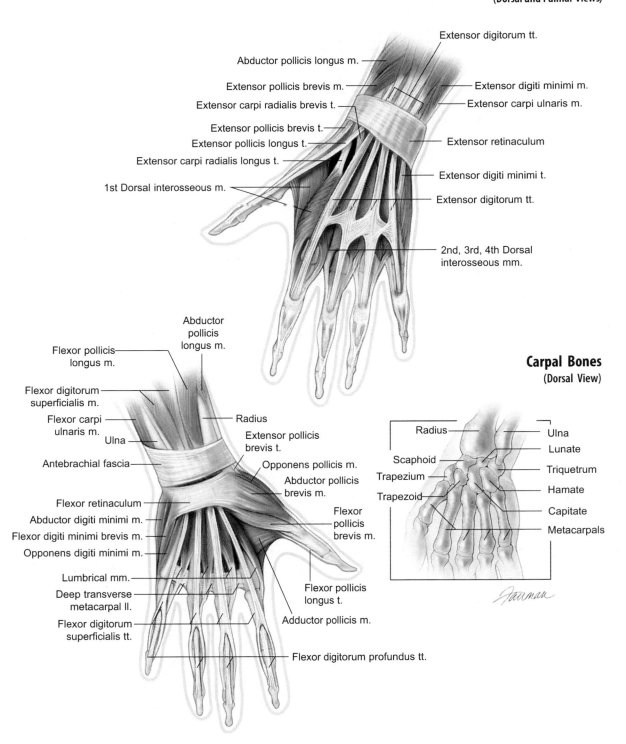

Extensor digitorum tt.

Abductor pollicis longus m.

Extensor pollicis brevis m.

Extensor carpi radialis brevis t.

Extensor pollicis brevis t.

Extensor pollicis longus t.

Extensor carpi radialis longus t.

1st Dorsal interosseous m.

Extensor digiti minimi m.

Extensor carpi ulnaris m.

Extensor retinaculum

Extensor digiti minimi t.

Extensor digitorum tt.

2nd, 3rd, 4th Dorsal interosseous mm.

Abductor pollicis longus m.

Flexor pollicis longus m.

Flexor digitorum superficialis m.

Flexor carpi ulnaris m.

Ulna

Antebrachial fascia

Flexor retinaculum

Abductor digiti minimi m.

Flexor digiti minimi brevis m.

Opponens digiti minimi m.

Lumbrical mm.

Deep transverse metacarpal ll.

Flexor digitorum superficialis tt.

Radius

Extensor pollicis brevis t.

Opponens pollicis m.

Abductor pollicis brevis m.

Flexor pollicis brevis m.

Flexor pollicis longus t.

Adductor pollicis m.

Flexor digitorum profundus tt.

Carpal Bones
(Dorsal View)

Radius

Scaphoid

Trapezium

Trapezoid

Ulna

Lunate

Triquetrum

Hamate

Capitate

Metacarpals

© Fairman Studios, LLC, 2002. All Rights Reserved.

Musculoskeletal System – Hip and Knee
(Anterior and Posterior Views)

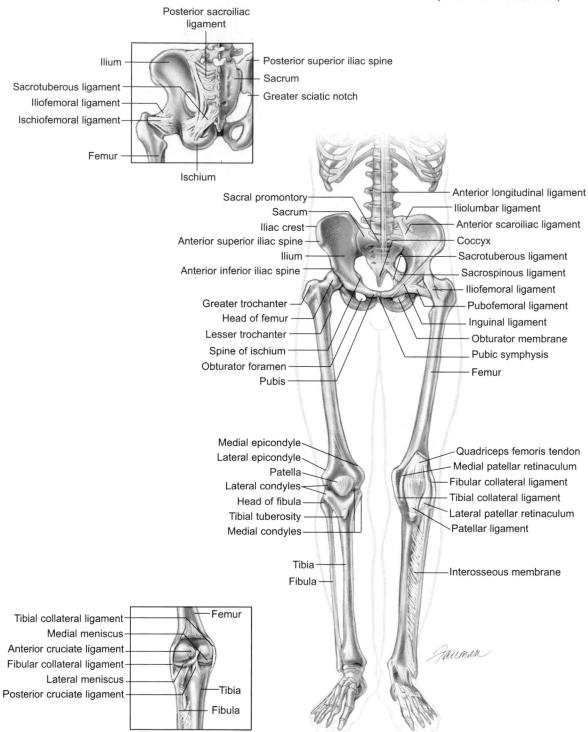

Posterior sacroiliac ligament

Ilium

Sacrotuberous ligament

Iliofemoral ligament

Ischiofemoral ligament

Femur

Ischium

Posterior superior iliac spine

Sacrum

Greater sciatic notch

Sacral promontory

Sacrum

Iliac crest

Anterior superior iliac spine

Ilium

Anterior inferior iliac spine

Greater trochanter

Head of femur

Lesser trochanter

Spine of ischium

Obturator foramen

Pubis

Anterior longitudinal ligament

Iliolumbar ligament

Anterior scaroiliac ligament

Coccyx

Sacrotuberous ligament

Sacrospinous ligament

Iliofemoral ligament

Pubofemoral ligament

Inguinal ligament

Obturator membrane

Pubic symphysis

Femur

Medial epicondyle

Lateral epicondyle

Patella

Lateral condyles

Head of fibula

Tibial tuberosity

Medial condyles

Tibia

Fibula

Quadriceps femoris tendon

Medial patellar retinaculum

Fibular collateral ligament

Tibial collateral ligament

Lateral patellar retinaculum

Patellar ligament

Interosseous membrane

Tibial collateral ligament

Medial meniscus

Anterior cruciate ligament

Fibular collateral ligament

Lateral meniscus

Posterior cruciate ligament

Femur

Tibia

Fibula

Musculoskeletal System – Foot and Ankle

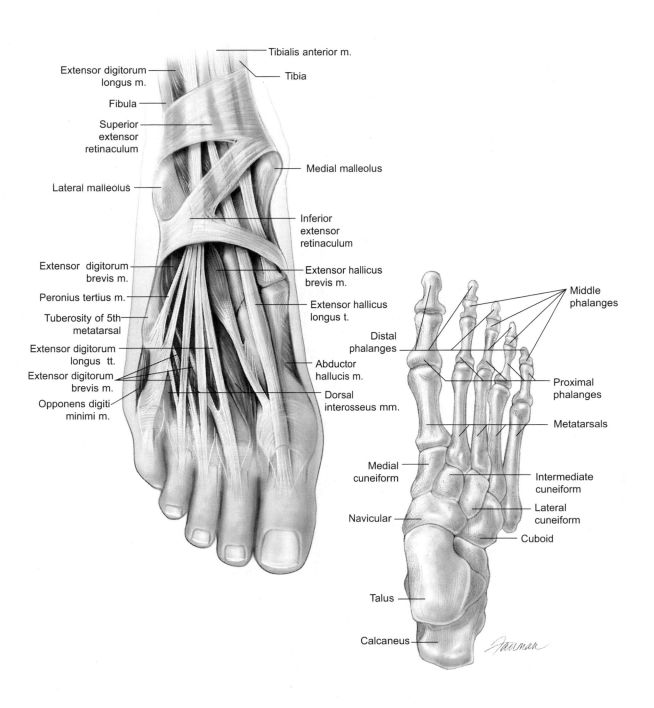

Tibialis anterior m.

Extensor digitorum
longus m.

Tibia

Fibula

Superior
extensor
retinaculum

Medial malleolus

Lateral malleolus

Inferior
extensor
retinaculum

Extensor digitorum
brevis m.

Extensor hallicus
brevis m.

Peronius tertius m.

Extensor hallicus
longus t.

Tuberosity of 5th
metatarsal

Extensor digitorum
longus tt.

Abductor
hallucis m.

Extensor digitorum
brevis m.

Opponens digiti
minimi m.

Dorsal
interosseus mm.

Middle
phalanges

Distal
phalanges

Proximal
phalanges

Metatarsals

Medial
cuneiform

Intermediate
cuneiform

Navicular

Lateral
cuneiform

Cuboid

Talus

Calcaneus

Vascular System

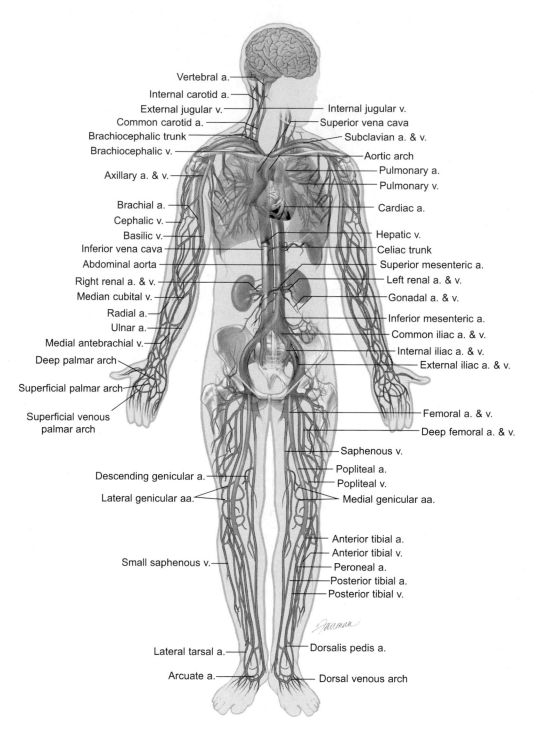

Vertebral a.
Internal carotid a.
External jugular v.
Common carotid a.
Brachiocephalic trunk
Brachiocephalic v.
Axillary a. & v.
Brachial a.
Cephalic v.
Basilic v.
Inferior vena cava
Abdominal aorta
Right renal a. & v.
Median cubital v.
Radial a.
Ulnar a.
Medial antebrachial v.
Deep palmar arch
Superficial palmar arch
Superficial venous palmar arch

Internal jugular v.
Superior vena cava
Subclavian a. & v.
Aortic arch
Pulmonary a.
Pulmonary v.
Cardiac a.
Hepatic v.
Celiac trunk
Superior mesenteric a.
Left renal a. & v.
Gonadal a. & v.
Inferior mesenteric a.
Common iliac a. & v.
Internal iliac a. & v.
External iliac a. & v.
Femoral a. & v.
Deep femoral a. & v.
Saphenous v.
Popliteal a.
Popliteal v.

Descending genicular a.
Lateral genicular aa.

Medial genicular aa.

Anterior tibial a.
Anterior tibial v.
Small saphenous v.
Peroneal a.
Posterior tibial a.
Posterior tibial v.

Lateral tarsal a.
Arcuate a.

Dorsalis pedis a.
Dorsal venous arch

ANATOMY

Heart
(External View)

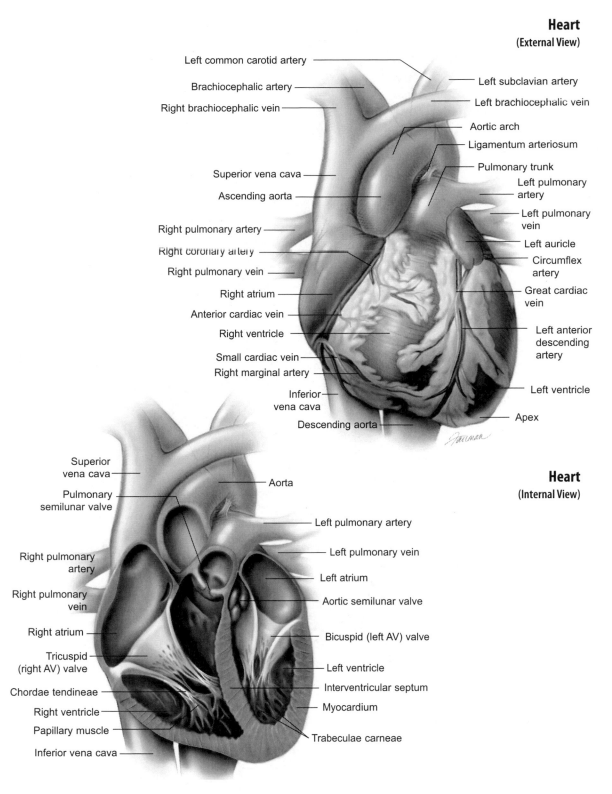

Left common carotid artery

Brachiocephalic artery

Right brachiocephalic vein

Left subclavian artery

Left brachiocephalic vein

Aortic arch

Ligamentum arteriosum

Superior vena cava

Ascending aorta

Pulmonary trunk

Left pulmonary artery

Left pulmonary vein

Right pulmonary artery

Right coronary artery

Right pulmonary vein

Left auricle

Circumflex artery

Right atrium

Anterior cardiac vein

Right ventricle

Great cardiac vein

Left anterior descending artery

Small cardiac vein

Right marginal artery

Inferior vena cava

Left ventricle

Apex

Descending aorta

Heart
(Internal View)

Superior vena cava

Pulmonary semilunar valve

Aorta

Right pulmonary artery

Left pulmonary artery

Right pulmonary vein

Left pulmonary vein

Left atrium

Aortic semilunar valve

Right atrium

Tricuspid (right AV) valve

Bicuspid (left AV) valve

Chordae tendineae

Left ventricle

Interventricular septum

Right ventricle

Myocardium

Papillary muscle

Trabeculae carneae

Inferior vena cava

© Fairman Studios, LLC, 2002. All Rights Reserved.

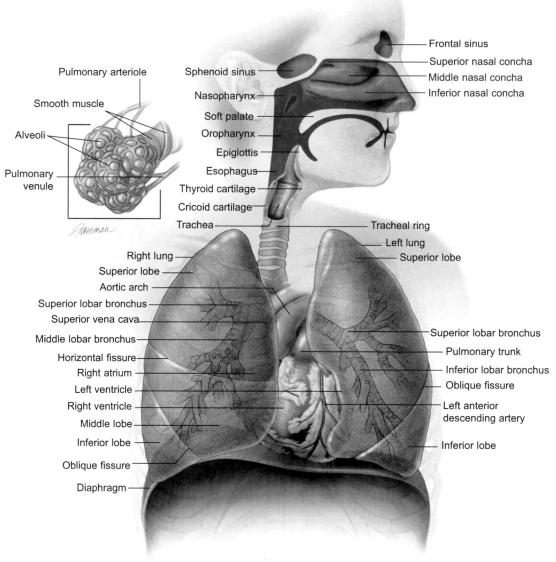

Respiratory System

Pulmonary arteriole

Smooth muscle

Alveoli

Pulmonary venule

Frontal sinus

Superior nasal concha

Middle nasal concha

Inferior nasal concha

Sphenoid sinus

Nasopharynx

Soft palate

Oropharynx

Epiglottis

Esophagus

Thyroid cartilage

Cricoid cartilage

Trachea

Tracheal ring

Left lung

Superior lobe

Right lung

Superior lobe

Aortic arch

Superior lobar bronchus

Superior vena cava

Middle lobar bronchus

Horizontal fissure

Right atrium

Left ventricle

Right ventricle

Middle lobe

Inferior lobe

Oblique fissure

Diaphragm

Superior lobar bronchus

Pulmonary trunk

Inferior lobar bronchus

Oblique fissure

Left anterior descending artery

Inferior lobe

© Fairman Studios, LLC, 2002. All Rights Reserved.

Digestive System

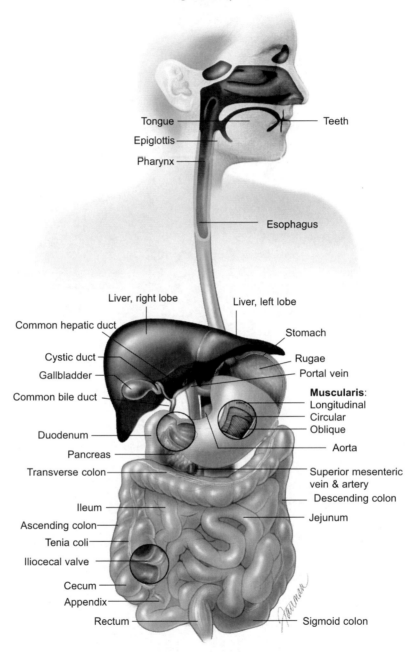

Tongue
Epiglottis
Pharynx
Teeth

Esophagus

Liver, right lobe
Liver, left lobe

Common hepatic duct
Stomach

Cystic duct
Rugae

Gallbladder
Portal vein

Common bile duct
Muscularis:
Longitudinal
Circular
Oblique

Duodenum
Pancreas
Aorta

Transverse colon
Superior mesenteric
vein & artery

Ileum
Descending colon

Ascending colon
Jejunum

Tenia coli
Iliocecal valve

Cecum
Appendix

Rectum
Sigmoid colon

© Fairman Studios, LLC, 2002. All Rights Reserved.

Nervous System

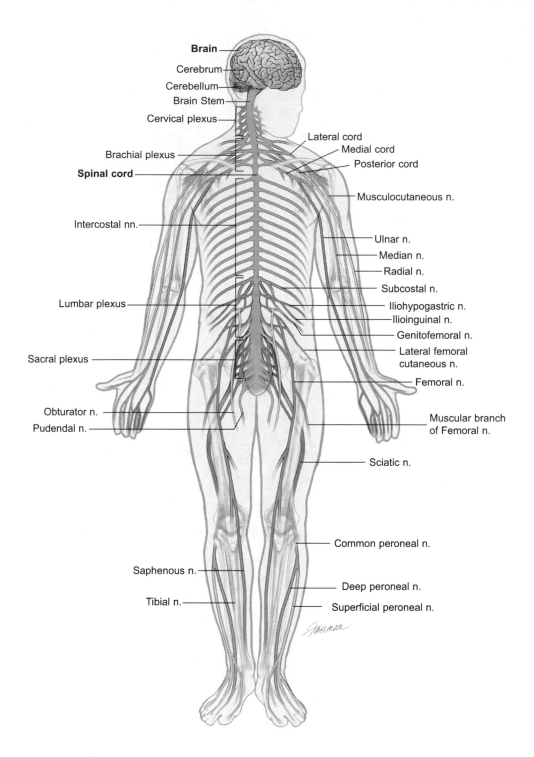

- Brain
- Cerebrum
- Cerebellum
- Brain Stem
- Cervical plexus
- Brachial plexus
- Spinal cord
- Intercostal nn.
- Lumbar plexus
- Sacral plexus
- Obturator n.
- Pudendal n.
- Saphenous n.
- Tibial n.

- Lateral cord
- Medial cord
- Posterior cord
- Musculocutaneous n.
- Ulnar n.
- Median n.
- Radial n.
- Subcostal n.
- Iliohypogastric n.
- Ilioinguinal n.
- Genitofemoral n.
- Lateral femoral cutaneous n.
- Femoral n.
- Muscular branch of Femoral n.
- Sciatic n.
- Common peroneal n.
- Deep peroneal n.
- Superficial peroneal n.

Brain
(Inferior View)

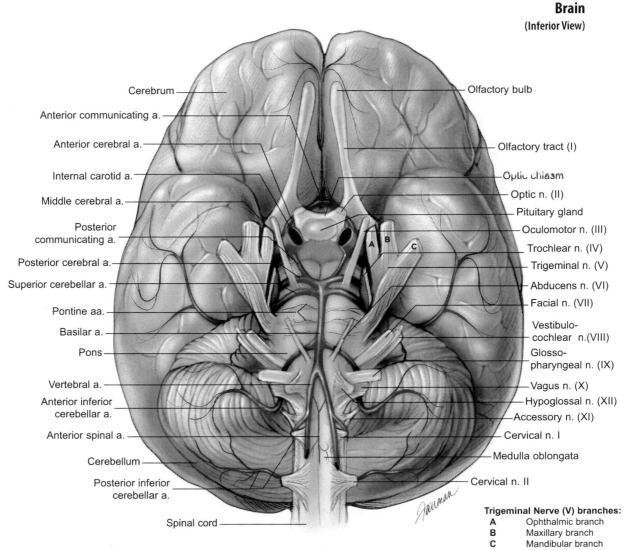

Cerebrum

Anterior communicating a.

Anterior cerebral a.

Internal carotid a.

Middle cerebral a.

Posterior communicating a.

Posterior cerebral a.

Superior cerebellar a.

Pontine aa.

Basilar a.

Pons

Vertebral a.

Anterior inferior cerebellar a.

Anterior spinal a.

Cerebellum

Posterior inferior cerebellar a.

Spinal cord

Olfactory bulb

Olfactory tract (I)

Optic chiasm

Optic n. (II)

Pituitary gland

Oculomotor n. (III)

Trochlear n. (IV)

Trigeminal n. (V)

Abducens n. (VI)

Facial n. (VII)

Vestibulo-cochlear n.(VIII)

Glosso-pharyngeal n. (IX)

Vagus n. (X)

Hypoglossal n. (XII)

Accessory n. (XI)

Cervical n. I

Medulla oblongata

Cervical n. II

Trigeminal Nerve (V) branches:
A   Ophthalmic branch
B   Maxillary branch
C   Mandibular branch

Female Breast

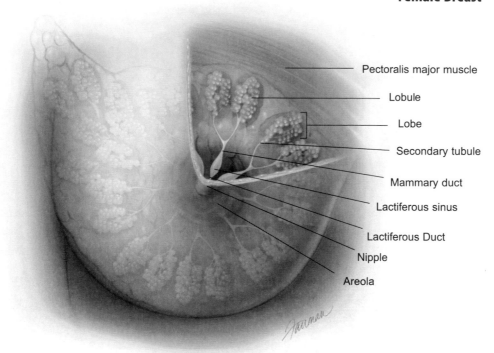

Pectoralis major muscle

Lobule

Lobe

Secondary tubule

Mammary duct

Lactiferous sinus

Lactiferous Duct

Nipple

Areola

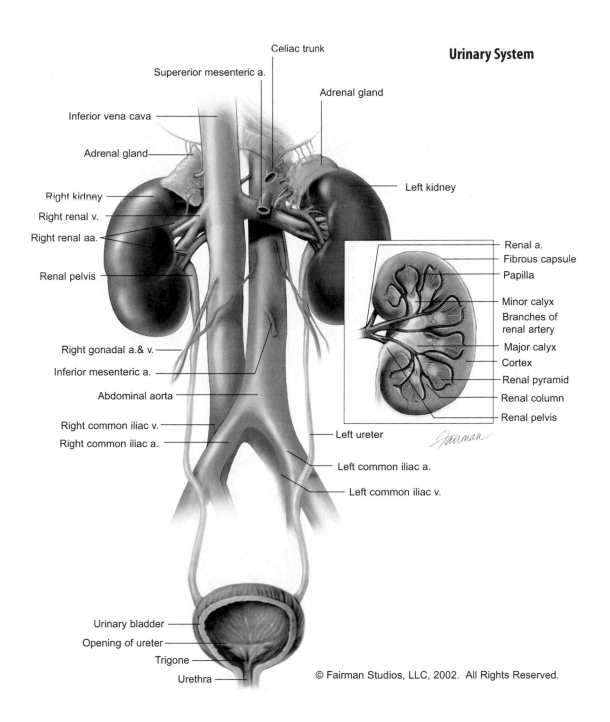

Urinary System

Celiac trunk

Supererior mesenteric a.

Adrenal gland

Inferior vena cava

Adrenal gland

Left kidney

Right kidney

Right renal v.

Right renal aa.

Renal pelvis

Renal a.

Fibrous capsule

Papilla

Minor calyx

Branches of renal artery

Major calyx

Cortex

Renal pyramid

Renal column

Renal pelvis

Right gonadal a.& v.

Inferior mesenteric a.

Abdominal aorta

Right common iliac v.

Right common iliac a.

Left ureter

Left common iliac a.

Left common iliac v.

Urinary bladder

Opening of ureter

Trigone

Urethra

© Fairman Studios, LLC, 2002. All Rights Reserved.

Male Genital System

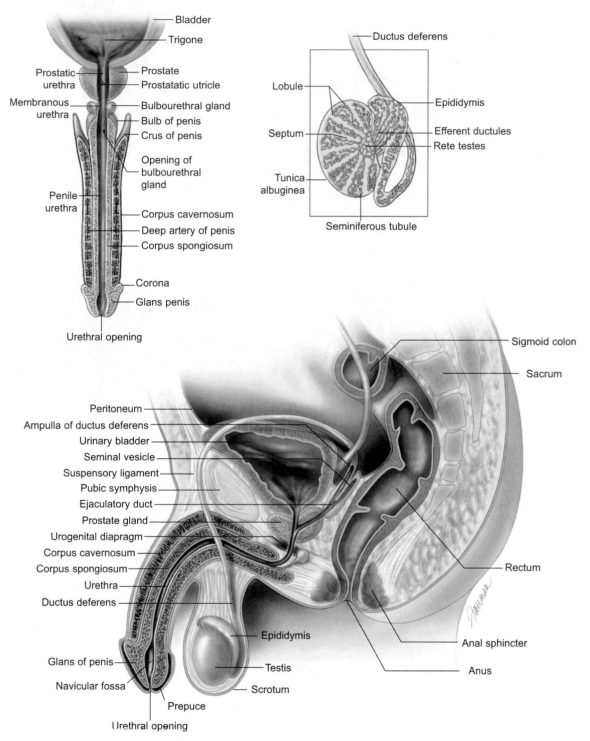

Bladder
Trigone
Prostatic urethra
Prostate
Prostatatic utricle
Membranous urethra
Bulbourethral gland
Bulb of penis
Crus of penis
Opening of bulbourethral gland
Penile urethra
Corpus cavernosum
Deep artery of penis
Corpus spongiosum
Corona
Glans penis
Urethral opening

Ductus deferens
Lobule
Epididymis
Septum
Efferent ductules
Rete testes
Tunica albuginea
Seminiferous tubule

Sigmoid colon
Sacrum
Peritoneum
Ampulla of ductus deferens
Urinary bladder
Seminal vesicle
Suspensory ligament
Pubic symphysis
Ejaculatory duct
Prostate gland
Urogenital diapragm
Corpus cavernosum
Corpus spongiosum
Urethra
Ductus deferens
Rectum
Epididymis
Glans of penis
Testis
Anal sphincter
Navicular fossa
Scrotum
Anus
Prepuce
Urethral opening

© Fairman Studios, LLC, 2002. All Rights Reserved.

Female Genital System

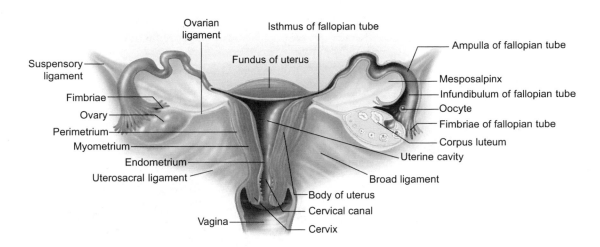

Ovarian ligament
Isthmus of fallopian tube
Fundus of uterus
Ampulla of fallopian tube
Suspensory ligament
Mesposalpinx
Fimbriae
Infundibulum of fallopian tube
Ovary
Oocyte
Perimetrium
Fimbriae of fallopian tube
Myometrium
Corpus luteum
Endometrium
Uterine cavity
Uterosacral ligament
Broad ligament
Body of uterus
Cervical canal
Vagina
Cervix

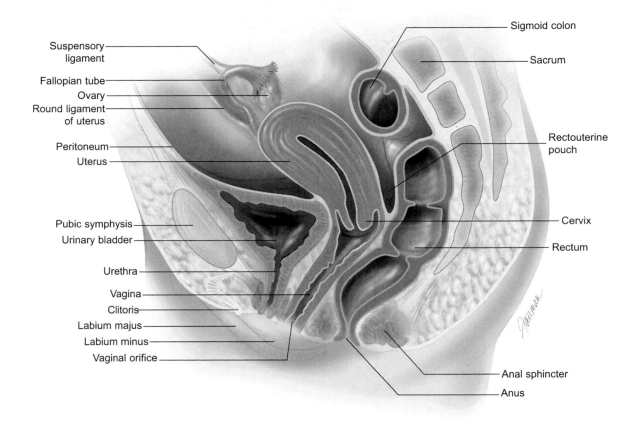

Suspensory ligament
Sigmoid colon
Fallopian tube
Sacrum
Ovary
Round ligament of uterus
Peritoneum
Rectouterine pouch
Uterus
Pubic symphysis
Cervix
Urinary bladder
Rectum
Urethra
Vagina
Clitoris
Labium majus
Labium minus
Vaginal orifice
Anal sphincter
Anus

© Fairman Studios, LLC, 2002. All Rights Reserved.

Anatomy

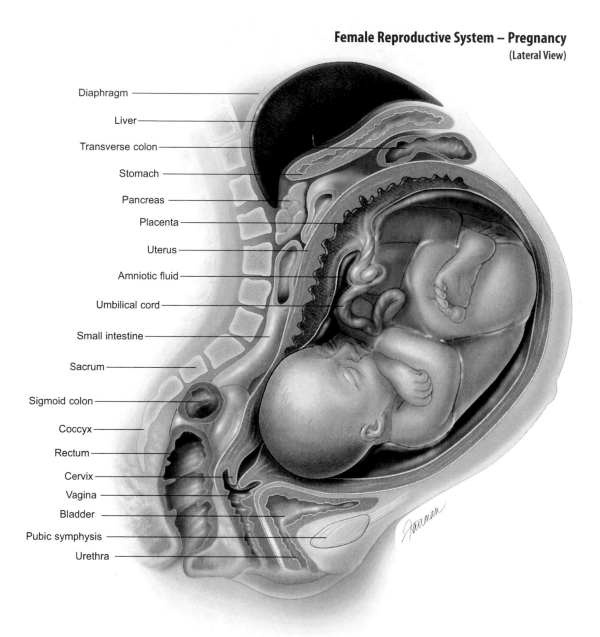

Female Reproductive System – Pregnancy
(Lateral View)

Diaphragm

Liver

Transverse colon

Stomach

Pancreas

Placenta

Uterus

Amniotic fluid

Umbilical cord

Small intestine

Sacrum

Sigmoid colon

Coccyx

Rectum

Cervix

Vagina

Bladder

Pubic symphysis

Urethra

A00 **Cholera**

Cholera is an acute intestinal infection caused by the bacterium *Vibrio cholerae* through the ingestion of contaminated food or water. Epidemics are often related to fecal contamination of drinking water and street vended foods, although eating raw or undercooked shellfish is also a source of infection as the bacteria found in marine water attach themselves easily to the shells. Cholera is rare in the United States and other industrialized nations, but still causes millions of cases each year globally. The disease may sometimes be mild and can even occur without symptoms. Severe disease strikes about 1 in 20 of those who are infected and is characterized by profuse, watery diarrhea, vomiting, and cramping. This leads to rapid loss of body fluids and electrolytes. Death can result within hours if not treated. Symptoms can appear within a few hours to a few days after infection. Treatment consists of immediate replacement of the lost fluid and salts. Rehydration is critical to survival. Patients are treated with oral rehydration solutions and/or intravenous fluids. With prompt treatment, mortality is reduced to less than 1% of infected patients.

A00.0 **Cholera due to Vibrio cholerae 01, biovar cholerae**

Vibrio cholerae has many serogroups, only two of which--serogroup 01 and serogroup 0139--can cause epidemic cholera when they produce the cholera toxin. Serogroup 01 contains both toxigenic strains that cause cholera disease and non-toxigenic strains that cause a cholera-like illness. Only the toxigenic strains are responsible for widespread epidemics. *Vibrio cholerae* 01 has two biotypes--biovar cholerae or 'classical,' and biovar eltor or 'El Tor.' Symptoms are the same; however the classical biotype is becoming rare and is seen mainly confined to areas in Bangladesh and India.

A00.1 **Cholera due to Vibrio cholerae 01, biovar eltor**

Vibrio cholerae has many serogroups, only two of which--serogroup 01 and serogroup 0139--can cause epidemic cholera when they produce the cholera toxin. Serogroup 01 contains both toxigenic strains that cause cholera disease and non-toxigenic strains that cause a cholera-like illness. Only the toxigenic strains are responsible for widespread epidemics. *Vibrio cholerae* 01 has two biotypes--biovar cholerae or 'classical,' and biovar eltor or 'El Tor.' Symptoms are the same; however the El Tor biotype displays a higher proportion of mild diarrhea or asymptomatic infections.

A00.9 **Cholera, unspecified**

An unspecified type of cholera reported here may actually be of a non-01 or non-0139 collective serogroup type that produces less severe diarrheal disease without epidemic potential. It may also be an unidentified subtype of the 01 serogroup. However, cholera that is identified as Asiatic cholera or malignant epidemic cholera is also reported here. This type is of the 0139 serogroup and is known only in Asia with the potential to cause epidemic cholera.

A01 **Typhoid and paratyphoid fevers**

Typhoid and paratyphoid fever present with high fever, abdominal pain, a rose-colored spotted rash on the chest and abdomen, constipation or diarrhea, and occasional intestinal hemorrhage. In most cases, the disease is spread through contaminated food or water.

A01.0 **Typhoid fever**

Salmonella typhi is a strain of the salmonella bacteria that causes typhoid fever.

A01.1 **Paratyphoid fever A**

Paratyphoid fever A is caused by the *Salmonella paratyphi* strain.

A01.2 **Paratyphoid fever B**

Paratyphoid fever B is caused by the *Salmonella schottmulleri* strain.

A01.3 **Paratyphoid fever C**

Paratyphoid fever C is caused by the *Salmonella hirschfeldii* strain.

A02 **Other salmonella infections**

This category includes salmonella infections other than *S. typhi* and *S. paratyphi*. Symptoms usually develop in 12-72 hours of infection and include diarrhea, abdominal cramps, fever, nausea, and/or vomiting, which can lead to severe dehydration in some cases. Salmonella bacteria live in the intestinal tracts of humans and other animals, such as birds and reptiles. Infection usually occurs by ingesting foods contaminated from an animal origin, such as milk, eggs, poultry, or beef, or by an infected food handler. In more severe cases, the salmonella infection may spread from the intestines to the bloodstream and to other parts of the body, causing salmonella sepsis and other localized infections, which have the potential for mortality. There is no long-term innoculation available.

A02.0 **Salmonella enteritis**

Salmonella enteritis is an intestinal infection with a strain of Salmonella bacteria, such as the serotype Enteriditis, which is common in the U.S. Diarrhea, fever, and abdominal cramping usually appear within 72 hours of infection and last about 5-7 days. Most people will recover without treatment except oral fluids; however hospitalization may be required for severe diarrhea. The young, elderly, and immunocompromised are most likely to have severe infections. It may take several months after recovery for bowel habits to return to normal. Because antibiotic treatment can actually prolong the time required to excrete non-typhoidal serotypes of salmonella, antibiotic treatment is usually given only to those with severe disease or those at high risk for complications. One complication is reactive arthritis that can last for months or years and lead to chronic arthritis.

A02.21 **Salmonella meningitis**

Salmonella meningitis is inflammation and infection of the meninges, the protective membrane covering the brain and spinal cord, with salmonella species other than *S. typhi* or *S. paratyphi*. When such an infection occurs, symptoms may range from a mild fever and headache to the more severe presentation of fever, drowsiness, confusion, severe headache, stiffness in the neck, painful sensitivity to bright lights, and nausea and vomiting. Most patients recover in 5 to 10 days without permanent adverse effects.

A03 **Shigellosis**

Shigellosis, a bacterial infection usually spread by ingesting contaminated food, presents with diarrhea (often with blood or mucus in the stool), fever, nausea, vomiting, abdominal cramps, and intestinal pain. Shigellosis usually takes 1-4 days to incubate, and symptoms generally last from 4-7 days. Group B and D Shigella account for almost all shigellosis infection in the United States.

A03.0 **Shigellosis due to Shigella dysenteriae**

Shigellosis due to *Shigella dysenteriae* is an infection by Group A Shigella (Schmitz bacillus). This form of dysentery is severe, and can be fatal to children.

A03.1 **Shigellosis due to Shigella flexneri**

Shigellosis due to *Shigella flexneri* is an infection by Group B Shigella.

A03.2 **Shigellosis due to Shigella boydii**

Shigellosis due to *Shigella boydii* is an infection by Group C Shigella.

A03.3 Shigellosis due to Shigella sonnei

Shigellosis due to *Shigella sonnei* is an infection by Group D Shigella, which is the most common strain of Shigella.

A04.0 Enteropathogenic Escherichia coli infection

Enteropathogenic strains of *E. coli* (EPEC) are divided into typical and atypical. The typical type relies only on humans as a reservoir and is the most common cause of infantile diarrhea in developing countries, but is rarely seen in industrialized nations. Atypical strains are seen in industrialized countries, and are more common among hospitalized infants and also in baby animals of different species. The main mechanism of disease is the formation of attaching and effacing (A/E) lesions, marked by destruction of the microvilli with bacterial adherence to the intestinal epithelium, causing a pedestal formation, and the accumulation of actin filaments under attached bacteria.

A04.1 Enterotoxigenic Escherichia coli infection

Enterotoxigenic *E. coli* (ETEC) is the name given to the strain of *E. coli* that causes intestinal disease specifically through the action of special toxins. The toxins affect the mucosal lining of the intestines and induce the production of excessive fluid, causing diarrhea. The enterotoxigenic strain is the most common cause of traveler's diarrhea and diarrhea afflicting people in developing nations, particularly children. It is spread through food or water contaminated with human or animal feces. Infection usually limits itself and is rarely life-threatening.

A04.2 Enteroinvasive Escherichia coli infection

Enteroinvasive serotypes of *E. coli* (EIEC) are related to Shigella and are common among children in developing countries. The bacteria invade the epithelial lining of the colon and cause dysentery. The infection may occur through food poisoning or through bacterial overpopulation that occurs during antibiotic therapy.

A04.3 Enterohemorrhagic Escherichia coli infection

In enterohemorrhagic *E. coli* the infection causes ulceration and bleeding so that blood appears in the stool.

A04.4 Other intestinal Escherichia coli infections

Other intestinal *E. coli* infections may include enteroadherent types (EAEC) that adhere to the mucosa in the intestines, forming colonies and causing chronic forms of watery diarrhea. This also includes enteritis caused by an unspecified strain of *E. coli,* a bacterium commonly found in the intestines of humans and warm-blooded animals as a normal part of the flora that helps digest food. Most *E. coli* is harmless and does not cause disease in humans but when the bacteria invade other areas of the body, or a person becomes infected with one of the dangerous strains, serious illness can result. The dangerous strains of *E. coli* cause severe cramping, nausea, and diarrhea, and can damage the lining of the intestines or the kidneys. The bacteria can be ingested through meat, unpasteurized milk or juice, fruits and vegetables, and contaminated water, including swimming pools or well water infected with human or animal feces. Cattle are the main source of *E. coli,* which can enter meat during the slaughtering process. The bacteria may also reside on fruits and vegetables that are fertilized with manure or irrigated with water contaminated by manure.

A04.5 Campylobacter enteritis

Infection of the small intestine by the *Campylobacter jejuni* bacteria is a common cause of food poisoning and diarrhea, particularly among travelers. Most infections occur from eating or drinking contaminated food and water, unpasteurized milk, and even some fresh produce. Infection can also occur by close contact with another infected person or animal. Stool sample with culture and/or complete blood count with differential may be done for identification. Symptoms of watery diarrhea, abdominal cramping, fever, nausea, and vomiting usually appear within 4 days of being exposed and last for about a week. Most infections will clear on their own. Treatment with antibiotics such as azithromycin or ciprofloxacin may be given in severe cases or to those with high risk of the infection spreading to the heart or brain.

A04.6 Enteritis due to Yersinia enterocolitica

Yersinia enterocolitica is a gram negative, rod-shaped bacteria that causes enterocolitis and terminal ileitis and is known to mimic appendicitis. Symptoms may vary depending on the patient's age. Common symptoms include diarrhea that may appear bloody in serious cases, abdominal pain often localized to the right lower quadrant in older children and adults, fever, and vomiting. The symptoms appear 4-7 days after exposure and can last up to 3 weeks or longer. Pigs are the most common source of infection in humans, although the bacteria are also found in other animals such as rabbits, sheep, and cattle. Infection occurs by ingesting contaminated food, especially undercooked pork, by drinking unpasteurized milk or untreated water, and sometimes by contact with infected animals or those who have handled raw pork products without proper hygienic measures. Enteritis due to *Yersinia enterocolitica* is generally diagnosed by detection in the stool. Uncomplicated cases usually resolve on their own without the use of antibiotics, which are used to treat severe or complicated infections.

Note: Long term consequences of infection include joint pain and/or the skin rash erythema nodosum on the legs and trunk that may develop about a month after initial infection and take longer to resolve. Yersiniosis caused by migration of the bacteria outside of the intestines is coded to A28.2.

A04.7 Enterocolitis due to Clostridium difficile

Clostridium difficile is a common strain causing serious enteric disease from the toxins it produces. *C. difficile* is the most common cause of bacterial diarrhea in hospitalized patients and is associated with antimicrobial drug therapy, particularly amoxicillin, clindamycin, and cephalosporins. Outbreaks have been reported worldwide with increased severity, relapses, and even death.

A04.8 Other specified bacterial intestinal infections

Other specified bacterial intestinal infections may be due to other types of bacteria identified as gram-negative. In a Gram stain, a bacteria culture is stained with a crystal violet dye and then washed with alcohol. Gram-negative bacteria will not retain the dark blue color of the dye after the alcohol wash, allowing them to take on the pink stain of a subsequent dye. Gram-negative bacteria are far more likely to cause disease than gram-positive bacteria.

A05.0 Foodborne staphylococcal intoxication

Food poisoning caused by *Staphyloccal aureus,* a common bacterium found on skin and in the nose of many healthy people. Food becomes infected through contaminated handling. The bacteria produce a toxin as they grow, particularly in foods such as ham and other sliced meats, eggs, puddings, cream-filled pastries, and foods that require no cooking or remain unrefrigerated. Gastrointestinal illness arises not from ingesting the bacteria, but from the effects of the toxins they produce. Symptoms can develop in 30 minutes to 6 hours after ingestion and include nausea, vomiting, stomach cramps, and diarrhea. Most patients recover in 1-3 days.

A05.1 Botulism food poisoning

Botulism is a serious, muscle-paralyzing disease that is a public health emergency. The disease is caused by ingesting the neurotoxins produced by the bacteria, *Clostridium botulinum.* Symptoms commonly appear within 12-36 hours, but can begin in as little as six hours or take up to 14 days. Symptoms include eyelid drooping, double or blurred vision, slurred speech, difficulty swallowing, and muscular weakness that moves down the neck affecting the shoulders and upper arms, and continuing downwards. Paralysis may occur in the respiratory muscles, leading to death unless ventilatory support is given. Infection requires an antitoxin to reduce the muscle paralyzing effects. Most patients eventually recover after requiring weeks or even months of supportive care.

A05.2 Foodborne Clostridium perfringens [Clostridium welchii] intoxication

Clostridium perfringens is a common cause of infectious foodborne illness, especially where cooked meat is the source. This ubiquitous, anaerobic, gram-negative bacillus lives through the high temperatures of initial cooking and the spores grow while the food is cooling. The dormant forms then begin multiplying when the food is held at under 125 degrees

Fahrenheit. Most cases are traced to ingesting the meat when it is no longer hot, and has not been adequately reheated. Symptoms include diarrhea and cramping.

A05.3 Foodborne Vibrio parahaemolyticus intoxication

Vibrio parahaemolyticus is a bacterium belonging to the same family as the cholera-causing bacteria. *V. parahaemolyticus* inhabits brackish coastal waters in high concentrations in the summer. Most people become infected by eating undercooked or raw seafood, especially oysters. Symptoms include watery diarrhea, abdominal cramps, fever, nausea, vomiting, and chills that appear within 24 hours of ingestion. The poisoning is usually self-limited, lasting about three days.

A05.4 Foodborne Bacillus cereus intoxication

Bacillus cereus is a type of bacteria present in food that multiplies quickly at room temperature and produces toxins. This bacteria is commonly found in soups, sauces, rice, and other prepared leftovers that have sat out too long. The toxins produce two kinds of illness--diarrheal and emetic. The emetic toxin produces nausea and vomiting within 30 min to 6 hours of ingestion. The diarrheal toxin produces watery diarrhea and abdominal cramping within 6-15 hours of ingestion. Illness from both types usually lasts about 24 hours. Usually the only treatment necessary is rest and drinking plenty of fluids.

A05.5 Foodborne Vibrio vulnificus intoxication

Vibrio vulnificus is a bacterium that lives in warm sea water and belongs to the same family as the cholera-causing bacteria. It causes vomiting, diarrhea, and abdominal pain in those who ingest contaminated seafood, especially oysters. Most cases are reported in the gulf coast states of Alabama, Mississippi, Texas, Florida, and Louisiana. Ingestion of *V. vulnificus* can become an infection of the bloodstream that leads to septic shock and blistering skin lesions in those with immunocompromising medical conditions.

A05.8 Other specified bacterial foodborne intoxications

Other specified bacterial food poisoning may include other strains of Clostridia, a heterogenous group of anaerobic, spore-forming, rod-shaped bacteria that usually test gram negative, which are part of the normal microflora found in the colon and throughout the environment, including: *C. clostridioforme, C. innocuum, C. ramosum, C. butyricum, C. septicum,* and *C. tertium.*

Note: Food poisoning and infection by *C. difficile*, the most common strain, is reported with A04.7.

A07 Other protozoal intestinal diseases

A protozoa is a single-celled, usually microscopic organism, such as an amoeba, ciliate, flagellate, or sporozoan.

A07.0 Balantidiasis

Balantidiasis is caused by the presence of *Balantidium coli* in the large intestine. Most balantidiasis infections pass without any noticeable infections at all; however, in acute cases, the victim may present with diarrhea, adominal cramps and pain, and even ulceration of the intestinal wall (which may be indicated by blood in the stool).

A07.1 Giardiasis [lambliasis]

Giardiasis is caused by the *Giardia lamblia* parasite. It may not present with any symptoms at all, or it may present with diarrhea, gas and bloating, abdominal cramps, nausea, loss of appetite, loss of weight, and fatigue. In most cases, these symptoms pass in 7-10 days without treatment, but in some cases, the symptoms may become chronic.

A07.2 Cryptosporidiosis

Cryptosporidiosis is most often transmitted by drinking water contaminated with *Cryptosporidium* parasites, which are resistant to chlorine and may live for several days in a swimming pool, for example. The most common symptoms are diarrhea, abdominal cramps, weight loss, and dehydration,

as well as a low-grade fever in children. These symptoms typically last 2-4 weeks.

A07.3 Isosporiasis

Coccidiosis is an infection of the intestine by the *Isospora belli* parasite and presents with symptoms ranging from mild diarrhea to rupture of the intestinal wall (indicated by blood in the stool). It is most often found in the Southeastern United States in patients with depressed immune systems (e.g., from HIV or AIDS).

A07.4 Cyclosporiasis

Cyclosporiasis is an infection of the small intestine by the *Cyclospora* parasite, which can be contracted by ingesting contaminated food or water. It commonly presents with symptoms of diarrhea, abdominal cramps, nausea and vomiting, low-grade fever, and fatigue. If left untreated, the illness may persist anywhere from a few days to more than a month.

A07.8 Other specified protozoal intestinal diseases

Other specified protozoal intestinal diseases includes intestinal microsporidiosis and trichomoniasis, sarcocystosis and sarcosporidiosis. Microsporidiosis is infection with a microscopic parasite that lives in other host cells and produces infective spores. This is rarely seen in people with normal immune systems. Intestinal microsporidiosis is more often seen primarily in those with HIV or other compromised immune systems. Symptoms include chronic diarrhea that can become debilitating to AIDS patients, malabsorption, wasting, and even gallbladder disease. Intestinal trichomoniasis is infection with the flagellate protozoan parasite Trichomonas. Infection can cause diarrhea with mucus, intestinal mucosal congestion with edema and inflammation, and even intestinal epithelial cell degeneration or necrosis. Intestinal sarcosporidiosis or sarcocystosis is infection with the intracellular protozoan parasite, Sarcocystis. Symptoms usually appear within a day of ingesting meat, particularly beef or pork, that is contaminated with oocysts, which reproduce in the intestinal tract, causing enteritis with diaphoresis, fever, chills, vomiting, and diarrhea. Most cases are seen in Southeast Asia.

A07.9 Protozoal intestinal disease, unspecified

Note: Unspecified protozoal intestinal disease includes any cases of diarrhea, colitis, or dysentery identified as being caused by flagellates or protozoa without more specification.

A08.0 Rotaviral enteritis

Rotaviruses are a group of wheel-shaped viruses that commonly infect the intestines. Rotaviral enteritis is most often seen in infants and young children and is the most common cause of severe diarrhea among this age group. Symptoms usually appear within 2 days of exposure and include copious amounts of watery stool causing dehydration, abdominal cramps, anorexia, low-grade fever, vomiting, and significantly decreased urine output which may be hard to identify in diapered infants and toddlers. Dehydration and loss of electrolytes may produce altered mental status and seizures. The highest risk factor for rotavirus infection is group daycare as the virus is spread by fecal-oral contact. Appropriate rehydration is crucial.

A08.11 Acute gastroenteropathy due to Norwalk agent

The Norwalk virus, the most prominent genus of a group called noroviruses, causes severe inflammation of the intestinal tract that usually clears up in 2-3 days.

A08.2 Adenoviral enteritis

Adenoviruses most commonly cause conjunctivitis and upper respiratory tract infections, but also infect the intestinal tract. Adenoviral enteritis most commonly affects infants and young children under age 2 by a direct fecal-oral route. The incubation period is 8-10 days and causes watery diarrhea associated with mild fever, abdominal pain, and vomiting. Diarrhea often lasts about 10 days, but the virus may take up to 14 days to be excreted in the stool. Some patients may develop secondary lactose intolerance or chronic diarrhea or are predisposed to intussusception. Oral or intravenous rehydration is necessary.

A08.3 Other viral enteritis

This code should be used to report an intestinal infection due to some other viral cause of enteritis, such as the Torovirus, Coxsackie virus, and Echovirus.

A08.31 Calicivirus enteritis

A calicivirus is a Norwalk-like virus which is among the most common causes of intestinal inflammation, but which is rarely diagnosed due to the lack of availability of the necessary test. An infection by this virus usually causes more nausea and vomiting than diarrhea and clears up within two days.

A08.32 Astrovirus enteritis

An infection by this virus typically causes a mild case of gastroenteritis which lasts for several days.

A09 Infectious gastroenteritis and colitis, unspecified

Use this code to report infection or inflammation of the colon (colitis), intestine (enteritis), stomach and intestines (gastroenteritis), or unspecified hemorrhagic or epidemic dysentery. This code should be used if the patient is suffering from diarrhea known to be infectious, but only if the condition is otherwise ill-defined; i.e., if the specific infectious agent is known, use the more specific code instead.

Note: Unspecified cases of colitis, enteritis, and gastroenteritis which are not known to be infectious should be reported with K52.9 and unspecified cases of diarrhea that are not known to be infectious should be reported with R19.7.

A15 Respiratory tuberculosis

Tuberculosis (TB) is a disease caused by *Mycobaterium tuberculosis* and is transmitted primarily through inhalation of infected air from those already infected.The most common site of tuberculous infection is within the lungs and other parts of the respiratory system, but the tubercles can spread to other locations in the body through the lymph and blood vessels. Symptoms of TB include a cough that goes on for two or more weeks (sometimes with small amounts of blood in the phlegm), fever, night sweats, and unexplained weight loss. Other symptoms may be present depending on the location of the infection; however, all of the symptoms mentioned are also caused by other pulmonary infections, so final diagnosis of the disease can only be made by further examination.

A17.0 Tuberculous meningitis

Tuberculous meningitis causes an inflammation of the protective membrane covering the brain and spinal cord by an infection with *Mycobacterium tuberculosis*. When such an inflammation occurs, symptoms may range from a mild fever and headache to the more severe presentation of fever, drowsiness, confusion, a severe headache, stiffness in the neck, a painful sensitivity to bright lights, and nausea and vomiting.

A17.1 Meningeal tuberculoma

Tuberculosis bacteria are not often destroyed following an active infection, but are contained instead within a covering of immune cells that walls off the bacteria and renders them inactive, resulting a nodule or swelling called a granuloma or tuberculoma. Use this code for a tuberculoma within the protective membrane covering the brain and/or spinal cord.

A18.0 Tuberculosis of bones and joints

Symptoms of tuberculosis infections of the bones and joints include joint pain and stiffness, as well as anemia when the bone marrow is infected. If left untreated, the infection may result in arthritic destruction of the bone, or even paralysis.

A19 Miliary tuberculosis

Tuberculosis (TB) is a disease caused by *Mycobacterium tuberculosis* and is transmitted primarily through inhalation of Infected air from those already Infected.In some instances, the tuberculosis bacilli may be passed between distant organs through the vascular or lymphatic systems, planting widely disseminated tubercles in various parts of the body. This spread, known

as miliary tuberculosis, can cause symptoms of profound toxemia (blood poisoning).

A20 Plague

Plague is caused by an infection with the *Yersinia pestis* bacillus and is most often transmitted by the bites of fleas, ticks, and lice. However, it can also spread by contact between infected material and the mucous membranes of the nose or throat. It comes in three distinct forms in humans: bubonic, septicemic, and pneumonic plague, and presents with a number of severe symptoms, including fever, chills, muscle pain and weakness, sore throat, headache, painfully swollen lymph nodes, abdominal pain, nausea and vomiting, constipation and/or diarrhea (often with blood in the stool), coughing, and shortness of breath. In the late stages it presents with convulsions, bleeding from the orifices, gangrene in the digits and limbs, and respiratory failure.

A20.0 Bubonic plague

Bubonic plague is the best known and most severe kind of the three forms of plague, and presents with massively swollen and bleeding lymph nodes, which appear as black swellings on the surface of the skin (called a bubo).

A20.1 Cellulocutaneous plague

Cellulocutaneous plague presents with severe inflammation and necrosis or death of skin cells.

A20.2 Pneumonic plague

Pneumonic plague is the most vicious form of plague, and has a 100% mortality rate if not treated within 24 hours of infection. In many cases, it may be mistaken for pneumonia. In primary pneumonic plague, the infection originates in the lungs. Secondary pneumonic plague occurs when the plague first sets in elsewhere and then spreads to the lungs.

A20.7 Septicemic plague

Septicemic plague results from the *Y. pestis* organism infecting the bloodstream and presents with abdominal pain and other gastrointestinal symptoms.

A21 Tularemia

Tularemia, also called deerfly fever and rabbit fever, is caused by an infection by the *Francisella tularensis* (also sometimes called the *Pasteurella tularensis*) bacterium. Symptoms vary depending on the site of the infection, but may include a slow-growing ulcer at the site where the bacteria entered the skin, swollen lymph nodes, sudden onset of chills, fever, aches, malaise, muscle pains, sore throat, abdominal pain, diarrhea and vomiting, and in rare cases, pneumonia.

A21.0 Ulceroglandular tularemia

Ulceroglandular tularemia presents with a lesion or ulcer on the surface of the skin where the bacillus first penetrated, often on the hands.

A21.1 Oculoglandular tularemia

In oculoglandular tularemia, the disease enters the conjunctiva (protective membrane over the white) of the eye, causing inflammation and the formation of pus (conjunctivitis) among other symptoms.

A22 Anthrax

Anthrax is a potentially deadly disease caused by *Bacillus anthracis*. It is most often spread to humans through handling contaminated animal products or breathing spores from infected animals (e.g., breathing in spores from the wool of an infected sheep). Anthrax is also a potential biological weapon, and is classified by the route of inoculation.

A22.0 Cutaneous anthrax

Cutaneous anthrax, an infection that enters through the skin, presents as a small sore that turns into a blister. The blister becomes an ulcer with a center of black, dead tissue, usually within 48 hours of the initial infection. None of the three stages are painful.

A22.1 Pulmonary anthrax

Pulmonary anthrax, also called inhalation anthrax, initially presents flu-like symptoms, including sore throat, mild fever, and muscle aches two to five days after exposure. Later symptoms include shortness of breath, coughing, and chest congestion. Anthrax is primarily a disease of herbivores such as cattle, sheep, goats, and horses. Infection may be cutaneous, respiratory, or intestinal and results from exposure, ingestion or inhalation of *Bacillus anthracis* spores. Humans are relatively resistant to invasion by *B. anthracis*, which must enter the skin through cuts or breaks, be swallowed, or be inhaled all the way into the lungs in a sufficiently large amount of spores to cause the disease. Casual contact does not necessarily mean development of the disease.

Pulmonary anthrax is very rare but is a most dangerous, rapidly fulminating disease that is almost always fatal. It begins like a common cold with low grade fever and cough, but rapidly turns into severe pneumonia requiring hospitalization. Inhalation anthrax and septicemic anthrax have the highest mortality rate at over 90 percent. Some patients improve before deteriorating rapidly into high fever, shortness of breath, tachypnea, cyanosis, profound sweating, and chest pain which may be confused with a myocardial infarction. Hemorrhagic pleural effusions also occur. Overwhelming septicemic infection occurs secondarily. Death is caused by the effects of lethal toxins with bleeding from orifices occurring at or near death.

A22.2 Gastrointestinal anthrax

Gastrointestinal anthrax is generally contracted by ingesting undercooked meat. It presents the symptoms of nausea, loss of appetite, diarrhea (often with blood in the stool), fever, and abdominal pain.

A22.7 Anthrax sepsis

Anthrax sepsis is a systemic infection throughout the body and bloodstream by the anthrax bacillus. Septic poisoning presents with a sudden onset of fever and chills, low blood pressure (which may result in pale or bluish limbs and lips), confusion or altered emotional state, and rash. If not treated immediately, sepsis can lead to septic shock and death.

A23 Brucellosis

Brucellosis is also known as Rock fever, Cyprus fever, Undulant fever, Mediterranean fever, Gibraltar fever, and Malta fever. It is far more common in animals than humans, and is usually contracted through ingesting undercooked meat or unpasteurized milk or cheese. The disease commonly presents the symptoms of fever with sweating and chills; muscle, joint, and back pain and weakness; headache; fatigue; abdominal pain with loss of appetite; and enlarged liver. This disease is classified according to the causative organism.

A23.0 Brucellosis due to Brucella melitensis

Brucellosis is caused by the *Brucella melitensis* bacteria and contracted through infected sheep and goats.

A23.1 Brucellosis due to Brucella abortus

Brucella abortus infection is contracted through infected cattle.

A23.2 Brucellosis due to Brucella suis

Brucella suis infection is contracted through infected swine.

A23.3 Brucellosis due to Brucella canis

Brucella canis infection is contracted through infected dogs.

A24.0 Glanders

Glanders, also known as Farcy and Malleus, is an infectious disease that is caused by the bacterium *Burkholderia mallei*, *Actinobacillus mallei*, *Malleomyces mallei*, or *Pseudomonas mallei*. Although rare in humans (the last known case of human infection in the United States was in 1945), in rare cases it can be transmitted by direct contact with infected animals, especially horses. Glanders commonly presents the symptoms of fever, chills, muscle aches and tightness, chest pain, headache, swollen glands, excessive tearing and light sensitivity, and diarrhea.

A24.9 Melioidosis, unspecified

Melioidosis is also known as Whitmore's disease and Pseudoglanders and is caused by an infection by the *Malleomyces pseudomallei* bacteria. It is mostly found in tropical climates, and can be transmitted by inhalation of infected particles or ingestion of contaminated water or food. It presents with fever, muscle ache, and headache. An infection of the lungs usually causes coughing, which may or may not bring up phlegm. In patients with weakened immune systems due to another disease or condition, melioidosis can infect the bloodstream. Symptoms vary depending on the site of the original infection, but may include difficulty in breathing, severe headache, fever, diarrhea, infected sores on the skin, muscle tenderness, and disorientation. Untreated, this form of melioidosis may result in severe shock and even death.

A25 Rat-bite fevers

Rat-bite fever is a disease transmitted via contact with an infected rodent's mucous or urine, most commonly through an open wound, such as a bite. Symptoms may vary depending on which type of the disease is contracted.

A25.0 Spirillosis

Spirillary fever, or spirillosis, is caused by the *Spirillum minus* bacteria. This form of rat-bite fever is common in Japan, where it is called sodoku, and presents with a skin rash of red and purple splotches, which may or may not cause the original wound to reopen.

A25.1 Streptobacillosis

Streptobacillary fever, which is caused by the *Streptobacillus moniliformis* bacteria, presents with a widespread rash that is particularly prominent on the arms and legs. It often spreads to one or more joints, causing them to become inflamed and painful. If left untreated it can also spread to the heart valves, causing potentially life-threatening complications.

A26.0 Cutaneous erysipeloid

An Erysipelothrix infection is a disease caused by the *Erysipelothrix insidiosa* bacteria (also called *Erysipelothrix rhusiopathiae*). The disease most commonly presents with tender, purplish sores on the skin, especially on the hands and between the fingers. If it spreads, it presents with more general symptoms such as fever, chills, weight loss, joint pain, cough, and headache, which may vary depending on which body systems are affected.

A27 Leptospirosis

Leptospirosis is a disease caused by a spirochete-type bacteria. The disease is spread to humans through the urine or tissue of infected animals. Infection produces flu-like symptoms 2 to 25 days after exposure and, if not treated, serious inflammation of the eyes, brain, and spinal cord can develop. Problems with the lungs and heart are less common but possible.

A27.0 Leptospirosis icterohemorrhagica

Leptospirosis icterohemorrhagica, also known as Weil's disease, is a severe form of leptospirosis that causes fever, muscle aches, jaundice, and hemorrhaging.

A27.81 Aseptic meningitis in leptospirosis

An inflammation of the protective membrane which covers the brain and/or spinal cord caused by leptospirosis. This inflammation is aseptic, meaning that bacteria does not grow in a culture taken from the inflamed tissue.

A28 Other zoonotic bacterial diseases, not elsewhere classified

Other zoonotic bacterial diseases are those caused by bacteria that can pass between animals and humans or vice-versa.

A28.0 Pasteurellosis

Pasteurellosis is a disease caused by the *Pasteurella multocida* bacteria, also called *Pasteurella septica*. It is most often transmitted by an animal scratch or bite, and presents with inflammation and drainage of blood and other fluids from the wound. If it spreads, symptoms can change depending on the system affected, e.g. in a respiratory infection, it can cause pneumonia.

A28.1 Cat-scratch disease

Benign lymphoreticulosis is commonly known as cat-scratch fever and is often caused by the *Bartonella henselae* bacterium. This disease gets its nickname due to often being transmitted by a scratch from a cat, usually a kitten. The disease is marked by a mild, flu-like infection with swollen lymph nodes and a fever. A pustule may form at the site of the scratch.

A30 Leprosy [Hansen's disease]

Leprosy, also called Hansen's disease, is caused by an infection by the *Mycobacterium leprae* bacteria. Its long incubation period often makes it difficult to pinpoint the time of the original infection, which most often takes place in childhood. Leprosy presents with sores on the skin that are of lighter color than the surrounding flesh and are numb to the touch, and which do not heal even after several weeks or months. As symptoms progress, numbness and muscle weakness usually spread to all four limbs. Foot drop, in which the patient drags a toe over the ground when walking, is a common sign.

A30.0 Indeterminate leprosy

Indeterminate (group I) leprosy presents with few to no symptoms.

A30.1 Tuberculoid leprosy

Tuberculoid (type T) leprosy is a localized infection that presents with small lesions and fewer bacteria.

A30.3 Borderline leprosy

Borderline (group B) leprosy, also called dimorphous leprosy, occupies the middle ground of severity between type L and type T leprosy.

A30.5 Lepromatous leprosy

Lepromatous (or type L) leprosy is characterized by widespread lesions and bacterial infections.

A31 Infection due to other mycobacteria

Other diseases that may occur due to a mycobacterial infection are categorized by the infected system and by the species of bacteria. Mycobacteria is a classification of non-motile bacteria (unable to move on their own) that are spread through the air and are most often contracted through inhalation or via an open wound. Symptoms vary depending on the type and extent of the infection, and the primary system affected.

A32 Listeriosis

Listeriosis is a disease caused by the *Listeria monocytogenes* bacteria. It is most often contracted from eating undercooked, contaminated food. The onset of the disease can begin anywhere from 11 to 70 days after exposure, and symptoms are very similar to those of the flu, including fever, headache, nausea and vomiting, tiredness, and diarrhea. In pregnant women, Listeriosis can cause miscarriage, premature labor, early rupture of the birth sac, and stillbirth. It can also be passed to an infant both in the womb and during delivery, and is far more dangerous to a newborn than to an adult.

A32.0 Cutaneous listeriosis

Listeriosis is a disease caused by the *Listeria monocytogenes* bacteria. It is most often contracted from eating undercooked, contaminated food. The onset of the disease can begin anywhere from 11 to 70 days after exposure, and symptoms are very similar to those of the flu, including fever, headache, nausea and vomiting, tiredness, and diarrhea. In pregnant women, listeriosis can cause miscarriage, premature labor, early rupture of the amniotic sac, and stillbirth. It can also be passed to an infant both in the womb and during delivery, and is far more dangerous to a newborn than to an adult.

A33 Tetanus neonatorum

Tetanus neonatorum is a tetanus infection in a newborn, usually acquired after the umbilical cord is severed with a non-sterile surgical instrument.

A35 Other tetanus

Tetanus, commonly called lock-jaw, is a disease caused by the bacterium *Clostridium tetani*, which enters the body via an open wound. Its symptoms begin with pain and cramping in the neck and jaw muscles. The symptoms appear two days to two months after infection (less than two weeks is average), and as a general rule, the shorter the time between infection and the onset of the disease, the more severe the symptoms will be.

As the tetanus progresses, the disease spreads to the body and limbs, causing cramping, partial paralysis, muscle spasms, and sometimes convulsions severe enough to affect the heart or even cause bone fractures. Since it can affect the heart, diaphragm, and throat, causing an irregular heartbeat and difficulty in breathing and swallowing, it is a potentially fatal disease.

A36 Diphtheria

Diphtheria is an infection by *Corynebacterium diphtheriae*, which is primarily spread through the air. One to six days after the initial infection the disease presents with a severe sore throat, swollen glands in the neck, and a low grade fever. If left untreated, it can infect other systems, causing potentially dangerous and chronic complications. Because of this, patients are usually hospitalized for treatment. This disease is classified by the primary location of the infection.

A36.0 Pharyngeal diphtheria

Faucial diphtheria is an infection of the tonsils. This type of infection can be dangerous due to a thick, gray membrane that forms over the tonsils and throat that can make swallowing difficult.

A36.1 Nasopharyngeal diphtheria

A nasopharyngeal diphtherial infection affects the soft tissues of the nose and pharynx (or throat). Like a faucial, or tonsillar infection, this type of infection can be dangerous due to a thick, gray membrane that forms over the throat that can make swallowing and breathing difficult.

A36.3 Cutaneous diphtheria

Cutaneous diphtheria is an infection of the skin and its underlying structures that presents with a painful, red rash or open sores.

A36.81 Diphtheritic cardiomyopathy

Diphtheritic myocarditis or cardiomyopathy is an infection of the wall of the heart by diphtheria bacteria which leads to inflammation, and is a potentially life-threatening disease. This form of the infection can cause serious and permanent damage to the heart muscles and even paralyze breathing.

A36.85 Diphtheritic cystitis

A diphtheritic infection of the bladder usually presents with a false membrane forming in the bladder that can result in difficulty urinating or a continuous urge to urinate.

A37 Whooping cough

Whooping cough, also called pertussis, is a highly contagious infection of the upper respiratory tract caused by *Bordetella pertussis*, *Bordetella parapertussis*, or other Bordetella species, such as *Bordetella bronchiseptica*. The bacteria are spread from person to person and infect the nasal passages at the back of the throat, causing irritation and severe coughing spells. There are three different stages which may last longer than 10 weeks. The first stage manifests as cold-like symptoms, the second stage sees the cough turn from dry and hacking to bursts of uncontrollable, violent coughing during which it is impossible to take a breath. Airways are narrowed by inflammation and gasping for air when finally able to breathe causes the typical 'whooping' sound. In the third stage, the patient may be getting stronger, but the cough may sound worse. Bacterial pneumonia is the most common complication resulting from whooping cough and is the most common cause of pertussis-related deaths when they occur, seen most often in children under one year of age who are hit the hardest by the pertussis. Adults have much milder cases and may not even know they are infected.

A38.9 Scarlet fever, uncomplicated

An infectious illness caused by the group A beta-hemolytic streptococcal bacteria that develops in some people who have strep throat. It most commonly affects children and causes the characteristic sore throat and bright red 'sandpaper' rash that covers most of the body, accompanied by a high fever. If left untreated, scarlet fever can cause the development of much more serious conditions affecting the eyes, kidneys, heart, or other organs.

A39   Meningococcal infection

Meningococcus is a bacterium that commonly resides in the human nose or throat without causing any symptoms, but which can be spread even by those who are not ill via sneezing, coughing, or kissing. If it enters the bloodstream, it can spread to other systems.

A39.0   Meningococcal meningitis

The most dangerous type of meningococcal infection is meningitis, an infection of the protective lining of the brain and spinal cord (meninges). This condition presents with a number of symptoms, including fever, a purplish rash, loss of appetite, headache, sensitivity to light, vomiting, stiffness in the neck, lethargy and/or drowsiness, irritability, and/or confusion. The patient may also lose consciousness and go into convulsions. In some cases, the patient may suffer long-term effects, such as deafness.

A39.1   Waterhouse-Friderichsen syndrome

Waterhouse-Friderichsen syndrome is a complete failure of the adrenal glands due to bleeding caused by Meningococcal bacteria. This infection is also known as meningococcal hemorrhagic adrenalitis and mengingococcic adrenal syndrome. The same characteristic purplish rash as seen in septicemia often appears on the patient's back. If not treated immediately, it can plunge the body into shock and cause death very quickly.

A39.2   Acute meningococcemia

Meningococcemia, or meningococcal septicemia, is an infection of the bloodstream caused by the bacterium *Neisseria meningitidis*. This bacteria is commonly found in the upper respiratory tract of humans without symptoms of illness. It is spread person to person by respiratory droplets. Symptoms of an acute infection can include high fever, headache, muscle pain, nausea, a a deep reddish or purplish petechial skin rash, and sometimes diarrhea and vomiting. A "glass test" may be used to test the severity of the infection: a glass is pressed against the rash, which will not fade or lose its color under pressure in a more serious infection.

A39.51   Meningococcal endocarditis

Meningococcal endocarditis is an inflammation of the membrane that lines the valves of the heart, and which may present with fever, fatigue, loss of appetite, and a heart murmur.

A39.52   Meningococcal myocarditis

Meningococcal myocarditis is an inflammation of the muscle of the heart which may present with fever, fatigue, chest pain, lung congestion and difficulty breathing, and a muffled pericardial friction rub.

A39.53   Meningococcal pericarditis

Meningococcal pericarditis is an inflammation of the heart's protective membrane, which may present with fever, fatigue, chest pain, and a peculiar scratching noise (which may be heard through a stethoscope) called a pericardial friction rub.

A39.81   Meningococcal encephalitis

Meningococcal encephalitis is an inflammation of the brain itself caused by the meningococcal bacteria. This inflammation can present with fever, headache, confusion, and in extreme cases, can cause brain damage, stroke, seizures, or even death.

A40   Streptococcal sepsis

Streptococcal sepsis is the most common form of infection in the bloodstream, which ususaly develops quickly and can be life threatening. Symptoms can include hypotension (low blood pressure), decreased tissue perfusion, change in mental status, increased heart and/or respiratory rate, temperature instability (fever and/or hypothermia) and skin rash. Streptococci are gram positive, aerobic organisms, most of which are sensitive to penicillin. The main streptococcal strains found causing sepsis

are *S. pyogenes* (Group A), *S. agalactiae* (Group B), *S. equi* (Group C), *S. faecalis* (Group D), *S. canis* (Group G), and *S. pneumoniae*. Although migration of these strains of bacteria into the bloodstream causes sepsis in any individual, some types of streptococcal sepsis are found occurring more commonly in particular populations, such as newborns.

Note: Neonatal and puerperal sepsis, as well as sepsis due to Streptococcus Group D are not coded within this category.

A40.0   Sepsis due to streptococcus, group A

S. pyogenes, or Group A streptococcus, is responsible for strep throat, and rheumatic and scarlet fever. Sepsis caused by Group A streptococcus is spread from the nasopharynx into the systemic circulation. It is also a common strain contracted in hospitals from those assisting with labor and delivery, and following surgical procedures, immunizations, and transfusions or other injections.

Note: When streptococcal sepsis, group A or other strains, occurs during labor or following a medical or surgical procedure, code first the specified situation with which or following which the streptococcal sepsis occurred, such as following immunization, code T88.0.

A40.1   Sepsis due to streptococcus, group B

S. agalactiae, a type of Group B streptococcus, is commonly found in the human gastrointestinal, reproductive, and urinary tracts. Although migration of these strains of bacteria into the bloodstream can occur in any individual, sepsis caused by *S. agalactiae* is most commonly seen in newborns who acquire the infection from their mothers during delivery while passing through the birth canal and is a very serious pathogen that can be deadly without early treatment.

Note: When Group B streptococcal sepsis occurs congenitally in a newborn, report with P36.0.

A40.3   Sepsis due to Streptococcus pneumoniae

This type of sepsis is caused by *Streptococcus pneumoniae*, gram-positive bacteria responsible for many other seriously acute pyogenic conditions, such as the most common form of lobar pneumonia. *S. pneumoniae* is commonly found within the nasopharynx of around 10 percent of healthy adults and up to 40 percent of healthy children. It attaches to the nasopharyngeal tissue and becomes pathogenic when the organisms are carried into other areas, where they activate the immune response. Once pneumococcal sepsis has occurred, the bacteria can spread quickly to the lining of the brain and spinal cord, joints, and bones, causing brain abscesses, meningitis, septic arthritis, and osteomyelitis.

A40.8   Other streptococcal sepsis

Note: This includes sepsis caused by *S. equi* (Group C), and *S. canis* (Group G).

Note: Sepsis caused by *S. faecalis* (Group D) is called enterococcal sepsis and is coded to A41.81.

A41   Other sepsis

Systemic response to an infection in the bloodstream caused by bacteria (other than streptococcus), virus, fungi, or parasites which trigger the body's immune system to release certain chemicals. Infection may originate in bone, bowel, urinary tract, brain, liver/gallbladder, lungs or skin and migrate into the bloodstream. Symptoms can include hypotension (low blood pressure), decreased tissue perfusion, change in mental status, increased heart and/or respiratory rate, temperature instability (fever and/or hypothermia) and skin rash.

A41.01   Sepsis due to Methicillin susceptible Staphylococcus aureus

Note: *Staphylococcus aureus* septicemia not otherwise specified as methicillin susceptible or resistant, is coded to susceptible for the default.

A41.02 Sepsis due to Methicillin resistant Staphylococcus aureus

A systemic infection throughout the bloodstream by a methicillin resistant strain of *Staphylococcus aureus*, known as MRSA. This strain is unaffected by the broad-spectrum antibiotics used to treat it. Most MRSA infections are acquired in hospitals, dialysis centers, and nursing homes with the elderly and immune compromised at greatest risk, but another type also occurs among otherwise healthy people in the community. Both community-associated and hospital-associated MRSA infections can be fatal.

A41.1 Sepsis due to other specified staphylococcus

Other species causing staphylococcal sepsis include *S. epidermidis*, *S. haemolyticus*, *S. hominis*, and *S. siumlans*. *S epidermidis* is commonly found as nonpathogenic flora on the skin, but may become a pathogenic cause of sepsis from secondary wound infections, particularly in a hospital environment from peritonitis and peritoneal dialysis. *S. haemolyticus* and *S. hominis* occur on human skin and are associated with wounds and infections of the urinary tract and conjunctiva, and are known to cause sepsis with an uncertain pathogenicity.

A41.3 Sepsis due to Hemophilus influenzae

H. influenzae is a very common, gram-negative, nonmotile bacillus that is generally aerobic, but can grow as a facultative anaerobe. Most strains are opportunistic pathogens that commonly live in the nasal mucus of most people, but only cause disease when another factor, such as a viral infection, reduces immunity and gives the bacteria the opportunity to invade other areas or the bloodstream, causing systemic infection, or sepsis. Because sepsis can be life-threatening, antibiotic treatment may be given even before the presence of *H. influenzae* is confirmed by laboratory results.

A41.4 Sepsis due to anaerobes

Anaerobes are microorganisms that live and grow within an environment that is completely or almost completely devoid of oxygen. Some of these bacteria can survive with oxygen in their environment, but cannot replicate; others are killed by oxygen and can only grow in its complete absence. Both aerobes and anaerobes are part of the normal bacterial flora in the gastrointestinal tract. Infection of the bloodstream can occur when the microflora leak from an injury or interruption in the continuity of the GI tract, possibly from trauma, surgery, or internal disease, causing sepsis.

A41.51 Sepsis due to Escherichia coli [E. coli]

E. coli is a facultative, anaerobic, gram negative bacillus that inhabits the intestinal tract as part of its normal flora. Infection of the bloodstream causing sepsis can occur when traumatic GI perforation, rupture of an abdominal abscess, spillage of colon contents, obstruction of bile ducts, or serious urinary tract infection leads to the presence of these bacteria in the blood. *E. coli* is a leading cause of nosocomial infections of the blood stemming from a gastrointestinal or genitourinary source. The bacteria produce endotoxins that can lead to disseminated intravascular coagulation and death.

A41.52 Sepsis due to Pseudomonas

Pseudomonas aeruginosa is a major opportunistic pathogen that almost never infects tissues that are not compromised. This gram-negative, aerobic, rod-shaped bacillus commonly inhabits soil, water, and the surface of both plants and animals, including humans. Blood stream invasion causing sepsis occurs from local sites of infection and is particularly a problem among patients with severe burns, cancer, cystic fibrosis, and AIDS. *P. aeruginosa* produces a toxin that has the same enzymatic action as diptheria toxin. Sepsis presents with the usual pathologic events of gram-negative invasion, including fever, hypotension, and intravascular coagulation.

A41.53 Sepsis due to Serratia

Serratia marcescens is the most frequently occurring Serratia species and lives in water, soil, and food. This gram-negative, motile, facultative anaerobe also occurs naturally in the intestines. It produces a kind or red-pigment stain and is an opportunistic pathogen associated with nosocomial bacteremia and sepsis, particularly in immunocompromised patients.

A41.59 Other Gram-negative sepsis

Poisoning of the bloodstream due to any other identified gram negative bacteria not specifically identified in another code. The typical microorganisms causing sepsis are gram-negative bacteria. They release toxins into the bloodstream that trigger immune responses, and in some cases, help to make the bacteria resistant to the action of phagocytosis and the serum immune response. Gram-negative sepsis presents with high fever, chills, weakness, a drop in blood pressure, excessive sweating, and disseminated intravascular coagulation from the action of the toxins, which can be deadly.

A42 Actinomycosis

Actinomycotic infection, also called actinomycosis, is an infection by rod-shaped bacteria called *Actinomycetales*. Its symptoms vary widely depending on the site of the infection. The disease is easy to treat with antibiotics, but if left untreated, it can become a chronic condition.

A42.0 Pulmonary actinomycosis

A pulmonary infection, also called thoracic actinomycosis, often presents as a chronic illness similar to pneumonia or tuberculosis with fever, cough (which may or may not produce phlegm), shortness of breath, fatigue, loss of appetite, and chest pain. Diagnosis of this disease is difficult because there are no symptoms or patterns of development unique to it.

A42.1 Abdominal actinomycosis

An abdominal infection that most often occurs as a complication of abdominal surgery, and is often misdiagnosed as a slowly growing tumor. In addition to a mass or lump that can be felt by pressing down on the abdomen, this disease presents a number of non-specific symptoms, including a low-grade fever, abdominal pain and discomfort, nausea and vomiting leading to weight loss, fatigue, and a change in bowel habits.

A42.2 Cervicofacial actinomycosis

Cervicofacial actinomycosis is the most common and easily recognized form of actinomycosis. It most commonly appears in patients with a history of injury to or surgery on the teeth or jaws, and those with poor oral hygiene habits. It presents as swellings on the jaw, which may or may not be painful. These swellings may be reddish or bluish in color, and may cause difficulty in chewing if they involve the muscle tissue. Over time, they will drain pus containing sulfur granules (particles). Unless treated with antibiotics, these swellings tend to recur on a regular basis.

A42.89 Other forms of actinomycosis

Cutaneous actinomycosis is another form of actinomycosis--an infection of the skin also known as erythrasma and trichomycosis axillaris. It presents as a mildly itchy, reddish-brown rash that may include scaly skin, most often appearing in the armpit, the groin, between the toes, and in other skin folds. It is easily misdiagnosed as a fungal infection because of the appearance of the disease.

A46 Erysipelas

Erysipelas is an airborne bacteria that can enter through a wound in the skin and become an active infection that most commonly appears as a raised, reddish rash on the face and/or legs. Blisters may appear on the affected area, and fever and chills are not uncommon. If left untreated, the disease may spread to the joints, bones, and even the heart valves, causing more severe complications.

Note: If classified as postpartum or puerperal erysipelas, see code O86.89.

A48.0 Gas gangrene

Gas gangrene is the result of a wound infected with Clostridium bacteria. The onset comes very quickly and spreads so quickly that it can be observed with the naked eye over a period of minutes. The disease presents with extremely painful swelling at the site of the wound, which may be pale or reddish-brown. Blisters filled with red-brown fluid and pockets of gas that feel "crackly" to the touch will also be evident. In addition, the patient may have a moderate to high fever, mood swings, a rapid heart beat (tachycardia), and may succumb to shock and die without treatment. The affected tissues are completely destroyed, and must be debrided (removed) to prevent the infection from spreading; in extreme cases, the affected limb may need to be amputated.

A48.1 Legionnaires' disease

Legionnaires' disease is pneumonia caused by *Legionella pneumophila* bacteria. The organisms are found in bodies of water and some in soil. In an aquatic environment, the bacteria attach to surfaces and form a biofilm. They also attach to and colonize on materials within the water system including plastic, rubber, and wood. The major source is water systems in large buildings and also humidifiers, whirlpools, spas, and hot springs. Symptoms appear about 10 days after exposure and include weakness, high fever, a cough that produces sputum, chest pain, and shortness of breath. Headaches, muscle aches, and gastrointestinal symptoms are also present, such as diarrhea, nausea, and vomiting. The infection is not contagious and is spread through contaminated water, not infected persons. When antibiotics are used near the onset of the disease, the outcome is very good.

A48.3 Toxic shock syndrome

Toxic shock syndrome (TSS) describes a set of symptoms that come from a severe infection, most often *Staphylococcus aureus* and *Streptococcus pyogenes*, and can lead to severe shock. Symptoms vary depending on the source of the infection. Both forms present with the symptoms of low blood pressure, decreased liver and kidney function with decreased urine output, bruising due to decreased platelet count, a widespread and reddish rash, and shedding of the skin in large sheets (especially from the palms and soles of the feet). In addition, the two forms of TSS have their own symptoms. TSS from a Staph infection also presents with a high fever over 102 degrees F, chills, headache, fatigue, vomiting and diarrhea, muscle pain, and confusion. Streptococcal toxic shock syndrome, or STSS, presents with shock and difficulty breathing. Since these symptoms can be found in similar illnesses (e.g. Rocky Mountain Fever), the final diagnosis must be made from a blood test or culture, a urine test, or a lumbar puncture. Treatment includes administering antibiotics and fluids via IV, blood transfusion, and surgical removal of infected tissues.

A48.5 Other specified botulism

Clostridium botulinum is an anaerobic, gram-positive bacillus which produces distinctive neurotoxins that cause weakness and paralysis, particularly of the respiratory system. *C. botulinum* spores are very heat resistant, and can survive boiling for several hours, although their toxins are readily destroyed by heat. In the body, toxins interfere with the release of acetylcholine at peripheral nerve endings, causing severe hyoptonia and paralysis. Symptoms usually begin with the cranial nerves and then descend. Patients require hospitalization with intensive care treatment to prevent mortality. With treatment, the mortality rate is under 10 percent.

Note: The type of botulism cases reported in this subcategory are not related to food poisoning or foodborne *C. botulinum* toxins, which is reported with code A05.1.

A48.51 Infant botulism

Infant botulism comes from the ingestion of *Clostridium botulinum* spores, which then colonize in the infant's large intestine and begin producing toxins. Although spores are commonly present in the environment, contraction by infants is usually idiopathic, occuring in babies under 6 months old, but it has sometimes been traced to ingesting certain kinds of honey that may contain spores. Constipation usually precedes the neuromuscular symptoms of poisoning and paralysis, marked by lethargy, slow feeding, severe hypotonia, and respiratory insufficiency.

A48.52 Wound botulism

Wound botulism is caused by *Clostridium botulinum* infecting traumatic injuries or deep puncture wounds, particularly abscessing sites of self-injected illegal drugs. The infection produces the neurological effects of severe hypotonia and paralysis, usually within two weeks, without the gastrointestinal symptoms.

Note: Another code should be assigned to identify the site of the complicated open wound.

A48.8 Other specified bacterial diseases

This includes rhinoscleroma, a chronic, upper respiratory infection caused by the bacterium *Klebsiella rhinoscleromatis*. It usually starts in the nasal passages, but can spread to the larynx and trachea. Rhinoscleroma presents in three distinct phases. In the first phase, the disease presents with an inflammation of the mucous membrane of the nose that discharges a foul-smelling pus. After several weeks or months, the disease progresses to the second stage, in which the inflammation of the mucous membrane becomes bluish red and small, rubbery knobs (or nodules) form inside the nose. These nodules can damage the cartilage of the nose, the nasal passages, and the soft palate, and may be mistaken at first for a malignant tumor. The patient's airway may become partially or even completely blocked by these growths. In the third stage, the affected tissue becomes hard and tough, and extensive scarring and constriction of the airways may occur. In the latter stages of the disease, surgical correction may be required to correct the damage.

A49.01 Methicillin susceptible Staphylococcus aureus infection, unspecified site

Note: A *Staphylococcus aureus* infection not otherwise specified as methicillin susceptible or resistant, is coded here as methicillin susceptible Staphylococcus aureus (MSSA) infection for the default.

A49.02 Methicillin resistant Staphylococcus aureus infection, unspecified site

Methicillin resistant Staph aureus, known as MRSA, is a strain that is resistant to, or unaffected by, the broad-spectrum antibiotics used to treat it. Most MRSA infections are acquired in hospitals, dialysis centers, and nursing homes with the elderly and immune compromised at greatest risk, but another type also occurs among otherwise healthy people in the community. Both community-associated and hospital-associated MRSA infections can be fatal.

A49.1 Streptococcal infection, unspecified site

Streptococcus is divided into many sub-types, or groups, each identified by a letter. While each group has symptoms and diseases more common to it than the others, they are similar enough that final diagnosis requires laboratory testing of a culture.

A49.2 Hemophilus influenzae infection, unspecified site

Hemophilus influenzae is a very common bacterium found in the nasal mucus of up to 90% of people. When it does infect the body, it usually causes a localized infection and/or inflammation of the sinuses, inner ear, heart, joints, conjunctiva of the eye, the covering of the brain, etc. Because some infections can be fatal, treatment by antibiotics is usually begun even before confirmation of the *H. influenzae* bacterium is verified by laboratory testing.

A49.3 Mycoplasma infection, unspecified site

Mycoplasma, also called Eaton's agent, is an infection by the *Mycoplasma pneumoniae* bacterium, which may be called Pleuropneumonia-like organisms (PPLO). It most commonly affects the lungs, usually causing a mild pneumonia over a course of one to three weeks.

A50 Congenital syphilis

In congenital syphilis, the spirochete *Treponema pallidum* is passed from an infected mother to her child during birth. Symptoms can include, but are not limited to, deformations of the teeth, mouth and/or nose, skin rash, anemia, jaundice, and enlargement of the lymph nodes. Death can result from pulmonary hemorrhage.

A50.0 Early congenital syphilis, symptomatic

Use this code for congenital syphilis in a child who is showing symptoms of the disease at less than two years of age.

A50.1 Early congenital syphilis, latent

Early congenital syphilis appears with a positive serological reaction before a child is two years of age. The latent form shows no symptoms or manifestation of the disease outside of the positive serological test with a negative spinal fluid test.

A50.2 Early congenital syphilis, unspecified

Use this code for a patient under two years old who is positive for syphilis when it is not specified whether or not they are showing symptoms.

A50.31 Late congenital syphilitic interstitial keratitis

Congenital syphilitic interstitial keratitis is a condition in which the corneal stroma (the middle layers of the cornea responsible for focusing light) of the eye becomes inflamed due to syphilitic infection. The disease usually develops in congenitally infected patients between ages 6-12. The disease usually begins unilaterally and becomes bilateral in 90% of cases.

A50.4 Late congenital neurosyphilis [juvenile neurosyphilis]

Juvenile neurosyphillis is a progressive and destructive infection of the brain or spinal cord which occurs in cases of untreated congenital syphilis.

A50.41 Late congenital syphilitic meningitis

In congenital syphilitic meningitis, the syphilis infection causes an inflammation of the lining of the brain and/or the spinal cord. When such an inflammation occurs, symptoms may range from a mild fever and headache to the more severe presentation of fever, drowsiness, confusion, a severe headache, stiffness in the neck, a painful sensitivity to bright lights, and nausea and vomiting. Most patients recover in 5 to 10 days without permanent injury.

A50.42 Late congenital syphilitic encephalitis

In congenital syphilitic encephalitis, the syphilis infection causes an inflammation of the brain, and presents with fever, headache, confusion, and in extreme cases, can cause brain damage, stroke, seizures, or even death.

A50.6 Late congenital syphilis, latent

Use this code for congenital syphilis diagnosed in patients age two or older who present without any symptoms. Late congenital syphilis without any clinical manifestations will appear with a positive serological reaction and a negative spinal fluid test.

A50.7 Late congenital syphilis, unspecified

Use this code for a patient two years or older who is positive for syphilis when it is not further specified whether or not they are showing symptoms.

A51 Early syphilis

Symptomatic early syphilis is an acquired syphilitic infection that presents with clinical manifestations in less than two years of the infection. Syphilis is contracted sexually, with the initial symptom being a painless chancre like a dull red, hard lesion at the site of the infection. This lesion may appear inside the vagina or rectum. Further symptoms of early syphilis include headache, fever, sore throat, patchy hair loss, and enlarged lymph nodes. Diagnosis is positive in a blood test.

A51.0 Primary genital syphilis

A single sore, or chancre first appears where syphilis entered the body on the external genitals or vagina. The sore is usually firm, round, and painless, and can often go unnoticed. The sore can last from 3 to 6 six weeks and heals whether or not the infected person is treated. If it remains untreated, the disease will progress to the secondary stage.

A51.1 Primary anal syphilis

A single sore, or chancre first appears where syphilis entered the body on the rectum or anus. The sore is usually firm, round, and painless, and can often go unnoticed. The sore can last from 3 to 6 six weeks and heals whether or not the infected person is treated. If it remains untreated, the disease will progress to the secondary stage.

A51.2 Primary syphilis of other sites

A single sore, or chancre first appears where syphilis entered the body on the lips, in the mouth, even on the fingers or breasts. The sore is usually

firm, round, and painless, and can often go unnoticed. The sore can last from 3 to 6 six weeks and heals whether or not the infected person is treated. If it remains untreated, the disease will progress to the secondary stage.

A51.3 Secondary syphilis of skin and mucous membranes

After the primary stage, when the chancre appearing at the site of the infection is healing or already healed, a secondary infection, in which syphilis spreads throughout the body, occurs without treatment. The second stage of syphilis is the most contagious. In secondary syphilis of the skin or mucous membranes, the patient presents with multiple sores and rashes often concentrated on the palms or soles of the feet, and may present with lesions in the mouth, vagina, or penis called syphilitic mucous patches, or warty lesions on the genitalia and moist skin folds called condylomata lata. Other symptoms include fever, loss of appetite, and fatigue.

A51.32 Syphilitic alopecia

Syphilitic alopecia is unusual hair loss due to syphilis.

A51.4 Other secondary syphilis

The secondary stage is the most infectious. In addition to the multiple sores and rashes that appear in the secondary stage as the primary sore is healing or already healed, the spirochetal bacteria infect other organs within the body, such as the eyes, liver, brain, kidneys, and bones causing nephritis, hepatitis, meningitis, oculopathy, osteopathy and lymphadenopathy along with other symptoms of fever, headaches, muscle aches, patchy hair loss, weight loss, and sore throat. The secondary symptoms then subside with or without treatment, but without it, the disease progresses to the latent (hidden) or even late stage. Complications can appear even 30 years later and include uncoordinated muscle movements, paralysis, progressive blindness, dementia, damage to internal organs including the brain, nerves, eyes, liver, bones, heart, and blood vessels.

A51.41 Secondary syphilitic meningitis

Syphilic meningitis is a secondary syphilitic inflammation of the protective lining of the brain and/or spinal cord. When such an inflammation occurs, symptoms may range from a mild fever and headache to the more severe presentation of fever, drowsiness, confusion, severe headache, stiffness in the neck, painful sensitivity to bright lights, and nausea and vomiting.

A51.45 Secondary syphilitic hepatitis

A secondary syphilitic infection of the liver will cause inflammation (hepatitis), which is characterized by fatigue, aching of the joints, abdominal pain, nausea and vomiting, unusually dark urine, loss of appetite, and fever.

A51.46 Secondary syphilitic osteopathy

A secondary syphilitic infection of the outer layer of bone can cause an inflammation called periostitis.

A51.5 Early syphilis, latent

Use this code to report acquired cases of syphilis in the early, latent form, showing no symptoms or manifestation of the disease outside of the positive serological test, with a negative spinal fluid test, less than two years after infection.

A52.10 Symptomatic neurosyphilis, unspecified

Neurosyphilis is a syphilitic infection of the nervous system that occurs in the later stage of the disease.

A52.11 Tabes dorsalis

Tabes dorsalis occurs when a syphilitic infection causes the hardening of the dorsal columns of the spinal cord. Symptoms of this condition include extreme weight loss, shooting pains in the legs and trunk, loss of muscular coordination, incontinence, and impotence.

A52.13 Late syphilitic meningitis

Late syphilitic meningitis is a syphilitic infection of the lining of the brain and/or spinal cord occurring two years or more after the initial acquired infection. Symptoms include fever, drowsiness, confusion, a severe headache, stiffness in the neck, painful sensitivity to bright lights, and nausea and vomiting.

A52.14 Late syphilitic encephalitis

Late syphilitic encephalitis is a syphilitic infection of the brain occurring two years or more after the initial acquired infection. The disease causes inflammation of the brain, which presents with fever, headache, confusion, brain damage, stroke, seizures, or even death.

A52.17 General paresis

General paresis, sometimes called Bayle's disease, is a syphilitic infection of the brain which causes dementia, weakness, and paralysis.

A52.8 Late syphilis, latent

Use this code to report acquired cases of syphilis in the late, latent form, showing no symptoms or manifestation of the disease outside of the positive serological test, with a negative spinal fluid test, more than two years after infection.

A53.0 Latent syphilis, unspecified as early or late

Use this code to report acquired cases of syphilis in the latent form, showing no symptoms or manifestation of the disease outside of the positive serological test, when it is not specified whether it is within two years or after two years of the infection.

A54 Gonococcal infection

This category classifies cases of gonorrhea, also called blenorrhagia or blenorrhea. Gonorrhea is a sexually transmitted disease caused by the *Neisseria gonorrhoeae* bacterium that may also be passed from an infected mother to the neonate at birth or to infants living in an infected household. Symptoms of a primary infection include painful urethritis, burning on urination, and a purulent discharge from the urinary tract, particularly in males. Men may also get painful or swollen testicles. Females often remain asymptomatic or are mild enough to be mistaken for a bladder or vaginal infection. Bacteremia occurs in both sexes. Lesions may appear on the mouth, genitals, or anus. The eyes may also become infected. The untreated disease can cause serious and permanent problems in both men and women. Women are particularly at risk for serious complications, regardless of the severity of symptoms, such as pelvic inflammatory disease which can cause abscesses, chronic pain, and permanent damage to fallopian tubes, resulting in infertility. Epididymitis in men can also lead to infertility. Gonorrhea may disseminate and spread to the blood or joints and become life-threatening.

A54.03 Gonococcal cervicitis, unspecified

Gonococcal infections in women can manifest primarily in endocervicitis as the vagina is infected. Retrograde spread of the disease will occur in about 20 percent of those with cervicitis, in which the bacteria will move from the cervix into the uterus and other organs, causing pelvic inflammatory disease and affecting the fallopian tubes, endometrium, or ovaries.

A54.23 Gonococcal infection of other male genital organs

After the male urethra has been infected, the gonococcal bacterium may move to areas of the genitourinary tract further up the body and infect the testicles or epididymis. Untreated infection of the testes and epididymis is a painful condition that can lead to permanent damage and result in infertility if left untreated.

A54.24 Gonococcal female pelvic inflammatory disease

Gonorrhea is a common cause of serious pelvic infection affecting the fallopian tubes. Symptoms include fever, foul-smelling discharge, lower abdominal pain, and painful intercourse and urination. Sometimes symptoms may be mild and remain unrecognized while serious damage is being done. Chronic infection of the fallopian tubes turns normal tissue into scar tissue, which then partially or completely blocks the tubes, interfering with the movement of sperm to egg or egg to the uterus. The scar tissue causes chronic pain. Even partial blockage or slight damage can result in infertility, or stop a fertilized egg from reaching the uterus, resulting in an

ectopic pregnancy, which can rupture the tube, cause internal bleeding, and even death.

A54.3 Gonococcal infection of eye

The *Neisseria gonorrhoeae* bacterium can infect the eyes where it grows very easily after contact is made with infected body fluids or areas, such as the penis, vagina, mouth, or anus, followed by touching the eye(s). It can also be passed from mother to child during birth.

A54.31 Gonococcal conjunctivitis

Conjunctivitis can occur in adults as well as in children after contamination with the *Neisseria gonorrhoeae* bacterium. The eyes are very red, have thick drainage, and swelling of the eyelids. Adults become infected by touching the eye after contact with an infected area such as the penis, vagina, mouth, or anus. Infants become infected with this kind of conjunctivitis by passage through the birth canal. Preventative eye drops are used in all infants of infected mothers. Gonococcal conjunctivitis is usually severe and can lead to blindness. IV antibiotics may be required for treatment.

A54.33 Gonococcal keratitis

Neisseria gonorrhoeae infections of the eye are severe. Keratitis occurs when the bacterium penetrates the intact corneal epithelium and infects the cornea, causing ulceration and perforation.

A54.42 Gonococcal arthritis

Gonococcal arthritis results from a disseminated gonococcal infection in a later stage and presents with symptoms that include fever, rash, and pain in the joints. Although the pathogenesis of articular infection is still in debate, it usually presents as either a bacteremic-arthritic-dermatitis syndrome with a migratory polyarthralgia, or as a localized septic or purulent arthritis with severe pain, swelling, effusion, and decreased mobility in a single joint, commonly the knee. To prevent joint destruction, patients sometimes require hospitalization for antibiotic therapy.

A54.49 Gonococcal infection of other musculoskeletal tissue

Gonococcal tenosynovitis is common in disseminated gonococcal infections. It causes redness and tenderness along an affected tendon sheath and pain with motion. This kind of tenosynovitis usually affects the smaller joints of the hands, but is also found in the lower extremities. Gonococcal bursitis is an inflammation of the tiny fluid-filled sacs that reduce friction at major joints and tendons. The bacteria may likewise infect the synovium and the bursa of a joint.

A54.5 Gonococcal pharyngitis

Gonococcal bacteria are highly infectious and can infect any mucosal surface. The bacteria colonize easily in the warm, moist areas of the body. Infection can come from a single contact. Besides genitourinary infection, gonorrhea also manifests in the pharyngeal mucosa in a significant percentage of people, causing pharyngitis, which is usually asymptomatic, but sometimes causes mild to severe pain in the throat upon swallowing.

A54.6 Gonococcal infection of anus and rectum

Rectal infection occurs with anal intercourse and by spread of the organism from another genitourinary site, particularly in women. The infection may be asymptomatic, but also causes rectal pain, itching, discharge, lesions, and bloody diarrhea.

A54.81 Gonococcal meningitis

Gonococcal meningitis is an inflammation of the protective membrane that covers the brain and/or spinal cord. When such an inflammation occurs, symptoms may range from a mild fever and headache to the more severe presentation of fever, drowsiness, confusion, severe headache, stiffness in the neck, painful sensitivity to bright lights, and nausea and vomiting.

A54.83 Gonococcal heart infection

Gonococcal pericarditis is an inflammation of the membrane that lines and protects the exterior of the heart. Endocarditis and myocarditis may also occur as a more rare complication of a disseminated gonococcal infection affecting the heart. These conditions appear more often in men.

Fever, chills, sweating, and fatigue may set in and patients may develop atypical chest pain, a new murmur, tachycardia, and dyspnea. Lesions from embolism may occur. Rarely, severe heart valve damage results that can lead to death if not recognized and treated.

A54.85 Gonococcal peritonitis

Gonococcal peritonitis occurs when the primary genital infection spreads in a retrograde fashion and infects the abdominal cavity and the membrane that protects the visceral organs.

A54.89 Other gonococcal infections

Gonococcal keratoderma is coded here. This is a pink or red maculopapular rash that may become pustular, pruritic, or necrotic over time and presents at different stages of development in a majority of patients with disseminated gonorrhea. The rash is often below the neck, sparing the face and scalp, and may also involve the palms and the soles of the feet in addition to the torso and limbs.

A55 Chlamydial lymphogranuloma (venereum)

This sexually transmitted disease is caused by three different subtypes of *Chlamydia trachomatis*-different bacteria than those involved in the more common cases of genital Chlamydia. Lymphogranuloma venereum (LGV) is seen more in Central and South America than in the U.S. It presents up to a month after infection with a painless ulcer on male genitalia or in the female genital tract. Inguinal and/or perirectal lymph nodes become swollen as the bacteria spread, causing buboes, which are abscessed nodes that can rupture and drain through the skin. Complications include perianal or rectovaginal fistula and long term swelling and inflammation of the genitalia.

A56 Other sexually transmitted chlamydial diseases

Chlamydia is the most frequently reported bacterial sexually transmitted disease in the United States with many more cases unreported. Many people do not know they are infected because symptoms can be mild or absent, with half of infected men and three quarters of infected women having no symptoms at all. The bacteria can cause silent damage, particularly to female reproductive organs, and infertility can result. Chlamydia can also be passed from mother to baby through vaginal childbirth.

A56.01 Chlamydial cystitis and urethritis

Chlamydia bacterial infections usually occur initially in the urethra, producing a burning sensation on urination when symptoms are present. Men may also have itching or burning at the opening of the urethra and penile discharge.

A56.09 Other chlamydial infection of lower genitourinary tract

In women, the initial chlamydial infection usually occurs in the cervix. Sexually active young women, whose cervix is not fully matured, are especially at high risk for infection. The bacteria spread from there, sometimes causing irreversible damage even without symptoms, although women may have an abnormal vaginal discharge.

A56.11 Chlamydial female pelvic inflammatory disease

The disease usually spreads from an initial infection of the urethra or cervix. When it is left untreated, it can spread through other reproductive organs, such as the fallopian tubes, ovaries, uterus, or uterine adnexa and throughout the pelvis, causing pelvic inflammatory disease and even permanent tissue damage in women. This happens in about 40 percent of untreated cases. When tissue damage occurs, it can cause chronic pain, ectopic pregnancy, and infertility.

A56.19 Other chlamydial genitourinary infection

This code includes other sites such as the testes or epididymis in men, although it is not as common as other sites of infection. Epididymo-orchitis causes pain, fever, and possibly sterility.

A56.3 Chlamydial infection of anus and rectum

Chlamydia infection of the cervix and vagina in females can spread to the rectum as well as through anal intercourse. Anal or rectal infections can manifest with rectal pain, discharge, and bleeding.

A56.4 Chlamydial infection of pharynx

Chlamydia bacteria grow in warm, moist mucosal surfaces. The pharynx and throat is a site of infection in those with infected partners, since it can be passed on by oral sex.

A56.8 Sexually transmitted chlamydial infection of other sites

When a genitourinary chlamydial infection spreads in a retrograde fashion through other reproductive organs and into the pelvis or abdominal cavity, it can spread far enough to infect the peritoneum, the membrane that protects the visceral organs. This can also affect the liver, called perihepatitis.

A57 Chancroid

This bacterial disease is spread only through sexual contact and is caused by the gram-negative *Haemophilus ducreyi* bacteria. Chancroid begins as a small bump on the genital area that ruptures and forms a painful, draining ulcer. Half of men infected have only one ulcer, while women commonly have four or more. Half of those infected will develop enlarged inguinal lymph nodes, which may progress to the point where they rupture through the skin, causing draining abscesses, caused buboes. Chancroid can resolve spontaneously, but may take months. Antibiotics are given to treat the lesions with minimal scarring. Most cases diagnosed in the U.S. are in individuals who have traveled outside the country to developing or third world nations, where it is more common.

A58 Granuloma inguinale

This venereal disease is caused by the bacteria *Calymmatobacterium granulomatis* and is rarely seen in the United States, but found in tropical and subtropical regions. Men are affected twice as much as women. The bacteria cause beefy-red, velvety nodules that destroy the skin and subcutaneous tissue of the genitalia and perianal area, replacing it with elevated granuloma formation. The nodules gradually spread, eroding the genital tissue. Untreated disease can leave permanent mutilation.

A59 Trichomoniasis

Trichomoniasis is a sexually transmitted disease caused by the protozoan *Trichomonas vaginalis*. The disease causes a urinary tract infection in women, along with urethral discharge. Men can carry the disease, but typically have no symptoms.

A66 Yaws

Yaws is a chronic infectious disease that occurs frequently in humid, tropical climates, almost always among children. Yaws is caused by the spirochete bacteria *Treponema pertenue*. Symptoms of infection begin with sores on the face, hands, feet, and genitals. A primary lesion, known as the mother yaw, forms at a cut or scratch on the skin where the bacteria first enters the body. Secondary lesions follow soon after. Infected patients may also complain of malaise and loss of appetite. If left untreated, yaws can destroy areas of skin, bones, and joints, leaving them deformed. In this stage of the disease, the palms and soles of the feet become thickened and painful.

A66.1 Multiple papillomata and wet crab yaws

Papillomatas and wet crab yaws are wet, wart-like lesions that typically form on the soles of the feet.

A66.2 Other early skin lesions of yaws

This code describes the secondary lesions which may form after the initial lesions in a case of yaws, that may last for up to 6 months.

A66.3 Hyperkeratosis of yaws

Hyperkeratosis is also known as ghoul hands. This occurs when yaws causes the skin on the palms of the hands to thicken and coarsen, impairing function of the hands and fingers.

A66.4 Gummata and ulcers of yaws

Gummata and ulcers occur when yaws lesions turn rubbery and begin to create patches of dead skin around them.

A66.5 Gangosa

Gangosa are large, disfiguring sores in the nose and mouth caused by yaws.

A67 Pinta [carate]

Pinta is a contagious skin disease that occurs in Central and South America. Pinta is caused by the spirochete bacterium Treponema carateum. Symptoms of the disease include extreme thickening and discoloration of the skin. These discolorations are white, red, or purple in appearance. Pinta is classified primarily by the stage of the infection.

A67.0 Primary lesions of pinta

The primary lesions are indicative of the early stage of infection, and appear 2-3 weeks after the initial infection, usually on an exposed part of the skin. These lesions are red and scaly.

A67.1 Intermediate lesions of pinta

The intermediate lesions, called pintids, occur 3-9 months after infection. They vary in size, location, and pigmentation.

A67.2 Late lesions of pinta

The late lesions of pinta result in a mottled appearance to the skin and other disfiguring pigmentary changes.

A67.3 Mixed lesions of pinta

Mixed lesions are characteristic of more than one stage of the disease present on the patient at the same time.

A69.0 Necrotizing ulcerative stomatitis

Vincent's angina, more commonly known as trench mouth, is a disease whose key symptom is the presence of painful ulcerations of the gums and membranes of the mouth. Other symptoms are foul breath and difficulty talking or swallowing. Cancrum oris is a condition in which the tissues of the mouth are afflicted with severe gangrene, which can be fatal if not immediately treated. This condition is found primarily in undernourished children in third-world countries afflicted by famine and disease.

A69.2 Lyme disease

Lyme disease is a potentially dangerous infection spread by the deer tick, which is primarily seen in the northeastern United States. Lyme disease is a chronic illness which causes skin inflammation, fever, joint pain, and headache. In later stages, chronic arthritis, and permanent damage to the nervous system and heart follow.

A70 Chlamydia psittaci infections

Ornithosis is an infectious disease caused by the bacterium *Chlamydia psittaci* transmitted to humans through contact with infected birds. Symptoms include high fever and headache, as well as other symptoms similar to pneumonia. Other names for the disease include psittacosis and parrot fever, as parrots are a common vector of infection. Mortality rates for ornithosis may be as high as 30%.

A71 Trachoma

Trachoma is a contagious disease which affects the conjunctiva and cornea of the eye, and is a leading cause of blindness in the third world. The infection is caused by the bacterium *Chlamydia trachomatis*. In the early stage, the eyelid becomes congested and swollen, causing vision problems, often followed by infection of the cornea. If not treated, scar tissue develops, which leads to partial or total blindness if the cornea is involved.

A74.0 Chlamydial conjunctivitis

Inclusion conjunctivitis is caused by the chlamydia virus. This disease can affect children born to mothers who are infected with chlamydia, or can affect adults when the eye is exposed to contaminated genital secretions. Rarely, the disease can be acquired through a poorly chlorinated pool or hot tub. Infection causes pustules and swelling on the inside of the eyelid, as well as a discharge of pus and mucus from the eye. The eye may turn red, and the cornea may become involved.

A75.0 Epidemic louse-borne typhus fever due to Rickettsia prowazekii

Louse-borne typhus is spread by rubbing contaminated lice feces into the skin, usually by scratching. Initial symptoms are severe headache, nausea, chills, and fever, followed by a rash over the entire body except the face, hands, and soles of the feet.

A75.1 Recrudescent typhus [Brill's disease]

Brill's disease is a condition in which epidemic typhus reoccurs in a milder form. This disease is caused by the *Rickettsia prowazekii* bacterium, and only occurs in patients who have previously been infected with epidemic typhus.

A75.2 Typhus fever due to Rickettsia typhi

Murine typhus, also known as fleaborne typhus, is caused by the *Rickettsia typhi* organism. This disease is most commonly found in rats and their fleas, although it can also be found in opossums, cats, and other mammals. This type of typhus is less severe than epidemic (louse-borne) typhus.

A75.3 Typhus fever due to Rickettsia tsutsugamushi

Scrub typhus is caused by *Rickettsia tsutsugamushi*. This variety of typhus most commonly appears in Asia.

A77.0 Spotted fever due to Rickettsia rickettsii

Spotted fevers, such as Rocky Mountain spotted fever, are usually spread through the bite of a tick. The most prominent symptom is a rash that covers most of the body, and is most prominent on the extremities. The rash frequently occurs on the palms and soles of the feet. Severe headache, high fever, and muscle pain are also possible symptoms.

A77.1 Spotted fever due to Rickettsia conorii

Boutonneuse fever usually occurs in India, Africa, and around the Mediterranean. Symptoms are similar to spotted fever, but milder.

A77.2 Spotted fever due to Rickettsia siberica

North Asian tick fever occurs in Siberia and parts of Mongolia. As with boutonneuse fever, symptoms are similar to spotted fever, but milder.

A77.3 Spotted fever due to Rickettsia australis

Choose this code to report Queensland tick typhus, which occurs in Australia. Symptoms are similar to spotted fever, but milder.

A77.41 Ehrlichiosis chafeensis [E. chafeensis]

Ehrlichiosis chaffeensis causes symptoms comparable to Rocky Mountain spotted fever with severe headache, high fever, and muscle pain, but without the rash.

A78 Q fever

Q fever, also known as Nine Mile fever and Quadrilateral fever, is an infectious disease caused by *Coxiella burnetii*. The bacteria is found in sheep, goats, cattle, and infected pets such as dogs and cats. When infected fluids from the animal are secreted and later dry out, the bacteria become airborne and are breathed into the lungs through contaminated barnyard dust, for instance. Symptoms of this disease include a high fever up to 105 degrees F, malaise, nausea, diarrhea, severe headache, cough, and muscular pain.

A79.0 Trench fever

Trench fever is a disease that is spread by lice and is characterized by fever and chills.

A79.1 Rickettsialpox due to Rickettsia akari

Rickettsialpox is an acute disease commonly spread by mites. Typical symptoms include fever, chills, backache, headache, sweating, and a papule--a small, solid, raised skin lesion or bump that appears at the site of the bite.

A80 Acute poliomyelitis

Acute poliomyelitis, more commonly known simply as polio, is a disease that has largely vanished from the Western world due to aggressive vaccination. In most patients, it manifests only as a mild to moderate upper respiratory or gastrointestinal infection with a headache and fever. However, in approximately 5% of patients, it attacks the nervous system, resulting in symptoms ranging from irritation and muscle weakness to complete paralysis.

A80.39 Other acute paralytic poliomyelitis

Acute paralytic poliomyelitis that is specified as bulbar, also called polioencephalitis and polioencephalomeylitis, is an attack by the virus on the rear section of the brain, which can cause total paralysis. It presents with hiccough, shallowness and slowing of respiration, a bluish tint to the skin and mucous membranes, restlessness, and anxiety. Other types of acute paralytic poliomyelitis result from a viral attack to the spinal cord. It initially presents with severe muscle pain and spasms, which degenerate into muscle weakness and paralysis over approximately 48 hours. The paralysis is asymmetrical (i.e., to different degrees on each side of the body) with the lower limbs more affected than the upper. The paralysis remains unchanged for days or weeks before slowly improving over months or even years.

A81.0 Creutzfeldt-Jakob disease

Jakob-Creutzfeldt disease, also called Creutzfeldt-Jakob disease (CJD), is a degenerative neural disease caused by a prion (an infectious protein) rather than a virus, and is the human form of what is popularly known as mad cow disease. In some cases (about 15%) the prion is inherited from one's parents. It presents with a loss of muscular control marked by an unsteady gait and twitching movements, loss of balance, loss of short- and long-term memory, nervousness and agitation, changes in personality, and dementia. As with other prion-based diseases, there is no cure to CJD and it is inevitably fatal to the host; however, the prion may reside in the host without causing the disease for many decades. Final diagnosis of the disease requires a biopsy or autopsy of the brain. However, since the disease is always fatal, a brain biopsy is rarely performed except to rule out other, treatable conditions.

A81.01 Variant Creutzfeldt-Jakob disease

Variant Creutzfeldt-Jakob (vCJD) disease is rare and fatal like other forms of Jakob-Creutzfeldt disease, but unlike traditional forms, it affects younger people, with an average age of 29, and has a relatively longer duration, about 14 months as opposed to 4.5 months. The variant type has also been classified as a transmissible spongiform encephalopathy due to the characteristic spongy like degeneration of the brain and its ability to be transmitted. It is strongly associated with exposure to bovine spongiform encephalopathy (of cattle) through food ingestion. Most people diagnosed with vCJD have lived in the UK. Clinical features include psychiatric symptoms, unusual sensory perceptions like the skin feeling sticky, unsteady gait, involuntary movements, and complete immobility and muteness preceding death.

A81.09 Other Creutzfeldt-Jakob disease

This code should be used to report the inherited, familial type, the iatrogenic type, sporadic type, and that classified as subacute spongiform encephalopathy. The familial type is associated with a gene mutation and the iatrogenic type is acquired from accidental transmission via contaminated surgical equipment, corneal or dura mater transplants, or human derived pituitary growth hormones. Sporadic cases have an unknown cause throughout the world.

A81.1 Subacute sclerosing panencephalitis

Subacute sclerosing panencephalitis, or SSPE, is a neural disease that results when a mutated form of the measles virus enters the brain, causing an inflammation. In rare instances, this disease may be acquired from a measles vaccine. SSPE usually develops 2-10 years after the original infection or vaccination, and presents with memory loss, irritability, seizures and involuntary muscle movements, and behavioral changes. As the disease progresses, the patient's mental and neurological functions continue to deteriorate, until death occurs 1-2 years after the initial symptoms. There

is presently no cure, though anti-viral drugs may slow the progression of the disease.

A81.2 Progressive multifocal leukoencephalopathy

Progressive multifocal leukoencephalopathy (PML) is an inflammation of the brain caused by the CJD virus. This virus resides without causing any symptoms or illness in up to 80% of the human population. PML tends to develop only in patients with depressed immune systems, and is commonly known among AIDS patients or those undergoing chemotherapy for cancer. PML presents with mental impairment, partial loss of vision, extreme weakness, paralysis on one side of the body, and speech impairment. Because of the similarity in its symptoms with other diseases such as multiple sclerosis, diagnosis can be difficult, requiring electronic imaging of the brain (e.g. a CAT or MRI scan) and/or testing the cerebrospinal fluid. There is currently no cure for PML, and death usually results in 2-6 months after the onset of symptoms.

A81.81 Kuru

Kuru is a degenerative neural disease caused by a prion (an infectious protein) rather than a virus, and is very similar to mad cow disease. It first surfaced in New Guinea and progresses in three distinct stages. In the first stage, the patient presents with unsteadiness in their movements, eyes, and speech, and may be seen to tremble slightly. In the second stage, the patient can no longer walk without support and the tremors become more pronounced. Patients also usually demonstrate emotional instability, inappropriate laughter, depression, and a decrease in mental ability. The third stage is terminal, and is marked by severe loss of motor control that prevents the patient from even sitting up without support, loss of urinary and bowel control, difficulty in swallowing, and the appearance of deep ulcers. The prion can lie dormant for as long as 30 years, but once symptoms appear, death nearly always occurs in less than a year (usually 3-6 months).

A81.82 Gerstmann-Sträussler-Scheinker syndrome

Gerstmann-Sträussler-Scheinker syndrome (GSS) is an extremely rare, slowly progressive, fatal disease of the brain that is almost always inherited and found only in a few families world-wide. The condition usually lasts between 2-10 years, with onset occurring between 35 and 55 years of age. A lack of muscle coordination and unsteady gait appear first, then become more pronounced as the patient develops dementia, slurred speech, nystagmus, spasticity, and sometimes blindness and deafness. The patient often becomes comatose before death. There is no cure or known treatment to slow the disease. GSS also belongs to the family of human and animal diseases known as transmissible spongiform encephalopathies to which kuru, Jakob-Creutzfeldt, and fatal familial insomnia belong.

A81.83 Fatal familial insomnia

Fatal familial insomnia is a very rare, autosomal dominant, inherited prion disease of the brain found in a few families in the world. The disease is caused by a dual mutation in a normally soluable prion protein that results in conversion to an insoluble prion protein. This conversion causes plaques made of aggregates of these insoluble proteins to form in the thalamus, which is the part of the brain responsible for sleep patterns. Insomnia then results and progresses to serious problems in four stages. Onset is anywhere from 30-60 years old. Insomnia leads to panic attacks and phobias. Noticeable panic attacks and hallucinations follow. Rapid weight loss occurs with complete inability to sleep. Dementia graduates to unresponsiveness or muteness preceding death, which occurs between 7-36 months.

A82 Rabies

Rabies is an acute, infectious viral disease carried by warm-blooded animals and is almost always transmitted through a bite. The virus attacks the central nervous system, and is almost always fatal if not treated immediately. Early warning symptoms of infection include anxiety, fever, and muscle pain. Eventually the brain and spinal cord will swell, resulting in seizure, paralysis, coma, and death.

A82.0 Sylvatic rabies

Rabies is an acute, infectious viral disease carried by warm-blooded animals and is almost always transmitted through a bite. The virus attacks the central nervous system, and is almost always fatal if not treated immediately. Early warning symptoms of infection include anxiety, fever, and muscle pain. Eventually the brain and spinal cord will swell, resulting in seizure, paralysis, coma, and death.

A83   Mosquito-borne viral encephalitis

Viral encephalitis is caused by a flavivirus, and is carried by insect parasites that latch on to a human host and transmit the disease into the bloodstream. Encephalitis causes an inflammation of the nerve cells in the brain. The disease most commonly presents as flu-like symptoms. Other symptoms include stiff neck, hallucinations, seizures, and partial paralysis, depending on the affected areas of the brain. Different strains of the flavivirus responsible for the infection are named after the geographic area in which they are found.

A83.4   Australian encephalitis

This type of encephalitis found in Australia is also sometimes referred to as Murray Valley encephalitis.

A84.8   Other tick-borne viral encephalitis

Louping ill is a strain of encephalitis spread to humans from sheep in the British Isles.

A87.0   Enteroviral meningitis

Meningitis, an infection and inflammation of the protective fluid and membranous covering (meninges) of the brain and spinal cord, may in some instances be caused by the migration of an enterovirus, a virus that normally resides in the intestines. When such an inflammation occurs, symptoms may range from a mild fever and headache to the more severe presentation of fever, drowsiness, confusion, a severe headache, stiffness in the neck, a painful sensitivity to bright lights, and nausea and vomiting. Most patients recover in 5-10 days without permanent injury. Enteroviruses originating in the intenstinal tract are very contagious, especially during summer and fall, but most of those infected do not show any symptoms or else come down with a mild cold or sore throat. Only 1 in 1000 infected develop meningitis. Enteroviruses that may cause meningitis include the Coxsackie virus and the echovirus.

A87.2   Lymphocytic choriomeningitis

Lymphocytic choriomeningitis, also called LCM or lymphocytic meningitis, is a disease most often spread by contact with rodents, including hamsters and gerbils. The first symptoms, which appear 8-13 days after exposure to the virus, are easily mistaken for the flu, including fever, tiredness, weight loss, muscle aches, headache, nausea, and vomiting, lasting for up to a week. The symptoms vanish for a few days before returning along with the usual symptoms of meningitis (an inflammation of the covering of the brain and spinal cord): headache, sensitivity to light, vomiting, stiffness in the neck, lethargy and/or drowsiness, irritability and/or confusion. In some cases, the virus may develop into encephalitis (an inflammation of the brain itself) and present with drowsiness, confusion, sensory disturbances, and/or motor abnormalities (e.g. paralysis). There is no effective treatment for LCM, but most patients fully recover, though they may suffer an extended period of dizziness, sleepiness, and fatigue.

A88.1   Epidemic vertigo

Epidemic vertigo is a disease usually found in young adults in which a virus impairs vestibular function, which governs the ability to balance. This disease usually goes away on its own in a few days.

A90   Dengue fever [classical dengue]

Dengue fever, also known as breakbone fever, is a viral disease carried by mosquitoes. Found exclusively in tropical regions, dengue fever presents primarily as fever, headache, and a bright red rash appearing most commonly on the lower limbs. Collectively, these symptoms are known as the dengue triad. Other symptoms include swollen glands and severe muscle and joint pains.

Note: This disease is similar to, and should not be confused with, dengue hemorrhagic fever (code A91).

A91   Dengue hemorrhagic fever

Hemorrhagic fevers are caused by viruses and develop rapidly, resulting in muscle and joint pain, fever, and blood loss, which can also result in shock. Bleeding is caused by ruptured capillaries in the internal organs and the mucous membranes, as well as the skin. Hemorrhagic fevers have a very high mortality rate. Dengue hemorrhagic fever is transmitted by mosquitos while several other types of hemorrhagic fever are transmitted by tick.

A92.2   Venezuelan equine fever

Venezuelan equine fever is a mosquito borne flavivirus that causes severe headache, back pain, prostration, and chills. This is a serious disease with a high mortality rate.

A92.3   West Nile virus infection

West Nile virus (WNV) is a mosquito-borne virus causing disease mainly in older persons and those with weakened immune systems. There are currently no vaccines to prevent WNV or medications to treat infection with the WNV. Protection from mosquito bites is the best preventative measure. Mosquitos become infected when they feed on infected birds and then pass the virus on the other animals and humans. Outbreaks have occurred in the US every summer since 1999. The incubation period is anywhere from 2 to 14 days, but can be longer. Most people who become infected will never develop any symptoms.

A92.30   West Nile virus infection, unspecified

Up to 80% of those who become infected with the West Nile virus do not develop any symptoms. About 1 in 5 will develop a fever and show general symptoms such as vomiting, diarrhea, rash, joint pain, headache, or body aches. Most people recover completely and have no complications although fatigue or weakness can linger for weeks or months.

A92.31   West Nile virus infection with encephalitis

Approximately 1% of people infected with the West Nile virus will develop serious neurologic complications, such as infection and inflammation of the brain and/or spinal cord. Symptoms of encephalitis or encephalomyelitis include headache, neck stiffness, high fever, disorientation, tremors, seizures, even coma and paralysis. Those most at risk for serious illness include the elderly, those with compromised immune systems, and people with certain other medical conditions such as cancer, diabetes, kidney disease, and even hypertension. Since there is no preventative vaccine or medication to treat the infection, supportive treatment includes intravenous fluids and pain medication. Some neurologic effects may become permanent. About 10% of people who do develop serious neurological illness, such as encephalitis will die.

A92.32   West Nile virus infection with other neurologic manifestation

Approximately 1% of people infected with the West Nile virus will develop serious neurologic complications. Other types of neurologic manifestations reported here may include optic neuritis or disorders of other cranial nerves, and polyradiculitis.

A93.1   Sandfly fever

Phlebotomus fever is a mild disease also known as sandfly fever or three-day fever. This disease is spread by the bite of the sandfly and is characterized by fever, malaise, eye pain, and headache.

A95   Yellow fever

Yellow fever is a viral disease found only in tropical regions of South America and Africa. The disease is spread by mosquitoes, and causes high fever and jaundice as the virus attacks the kidneys, liver, and other body systems. The yellow appearance of jaundiced victims is what gives yellow fever its name, as the French word for yellow is "jaune." Severe infections can be fatal.

A95.0   Sylvatic yellow fever

Sylvatic, or jungle, yellow fever is primarily spread to humans by mosquito bite.

A95.1 Urban yellow fever

Urban yellow fever is spread from humans to other humans.

A96 Arenaviral hemorrhagic fever

Arenaviral hemorrhagic fever is a class of diseases transmitted to humans by rodents. Each type of this virus is associated with the specific rodent that carries it. These diseases can cause severe hemorrhagic fevers and are frequently fatal.

A98.5 Hemorrhagic fever with renal syndrome

Hemorrhagic nephrosonephritis is a viral infection characterized by bleeding and severe kidney problems. Symptoms typically last 1-2 weeks, and may result in death.

B00 Herpesviral [herpes simplex] infections

Herpes simplex is caused by one of two variants of the herpes simplex virus, HSV-1 or HSV-2. The disease is usually localized, with HSV-1 commonly affecting the mouth, lips, and conjunctiva (the covering of the whites of the eyes), and HSV-2 commonly affecting the genitals and being passed by sexual contact; however, these locations are not ironclad, and either form of the virus can appear in any location. The disease presents as painful and itchy sores that appear on the affected area of the body for short periods of time. The first outbreak, occurring 2-20 days after exposure to the virus, is usually the worst, lasting up to several weeks, with each successive outbreak lasting 2-10 days each. During each outbreak, the patient presents with the characteristic sores as well as flu-like symptoms, the discharge of fluid from the vagina, painful urination, and a swelling of the lymph nodes in the groin area. An outbreak may be triggered by stress, another illness, sunburn, menstruation, and sexual intercourse. Many patients can anticipate an outbreak by a tingling sensation that appears in the infected area, and most have 5-8 outbreaks a year. Herpes outbreaks can be treated, but the virus cannot be cured. While it can be transmitted more easily when the carrier exhibits open sores, it can also be transmitted even when the person has no symptoms, in fact, the most contagious period is just before an outbreak occurs. The most common way to spread the virus is through sexual intercourse. Herpes simplex infections that affect the anal region or the genitals are coded to category A60.

B00.0 Eczema herpeticum

Ezcema herpeticum is a serious and potentially fatal infection by HSV-1 in an area of skin that is already inflamed due to an allergic reaction, most commonly appearing in the head, neck, and trunk. It presents with an unusually severe rash, often accompanied by fever and fatigue. Without treatment by antiviral medications (usually acyclovir), the mortality rate is as much as 75%.

B00.1 Herpesviral vesicular dermatitis

This code includes vesicular dermatitis of the face, ear, and lip. Herpes simplex otitis externa is marked by inflammation and pain in the ear (which may grow worse when tugging on the ear lobe), discharge of pus and/or fluid from the ear, and temporary hearing loss in addition to the typical herpes outbreak.

B00.3 Herpesviral meningitis

Herpes infection of the lining around the brain and/or spinal cord presents with a number of symptoms, including fever, a purplish rash, loss of appetite, headache, sensitivity to light, vomiting, stiffness in the neck, lethargy and/or drowsiness, irritability and/or confusion. The patient may also lose consciousness and go into convulsions. In some cases, the patient may suffer long-term conditions, such as deafness.

B00.4 Herpesviral encephalitis

Herpesviral encephalitis is an inflammation of the brain by herpes simplex. This also includes meningoencephalitis, which is an inflammation of the brain as well as its protective membranes. This condition presents with a number of symptoms, including fever, a purplish rash, loss of appetite, headache, sensitivity to light, vomiting, stiffness in the neck, lethargy and/or drowsiness, irritability and/or confusion. The patient may also lose consciousness and go into convulsions. In some cases, the patient may suffer long-term effects, such as deafness.

B00.51 Herpesviral iridocyclitis

Iridocyclitis is an inflammation of the iris and ciliary body, the hair-like structures that support the lens, causing sensitivity to light and/or an inability to focus vision in the affected eye(s). This condition can cause permanent damage if not treated promptly.

B00.52 Herpesviral keratitis

A herpesviral infection or the cornea presents with inflammation, open sores, or swelling in the cornea that can cause permanent damage to vision and the need for a transplant.

B00.59 Other herpesviral disease of eye

This includes herpes simplex dermatitis of the eyelid, and other herpes simplex viral diseases of the eye not specifically listed above, leading to ocular complications such as posterior uveitis and chorioretinitis.

B00.7 Disseminated herpesviral disease

Disseminated herpesviral disease includes herpetic sepsis, or systemic-wide infection throughout the bloodstream. Disseminated infection presents with the sudden onset of fever and chills, low blood pressure (which may result in pale or bluish limbs and lips), confusion or altered emotional state, and rash. If not treated immediately, sepsis can lead to shock and death.

B00.81 Herpesviral hepatitis

Hepatitis caused by the herpes simplex virus (HSV) is a rare and potentially fatal complication of HSV infection that leads to acute liver failure and the need for transplantation. This mainly occurs in those with impaired immunity. Diagnosis of HSV hepatitis is difficult as it presents with a wide range of clinical signs and symptoms and often remains unsuspected. It may mimic serious HIV infection or acute liver failure from other causes. The main features it presents with are fever, coagulopathy, and encephalopathy. Many cases are diagnosed at autopsy. Early detection and the use of viral DNA identification tools, as well as antiviral (acyclovir) treatment even when there is still only the suspicion of herpes simplex hepatitis, can have a dramatic effect on improving the outcome for patients.

B00.82 Herpes simplex myelitis

Herpes simplex myelitis is an inflammation of the spinal cord, which occurs as a secondary disorder following infection with the human herpes simplex virus (HSV) type 1 or 2 that has established latency in the dorsal root ganglia. The spinal cord becomes inflamed when the virus reactivates, usually associated with physical and emotional stress, tissue damage, or immune suppression and then spreads to the spinal cord. Herpes simplex myelitis presents as rapidly progressing symmetrical paralysis accompanied by acute lower leg pain, loss of sphincter control with a dysfunctioning bladder and bowels, and loss of deep tendon reflexes. HSV-2 has been known to cause rapidly ascending necrotizing myelitis.

B00.89 Other herpesviral infection

This includes herpetic whitlow, which presents with a painful, blistery eruption of the herpes sore that appears on the fingertip, sometimes called a herpetic felon.

B01 Varicella [chickenpox]

Chickenpox, caused by the varicella zoster virus, is a common childhood disease that presents with an itchy, blistered rash 10-21 days after exposure. This rash normally scabs and vanishes in 7-10 days. The disease is highly contagious, so that up to 90% of the non-immune family members living in a house with an infected person will become infected themselves, but once the disease has run its course, the person is normally immune to it for life afterwards. Once a person contracts chickenpox, the virus normally remains dormant in the nervous system for the rest of the person's life. However, if the person's immune system becomes compromised or stressed, the virus can become active again and cause shingles, also called herpes zoster.

B01.0 Varicella meningitis

Meningitis is an infection and inflammation of the protective membrane that covers the spinal cord and brain. Viral cases of meningitis are usually less severe than bacterial cases, which can be fatal. Identification of the virus is important in cases of meningitis and is normally done by testing samples of blood or cerebrospinal fluid. Varicella is the same virus that causes chicken pox and shingles. The varicella virus can be spread through direct or indirect contact with infected saliva, sputum, or mucus. Even after a person becomes infected with the varicella virus, it is unlikely to cause meningitis. Although it can affect anyone, children and those with weakened immune systems are at higher risk for complications. In addition to the normal symptoms of chicken pox, varicella meningitis presents with sudden appearance of high fever, severe headache, and stiff neck, that is often accompanied by light sensitivity, nausea, vomiting, and trouble waking up. Children may display irritability, poor eating, and sleepiness from which it is difficult to arouse the child. Symptoms usually last 7-10 days and those with healthy immune systems usually recover fully on their own. Hospitalization may be necessary in some cases.

B01.11 Varicella encephalitis and encephalomyelitis

Postvaricella encephalitis and encephalomyelitis is an inflammation of the brain or the brain and spinal cord due to the chickenpox virus. In addition to the normal symptoms of chickenpox, it usually presents with fever, headache, and confusion, and can cause brain damage, stroke, seizures, or even death in extreme cases.

B01.12 Varicella myelitis

Postvaricella myelitis is an inflammation of the spinal cord occurring as a sequela of infection with the chickenpox virus. Although complications of the varicella virus are rare, serious morbidity may develop in both normal and immunocompromised patients, even those who had an uneventful course of chickenpox. Postvaricella myelitis is characterized by symptoms of paraplegia, normal sensory loss, urinary and fecal incontinence, and increased sensitivity or pain sensations from normally painless stimuli.

B01.2 Varicella pneumonia

Varicella pneumonia is a lung infection caused by the chickenpox virus. This is a rare complication that occurs when the virus travels to the lungs. Pneumonia can develop anywhere from 2-10 days after the initial chickenpox rash appears. The first signs of pneumonia complication are fever, cough, and abnormally rapid breathing. Teens and adults are at higher risk for this particular complication of chickenpox than children. Others at risk are smokers and those with chronic lung disease or impaired immune systems. Pregnant women who contract chickenpox in the last trimester are also at risk for varicella pneumonia, in which cases, it can be severe. Most people will recover, although the symptoms can last for weeks. Long term consequences include lung scarring that can impair gas exchange over many months. Treatment may require oxygenation and antiviral medication, such as acyclovir.

B01.81 Varicella keratitis

Varicella keratitis is an infection of the cornea with the chickenpox virus. Although ocular complications of this viral infection are rare, it has been known to occur weeks or months after the resolution of the acute phase rash of chickenpox. This tends to occur more in children when either the live virus or retained positive antigen to the varicella zoster virus (VZV) are still present. Varicella ocular infection tends to be self-limiting. Epibulbar conjunctival and corneal pock marks may persist for 1-2 weeks before resolving spontaneously. The pock marks may leave corneal scarring and vascularization. Different forms of keratitis can be caused by varicella, including punctate or dendritic, nummular, and disciform. Varicella dendritic keratitis is marked by the presence of rounded up dendrite lesions of epithelium that can be debrided. Varicella disciform keratitis tends to be the shortest lived and mildest of the viral disciform types lasting about 2-5 months with less corneal scarring. Treatment may include both topical and oral antiviral medications as well as topical steroids, or even supportive antibiotics.

Note: Ocular manifestations of varicella zoster virus complications are differentiated as sequelae of the varicella virus and sequelae of the herpes zoster virus. Varicella ocular infections tend to occur in childhood and are shorter lived. The other tends to occur later in life as herpes zoster infections--developed from a reactivation of the latent varicella zoster virus. This is known as herpes zoster ophthalmicus and is reported with

codes from subcategory B02.3. These types tend to cause protracted ocular complications accompanied by chronic neurogenic pain.

B02 Zoster [herpes zoster]

Herpes zoster is an acute infectious disease caused by the reactivation of human herpes 3 virus, called the varicella-zoster virus, which causes chickenpox. After the initial attack of chickenpox, the body may be rendered partially immune and the virus lies dormant in the nervous system for many years. Herpes zoster, also called shingles, commonly reappears after age 50 and the risk increases with age, stress, or a weakened immune system. Shingles appears with numbness, itching, intense pain, and the eruption of clusters of blister-like lesions, usually on one side of the body. The eruptions appear along a strip or track of skin following the path of the affected nerve fibers from a spinal root. Neurological manifestations from reactivation of the varicella zoster virus may appear across a spectrum of disease even without the characteristic rash or skin eruptions of shingles. Herpes zoster or shingles is contagious to those who have never had chickenpox. These non-immune people can catch chickenpox by close proximity to another person with shingles; however, shingles itself cannot be passed from person to person, but is contracted only though one's own dormant chickenpox virus.

B02.1 Zoster meningitis

Herpes zoster reactivation may cause meningitis, an inflammation of the covering of the brain and/or spinal cord. This presents with a number of symptoms, including fever, a purplish rash, loss of appetite, headache, sensitivity to light, vomiting, stiffness in the neck, lethargy and/or drowsiness, irritability, and/or confusion. The patient may also lose consciousness and go into convulsions. In some cases, the patient may suffer long-term conditions, such as deafness.

B02.21 Postherpetic geniculate ganglionitis

This herpes zoster infection includes Ramsay-Hunt syndrome and postherpetic geniculate neuralgia. Ramsay-Hunt syndrome, also called postherpetic geniculate ganglionitis (or oticus), is an inflammation of the facial and vestibular nerves, (VII and VIII cranial nerves) possibly involving other cranial nerves, with the herpetic eruption occurring along the external auditory meatus or tympanic membrane. It presents with ipsilateral facial palsy, severe pain in the ear, vertigo, tinnitus, deafness, and inflammation of the pinna. Pain that persists along the area after the eruption or inflammation has healed is known as postherpetic neuralgia.

Note: Postherpetic neuralgia specific to the trifacial, or trigeminal, nerve is coded to B02.22.

B02.22 Postherpetic trigeminal neuralgia

Use this code to report severe pain that persists along the distribution of the trigeminal nerve pathway (cranial nerve V) after the herpetic vesicle eruption and inflammation of shingles has healed. The trigeminal nerve sensory root supplies the face, mouth, nasal cavity, and teeth, while the motor root supplies the muscles used for chewing.

B02.23 Postherpetic polyneuropathy

This code reports the chronic pain that follows an acute herpes zoster infection and neuron damage in multiple affected peripheral regions after the herpetic vesicle eruption has healed. This may be facilitated in part by an underlying, pre-existing impairment, or polyneuropathy of afferent nerve fibers.

B02.24 Postherpetic myelitis

Herpes zoster myelitis is an inflammation of the spinal cord caused by a virus identical to the varicella (chickenpox) virus, which occurs when the dormant infection in a previously exposed, immune person becomes active and migrates to the central nervous system in response to altered immunity, neoplastic disease, drugs, trauma, radiation, or even by chance. The virus causes a rare lesion on the spinal cord that presents clinically with acute onset of paraplegia.

B02.29 Other postherpetic nervous system involvement

This code includes postherpetic neuralgia affecting the ophthalmic nerve and is used to report any other postherpetic neuralgia that is not classified elsewhere specifically as geniculate, trigeminal, or postherpetic polyneuropathy of multiple peripheral nerves. Postherpetic neuralgia is severe pain that persists along the distribution of the nerve pathway after the herpetic vesicle eruption and inflammation of shingles has healed. The pain may persist for weeks, months, or even years, though rare, and is thought to be caused by damage to the nerve fibers from the herpes zoster virus, leaving the nerve fibers unable to transmit electrical signals as they normally do to and from the brain. Some patients experience excruciating pain even from gentle touch due to hypersensitive pain detection and/or the formation of new connections of central pain transmitting neurons. Other patients experience severe pain spontaneously.

B02.32 Zoster iridocyclitis

Infection of the iris and the ciliary body caused by migration of the herpes zoster virus into the eye from shingles that have erupted on the same side of the face. The iris is the colored, circular membrane behind the cornea and the ciliary body is composed of the hair-like structures that support the lens. The infection causes swelling, pain, sensitivity to light, inability to focus vision in the affected eye, and possibly permanent damage.

Note: Herpes zoster iridocyclitis may also be called herpes zoster anterior uveitis, or uveokeratitis.

B02.33 Zoster keratitis

Zoster keratitis is a shingles eruption of the face that infects the cornea with the herpes zoster virus. This occurs when a latent varicella zoster virus is reactivated within the ophthalmic division of the trigeminal nerve. Most patients present with a classic vesicular, pustular rash around the orbital area distributed along the affected dermatome, but some may have only ocular manifestations limited to the cornea. Some patients will also experience a prodromal phase with an influenza-type illness, fatigue, general malaise, and a low grade fever that persists for about a week before the outbreak of the rash and pain along the ophthalmic nerve. The virus causes inflammation of the cornea, or both the cornea and conjunctiva, resulting in itching, burning, swelling, light sensitivity, and even numbness in the cornea, which can lead to permanent damage such as chronic ocular inflammation, vision loss, and debilitating neurologic pain. Antiviral medications are the key therapy and are most effective when they are begun within 72 hours of rash onset. Timely diagnosis and treatment is a critical factor for preventing permanent loss of vision.

B02.39 Other herpes zoster eye disease

Use this code when a shingles eruption affecting the face infects the skin of the eyelid (blepharitis) with the herpes zoster virus, causing inflammation, pain, and redness. This code includes all other cases of herpes zoster eye infection affecting other specified structures of the eye, caused by migration of the virus from a shingles eruption occurring on the same side of the face.

Note: This may include herpes zoster posterior uveitis and chorioretinitis.

Note: Reactivation of the dormant herpes zoster virus along the ophthalmic nerve itself, causing the characteristic eruption of shingles is coded to B02.29 Other postherpetic nervous system involvement.

B02.8 Zoster with other complications

Herpes zoster otitis externa is an inflammation of the ear canal similar to swimmer's ear. This condition is marked by inflammation and pain, which may grow worse when touching or tugging on the ear lobe, discharge of pus and/or fluid from the ear, and temporary hearing loss caused by infection with the herpes zoster virus from an eruption of shingles on the same side of the face.

B02.9 Zoster without complications

This code reports an eruption of shingles at any site in the body that is not specifically classified elsewhere in category B02 when there is no mention of any complication. Shingles is an acute infectious disease caused by the reactivation of the varicella-zoster virus, which causes chickenpox. After the initial attack of chickenpox, the virus lies dormant in the nervous system for many years and may then reappear, commonly after age 50. The risk increases proportional to age, stress, or a weakened immune system. Shingles causes intense pain with a characteristic eruption of blister-like lesions, usually on one side of the body along an area of skin in the path of the affected nerve.

B03 Smallpox

Smallpox is a potentially fatal, highly-contagious disease that has not been seen in the United States since 1949 thanks to an aggressive immunization program. However, it is still a possible agent for a biological weapon. The B03 category is maintained for surveillance purposes. The name "smallpox" comes from a Latin word that means "spotted," and refers to the disease's distinctive rash. Symptoms also include high fever, fatigue, body aches, and sometimes vomiting.

The rash appears on the patient's skin, concentrating on the face, arms, and legs within 24 hours of the initial infection. By the third day, the rash changes into raised bumps, which fill with a thick, opaque liquid by the fourth day. These bumps often become depressed in the center so that they almost appear as little bellybuttons. Next, these bumps become firm to the touch, feeling almost as if tiny firm pellets were embedded under the skin. This condition lasts for about 4-5 days, after which the hardened bumps, called pustules, begin to scab over. The scabs last about six more days before falling off.

Smallpox vaccination is no longer routinely administered due to the expense and the risk of adverse effects since the disease has been virtually eradicated. However, it can be administered 2-3 days after the initial exposure to the disease and provide complete protection, and administration up to 4-5 days after the initial exposure will usually save the patient's life. Variola major is the more severe and common form of smallpox, having a more extensive rash, higher fever, and higher mortality rate than other smallpox variants. The Alastrim virus, or variola minor, causes a less severe variant of smallpox than variola major. Modified smallpox, also called varioloid smallpox, is a minor type of the disease that can occur after vaccination.

B04 Monkeypox

Monkeypox is a rare disease occurring mainly in central and western Africa. In the U.S., monkeypox has occurred among people having contact with infected pet prairie dogs or monkey handlers in special settings. The disease can also spread from person to person through prolonged face-to-face contact or contaminated fluids or clothing. The disease presents like smallpox, only milder, with fever, aches, swollen lymph nodes, and a rash that turns into fluid-filled bumps that crust, scab, and fall off. The disease usually lasts up to 4 weeks.

B05 Measles

Measles is a common childhood disease caused by the paramyxovirus, which is spread via airborne droplets. Infants normally inherit immunity from the disease from the mother that lasts for 6-8 weeks after birth, and after that, most children in the United States are vaccinated. As a result, outbreaks of the disease are most common in college students who either did not receive immunizations, or in whom the immunizations have worn off since childhood. The disease initially presents with irritability, high fever, a runny nose, sensitivity to light, and a flat, reddish rash that begins at the forehead. This rash then spreads down over the face, neck, and body to the feet over the next three days. The disease usually lasts about two more days after the rash has reached the legs and feet. Sometimes, the skin may retain a brownish color as it heals, with the brown patches peeling off after several days. In some cases, measles may present with Koplik's spots along with fever and coughing one or two days before the rash appears. Koplik's spots appear in the mouth, and are red with bluish or white centers. Measles can cause a number of complications that can present after the primary symptoms have begun to fade.

B05.0 Measles complicated by encephalitis

Postmeasles encephalitis is an inflammation of the brain that takes place after the primary measles infection has passed. It presents with one or more of the following flu-like symptoms, which usually last for two to three weeks: fever, fatigue and/or drowsiness, sore throat, stiff neck and back, headache, confusion and irritability, loss of balance, vomiting, and sensitivity to light. In more severe cases, it can also present with seizures, muscle weakness and paralysis, loss of responsiveness, memory loss, and impaired thinking and judgment.

B05.2 Measles complicated by pneumonia

Postmeasles pneumonia is a condition in which one or both lungs fill with fluid after the primary measles infection has passed, causing shortness of breath and a sensation of drowning.

B05.3 Measles complicated by otitis media

Postmeasles otitis media is an inflammation of the middle ear, often accompanied by a buildup of fluid, which occurs after the primary measles infection has passed.

B05.81 Measles keratitis and keratoconjunctivitis

Measles keratitis and keratoconjunctivitis is an inflammation of the cornea or the corneal and the conjunctiva, the covering of the white of the eye that occurs as a complication of measles. Symptoms include itching, burning eyes, sensitivity to light, and enlarged preauricular lymph nodes.

B06 Rubella [German measles]

Rubella, also called German measles or three-day measles, is a highly contagious but mild disease. It presents with a low-grade fever, fatigue, and muscle/joint pain, headache, a runny nose, red and inflamed eyes, and a reddish rash in about half of those infected. Though rarely dangerous to most patients, it can cause complications, congenital defects, and stillbirth when infecting a pregnant woman, and as a result is considered a serious health risk.

B06.01 Rubella encephalitis

Encephalitis is an inflammation of the brain. This also includes meningoencephalitis affecting the brain and its protective covering. It commonly presents with fever, fatigue and/or drowsiness, sore throat, stiff neck and back, headache, confusion and irritability, loss of balance, vomiting, and sensitivity to light. In more severe cases, it can also present with seizures, muscle weakness and paralysis, loss of responsiveness, memory loss, impaired thinking and judgment, and even coma.

B07.0 Plantar wart

Plantar warts, also called verruca plantaris, are noncancerous skin growths that appear on the soles of the feet, caused by the human papilloma virus (HPV). The virus enters through tiny cuts or cracks in the skin. The warts can be painful as they often develop under pressure points, like the ball of the foot. They may need to be removed by a physician, if they prove to be resistant to other treatment.

B07.8 Other viral warts

Other viral warts includes common warts, also known as verruca vulgaris, and flat warts, also called verruca plana. A flat wart is a skin-colored, pink, yellow, or light-brown colored papule about 2-5 mm across that is well demarcated in its margins, slightly raised but flat-surfaced, and smooth, often flush with the skin. They usually appear grouped together on the face, neck, and legs, sometimes in lines or circles. Flat warts are smaller than common warts, which are raised, dome-shaped, rough lesions that usually appear on the fingers, hands, toes, and knees. Both types of warts are caused by an infection with the human papillomavirus that is spread by direct contact or autoinoculation, such as when the wart is scratched or shaved. Treatment can include simply covering the wart 24 hours a day; stimulating the body's own immune response by painting the wart with a chemical treatment or topical antiviral cream applications; freezing the wart with liquid nitrogen cryotherapy; and laser vaporization or electrosurgical curettage and cautery.

B08.0 Other orthopoxvirus infections

Orthopox viruses include the vaccinia virus, and the cowpox virus, which are coded here, as well as the variola virus that causes smallpox, and other rare diseases such as monkeypox, which are coded elsewhere. Orthopoxviruses cause systemic infections in humans that require treatment as well

as infection control precautions that are different from other poxvirus infections that normally remain compartmentalized within the skin.

B08.010 Cowpox

Cowpox is a disease of the skin similar to smallpox, only much milder. The cowpox virus is closely related to the vaccinia virus and previously thought to be one and the same. Today, cowpox is rare, usually confined to small mammals in Europe and Great Britain. Humans usually contract it through contact with an infected cat that aquired it from smaller animals. The disease manifests as small, red, fluid-filled pustules localized to the site of introduction, usually the hands and face. The blisters appear after 9-10 days and last for weeks before scabbing with a black eschar and then healing. Cowpox is not endemic in the U.S. but may be imported through animals or infected travelers.

B08.011 Vaccinia not from vaccine

Vaccinia is a large, complex poxvirus that is closely related to the cowpox virus, and previously thought to be one and the same. Vaccinia is also so closely related to the variola virus, the causative agent of smallpox, that vaccinia has become famous for its role as the vaccine that eradicated smallpox and is still used as the live virus in the smallpox vaccine. A vaccinia infection is normally mild and produces a rash, fever, head and body aches; but in some cases, complications can be severe. The immune response generated by this infection protects from lethal smallpox infection. Vaccinia is spread by touching skin or clothing contaminated with the live virus, which may occur in individuals who touch an unhealed injection site, bandage, or clothing of another person. Humans may also be infected with a dairy-associated wild strain version of vaccinia.

Note: Vaccinia that occurs in an individual who was vaccinated is coded to T88.1.

B08.02 Orf virus disease

Contagious pustular dermatitis, sometimes called Ecthyma contagiosum, sore-mouth, or orf, is a variant on the poxvirus that is found in sheep and goats. The blisters tend to congregate around the eyelids, ears, nostrils, and lips and last for 2-4 weeks.

B08.03 Pseudocowpox [milker's node]

Pseudocowpox, also called Milker's node, is similar in presentation to cowpox. Hand blisters tend to exhibit a grayish coating in the early phases, become red or purplish in the middle stages, and become wart-like in appearance towards the end of its nominal 5-7 week course. The disease normally resolves itself without any treatment.

B08.1 Molluscum contagiosum

Molluscum contagiosum is a skin disease caused by the Poxviridae family of viruses. The primary symptom is the formation of small, white, round papular lesions on the skin. The disease is usually transmitted sexually.

B08.2 Exanthema subitum [sixth disease]

Roseola infantum, also called sixth disease and exanthum subitum, is a common childhood disease of mild viral illness affecting those between 6 months and two years of age. The causative organism is the human herpes virus, types 6 and 7, which is spread through tiny droplets from the nose and throat of infected people. HHV-6 infection is nearly universal in the U.S. among older children. HHV-7 is not common and has only been identified in a few cases of roseola. The child typically develops some mild upper respiratory symptoms, swollen glands, decreased appetite, and a high fever that may be over 103 degrees Fahrenheit, lasting three days to a week. The fever may cause a febrile convulsion or seizure and will typically end abruptly, followed by a rash breaking out with small, pale pink raised papules or flat macules that blanch white when touched. The rash then lasts a few hours to a few days, sometimes with red papules on the soft palate mucosa.

B08.21 Exanthema subitum [sixth disease] due to human herpesvirus 6

The human herpes virus 6 (HHV-6) has two recognized, distinct variants--A and B. Primary infection with HHV-6B causes roseola infantum. In most cases, the virus goes into latency or even remains asymptomatic.

B08.22 Exanthema subitum [sixth disease] due to human herpesvirus 7

The human herpes virus 7 (HHV-7) is not very common or well understood, although it is genetically similar to HHV-6. It has been identified as causing some cases of roseola. The virus can reactivate and cause repeated or concomitant disease in immunocompromised patients and is thought to be associated with reactivation of HHV-6.

B08.3 Erythema infectiosum [fifth disease]

Erythema infectiosum, also called slapped-cheek disease or fifth disease, initially presents as a mild flu, with fever and fatigue, and often passes with no further symptoms at all. An itchy, reddish rash may also appear on the cheeks and spreads to the arms and legs in a few days; this rash only rarely afflicts the whole body. In some adults (more commonly in female patients), the disease also presents with painful, swollen joints. Symptoms usually vanish within a week. The most serious risk from erythema infectiosum is in pregnant women. In about 5% of cases, the disease can be passed to the fetus just as rubella can, which may cause miscarriage or stillbirth. In some cases, it can simply cause anemia in the child, which may require a blood transfusion in the uterus to treat.

B08.4 Enteroviral vesicular stomatitis with exanthem

Hand, foot, and mouth disease is a mild variant of coxsackie that causes fever and a rash on the hands, feet, and mouth. This disease occurs primarily in children.

B08.5 Enteroviral vesicular pharyngitis

Herpangina is a viral infection primarily found in children which is marked by sore throat, headache, pustules in the throat and mouth, and abdominal pain.

B08.6 Parapoxvirus infections

Parapoxviruses include bovine papular stomatitis virus and the sealpox virus. These are zoonotic and endemic within the U.S. These infections are generally self-limiting and confined to the skin. The clinical picture for different parapoxvirus infections is very similar one to another and generally consists of a solitary or multiple, fairly painless cutaneous lesions that heal slowly, normally without complications. Sometimes, they may also be mistaken for life-threatening zoonotic infections, such as cutaneous anthrax.

B08.61 Bovine stomatitis

Foot and mouth disease is a highly contagious viral disease usually found in cloven-hoofed animals, but very rarely transmitted to humans. This disease causes fever and the eruption of vesicles around the mouth. This virus is associated with contact with infected beef cattle.

B08.62 Sealpox

Sealpox is seen among marine mammal handlers and is associated with contact with infected sea lions, harbor seals, and gray seals.

B08.7 Yatapoxvirus infections

Yatapoxvirus infections are endemic to sub-Saharan Africa and are mainly a concern to travelers and special animal handlers involved with research.

B08.71 Tanapox virus disease

Tanapox virus is mostly documented in Kenya and Zaire and was first seen among the flood plain of the Tana River in Kenya. It presents with a pre-eruptive febrile illness, severe headaches and backaches, followed by a solitary or multiple skin nodules that enlarge and ulcerate in the third week and gradually heal with a scar.

B08.72 Yaba pox virus disease

The yaba monkey virus is a tumor-producing DNA virus of primates that was discovered in monkeys near Yaba, Nigeria. It causes histiocytomas in both monkeys and humans.

B10 Other human herpesviruses

The human herpes viruses (HHV) are classified into alpha, beta, and gamma groups. The alpha herpes viruses are the familiar herpes simplex types 1 and 2 and the varicella-zoster virus. This category makes provision for classifying infection by HHV-6, 7, and 8 within the other two groups of human herpes viruses.

The gamma herpes viruses often lie dormant in lymphatic tissue and include Epstein-Barr and HHV-8, the Kaposi's sarcoma-associated virus that is also linked to other neoplastic disease and lymphomas.

The beta group consists of HHV-6 and HHV-7. HHV-6 is very neuroinvasive and is connected with encephalitis, pediatric febrile seizures, and possibly with multiple sclerosis and chronic fatigue. HHV-7 is genetically similar to HHV-6 and is also known to cause roseola and encephalitis. The virus is tropic for human T-lymphocytes and infects almost all children by age 3, remaining in the body. It has been associated with the reactivation of HHV-6, but the pathogenesis and sequelae of HHV-7 are not well understood.

Note: Infections with the Epstein-Barr virus are coded to B27.0- and roseola infantum (sixth disease) is coded to B08.2.

B10.0 Other human herpesvirus encephalitis

Encephalitis is an inflammation of the brain that can present with headache, lethargy, fever, confusion, changed mental status, vomiting, delirium, seizure, and even coma.

B10.01 Human herpesvirus 6 encephalitis

HHV-6 infection of the brain is a rare consequence of immunosuppressive treatment, especially in transplant patients, and a complication of AIDS. Subacute cases have occurred with bone marrow and stem cell transplants, particularly when no prophylactic antiviral therapy was given. HHV-6 is very neuroinvasive. Some sporadic cases of encephalitis have been documented in primary infection of infants with roseola as well as by reactivation of the virus in transplant patients. HHV-6 encephalitis is associated with drug hypersensitivity syndrome, organ failure, bone marrow suppression, and rash. There have been rare cases of HHV-6 encephalitis in immunocompetent adults. Infection outcomes can range anywhere from full recovery to mortality.

B10.09 Other human herpesvirus encephalitis

This code includes infection of the brain with human herpes virus 7 (HHV-7), which is less common than HHV-6 and not as well understood, although it is genetically similar to HHV-6. HHV-7 can reactivate HHV-6 and cause repeated or concomitant disease is patients who are already immunocompromised.

B10.81 Human herpesvirus 6 infection

Human herpes virus 6, HHV-6, is an immunosuppressive, neurotropic virus known to cause encephalitis, roseola, and seizures in primary infections or when reactivated. Recent research finds that HHV-6 may also play a role in chronic neurological conditions, such as multiple sclerosis, chronic fatigue, temporal lobe epilepsy, and status epilepticus. HHV-6 has two distinct variants--A and B. HHV-6B causes roseola infantum and occasionally febrile seizures and encephalitis in infants; it infects almost all children universally after age 2 and can reactivate from its latent state in transplant or other immunocompromised patients. HHV-6A is more likely to be found in multiple sclerosis, AIDS, and cancer patients. HHV-6 infection can persist in its active state at low or subacute levels for years, causing CNS dysfunction. This virus also causes selective immune suppression, making it difficult for the body to ward off cancer, other viruses, and bacteria, while transactivating related viruses like Epstein-Barr, HHV-8, and cytomegalovirus.

B10.82 Human herpesvirus 7 infection

Human herpes virus 7, HHV-7, is genetically similar to HHV-6 and is also known to cause roseola and encephalitis. The virus is tropic for human T-lymphocytes and infects almost all children by age 3, remaining with infectious shedding of the virus in saliva. It is reported to be associated with the reactivation of HHV-6, but the pathogenesis and sequelae of HHV-7 are poorly understood. It differs from HHV-6 in that it binds to the cell surface molecule CD4 protein of T-lymphocytes as part of its receptor.

B10.89 Other human herpesvirus infection

This code reports other human herpesvirus infections with HHV-8 or the Kaposi's sarcoma-associated herpesvirus. This virus is connected to some neoplastic disease and lymphomas. It belongs to the gamma group of herpesviruses and is closely related to the Epstein-Barr virus.

B15 Acute hepatitis A

Viral hepatitis causes an inflammation of the liver. Symptoms include jaundice, fatigue, headache, fever, diarrhea, nausea, vomiting, diffuse abdominal pain, and loss of appetite. There are five different hepatitis viruses: A, B, C, D, and E. All varieties of the virus can cause acute hepatitis, and B, C, and D viruses can also cause chronic hepatitis. If left untreated, patients suffering from chronic infection often develop severe liver problems, such as cirrhosis. All varieties of the virus can be spread through sexual contact or IV drug use (sharing needles).

Hepatitis A is most commonly passed through food or water that has been contaminated with fecal matter from an infected individual. The infection usually resolves on its own over several weeks.

Hepatitis B is acquired through contact with infected blood. IV drug use and sexual transmission are the usual vectors of infection, though infected mothers can pass the disease onto a child. The disease usually resolves on its own, but can be chronic.

Hepatitis C is usually transmitted from person to person through shared needles and sexual contact. Acute infections will usually resolve within a few months, but the disease is often chronic.

Hepatitis D occurs only in patients who are already infected with hepatitis B, and is usually seen in populations of IV drug users who are suffering from chronic hepatitis B. The hepatitis D virus can cause both acute and chronic infections.

Hepatitis E is spread through food or water contaminated by feces from an infected individual, and is usually seen in countries where sanitary conditions are poor. Infections with this virus usually resolve on their own in a matter of weeks or months. Hepatitis E is rarely found in the United States.

Note: Accurate coding for viral hepatitis depends on knowing the variety of virus that is causing the infection, whether the condition is acute or chronic, and whether the patient presents with hepatic coma, a symptom of severe liver disease.

B17.0 Acute delta-(super) infection of hepatitis B carrier

Hepatitis D occurring without mention of a hepatitis B infection, but with hepatitis B carrier state.

B20 Human immunodeficiency virus [HIV] disease

Human immunodeficiency virus (HIV) causes Acquired Immune Deficiency Syndrome, or AIDS. HIV must be transferred through direct fluid exchange (e.g. blood, semen, etc.) and does not survive transfer through the air. The most common vector of infection is sexual contact, so it is classified as a sexually transmitted disease. Within days or weeks after entering the bloodstream, HIV bonds to the patient's white blood cells. During this initial period of infection, called primary or acute HIV infection, the patient may develop flu-like symptoms as the body's natural defenses try to create antibodies to fight off the virus. After this, all symptoms vanish and the patient enters a "window period" of two weeks to six months, during which standard blood tests are ineffective in detecting the virus. After the window period, the virus settles into a period of latency of varying length, during which standard blood tests for HIV will show a positive result. Even without

drug therapy, this latent period may last 10 years or longer before the patient develops active AIDS. Before then, the patient may exhibit a variety of symptoms including painful boils, rashes, and blisters on the body, a thick white coating in the mouth, herpes, fevers and night sweats, weight loss, and severe fatigue.

AIDS is the final stage of the disease. At the onset, most of the immune system is still intact, but the patient often experiences one or two persistent infections that have to be treated with massive doses of antibiotics, as the body can no longer fight them off without aid. Chest infections are the most common, but infections of the brain and nervous system are also normal. In addition, HIV can bond directly to the brain itself, causing permanent damage. Full-blown AIDS usually leads to the death of the individual in 5-7 years, most often from a secondary infection rather than from the virus itself.

B25 Cytomegaloviral disease

Cytomegaloviral disease is characterized by the presence of inclusion bodies in infected cells. Other symptoms may include jaundice, fever, and enlargement of the liver and spleen. This disease is usually seen in newborns, who acquire it from the birth canal of the mother during delivery, or in patients with compromised immune systems. Cases of cytomegalic inclusion body disease are very rare in adults; those who contract the disease usually have predisposing factors such as Wegener's granulomatosis or Hodgkin's disease and acquire cytomegalic inclusion disease as a complication. The drugs used to treat the underlying condition also predispose for cytomegalic inclusion body disease. The virus produces inclusion bodies within the nucleus or cytoplasm of infected cells. Affected cells can be up to four times their normal size and the patient will have any number of clinical symptoms, depending on age and immune system condition. In infants, the disease tends to be localized to the salivary glands and is of little clinical importance, but it can become generalized and affect the kidneys and lungs among other organs. In adults, the disease is most often generalized and affects many organs, including the lungs; but it may also be localized to a definite lesion or even confined to the lungs. In these cases, pneumocystis pneumonia, caused by *Pneumocystis carinii* tends to be present.

B26 Mumps

Mumps is a viral disease that primarily infects the parotid salivary glands at the back of the cheeks. The glands become swollen and painful until the infection passes in about a week. Other symptoms include fever and painful swallowing.

B26.0 Mumps orchitis

Mumps may be accompanied by orchitis, which is a swelling of one or both testicles. This usually occurs in males 13 or older who contract mumps.

B26.1 Mumps meningitis

Mumps occurring with meningitis, an inflammation of the protective membrane that lines the brain and spinal cord. When such an inflammation occurs, symptoms may range from a mild fever and headache to the more severe presentation of fever, drowsiness, confusion, a severe headache, stiffness in the neck, a painful sensitivity to bright lights, and nausea and vomiting. Most patients recover in 5-10 days without permanent injury.

B26.2 Mumps encephalitis

Mumps accompanied by encephalitis, an inflammation of the brain itself. This inflammation presents with fever, headache, confusion, and in extreme cases, can cause brain damage, stroke, seizures, or even death.

B27.9 Infectious mononucleosis, unspecified

Infectious mononucleosis, commonly known as mono, is caused by the Epstein-Barr virus. 95% percent of people will be infected by the virus before age 40. Typical symptoms include fever, sore throat, and swollen lymph nodes. When occurring in adolescents, lethargy may be a pronounced symptom. More severe effects such as heart problems, swelling of the spleen and liver, and involvement of the CNS are possible but rare. The disease usually runs its course in 1-2 months.

B30 Viral conjunctivitis

The conjunctiva is the thin, clear membrane that lines the inner, pink surface of the eyelid and covers the white part of the eye. Viral cases of conjunctivitis are most often caused by contagious viruses associated with the common cold and are transmitted through coughing and sneezing, or migration within the body's own mucous membranes. There are no eye drops or ointments that can eradicate the infecting virus as in cases of bacterial conjunctivitis. The infection must run its course, sometimes lasting up to three weeks. In cases of extreme inflammation, topical steroids may be used to reduce the pain.

Note: There are three main causative types of conjunctivitis: allergic, infectious, and chemical. This category reports viral infectious cases of conjunctivitis. Bacterial cases are reported under the specific bacterial infection. Allergic cases are reported as acute (H10.1-), chronic (H10.45), or vernal (H10.44). See category H10.21- for chemical cases. Newborn cases must be reported with P39.1 and the code that reports the specific infecting organism.

B30.0 Keratoconjunctivitis due to adenovirus

Epidemic keratoconjunctivitis is the most serious type of ocular infection caused by a group of adenoviruses with different serotypes. It is highly contagious, most often associated with adenovirus serotypes 8 and 19, and causes infection of both the cornea and the conjunctiva that can last up to a month. Epidemic cases occur most often in places of close human contact, such as schools and offices. The most common route of infection is by direct contact with infected ocular fluid or tears. When instruments are not properly disinfected, even the eye doctor's office can become a common place of infection. Symptoms include sudden onset of redness, soreness, itching, and swelling of the eye and lid with the sensation of sand in the eye, sensitivity to light, and excessive tearing. A few days later, subepithelial infiltrates often appear as whitish spots on the cornea that affect vision, and the lymph nodes in front of the ears often become swollen. Some patients may also develop a mucus-like pseudomembrane on the conjunctival tissue under the lower eyelid that may need to be removed. Diagnosis is made by review of symptoms, biomicroscopic slit lamp examination, and a test for the adenovirus, called the RPS Adeno Detector that can give an accurate result within 10 minutes. Treatment for epidemic keratoconjunctivitis focuses on alleviating the uncomfortable symptoms with the use of artificial tears, cold compresses, vasodilators, and steroid eye drops in severe cases. Long-term consequences include persistent dry eye and conjunctival scarring.

Note: The same causative viral infecting agents responsible for epidemic keratoconjunctivitis also cause similar disease such as pharyngoconjunctival fever reported with B30.2.

B30.1 Conjunctivitis due to adenovirus

Conjunctivitis caused by adenoviruses is highly contagious and results in the self-limiting infection of the membrane lining the eyelid commonly known as 'pinkeye.' Symptoms include red, itchy, tearing eyes with the sensation of a foreign body in the eye. There may be watery discharge and swelling of the lymph nodes in front of the ears. The infection resolves within 2-4 weeks and remains highly contagious for about 12 days, or as long as the eye is red. The virus may be spread by shaking hands, sharing towels, and inoculation by contact with infected respiratory droplets, or swimming pools. There are multiple serotypes of adenoviruses that can result in infection. Acute adenoviral follicular conjunctivitis may be caused by many of the same serotypes that result in epidemic keratoconjunctivitis and pharyngoconjunctival fever, but do not affect the cornea. It presents with extreme redness of the eye, watery discharge, photophobia, and periorbital pain. The follicles appear as gray or white, rounded elevations with an irregular or velvety appearance, mainly in the tarsal conjunctiva, but also in the bulbar or limbal conjunctiva.

B30.2 Viral pharyngoconjunctivitis

Viral pharyngoconjunctivitis, or pharyngoconjunctival fever, is caused by the same group of adenoviruses responsible for epidemic keratoconjunctivitis. Viral pharyngoconjunctivitis is most commonly seen in smaller outbreaks among school children caused by adenovirus serotype

3, when the highly contagious virus infects not only the conjunctiva lining the eye, but the respiratory tract as well. The incubation period is about 5-12 days. Symptoms appear as redness of the eyes with itching, burning, tearing, and lid swelling, severe sore throat, and a fever that may be sudden or gradual ranging from 100-104 degrees. The fever often lasts up to 10 days, although the infection often takes a few weeks to run its course, during which time, the patient remains highly contagious. In some cases, punctate keratitis may develop days after initial symptoms appear, followed by corneal infiltrates. Treatment focuses on alleviating the symptoms with cold compresses and artificial tears, since there is no medication effective against the virus as there is for bacteria.

Note: Serotypes 1, 4-7, and 14 have also been associated with pharyngoconjunctival fever.

B30.8 Other viral conjunctivitis

Other viral conjunctivitis includes Newcastle conjunctivitis, caused by exposure to the Newcastle virus, an avian paramyxovirus that is deadly to infected birds and particularly affects domestic poultry. In humans, it causes only mild conjunctivitis, or pinkeye, and mild flu-like symptoms. Newcastle conjunctivitis usually occurs in laboratory, farm, and poultry packing workers who are not wearing protective eyewear or gloves, or washing with soap and water. The conjunctivitis results in redness, itching, watery or sensitive eyes and is usually mild and self-limiting.

B33.0 Epidemic myalgia

This includes epidemic pleurodynia, also known as Bornholm disease, a rare condition in which the coxsackie virus attacks the pleura around the lungs. This presents with severe chest and abdominal pain that increases with deep breathing, fever, and sore throat.

B33.1 Ross River disease

Ross River fever is a mosquito-borne infectious disease caused by the Ross River virus endemic to Australia, New Guinea, and other South Pacific islands. The virus causes joint pain and swelling, muscle aches, fatigue, and rash. Some people develop symptoms within 3-11 days, while others do not show any symptoms until 21 days after exposure. Although nearly everyone recovers, some people will have intermittent symptoms lasting a year or more. Arthritis caused by the Ross River virus can last days or months, with transient symptoms that continue to appear for a year or more while becoming less severe. The joints most commonly affected are the wrist, knees, ankles, and small joints of the hand.

B33.4 Hantavirus (cardio)-pulmonary syndrome [HPS] [HCPS]

Hantavirus is a grouping of RNA viruses that are carried by rodents. Humans contract the disease by inhaling the vapors of contaminated urine, feces, or saliva. Hantaviruses can cause hemorrhagic fever and severe pulmonary diseases.

B33.8 Other specified viral diseases

Sweating fever, also known as miliary fever, is a viral disease that causes the eruption of skin vesicles and blisters, which in turn aggravate the sweat glands, and result in profuse sweating.

B34.0 Adenovirus infection, unspecified

An infection caused by an adenovirus, a group of viruses that infect the membranes of the repiratory tract, eyes, intestines, and urinary tract. Children are affected by adenoviruses more often than adults.

B34.3 Parvovirus infection, unspecified

Parvovirus B19 is the only parvovirus causing disease in humans. It can cause a false positive on hepatitis B surface antigens and is known to cause erythema infectiosum, also known as fifth disease, as well as acute symmetrical polyarthropathy, pure red blood cell aplasia, or transient aplastic crisis of temporary red blood cell failure, chronic anemia, hydrops fetalis, and congenital anemia.

Note: Although this virus is responsible for causing erythema infectiosum, a definitive diagnosis of such is not coded here as parvovirus B19 infection, but to its own specific code.

B35 **Dermatophytosis**

Dermatophytosis is a fungal infection of the skin. The most common site of infection is the feet, causing a condition known as athlete's foot. The infection usually occurs on skin covered by moist clothing and causes redness, fissures, scaling, and small papular vesicles. Dermatophytosis is classified by the affected area.

B35.0 **Tinea barbae and tinea capitis**

Tinea barbae is a superficial dermatophyte fungal infection of the bearded, or hair-covered parts of the face and neck, also known as ringworm of the beard. This mostly affects adult male farmers by direct contact with an infected animal, and is more common than tinea capitis, the dermatophytic fungal infection of the scalp. The fungus responsible is most often a zoophillic, or animal fungus from cattle (T. verrucosum) or horses (T. equinum). The fungal filaments and spores usually cover the outside of course facial hair. The infected area appears very inflamed with red, lumpy areas, pustules, and crusting and the hair can be pulled out easily. Diagnosis is confirmed by microscopy of the hair pulled out from the roots and infected skin scraping. Bith topical and oral antifungals may be used in treatment

B35.1 **Tinea unguium**

Tinea unguium is a fungal infection of a nail, also known as dermatophytic onychomycosis. It is the most common disease affecting nails, and affects toenails more frequently than fingernails. The surface, lateral, and distal edges of the nail are often infected first. The nail becomes thickened, discolored, and brittle. Pieces of the nail may break off or come away completely. Later the tissue of the nail bed underneath the nail plate becomes infected and the nail may be lost.

B35.5 **Tinea imbricata**

Tinea imbricata is a fungal infection of the skin areas that contain few or no hair follicles, usually seen in humid climates. The lesions are ring-like and appear with a circle of scales around the outer boundary.

B35.8 **Other dermatophytoses**

A deep seated dermatophytosis sometimes occurs following mild skin trauma, such as when women continuously shave their legs. Oval patches of papules may appear, as well as patches of scaling.

B36.0 **Pityriasis versicolor**

Pityriasis versicolor is a fungal infection of the skin that causes spots lighter than the surrounding skin to appear on the chest, back, shoulders, and other areas of the body with many oil glands.

B36.1 **Tinea nigra**

Tinea nigra is a fungal infection that occurs primarily on the palms of the hands and manifests as a dark spot on the skin.

B36.2 **White piedra**

Tinea blanca is a fungal infection of the skin that usually occurs on the scalp, but can occur on any hairy surface of the body. The telltale sign is a pale patch on the skin. After the disease clears, there will be a permanent bald spot where the infection occurred.

B36.3 **Black piedra**

Black piedra is a superficial infection of the hair shaft. It presents as hard black nodules which appear on the shafts of infected hairs.

B37 **Candidiasis**

Candidiasis is an infection by the candida fungus, which is usually found on the mucous membranes of the mouth, vagina, or digestive tract. The candida fungus can also enter the bloodstream. Typical symptoms are an itching and/or burning sensations, and a white or gray discharge may be present.

B37.0 **Candidal stomatitis**

Candidiasis of the mouth is more commonly known as thrush.

B37.5 **Candidal meningitis**

Candidal meningitis, which occurs when candida enters the bloodstream and causes inflammation of the protective membrane which covers the brain and/or spinal cord. When such an inflammation occurs, symptoms may range from a mild fever and headache to the more severe presentation of fever, drowsiness, confusion, a severe headache, stiffness in the neck, a painful sensitivity to bright lights, and nausea and vomiting.

B37.7 **Candidal sepsis**

Disseminated candidiasis occurs when the infection enters the bloodstream. Many body systems can be infected once this stage of infection is reached, causing a wide array of symptoms that can be difficult to identify as candidiasis.

B37.84 **Candidal otitis externa**

Candidal otitis externa is a condition more commonly known as swimmer's ear that occurs when candida infects the skin covering the outer ear canal.

B38 **Coccidioidomycosis**

Coccidioidomycosis is a respiratory disease caused by inhaling the fungus *Coccidioides immitis*. Primary symptoms are present in only a fraction of infected people and include cough, fever, headache, swelling of the knees, and other symptoms associated with respiratory illness. If left untreated, the infection can spread to the bones and central nervous system, where it can be fatal.

B38.4 **Coccidioidomycosis meningitis**

Coccidioidal meningitis is an infection that causes inflammation of the protective membrane that covers the brain and/or spinal cord. When such an inflammation occurs, symptoms may range from a mild fever and headache to the more severe presentation of fever, drowsiness, confusion, severe headache, stiffness in the neck, painful sensitivity to bright lights, and nausea and vomiting.

B39 **Histoplasmosis**

This category is used to report an infection caused by the Histoplasma family of fungi. Infection is the result of inhaling the fungus, which then infects the pulmonary system. If left untreated, the infection can spread to other parts of the body.

B41 **Paracoccidioidomycosis**

Paracoccidioidomycosis is a chronic, often severe infection caused by the *Paracoccidioides brasiliensis* fungus. Symptoms include skin lesions, fever, weakness, and weight loss. If the lungs are involved, shortness of breath and chest pain may occur. The mucous membranes of the nose and/or mouth may also be infected.

B42 **Sporotrichosis**

Sporotrichosis is an infection by the fungus *Sporothrix schenckii*. The most common form of the disease produces skin lesions on the affected part of the body. Advanced stages of the disease can infect the bones, the pulmonary system, or even cause meningitis, an inflammation of the protective membrane that covers the brain and/or spinal cord. The disease can also disseminate via the bloodstream to infect multiple body systems.

B43.0 **Cutaneous chromomycosis**

Chromoblastomycosis is a chronic, localized infection of the skin that results in visible lesions. Many different fungi can cause an outbreak of this disease. Infection follows the traumatic implantation of the responsible fungus. The disease may spread through the bloodstream in patients with compromised immune systems.

B44 **Aspergillosis**

An aspergillosis infection is caused by fungi of the family Aspergillus. This disease usually invades the lungs and sinuses, but can also attack burns, post-surgical wounds, the urinary tract, and other areas. Aspergillus is a species of molds found in organic matter. Infection almost always appears only in those who have an underlying lung disease or immunodeficiency. Those types causing human illness include *Apergillus fumigatus*, *A. niger*,

A. *flavus,* and *A. clavatus,* which are transmitted by inhalation and cause a broad spectrum of disease primarily infecting the lungs.

B44.0   Invasive pulmonary aspergillosis

Invasive aspergillosis-a rapidly progressing fatal infection occurring in the severely immunocompromised, characterized by blood vessel invasion and cavitary, multifocal infiltrates; and also chronic necrotizing aspergillus pneumonia. This kind of pneumonia is a subacute process that is unresponsive to antibiotics and antituberculous therapy, occurring in immunosuppressed patients, those with an underlying lung disease, alcoholism, or long-term corticosteroid therapy. The pneumonia often remains unidentified for weeks and cavitates over time, causing progressive lung infiltrates with granuloma formation and alveolar consolidation.

B44.1   Other pulmonary aspergillosis

Aspergillus is a species of molds found in organic matter. Infection almost always appears only in those who have an underlying lung disease or immunodeficiency. Those types causing human illness include *Aspergillus fumigatus, A. niger, A. flavus,* and *A. clavatus,* which are transmitted by inhalation and cause a broad spectrum of disease primarily infecting the lungs such as aspergilloma--a ball of fungus within a pre-existing pulmonary cavity from underlying disease such as treated tuberculosis or sarcoidosis.

B44.81   Allergic bronchopulmonary aspergillosis

Allergic bronchopulmonary aspergillosis is a hypersensitivity reaction to *Aspergillus fumigatus* in the tracheobronchial tree occurring with asthma and cystic fibrosis. Aspergillus is a species of molds found in organic matter. Infection almost always appears only in those who have an underlying lung disease or immunodeficiency. Those types causing human illness include *Aspergillus fumigatus, A. niger, A. flavus,* and *A. clavatus,* which are transmitted by inhalation and cause a broad spectrum of disease primarily infecting the lungs.

B44.9   Aspergillosis, unspecified

Unspecified aspergillosis includes pneumonia in aspergillosis.

B45   Cryptococcosis

Cryptococcosis is an infection caused by the fungus *Cryptococcus neoformans.* The infection can target any organ in the body, including the lungs, skin, bones, and the brain and its protective surrounding tissues.

B45.1   Cerebral cryptococcosis

Cerebral cryptococcosis is caused by a fungus called *Cryptococcus neoformans.* This infection is uncommon outside of those whose immune systems are already weakened by another disorder such as HIV or chemotherapy for cancer. The infection causes hydrocephalus and intracerebral cysts.

B46.9   Zygomycosis, unspecified

Zygomycosis is a fungal infection caused by a fungus of the class Zygomycetes. The disease usually attacks the blood vessels.

B47.0   Eumycetoma

Maduromycosis, or mycotic madura foot, is a chronic, progressive fungal infection that typically attacks the foot or leg. The primary symptom is the presence of pus-filled nodules on the infected limb and/or extremity, following long-term swelling. The swelling may remain for years before becoming a small, hard knob, or lesion. This knob (or nodule) may again last for several years before rupturing and leaking pus. The infection may also cause multiple draining sinuses and spread to other body parts, causing similar swellings there.

Note: Madura foot can also be caused by a bacteria with identical symptoms. A biopsy of the affected area must be taken to determine whether the cause is bacterial or fungal. Bacterial, or unspecified madura foot is reported with B47.9.

B47.9   Mycetoma, unspecified

Madura foot (NOS) is named for the region of India in which it was first diagnosed. It is a chronic condition that initially presents with a painless swelling on the skin of the foot that only occasionally causes pain and/or itching. That swelling may remain for years before becoming a small, hard knob, or lesion. This knob (or nodule) may again last for several years before rupturing and leaking pus. The infection may also cause multiple draining sinuses and spread to other body parts, causing similar swellings there.

Note: Madura foot can also be caused by a fungus with identical symptoms. A biopsy of the affected area must be taken to determine whether the cause is bacterial or fungal. Fungal, or mycotic madura foot is reported with B47.0.

B48.0   Lobomycosis

Lobomycosis is a rare infection which causes keloids and nodules to form beneath the skin, that must be removed surgically. Relapse is frequent.

B48.1   Rhinosporidiosis

Rhinosporidiosis is a disease caused by the *Rhinosporidium seeberi* fungus. The disease affects the conjunctivae of the eyes and the mucous membranes inside the nose. Painless polyps form at the site of infection. In rare cases, the fungus may enter the bloodstream and infect multiple body systems.

B48.2   Allescheriasis

Allescheriosis is an infection of the lungs caused by the fungus *Allescheria boydii.*

B48.8   Other specified mycoses

Dematiacious fungi cause a variety of severe infections known collectively as phaeohyphomycosis, which most often affect the skin and eyes.

B50   Plasmodium falciparum malaria

Plasmodium falciparum malaria is recognized as the most dangerous type of malaria. The disease is usually spread to humans via mosquito bites. The most common symptoms are malaise, headache, chills, fever, sweating, vomiting, and diarrhea. In this type of malaria, microinfarctions — tiny areas of dead tissue caused by a loss of blood supply — form throughout body systems as red blood cells become infected, which can lead to death in just hours after infection.

B50.8   Other severe and complicated Plasmodium falciparum malaria

Blackwater fever is a serious, often fatal complication of a falciparum malaria infection in which the kidneys become severely damaged. The telltale symptom is the passage of bloody urine in combination with the other symptoms of falciparum.

B51   Plasmodium vivax malaria

Plasmodium vivax malaria is a more common and milder type of malaria than falciparum. While it shares common symptoms with other forms of malaria, the symptoms occur in attacks every three days or so instead of continuously. The disease normally runs its course in about two months.

B52.9   Plasmodium malariae malaria without complication

Quartan malaria, like vivax, is a relatively benign form in which a recurrence of symptoms happens on a 72 hour cycle. Mixed malaria is a condition in which multiple strains of malaria combine in one infection. The symptoms and severity vary depending on the strains involved.

B53.0   Plasmodium ovale malaria

Ovale malaria is similar to vivax and quartan malaria, with relatively mild symptoms recurring every three days.

B53.8   Other malaria, not elsewhere classified

In therapeutically induced malaria, the patient is intentionally given malaria (e.g., via injection) in order to treat another disease. Note that this code should not be used to report accidental infection from a syringe or blood transfusion.

B54 Unspecified malaria

Malaria is a disease caused by a protozoan of the genus Plasmodium, which affects the red blood cells. The disease is usually spread to humans via mosquito bites. The most common symptoms are malaise, headache, chills, fever, and sweating. Vomiting, diarrhea, and jaundice may also occur.

B55 Leishmaniasis

Leishmaniasis is a disease caused by protozoans of the genus Leishmania. These diseases are usually spread to humans via the bite of the sand fly.

B55.0 Visceral leishmaniasis

Visceral leishmaniasis, also known as kala-azar, is the most serious form of leishmaniasis, causing widespread damage to the internal organs and discoloration of the skin as well as fever and anemia. This strain of the disease can be fatal if untreated.

B55.1 Cutaneous leishmaniasis

Urban cutaneous leishmaniasis is a disease that leaves dry, deep, disfiguring sores at the site of the sand fly bite, but is not usually dangerous.

Asian desert cutaneous leishmaniasis is similar to the urban cutaneous variety but produces wet, necrotizing (i.e., filled with dead tissue) sores at the spot of infection.

Ethiopian cutaneous leishmaniasis is a disease that produces widespread skin lesions which may be mistaken for leprosy.

American cutaneous leishmaniasis most commonly occurs in Mexico and produces skin lesions that may be either hard and raised (nodular) or open and inflamed (ulcerative).

B55.2 Mucocutaneous leishmaniasis

Mucocutaneous leishmaniasis produces ulcers on this skin. These ulcers can cause damage to the membranes of the nose and mouth if they spread into those orifices.

B56 African trypanosomiasis

African trypanosomiasis is a disease spread by the tsetse fly, causing an infection by the *Trypanosoma brucei* protozoa, known as sleeping sickness. It presents with symptoms of swollen lymph glands and spleen, aching muscles and joints, drowsiness and an uncontrollable urge to sleep. This infection is almost always fatal if untreated, and requires long-term monitoring after the initial occurrence.

B56.0 Gambiense trypanosomiasis

Gambian trypanosomiasis, also known as chronic sleeping sickness, or West African sleeping sickness, is characterized by enlargement of the spleen, drowsiness, an uncontrollable urge to sleep, and the development of personality changes. In its later stages, the disease progresses to a wasting away due to loss of appetite, which gradually leads to coma and eventual death. It is most often spread by the tsetse fly.

B56.1 Rhodesiense trypanosomiasis

Rhodesian trypanosomiasis, also known as East African sleeping sickness, is an acute illness similar to Gambian trypanosomiasis with a more rapid onset. It is also spread by the tsetse fly.

B57 Chagas' disease

American trypanosomiasis is a disease caused by the *Trypanosoma cruzi* protozoa, which is most often spread via insect bites. The diseases caused by this organism are usually chronic, and over time can result in the enlargement of the spleen, liver, and lymph nodes, as well as damage to the internal organs. The primary symptoms of this disease are red lesions on the skin, as well as headache and fever.

B57.0 Acute Chagas' disease with heart involvement

Chagas' disease involving the heart is a serious condition that is spread via the bite of an insect known as the vinchuca, which is found in Latin and South America. The primary symptoms of the disease are a red, inflamed lesion at the site of the bite, as well as headache, fever, and shortness of breath. Convulsions and rigidity of the neck are symptoms of the acute generalized form of the illness which may result in rapidly progressive heart disease.

Note: Code chronic cases of Chagas' disease with heart involvement to B57.2.

B57.1 Acute Chagas' disease without heart involvement

Use this code if an acute case of Chagas' disease does not involve the heart. Patients with non-complicated Chagas' disease will still have the telltale inflammation at the site of the bite, headache, and possibly a fever. Other symptoms are less common without heart or other organ involvement.

B58 Toxoplasmosis

Toxoplasmosis is a disease caused by the single-celled parasite *Toxoplasma gondii*. The most common way the disease is passed to humans is through the accidental ingestion of contaminated cat feces. Toxoplasmosis may also be acquired through the consumption of undercooked meat products.

B58.2 Toxoplasma meningoencephalitis

Meningoencephalitis due to toxoplasmosis is inflammation in the brain and the protective membrane surrounding the brain caused by infection with the toxoplasma parasite. This inflammation presents with fever, headache, confusion, and may be accompanied by pain and stiffness in the neck. In extreme cases, this inflammation can cause brain damage, stroke, seizures, or even death.

B59 Pneumocystosis

Pneumocystosis is pneumonia resulting from an infection of *Pneumocystis carinii* or *Pneumocystis jiroveci*.

B60.0 Babesiosis

Babesiosis is another tick-borne disease found in the same area as lyme disease, but which is more likely to damage the liver and kidneys than the heart and nervous system. Symptoms include fever, malaise, and anemia.

B60.1 Acanthamebiasis

Acanthamoeba is a microscopic, free living amebae commonly found in the environment in water, soil, sewage systems, and the air (in association with heating and cooling ventilation systems). Almost everyone is exposed to the amoeba, but infections occur mainly in the immunocompromised and those who wear contact lenses.

B60.11 Meningoencephalitis due to Acanthamoeba (culbertsoni)

This code includes meningoencephalitis due to *Acanthamoeba (culbertsoni)*, which is a ubiquitous free-living amoeba found in soil, fresh water, sea water, swimming pools, and heating, ventilation, and air conditioning systems. The organism enters the body through various routes, such as through the eyes, nose, and broken skin. When it migrates to the meninges protecting the brain, it disseminates, causing granulomatous amebic meningoencephalitis.

B60.13 Keratoconjunctivitis due to Acanthamoeba

An eye infection caused by improper storage, handling, or disinfecting of contact lenses, or in those with corneal damage, is called acanthamoeba keratitis or keratoconunctivitis. Symptoms include eye pain, redness, blurred vision, light sensitivity, sensation of something in the eye, and excessive tearing. The symptoms are similar to other infections and early diagnosis and treatment with the right medications to prevent permanent visual impairment or blindness is needed.

B60.2 Naegleriasis

This code includes primary amebic meningoencephalitis due to *Naegleria fowleri*, which is a ubiquitous free-living amoeba that rarely causes disease, but is fatal in 95% of cases. Most infections occur in the young who are exposed through swimming in warm, fresh water. The organism enters through the nose and migrates to the subarachnoid space where the cerebrospinal fluid supports its growth. *N. fowleri* causes hemorrhagic meningoencephalitis with purulent meningitis that mostly affects the cortical grey matter. Edema of the brain is severe and causes herniation of the cerebellum.

B60.8 Other specified protozoal diseases

Psorospermiasis is a disease caused by psorosperms, the lowest form of protozoa, usually affecting the kidneys and liver. Symptoms include nausea, vomiting, diarrhea, and the formation of papules on the face and skin.

B65 Schistosomiasis [bilharziasis]

Schistosomiasis is a disease caused by an infestation of schistosomes, which are trematode worms (a type of flat-worm). The parasites enter the body through contaminated drinking water and attack the kidneys, liver, and other organs.

B65.0 Schistosomiasis due to Schistosoma haematobium [urinary schistosomiasis]

Schistosoma haematobium is a type of fluke found in Africa and the Middle East that primarily attacks the bladder and rectum.

B65.1 Schistosomiasis due to Schistosoma mansoni [intestinal schistosomiasis]

Schistosoma mansoni is a trematode found throughout Africa, South America, and the Caribbean that attacks the intestines.

B65.2 Schistosomiasis due to Schistosoma japonicum

Schistosoma japonicum is a fluke found in Eastern Asia that attacks the digestive system, causing symptoms that include abdominal pain, bloody diarrhea, and fever.

B65.3 Cercarial dermatitis

An itching inflammation of the skin caused by the cutaneous penetration of larval forms of schistosomes or parasitic worms that occurs in those who bathe in infested waters.

B66.0 Opisthorchiasis

Opisthorchiasis is a trematode infestation contracted by eating raw or undercooked fish. The nematode infests the biliary ducts. This parasite is usually found in Southeast Asia.

B66.1 Clonorchiasis

Clonorchiasis is a trematode infestation of the biliary ducts usually contracted by eating raw or undercooked fish. This parasite is usually found in Korea, China, and Southeast Asia.

B66.3 Fascioliasis

Fascioliasis is a trematode infestation contracted by eating certain types of freshwater plants, usually affecting the biliary ducts. The fluke responsible for the infection can be found throughout Europe, the Middle East, and Asia.

B66.4 Paragonimiasis

Paragonimiasis is a trematode infestation contracted by eating raw or undercooked crustaceans that usually then infests the lungs. This infection is the most common fluke infection, and can be found throughout Asia, Africa, and the Americas.

B66.5 Fasciolopsiasis

Fasciolopsiasis is a trematode infestation of the intestines contracted by eating certain types of freshwater plants. The fluke responsible for the infection can be found throughout India and Asia, and is especially common in areas where pigs are raised.

B66.8 Other specified fluke infections

Metagonimiasis is a trematode infestation of the small intestine usually contracted by eating raw or undercooked fish. This particular fluke is found primarily in Eastern Asia, as well as Israel, Spain, and the Balkans. Heterophyiasis is a fluke infestation of the small intestine that is contracted

by eating raw or undercooked fish. This infestation is found in Egypt, The Middle East, and Eastern Asia.

B67 Echinococcosis

Echinococcosis is an infestation by one of several parasitic tapeworms that infest the lungs, liver, or other organs and form large cysts. The echinococcus genus of tapeworms live in the stomachs of dogs, and their larvae are passed through fecal matter. The disease spreads to humans who eat food contaminated with fecal larvae. Once ingested, the worm latches onto an organ and forms a cyst, which can grow to a very large size. If the cyst is ruptured, new cysts can form at different locations in the body. Each smaller section contains several juvenile worms. The diseases caused by these infestations are serious and often fatal if not promptly treated.

B68.0 Taenia solium taeniasis

Taenia solium is a tapeworm contracted by eating undercooked pork. The tapeworm latches onto the intestines.

B68.1 Taenia saginata taeniasis

Taenia saginata is a tapeworm that latches onto the intestine. This parasite is acquired by the consumption of undercooked beef.

B69 Cysticercosis

Cysticercosis is an infestation of the larvae of *Taenia solium*, the pork tapeworm, which can affect the muscles, eyes, brain, and spinal cord and form cysts.

B69.0 Cysticercosis of central nervous system

Cysticercosis is an infestation of the larvae of the pork tapeworm, *Taenia solium*, when it enters the brain and forms cysts, causing confusion, difficulty balancing, and swelling of the brain.

B70.0 Diphyllobothriasis

Diphyllobothriasis is a tapeworm contracted by humans through eating undercooked or raw fish. The tapeworm latches onto the small intestine.

B70.1 Sparganosis

Sparganosis is an infection caused by tapeworm larvae, often occurring in the skin.

B71.0 Hymenolepiasis

Hymenolepiasis is a tapeworm found in rats. Humans may contract the parasite by ingesting anything contaminated with feces. The tapeworm then infests the small intestine.

B72 Dracunculiasis

Dracontiasis is an infestation of *Dracunculus medinensis filaria*. This infection is also known as Guinea worm disease. The worm enters the body through ingestion of contaminated water and lurks in the body cavity until maturation occurs about a year later. The worm then protrudes out of the body through a painful sore.

B73.00 Onchocerciasis with eye involvement, unspecified

Onchocerciasis, also called river blindness, is an infestation of filarial worms of the genus Onchocerca. It occurs in tropical regions of Africa and South America, and causes lesions on the skin and eyes.

B74 Filariasis

A filarial infection is an infestation of small, threadlike nematode worms called filaria.

B74.0 Filariasis due to Wuchereria bancrofti

Bancroftian filariasis, commonly known as elephantiasis, is a disease found primarily in tropical and subtropical Asia, South America, Africa, and some Pacific Islands. Early symptoms include fever, chills, headache, and skin lesions. If left untreated, the immune response to the disease can cause gross enlargement of the limbs and genitals.

B74.3 Loiasis

Loiasis is a chronic parasitic infection spread by the horsefly, which implants the larvae in the skin. Once maturation occurs, the adult worm moves through the fascial layers of the skin, causing a creeping sensation and intense itching if they approach the skin surface. The worms often emerge near the eye, where they can be easily removed.

B74.4 Mansonelliasis

A *Mansonella ozzardi* infection may occur in the Caribbean, Central America, and parts of South America. Infected patients are usually symptomless, but may experience headaches, joint pain, or itchy red spots.

B74.8 Other filariases

Dipetalonemiasis is a rare tropical disease caused by *Acanthocheilonema perstans* which is usually found in Africa. Symptoms include irritated skin, chest and/or abdominal pain, and edema. If left untreated, the liver and spleen may become enlarged.

B75 Trichinellosis

Trichinosis, or trichiniasis, is caused by a parasite that is usually acquired by eating undercooked pork or wild game. The worm *Trichinella spiralis* infests the digestive system.

B76.0 Ancylostomiasis

The hookworm *Ancylostoma duodenale* causes gastrointestinal pain, diarrhea, and blood loss. The parasites latch onto the intestines and consume blood, causing anemia. *Ancylostoma braziliense* is a hookworm that uses dogs and cats as a host, where their larvae are passed in feces. While the larvae cannot develop in humans, they can burrow into the skin when contact is made and cause skin infections. *Ancylostoma ceylanicum* is a hookworm acquired by humans from hamsters. The parasites also latch onto the intestines and consume blood, causing anemia.

B77 Ascariasis

Ascariasis is an intestinal infection caused by the roundworm *Ascaris lumbricoides* that mainly affects the lungs and/or the intestines. Symptoms include coughing up worms or finding worms in the feces, fever, and loss of appetite, but not all infected patients have symptoms. Severe infestations of multiple worms can produce symptoms such as vomiting, shortness of breath, severe stomach and abdominal pain, intestinal blockage, and distension of the abdomen.

B78 Strongyloidiasis

Strongyloidiasis is an infection by the nematode *Strongyloides stercoralis*. Patients are frequently asymptomatic. The most common symptoms are abdominal pain and diarrhea, but other symptoms may present if the worms invade the lungs or skin.

B79 Trichuriasis

Trichuriasis is an infestation of nematodes of the genus Trichuris. Patients are usually asymptomatic, but massive infections may cause diarrhea or rectal prolapse.

B80 Enterobiasis

Enterobiasis is an infestation of pinworms. These parasites live in the rectum and emerge at night to lay eggs around the anus. The eggs can remain in clothing or bedding for weeks, and infect a new host when they are accidentally swallowed. Infections occur most often in daycare centers or other settings with a large numer of small children. Symptoms include itching around the anus and insomnia, but some patients will be asymptomatic.

B81.0 Anisakiasis

Anisakiasis is an infestation of the intestines caused by the larvae of the nematode *Anisakis marina*. The infestation is usually acquired by eating raw or undercooked fish. Symptoms include violent abdominal pain, nausea, and vomiting, during which the larvae are usually coughed up.

B81.1 Intestinal capillariasis

Capillariasis is an infestation caused by the nematode *Capillaria philippinensis*, which is acquired by eating raw or undercooked fish. Primary symptoms include abdominal pain and diarrhea. As new larvae hatch and reinfect the intestines, a massive infestation may occur, making symptoms more intense.

B81.2 Trichostrongyliasis

Trichostrongyliasis is an acute infection caused by the nematode *Trichostrongylus orientalis*. Patients are usually asymptomatic, but may present with cramps and diarrhea.

B83.0 Visceral larva migrans

Toxocariasis is an infection caused by a nematode of the genus Toxocara. This parasite is transmitted to humans who ingest soil or another substance contaminated by dog or cat feces. The larvae initially live in the human intestine, but may migrate to the muscles, liver, lungs, and occasionally to the brain and eyes, resulting in blindness in the latter case. Primary symptoms include weakness, rash, and abdominal pain, with other symptoms presenting depending on which organs are affected.

B83.1 Gnathostomiasis

Gnathostomiasis is an infection by a nematode of the genus Gnathostoma, which is transmitted to humans who eat infected raw or undercooked fish. The larvae migrate under the skin, causing intermittent, painful swellings. Depending on the organs the parasite infests, coughing, hematuria, meningitis, encephalitis, or ocular involvement may occur.

B83.4 Internal hirudiniasis

Internal hirudiniasis is a scientific term for an infestation by a leech or leeches. This term is especially identifies when they are inside a body cavity, such as the nose or mouth.

B85.0 Pediculosis due to Pediculus humanus capitis

Pediculus capitis is a species of louse that primarily infests the head.

B85.1 Pediculosis due to Pediculus humanus corporis

An infestation of the *Pediculus corporis*, also known as the body louse.

B85.3 Phthiriasis

Infestation with *Pediculus pubis*, the pubic louse, is often called crabs or phthiriasis pubis.

B86 Scabies

Scabies is an infestation of the microscopic parasite *Sarcoptes scabei*, which can spread quickly among people in crowded conditions. The primary symptoms are pimple-like irritations, intense itching, and sores on the body caused by scratching, which can become infected. Prolonged contact with an infected person is required to acquire scabies. Sexual contact is a common vector of infection.

B87 Myiasis

Myiasis is an infestation of body tissues by fly larvae, more commonly known as maggots.

B87.0 Cutaneous myiasis

Cutaneous myiasis is an infestation by the fly larvae (maggots) of the genus Oestrus, causing inflamed furuncles where the larvae are maturing beneath the skin.

B88.0 Other acariasis

Note: This code should be used for other mite infestations besides scabies in which the species of the mite is known.

B88.3 External hirudiniasis

External hirudiniasis is an infestation by leeches attached anywhere on the outside of the patient's body.

Note: Internal hirudiniasis is reported with B83.4 when leeches are inside a body cavity, such as the nose or mouth.

B95.0 Streptococcus, group A, as the cause of diseases classified elsewhere

Group A Streptococcus, sometimes abbreviated GAS, is an infection by the *Streptococcus pyogenes* bacterium, which spreads via skin-to-skin contact rather than through the air. This type of Streptococcus responds well to the antibiotic bacitracin; because most other groups are highly resistant to this antibiotic, a bacitracin test (exposing a culture to this antibiotic) is often used to diagnose GAS.

B95.1 Streptococcus, group B, as the cause of diseases classified elsewhere

Group B Streptococcus indicates an infection by the bacterium *Streptococcus agalactiae*. This bacterium commonly resides in the gastrointestinal and vaginal tracts of healthy women, and may be passed to newborn children during delivery. It is extremely unusual for a healthy adult to develop a group B infection, so it often serves as an indicator of another infection or condition that has depressed the immune system (e.g., diabetes).

B95.2 Enterococcus as the cause of diseases classified elsewhere

Group D Streptococcus is also known as Enterococcus, usually lives in the gastrointestinal tract without causing an infection. The antibiotic Vancomycin is the most common treatment for Enterococcus.

B95.3 Streptococcus pneumoniae as the cause of diseases classified elsewhere

Pneumococcus, also called *Streptococcus pneumoniae*, is a bacterium that lives harmlessly in the nasal passages or throat of up to 70% of healthy adults, but which can invade and infect the lungs, causing pneumococcal pneumonia. This disease presents with high fever, coughing and shortness of breath leading to rapid breathing and chest pains, and sometimes includes nausea, vomiting, head and muscle aches, and weariness.

B95.4 Other streptococcus as the cause of diseases classified elsewhere

Group C Streptococcus is primarily an animal disease, and rarely causes disease in humans. The most common type C bacillus responsible for human infection is *Streptococcus equisimilis*. Group G Streptococci are common on the skin, the throat, and the gastrointestinal system, and do not normally cause infection.

B95.61 Methicillin susceptible Staphylococcus aureus infection as the cause of diseases classified elsewhere

Note: A *Staphylococcus aureus* infection not otherwise specified as methicillin susceptible or resistant, is coded as susceptible for the default.

B95.62 Methicillin resistant Staphylococcus aureus infection as the cause of diseases classified elsewhere

Methicillin resistant *Staphylococcus aureus*, known as MRSA, is a strain that is resistant to, or unaffected by, the broad-spectrum antibiotics used to treat it. Most MRSA infections are acquired in hospitals, dialysis centers, and nursing homes with the elderly and immune compromised at greatest risk, but another type also occurs among otherwise healthy people in the community. Both community-associated and hospital-associated MRSA infections can be fatal.

B96.0 Mycoplasma pneumoniae [M. pneumoniae] as the cause of diseases classified elsewhere

Mycoplasma, also called Eaton's agent, is an infection by the *Mycoplasma pneumoniae* bacterium, which may be called Pleuropneumonia-like organisms (PPLO). *Mycoplasma pneumoniae* is a very small bacterium that can cause an atypical pneumonia and most commonly affects the lungs. This organism lacks a peptidoglycan cell wall, instead it has a cell membrane incorporating a sterol compound. The lack of a cell wall makes *Mycoplasma pneumoniae* resistant to many antibiotics.

B96.1 Klebsiella pneumoniae [K. pneumoniae] as the cause of diseases classified elsewhere

Klebsiella pneumoniae, also called Friedlander's bacillus, is another pneumonia-causing bacterium that presents with signs similar to Pneumococcus.

B96.21 Shiga toxin-producing Escherichia coli [E. coli] (STEC) O157 as the cause of diseases classified elsewhere

This is a type of enterohemorrhagic *E.coli* bacteria contracted by ingesting infected, undercooked meat, raw milk, unpasteurized juices, contaminated water, and raw produce. *E. coli* is also transmitted through the fecal-oral route by not washing hands after changing diapers or using the bathroom. Infection with Shiga toxin-producing strains typically presents with abdominal pain and cramping, sudden bloody, watery diarrhea, low-grade fever, and sometimes vomiting. The infection can cause illness from mild intestinal disturbance to severe cases with hemorrhagic colitis and hemolytic uremic syndrome. The illness is usually self-limiting and runs its course; antibiotics are ineffective against the milder cases and can make it worse, although serious cases require hospitalization. *E coli* includes many different serotypes, of which the 0157 is the most important. Serotype 0157:H7 is the most common strain in North America. When the H7 antigen is expressed, the strain always produces Shiga toxin. Other 0157 strains where the antigen is not known to be H7 also produce Shiga toxin, but require additional non-culture testing to identify them as Shiga toxin-producing.

B96.22 Other specified Shiga toxin-producing Escherichia coli [E. coli] (STEC) as the cause of diseases classified elsewhere

Infection with Shiga toxin-producing *E. coli* may be from many different possible serotypes. Use this code when the infection is not shown to be caused by the relatively important serotype, 0157, but by one of the more than 100 other non-0157 strains of *E. coli* such as 0111 and 026, still known to be of the O group. These non-0157 Shiga toxin-producing strains are more uncommon but are also recognized as producing hemolytic uremic syndrome.

B96.23 Unspecified Shiga toxin-producing Escherichia coli [E. coli] (STEC) as the cause of diseases classified elsewhere

Use this code to report an unspecified type of *E. coli* that is known to produce Shiga toxin (STEC) but is unspecified otherwise or as to the particular O type.

B96.29 Other Escherichia coli [E. coli] as the cause of diseases classified elsewhere

This code for other *E. coli* is reported for any *E.coli* infection with no other specification, or for non-Shiga toxin-producing forms of *E. coli*.

B96.3 Hemophilus influenzae [H. influenzae] as the cause of diseases classified elsewhere

Hemophilus influenzae is a very common bacterium found in the nasal mucous of up to 90% of people. This bacterium has six encapsulated strains (a–f) and some untypable, unencapsulated strains. *H. influenzae* is an opportunistic pathogen and when it infects the body, it usually causes a localized infection and/or inflammation of the sinuses, inner ear, heart, joints, conjunctiva of the eye, the covering of the brain, etc. Because some infections can be fatal, treatment by antibiotics is usually begun even before confirmation of the *H. influenzae* bacterium is verified by laboratory testing.

B96.4 Proteus (mirabilis) (morganii) as the cause of diseases classified elsewhere

Proteus can be caused by either the *Proteus mirabilis* or *Proteus morganii* bacteria. Symptoms vary depending on the site of the infection, so the disease must be diagnosed by a routine lab culture. The disease responds well to antibiotics.

B96.5   **Pseudomonas (aeruginosa) (mallei) (pseudomallei) as the cause of diseases classified elsewhere**

Pseudomonas is a common bacteria found in soil, water, and on the skin of both humans and animals. If it penetrates the skin, usually through a wound, it can cause illness ranging from minor skin inflammation or swimmer's ear to a potentially life-threatening infection of the blood (sepsis) or heart.

B96.6   **Bacteroides fragilis [B. fragilis] as the cause of diseases classified elsewhere**

Bacteroides fragilis includes both the *B. fragilis* bacterium itself and the *B. fragilis* group, which also includes *Bacteroides distasonis, Bacteroides ovatus, Bacteroides thetaiotaomicron,* and *Bacteroides vulgatus.* These are all common bacteria in the intestinal tract; in fact, as much as 50% of all fecal matter is actually B. *fragilis* cells. However, if these bacteria escape the intestinal tract, they can cause infections elsewhere in the body. B. *fragilis* is resistant to penicillin, but responds to other antibiotics.

B96.7   **Clostridium perfringens [C. perfringens] as the cause of diseases classified elsewhere**

Clostridium perfringens usually dwell in small numbers without causing illness in the intestines of both humans and animals, as well as in soil and sediment. Infection is usually acquired by eating infected, undercooked meat, with symptoms that vary from intense abdominal cramps and diarrhea that are over within 24 hours to (in rare cases) destruction of the intestinal tissue and even death.

B96.81   **Helicobacter pylori [H. pylori] as the cause of diseases classified elsewhere**

Helicobacter pylori is a bacterium that lives in the mucous lining of the stomach and the duodenum, the section of the small intestine just below the stomach. It most often presents as an ulcer in the stomach or duodenum, and is easily treated by antibiotics.

B97.0   **Adenovirus as the cause of diseases classified elsewhere**

An infection caused by an adenovirus, a group of viruses that infect the membranes of the repiratory tract, eyes, intestines, and urinary tract. Children are affected by adenoviruses more often than adults.

B97.11   **Coxsackievirus as the cause of diseases classified elsewhere**

There are two types of the coxsackie virus, which is a type of enterovirus, meaning it lives in the digestive tract and is a common human pathogen. Group A coxsackievirus most often infects the skin and mucous membranes and can include hemorrhagic conjunctivitis, hand-foot-mouth disease, febrile illnesses, rashes, upper respiratory infections, and aseptic meningitis.

Group B coxsackievirus more often infects the heart, pleura (lungs), pancreas, and liver. Both types can cause meningitis, pericarditis, and acute onset juvenile diabetes.

B97.12   **Echovirus as the cause of diseases classified elsewhere**

ECHO viruses are most commonly found in children and can cause a variety of diseases such as rashes, respiratory problems, and fevers. This is a group of DNA-containing viruses that affect the tissue lining of the respiratory tract, eyes, intestines, and urinary tract. There are many different serotypes.

B97.21   **SARS-associated coronavirus as the cause of diseases classified elsewhere**

A coronavirus is an RNA virus that attacks the respiratory system. The SARS-type virus is a newly discovered virus that causes severe symptoms, and can be fatal. Common symptoms are headache, stiffness, malaise, confusion, diarrhea, and a high fever.

B97.3   **Retrovirus as the cause of diseases classified elsewhere**

A retrovirus is a type of RNA virus that spreads by transcribing itself onto DNA. Some retroviruses then destroy the cell onto which the DNA was copied, which causes disease. Retroviruses are transmitted through the same vectors as HIV.

B97.33   **Human T-cell lymphotrophic virus, type I [HTLV-I] as the cause of diseases classified elsewhere**

HTLV-I is a retrovirus that causes diseases similar to multiple sclerosis. This virus is a known cause of cancer.

B97.34   **Human T-cell lymphotrophic virus, type II [HTLV-II] as the cause of diseases classified elsewhere**

HTLV-II is a virus that causes no specific disease on its own, but has been linked to some neurological diseases.

B97.35   **Human immunodeficiency virus, type 2 [HIV 2] as the cause of diseases classified elsewhere**

HIV-2 is a form of the HIV virus which occurs mostly in Africa. While basically similar to HIV-1, this virus seems to work more slowly on the immune system. Viral load tests for HIV-1 are not reliable for HIV-2.

B97.7   **Papillomavirus as the cause of diseases classified elsewhere**

The human papillomavirus is a group of many viruses that can cause warts on the hands, feet, and genitals, and may contribute to the development of cancers of the female reproductive organs.

C00 Malignant neoplasm of lip

A neoplasm, more commonly known as a tumor, is an abnormal tissue that grows more rapidly than normal, and which lacks the organization and functionality of the tissue around it. Ordinary cells receive feedback that limits the creation of new cells after a certain number of divisions so that new cells are generated properly for tissue repair and growth. Tumors develop when cells cease responding to the feedback and grow without control, causing damage to the surrounding cells, and disrupting the normal function of the body.

A neoplasm can be classified as either malignant, benign, or as a carcinoma in situ. A malignant tumor is one that grows quickly and destructively invades the surrounding tissue. A benign neoplasm is one that is neither growing excessively nor causing destruction in the surrounding cells. Even so, it may cause dysfunction due to its size or its effect on adjacent tissue. A carcinoma in situ is a contained neoplasm which is undergoing malignant changes but has not invaded the surrounding tissue.

The primary neoplasm is the site where the cancerous cells are believed to have originated. A secondary neoplasm is one where the neoplastic cells from another primary site were transported through the lymphatic or circulatory system to another location. This process of spreading cancerous cells is called metastasis. In some cases, a primary site other than the known neoplasm cannot be found, but the attending physician will rule that a tumor may be a secondary one because its characteristics are inconsistent with a primary tumor at that site. Neoplasms are organized by the level of malignancy, whether the tumor in question is a primary or a secondary site, and by location.

C02.0 Malignant neoplasm of dorsal surface of tongue

This code is used for a tumor on the dorsal (top) surface in the forward two-thirds of the tongue (that is, the mobile portion).

C02.3 Malignant neoplasm of anterior two-thirds of tongue, part unspecified

Select this code if the tumor is in the forward, mobile two-thirds of the tongue, but the exact location is either unspecified or overlaps the areas covered by two or more other of the above codes.

C02.4 Malignant neoplasm of lingual tonsil

This code is appropriate if the tumor is in the lingual tonsil, the collection of lymph nodes in the back of the tongue.

C04 Malignant neoplasm of floor of mouth

Malignant neoplasms of the floor of the mouth involve the lymph nodes and risk spreading to other parts of the body even more quickly than other cancers of the mouth. These types of cancers are most common in patients with a history of tobacco and/or alcohol abuse.

C05.2 Malignant neoplasm of uvula

Select this code to describe a tumor on the roof of the mouth in the uvula, the small, roughly conical flesh that is visible dangling in the back of the mouth.

C06.1 Malignant neoplasm of vestibule of mouth

This describes a tumor in either vestibule of the mouth, the slit-like space between the lips and cheeks and the teeth and gums.

C07 Malignant neoplasm of parotid gland

This code is used to describe a tumor in the parotid gland, which is the large salivary gland in the cheek just in front of the ear and along the jawbone.

C10.0 Malignant neoplasm of vallecula

The epiglottis is a fold of cartilage and tissue that folds down to cover the trachea as one swallows to prevent food from going down the wrong tube. The vallecula is the crevice between the root of the tongue and the epiglottis.

C11 Malignant neoplasm of nasopharynx

The nasopharynx area lies behind the nasal cavity and the soft palate. In addition to connecting the nasal cavity and throat, the nasopharynx also contains two openings to the ears, called Eustachian tubes. The nasopharynx is bounded in front by the rear edge of the nasal septum, the body of cartilage that separates the two nasal passages.

C12 Malignant neoplasm of pyriform sinus

The pyriform sinus, sometimes referred to as the pyriform fossa, is comprised of a pair of cul-de-sac-like depressions in the esophagus which are nestled against the trachea.

C13.0 Malignant neoplasm of postcricoid region

This code describes a malignant neoplasm involving the cricoid (a ring-shaped cartilage that protects the trachea just below the thyroid cartilage) and the postcricoid area (the lowest part of the hypopharynx, just below the separation of the larynx and pharynx).

C13.1 Malignant neoplasm of aryepiglottic fold, hypopharyngeal aspect

This code represents a malignant neoplasm in the aryepiglottic fold, which is a fold in the mucous membrane of the throat and a muscle in it that aids in the function of the epiglottis in preventing food from entering the trachea.

C14.2 Malignant neoplasm of Waldeyer's ring

This code depicts a malignant neoplasm in Waldeyer's ring, a ring of lymph nodes and lymphatic tissue that surrounds the pharynx and connects to the tonsils and adenoids.

C16.1 Malignant neoplasm of fundus of stomach

A malignant neoplasm found in the fundus (the upper portion of the stomach that rises above the cardia), is applicable to this code.

C16.4 Malignant neoplasm of pylorus

This details a malignant neoplasm where the stomach connects to the small intestine at the pylorus. A sphincter muscle regulates the passage of food through the two areas.

C17.1 Malignant neoplasm of jejunum

The jejunum is a segment that comprises approximately 40% of the small intestine, and is primarily located to the left side of the abdomen.

C17.2 Malignant neoplasm of ileum

The ileum comprises the remaining 60% of the small intestine and wraps around the right side of the abdomen and pelvic cavity before connecting to the large intestine at the cecum.

C17.3 Meckel's diverticulum, malignant

Meckel's diverticulum is a congenital abnormality in which the connection between the small intestine and umbilical cord does not close correctly, resulting in a small cul-de-sac-like pouch forming in the small intestine. In most patients, this condition causes no complications, but the pouch can potentially become infected, cause a bowel obstruction, or cause bleeding into the intestine.

C18.0 Malignant neoplasm of cecum

On the right side of the body, the cecum is a pouch-shaped section that hangs below the ileum of the small intestine.

C18.3 Malignant neoplasm of hepatic flexure

The hepatic flexure is the connecting turn between the transverse colon and the descending colon.

C18.4 Malignant neoplasm of transverse colon

The transverse colon is the upper third of the large intestine that crosses the abdomen from right to left.

C18.5 Malignant neoplasm of splenic flexure

The splenic flexure is in the large intestine between the ascending colon and the transverse colon.

C21.1 Malignant neoplasm of anal canal

A malignant neoplasm in the anal canal, which includes the anal sphincter muscle, is outlined by this code.

Note: This category includes malignant neoplasms of the anal canal, but does not include malignancies of the skin of the anus, such as melanoma, basal cell, or squamous cell carcinoma of the anus.

C23 Malignant neoplasm of gallbladder

Cancer of the gallbladder is rare and is usually found only in the elderly.

C24.1 Malignant neoplasm of ampulla of Vater

The common bile ducts connect with the duodenum of the small intestine by way of the ampulla of Vater, a juncture of the bile and pancreatic ducts.

C25.3 Malignant neoplasm of pancreatic duct

The pancreatic ducts are sometimes called the Santorini or Wirsung ducts, which run the length of the organ.

C30.0 Malignant neoplasm of nasal cavity

The upper respiratory system starts with the nasal cavities, which include the nasal cartilage and septum, the conchae (the bony protrusions into the nasal cavities that protect the openings to the sinuses and help to filter inhaled air), and the mucosa (the membrane that covers the interior tracts).

C31.0 Malignant neoplasm of maxillary sinus

The maxillary sinuses rest to either side of the nasal cavities behind the cheekbones.

C31.1 Malignant neoplasm of ethmoidal sinus

A malignant neoplasm in the ethmoidal sinuses is depicted with this code. The ethmoidal sinuses are to either side of the nasal cavities alongside the eyes, and are divided into numerous small chambers.

C31.2 Malignant neoplasm of frontal sinus

This depicts a malignant neoplasm in the frontal sinus in the forehead directly between the eyes.

C31.3 Malignant neoplasm of sphenoid sinus

The sphenoidal sinus is a chamber centered behind the eyes and beneath the brain.

C32.3 Malignant neoplasm of laryngeal cartilage

The laryngeal cartilages include nine cartilages of the larynx: the cricoid, thyroid, and epiglottic cartilages, and two each of arytenoid, corniculate, and cuneiform cartilages.

C38.1 Malignant neoplasm of anterior mediastinum

The mediastinum is the cavity between the lungs in which the heart, thymus, and parathyroid gland reside.

C38.4 Malignant neoplasm of pleura

The parietal pleura is the outermost layer of the pleural membranes. The visceral pleura is the innermost layer of the membranes that connects directly to the lungs.

C43 Malignant melanoma of skin

A malignant neoplasm of the skin may come as either a melanoma or another form. A melanoma appears as an irregular pigmented area that spreads rapidly across surrounding skin and metastasizes quickly to other parts of the body. It usually begins as a suspicious mole of irregular shape — not circular or ovoid, but a random shape with no symmetry — and an odd or splotchy color, often almost black. Moles that develop late in life, especially after early adulthood, or moles larger than one cm in diameter, should be tested through biopsy. A malignant melanoma is classified according to where it appears.

C44 Other and unspecified malignant neoplasm of skin

This category reports basal cell carcinomas, squamous cell carcinomas, and other specified malignant neoplasms of the skin by site on the face, ear, scalp and neck, trunk, and limbs. Basal cell carcinomas (BCC) and squamous cell carcinomas (SCC) begin from the keratinocytes or keratin producing cells found in the outer layer of skin and arise most commonly in areas exposed to the sun. Rarely, BCC tumors may develop on nonexposed areas. Basal cell carcinomas begin in the lowest layer of the epidermis where the cells divide and mature into keratinocytes. This type is the most common skin cancer and accounts for about 8 out of 10 skin cancers. They rarely metastasize and are very slow growing, but can damage surrounding tissue, causing destruction or disfigurement when tumors are large or more aggressive. Basal cell carcinomas can sometimes resemble other noncancerous skin conditions such as psoriasis or eczema.

Squamous cell carcinomas (SCC) are the second most common type of skin cancer. Squamous cell carcinomas begin in the cells of the upper layer of the epidermis and in mucous membranes. SCC also arises most commonly from chronically sun-exposed areas but can occur on any area of the body, particularly from burns, scars, areas of chronic inflammation or open sores, and areas exposed to radiation or chemicals like petroleum by-products. Up to 60% of SCCs begin from untreated actinic keratoses. These carcinomas typically look like a persistent, thick, rough, scaly patch, a wart-like growth, and a raised growth with central depression, that all occasionally bleed or crust.

Note: Merkel cell carcinoma of the skin is not coded to this category.

C46 Kaposi's sarcoma

Kaposi's sarcoma is a type of cancer that is very unusual in how it develops. Most forms of cancer start in one part of the body and then travel, or metastasize, to other parts through the blood vessels or lymphatic system. Kaposi's sarcoma can appear in multiple locations at once. This disease was once most common in older men of Jewish, Mediterranean, or African descent and organ transplant patients, but since the 1980s has most commonly developed as a complication in HIV and AIDS patients. This kind of cancer is rarely seen in patients with normal immune systems.

C46.0 Kaposi's sarcoma of skin

The most common presentation of this disease is small tumors that appear as raised blotches or nodules of a reddish, purplish, or browning color on the skin.

C46.1 Kaposi's sarcoma of soft tissue

This code depicts tumors in the soft tissue just beneath the skin, such as the blood and lymph vessels, muscle, fasica, and/or ligaments, or other connective tissue.

C4A Merkel cell carcinoma

Merkel cell carcinoma is an aggressive and lethal neuroendocrine cancer of the skin with a mortality rate much higher than that of melanoma. Although the exact function of Merkel cells in the skin is unknown, they are thought to be touch receptors. The uncontrolled growth of Merkel cells does not have a distinctive appearance but grows rapidly as a painless, firm bump that may be flesh-colored, red, or bluish in appearance with overlying skin breaking down. Merkel cell carcinoma occurs mainly in the elderly (average age of 74) with fair skin, a history of extensive sun exposure, and chronic immunosuppression, such as transplant or HIV. The tumors appear most commonly on the most sun-exposed skin, such as the head, neck, and arms. Prompt and aggressive treatment is required.

C53   Malignant neoplasm of cervix uteri

The cervix uteri is the "neck" of the uterus which comprises the lower third of the organ and joins it to the vagina.

C54   Malignant neoplasm of corpus uteri

A primary, malignant neoplasm of the corpus uteri, which literally means "body of the uterus."

C55   Malignant neoplasm of uterus, part unspecified

A primary, malignant neoplasm, or tumor, of the uterus in which the exact area is unspecified. Uterine malignancies commonly present with abdominal bleeding. In post-menopausal women, any bleeding from the uterus is considered to be cancerous until proven otherwise by a biopsy.

C57.1   Malignant neoplasm of broad ligament

The ovaries and fallopian tubes are suspended and connected to the uterus by a broad connective tissue called the broad ligament. The broad ligament is comprised of three major parts: the mesometrium, the mesosalpinx, and the mesovarium.

C57.2   Malignant neoplasm of round ligament

The round ligament anchors the uterus to the abdominal wall, and passes beneath and in front of the fallopian tubes.

C57.20   Malignant neoplasm of unspecified round ligament

The round ligament further anchors the uterus to the abdominal wall, and passes beneath and in front of the fallopian tubes.

C61   Malignant neoplasm of prostate

The prostate is a gland positioned around the urethra just beneath the bladder in men. It is responsible for the production of the milky fluid that accompanies the semen during ejaculation. Symptoms of prostate cancer include: frequent urination, especially at night, or an inability to urinate; trouble starting or holding back urination; a weak or interrupted flow of urine; painful or burning urination, blood in the urine or semen, painful ejaculation; and frequent pain in the lower back, hips, or upper thighs. However, it should be noted that while these can be symptoms of cancer, more often they are symptoms of noncancerous conditions.

C62   Malignant neoplasm of testis

The testicle, or testes, is responsible for production of both the male hormone (testosterone) and sperm. It begins development high in the abdomen and then normally descends to it's normal position in the scrotum before birth. However, in some cases, the testes' descent is either delayed or does not occur at all.

C63.0   Malignant neoplasm of epididymis

The epididymis is a narrow, tightly coiled tube that connects each testicle to the spermatic cord and provides a place for immature sperm to develop.

C63.1   Malignant neoplasm of spermatic cord

The spermtic cord, or vas deferens is a muscular tube surrounded by smooth muscle that connects the left and right epididymis to the ejaculatory duct.

C63.2   Malignant neoplasm of scrotum

The scrotum is the pouch of skin and connective tissue that contains the testicles, epididymis, and the first segment of the spermatic cords.

C65.1   Malignant neoplasm of right renal pelvis

The renal pelvis is the chamber that unites the major calices, the tubes through which urine leaves the kidneys.

C67.0   Malignant neoplasm of trigone of bladder

The trigone is a smooth, triangular area at the base of the bladder between the ureters and the urethra.

C67.1   Malignant neoplasm of dome of bladder

The dome is the "ceiling" of the chamber of the bladder.

C67.7   Malignant neoplasm of urachus

The urachus is a tube that connects the bladder to the umbilicus during prenatal development. It normally closes off after birth, but in some cases it does not, and the remaining tract is easily infected and a frequent site for neoplasms.

C68.1   Malignant neoplasm of paraurethral glands

The paraurethral glands surround the urethra in most, but not all women. They are believed to be similar to the prostate gland in men, but serve no vital function in the female and may be removed without affecting the body's function.

C69   Malignant neoplasm of eye and adnexa

A malignant tumor of the eye can have varying symptoms, including vision loss; "floaters," spots, or squiggles in the field of vision; flashes of light; a growing dark spot on the iris; or a change in the position and/or shape of the eyeball.

Note: Codes in this category do not include retinal freckle or dark area on the retina and choroid.

C69.1   Malignant neoplasm of cornea

The cornea is the protective lens over the iris and lens, which works together with them to focus light on the retina.

C69.2   Malignant neoplasm of retina

The retina is the portion on the back of the eye where light is focused and a dense cluster of nerves convey the information back to the brain.

C69.5   Malignant neoplasm of lacrimal gland and duct

The lacrimal gland, better known as the tear gland, lies to the side of the eye facing the nose. The lacrimal duct carries tears from the lacrimal sac into the nasal cavity.

C69.6   Malignant neoplasm of orbit

The orbit is the cavity of the skull that contains the eye, and includes the muscles and connective tissue.

C71.0   Malignant neoplasm of cerebrum, except lobes and ventricles

The cerebrum is the largest part of the brain, and is responsible for conscious thought. It is divided into two halves connected by the corpus stratatum and includes: the basal ganglia, which handles the coordination of habitual but acquired skills like chewing; the thalamus, which processes sensory input and the hyopthalamus, which regulates the heartbeat, body temperature, and fluid balance. The cerebral cortex, the outer layer of the cerebrum, processes information.

C72.59   Malignant neoplasm of other cranial nerves

The cranial nerves are composed of twelve pairs of nerves that emanate directly from the brain (rather than the spinal cord, as all other nerves) and control and receive information from the sensory organs and muscles in the head. A malignant neoplasm located in a cranial nerve other than the olfactory, optic, or acoustic nerves should be reported using this code.

C73   Malignant neoplasm of thyroid gland

A tumor of a gland may be defined as "functioning," in which it is meant that the tumor is causing an overproduction of one or more hormones, or "nonfunctioning," in which case it is not. This distinction does not affect the coding of the neoplasm itself, but it may affect the coding of secondary complications.

C74   Malignant neoplasm of adrenal gland

The adrenal glands lie on top of the kidneys and produce adrenaline along with other hormones. Symptoms vary depending on whether the tumor is functioning or not, and which hormones are being overproduced.

C74.00 Malignant neoplasm of cortex of unspecified adrenal gland

The adrenal glands rest atop the kidney, and produce adrenaline along with other hormones. Symptoms vary depending on whether the tumor is functioning or not, and if so, which hormones are being overproduced.

C75.0 Malignant neoplasm of parathyroid gland

The parathyroid glands are two pea-sized glands to either side of the thyroid in the neck. The parathyroid hormone controls the release of calcium into the bloodstream, which is obtained either from the bones, or from absorbing more calcium from food in the digestive tract. The malignant neoplasm may present with a small lump on the neck, kidney stones and/or failure, aching in the bones or osteoporosis, hoarseness, constipation, muscular weakness, and/or vomiting.

C75.1 Malignant neoplasm of pituitary gland

The pituitary gland is a gland about the size of a pea that is in the center of the brain and produces hormones responsible for regulating the body's growth. In young people, a functioning pituitary tumor can cause abnormal growth in the hands and feet. In adults, a pituitary tumor can cause what is known as Cushing's disease, which presents with an accumulation of fat in the face, high blood sugar, and muscular weakness. Other symptoms of either a functioning or non-functioning pituitary tumor include headaches, difficulty seeing, and nausea and vomiting due to pressure by the tumor on the surrounding nerves.

C75.3 Malignant neoplasm of pineal gland

The pineal gland is a small organ set in the ventricles of the brain. Its function is not entirely understood, but one thing it is known to do is produce melatonin, which regulates how much and when we sleep. A malignant neoplasm of thepineal gland may present with increased cerebrospinal fluid due to the increased size blocking the ventricles, causing headaches, vomiting, balance loss, and vision problems similar to those found in pituitary cancer. A functioning pineal tumor may also cause sleep disorders.

C75.4 Malignant neoplasm of carotid body

The carotid body comprises the division of the carotid artery into numerous smaller arteries that supply blood to both the inside and outside of the cranium. Tumors in this site, called chemodectomas, are malignant only about 10-15% of the time, and usually present with blockage and decreased blood flow to the brain, as well as increased blood pressure below the blockage.

C75.8 Malignant neoplasm with pluriglandular involvement, unspecified

Use this code in instances where a malignant neoplasm affects a pluriglandular area (that is affecting one or more glands) that is not otherwise specified. If the neoplasm affects multiple glandular sites that are known, these should be coded separately.

C77 Secondary and unspecified malignant neoplasm of lymph nodes

Secondary neoplasms are those which have metastatized, or spread, from other areas of the body, usually through the blood vessels or lymph nodes. These neoplasms can be every bit as malignant as the primary tumors from which they seeded. One of the most common systems in which to find secondary malignant neoplasms is in the lymphatic system. The lymphatic system carries excess water and other liquid from the body back to the bloodstream near the heart, using interconnected bean-shaped pods called lymph nodes to trap foreign material such as bacteria, viruses, and cancerous cells. White blood cells also flow through the lymphatic system, neutralizing infections. Secondary tumors are coded by their location in the body.

Note: This category excludes secondary neuroendocrine or carcinoid tumors, which are coded to C7B.-.

C7A Malignant neuroendocrine tumors

Both malignant and benign neuroendocrine tumors are generally classified as carcinoid tumors. These tumors represent a broad spectrum of biologically diverse malignant tumors that arise from hormone-producing cells throughout the body that makes them clinically diverse. They are characterized by functional activity that produces hormonal syndromes, such as carcinoid syndrome or medulloadrenal hyperfunction. Rarely, the occurrence of neuroendocrine tumors may also be associated as a part of multiple endocrine neoplasia [MEN] syndrome, type 1. Carcinoid tumors arise from three areas that are grouped according to the embryonic site of origin: the foregut = bronchi, lungs, stomach, proximal duodenum, thymus; the midgut = second portion of duodenum, jejunum, ileum, cecum, ascending colon, and appendix; hindgut = transverse, descending, and sigmoid colon, rectum, and organs of the genitourinary tract, such as the ovaries and testes.

These tumors are usually diagnosed between ages 50 and 70. They are slow growing, difficult to diagnose, and often do not produce symptoms, especially in early, benign stages, often remaining asymptomatic for years until they have metastasized. The signs of tumor vary with the organ of origin and are usually found incidentally during other procedures, such as an appendectomy or colonoscopy. Symptoms that actually cause people to seek medical attention are uncommon and tend to be vague, such as abdominal discomfort, flushing, telangiectastia, or spider-like veins on the face, diarrhea, hypotension, tachycardia, and pellagra.

Because these tumors arise from hormone-producing tissue, side effects in later stages are caused by the inappropriate release of hormones that may cause carcinoid syndrome, Zollinger-Ellison syndrome, atrophic gastritis, and ovarian teratoma. Surgery is the main treatment and can often cure the cancer if it has not spread.

Note: When multiple endocrine neoplasia syndrome is associated with any carcinoid tumor, the MEN syndrome should also be coded. Other associated endocrine syndromes, such as carcinoid syndrome, should be listed as an additional code.

C7A.01 Malignant carcinoid tumors of the small intestine

Over a dozen types of neuroendocrine cells exist in the gastrointestinal tract, all of which secrete specialized bioactive amines or peptides. Malignant carcinoid tumors arising in the small intestine are more likely to display secretory activity than elsewhere in the GI tract, although all gastrointestinal neuroendocrine tumors can cause nonspecific symptoms that are usually attributed to other more common conditions, such as irritable bowel syndrome. This makes them challenging to diagnose.

C7A.02 Malignant carcinoid tumors of the appendix, large intestine, and rectum

Over a dozen types of neuroendocrine cells exist in the gastrointestinal tract, all of which secrete specialized bioactive amines or peptides. Malignant carcinoid tumors arising in the large intestine, particularly the distal part of the colon and the rectum are more likely to remain nonfunctional in secretory activity than elsewhere in the GI tract, and to cause symptoms that are related to a tumor of increasing mass. However, all gastrointestinal neuroendocrine tumors can cause nonspecific symptoms that are usually attributed to other more common conditions, such as irritable bowel syndrome. This makes them challenging to diagnose.

C80.0 Disseminated malignant neoplasm, unspecified

Cases of carcinomatosis or generalized malignancy are reported here, whether specified as primary or secondary, although this condition usually arises when multiple secondary carcinomas develop at the same time by metastatic spread from a primary site. Disseminated malignancy can spread in either a generalized manner or hold to a certain defined pattern. Carcinomatosis generally referred to cancerous tumors arising from an epithelial source, called adenocarcinomas, and not those from lymphomas or sarcomas (sarcomatosis), but now covers all of those cancers with a metastatic spread. Manifestations of carcinomatosis differ according to the body parts affected.

C81 Hodgkin lymphoma

Hodgkin lymphoma is a form of lymphoma characterized by the presence of malformed cells with two nuclei called Reed-Sternburg cells. Unlike most lymphomas, which become more common with age, incidences of Hodgkin lymphoma increase in the 15-35 year age range as well as in the over 50 age range and affect more men than women. It presents with swollen, but not painful, lymph nodes, particularly (but not always) in the neck. Symptoms include low-grade fever, night sweats, weight loss, itchiness (especially in the area of the swollen nodes), and fatigue. Historically, there have been many, many histological classifications of Hodgkin lymphoma. The nomenclature and classification used for different types of Hodgkin lymphoma continues to evolve today as a greater understanding of cell types, immunophenotypes, and disease progression and prognosis help form the criteria used for subdividing the disease.

The subdivisions of paragranuloma, granuloma, and sarcoma date back to one of the first major steps taken in disease classification by Jackson and Parker in 1944, in which three stages were identified: the early stage (later called paragranuloma), granuloma, and sarcoma. In 1966, Lukes and Butler proposed a classification based on predominant histological features. They recognized other nodular and diffuse lymphocytic and/or histiocytic types within these cases and added a third and fourth group for nodular sclerosis and mixed cellularity. The Rye classification of 1965 modified that of Lukes and Butler with concepts of lymphocytic predominance and depletion. Predominant types included the paragranuloma type of Jackson and Parker and the lymphocytic/histiocytic types, both nodular and diffuse, of Lukes and Butler.

Pathologists today use the World Health Organization's (WHO) modification of the Revised European-American Lymphoma (REAL) classification, which divides Hodgkin lymphoma classification of adults into the two broad pathological classes of classical Hodgkin lymphoma, having four subtypes, and nodular lymphocyte predominant Hodgkin lymphoma. The four classical subtypes include lymphocytic rich, lymphocyte depleted, nodular sclerosis, and mixed cellularity types.

C81.0 Nodular lymphocyte predominant Hodgkin lymphoma

Nodular lymphocyte predominance type Hodgkin lymphoma is distinguished from classical types of Hodgkin lyphoma cases as having a different clinical pathology. This type has a differing immunophenotype, or B cell antigen expression, as well as oncogene expression that are not present in classical Hodgkin cases. It is often seen in young males, who are asymptomatic at diagnosis, with localized cervical or inguinal node involvement, usually without mediastinal nodes. The outcome has a longer survival with more treatment success.

C81.1 Nodular sclerosis classical Hodgkin lymphoma

Nodular sclerosis is a type of classical Hodgkin lymphoma with a low grade of malignancy and is the only form that affects more young women than men. This is the more common form of the disease, comprising up to 80% of Hodgkin lymphoma cases diagnosed in older children and adolescents. It usually arises in lymph nodes of the chest and mediastinum with bulky tumor growth. This type is characterized by bands of collagen that divide the lymph nodes into nodules as well as the presence of Reed-Sternberg cells appearing in a variant called lacunar cells. Lymphocytes are present in varying numbers.

C81.2 Mixed cellularity classical Hodgkin lymphoma

Mixed cellularity classical Hodgkin lymphoma is more common in younger children than in adolescents or adults. There are plentiful numbers of Reed-Sternberg cells that occur in the presence of abundant normal, reactive cells, too, such as lymphocytes, eosinophils, plasma cells, and histiocytes. These inflammatory type cells may be present more than in the lymphocyte rich types and is often confused with peripheral T-cell lymphoma.

C81.3 Lymphocyte depleted classical Hodgkin lymphoma

Lymphocyte depleted Hodgkin lymphoma is the least common form, accounting for less than one percent of cases. It appears mostly in older, immuno-compromised patients as an advanced stage of disease, usually beginning in the abdominal and pelvic lymph nodes. There are numerous Reed-Sternberg cells, not very many lymphocytes, and disorganized fibrosis. There may be necrosis in the center of the lymph tissue, surrounded by the R-S cells and very bizarre, or atypical cells.

C82 Follicular lymphoma

Follicular lymphoma is a type of non-Hodgkin lymphoma (NHL) that accounts for about 20-30% of all NHL cases in the U.S. This is an indolent, or slow-growing, B-cell lymphoma. Many patients have no symptoms of the disease at diagnosis, although symptoms may consist of lymph node enlargement in the neck, underarms, groin, or stomach along with fatigue, night sweats, weight loss, and shortness of breath. The follicular designation means that the cells tend to grow in a circular pattern within the lymph nodes. When patients are asymptomatic, or have very few symptoms, treatment may be delayed in favor of a watch and wait approach. Follicular lymphoma is normally very responsive to radiation and chemotherapy. In those with very limited disease, radiation has affected a cure; but although it is responsive to therapy, it remains nearly incurable. Because it can be managed well, many consider follicular lymphoma a chronic disease as opposed to a terminal one. The median age of onset is around 60 and remains rare in the very young, although those under age 40 have a more promising survival rate. Approximately one third of all follicular lymphomas will turn into a more aggressive, fast-growing diffuse B-cell lymphoma.

C82.0 Follicular lymphoma grade I

Follicular lymphoma is divided into three main grades. The grade refers to the number of large cells, called centroblasts, that are present within the neoplastic follicles under a microscope per high power field. Grade I is defined as a predominance of small centrocytes with 0-5 large centroblasts per high power field. Grade I remains slow growing and manageable.

C82.1 Follicular lymphoma grade II

Follicular lymphoma is divided into three main grades. The grade refers to the number of large cells, called centroblasts, that are present within the neoplastic follicles under a microscope per high power field. Grade II is defined as 6-15 centroblasts per high power field. Although grade II does have more large cells present than grade 1, it is still considered the same in terms of treatment and prognosis.

C82.2 Follicular lymphoma grade III, unspecified

Follicular lymphoma is divided into three main grades. The grade refers to the number of large cells, called centroblasts, that are present within the neoplastic follicles under a microscope per high power field. Grade III is defined as over 15 centroblasts per high power field and was previously referred to as follicular large cell lymphoma. The larger cells generally behave more aggressively, and Grade III has been associated with a worse overall survival rate.

C82.3 Follicular lymphoma grade IIIa

Grade III follicular lymphoma is subdivided into IIIa and IIIb. The grade refers to the number of large cells, called centroblasts, that are present within the neoplastic follicles under a microscope per high power field. Grade III is defined as over 15 centroblasts per high power field. Grade IIIa, however, shows a mix of smaller centrocytes and centroblasts within the follicles, while grade IIIb demonstrates sheets of large centroblasts without centrocytes. Dividing grade III into IIIa and IIIb is somewhat controversial, as studies have shown that grade IIIa is more accurately part of the indolent grade spectrum and has an outcome similar to grades I and II, and is not clinically an aggressive grade in regard to prognosis, behavior, or treatment.

C82.4 Follicular lymphoma grade IIIb

Grade III follicular lymphoma is subdivided into IIIa and IIIb. The grade refers to the number of large cells, called centroblasts, that are present within the neoplastic follicles under a microscope per high power field. Grade III is defined as over 15 centroblasts per high power field. Grade IIIb demonstrates sheets of large centroblasts without smaller centrocytes. Some data suggests that it is the presence of diffuse areas within a neoplastic follicle that determines more aggressive clinical behavior. This has led to controversy in dividing grade III into IIIa and IIIb, as studies have shown that grade IIIa, which shows a mix of smaller centrocytes with large centroblasts (or grade III with less than 50% diffuse component) is more accurately part of the indolent grade spectrum that has an outcome similar to grades I and II; while IIIb (or grade III with greater than 50% diffuse component) is more clinically aligned with the aggressive diffuse large B-cell lymphoma and is more accurately a grade III in clinical significance. Grade IIIb is treated aggressively with radiation and chemotherapy and has a poor prognosis.

C82.5 Diffuse follicle center lymphoma

Diffuse follicle center lymphoma is defined as a lymphoma with the same cell population as follicular lymphoma grade I and II, but without the characteristic follicular, or circular pattern. It displays the same outward observable characteristics as follicular lymphoma. It must sometimes be distinguished by cytological and immunological evidence.

Note: When diffuse follicle center lymphoma is identified as grade III, it is actually designated as diffuse large B-cell lymphoma and coded to C83.3-.

C83.0 Small cell B-cell lymphoma

Marginal zone lymphomas are actually a group of uncommon, small cell B cell non-Hodgkin lymphomas that involve the marginal zone portion of the lymph node, or patchy area outside of the follicular mantle zone. They can be either 'nodal' or 'extranodal.' These are indolent, or low-grade, slow-growing cancers that are not strongly responsive to traditional cancer therapies. There are at least three distinct subtypes of marginal zone B cell lymphomas: nodal, splenic, and mucosa associated lymphoid tissue. Nodal marginal zone B cell lymphoma is rare and used to be called monocytoid B cell lymphoma. It's cause is unknown and is usually found in the middle aged and elderly, more often in women. Painless swelling usually appears first in enlarged nodes of the neck, armpit, or groin and may involve nodes in other areas. Loss of appetite, weight loss, tiredness, fever, and profuse night sweats are also symptoms.

C83.07 Small cell B-cell lymphoma, spleen

Splenic marginal zone B-cell lymphoma is a very rare and distinct form of marginal zone lymphoma confined to the spleen. Symptoms may appear years after the first actual biological presence and manifest as huge splenic enlargement with involvement of the bone marrow and peripheral blood, but usually without lymph node enlargement.

C83.09 Small cell B-cell lymphoma, extranodal and solid organ sites

Mucosa associated lymphoid tissue (MALT) is a distinct type of marginal zone, or small cell B-cell lymphoma involving lymphatic tissue outside the lymph nodes in solid organs, such as the stomach, thyroid gland, lungs, and intestines. The stomach is the most common site, connected with *H. pylori* infection. Symptoms vary depending on the organ affected.

C83.1 Mantle cell lymphoma

Mantle cell lymphoma arises from malignant B lymphocytes in the 'mantle zone' portion of the lymph node. The boundaries are obliterated as the cancerous cells grow, appearing diffusely spread out under the microscope. Although the cause is unknown, many patients have an acquired translocation of genetic material on chromosomes 11 and 14, causing overexpression of a protein that results in excessive formation of B lymphocytes. Even though it is a low-grade, indolent class of lymphoma, it tends to grow more quickly than other forms.

The median age at diagnosis is 58 and it occurs more often in males. Symptoms include loss of weight and appetite, nausea, abdominal pain, bloating, vomiting, and an enlarged liver and spleen causing discomfort. Lymph node enlargement occurs particularly in the nodes at the back of the throat, including tonsils and adenoids. Lymphoma cells may also invade the

brain, spinal cord, gastrointestinal tract, and bone marrow, suppressing red blood cell production and causing anemia.

C84.0 Mycosis fungoides

This type of lymphoma is also called granuloma fungoides. The name is misleading as it was once believed to be a fungal-caused skin condition, but is actually a rare, progressive form of a slow-growing cutaneous T-cell lymphoma associated with a chromosome abnormality that evolves into a generalized, high grade, aggressive systemic form of lymphoma. Most cases present with successive stages of intensely itching red skin eruptions resembling eczema or psoriasis; then a stage of infiltrated plaques with abnormal mononuclear Sezary cells; and then a tumor stage in which mushroom-like tumors may begin to ulcerate.

Note: Peripheral T-cell lymphoma that is not classified is coded to C84.4-.

C84.1 Sézary disease

Sézary disease is a very rare type of cutaneous T-cell lymphoma, like an advanced progression of mycosis fungoides. In the early stage, only the skin is affected. Intensely itchy, exfoliative erythroderma becomes generalized from initial eczema or psoriasis-like lesions. Skin tumors appear in stage II, with enlarged lymph glands in the neck, armpit, and groin, and blood abnormalities in stages III and IV. T-lymphocytes increase to very large numbers in the blood. Sezary cells, which are abnormal, hyperchromatic, mononuclear cells of different shape infiltrate the skin, lymph nodes, and blood. Multiple therapies are used, but only early stages are promising for a complete cure. Nitrogen mustard is applied to the skin daily for up to a year, then less frequently. Different treatments used include electron beam radiation therapy; photopheresis, combining ultraviolet light therapy with the filtering of Sezary cells out of the blood; and systemic chemotherapy in later stages.

C84.4 Peripheral T-cell lymphoma, not classified

Also called mature T cell lymphoma and post-thymic T cell lymphoma, peripheral T cell lymphomas are a group of non-Hodgkin lymphomas that derive from neoplastic T lymphocytes that have already matured in the thymus gland and moved on to other lymphatic tissue sites throughout the body. These are fast growing, aggressive cancers that have diverse presentations, depending on the affected site(s), but usually appear with generalized as well as retroperitoneal lymphadenopathy, weight loss, fever, and profuse night sweats. The age range includes children, although the median age is 60. Extranodal sites affected include the bone marrow, spleen, liver, and skin, with lesions varying from plaques to papulosquamous changes to nodules. Rare extranodal sites for peripheral T cell lymphomas include gastrointestinal and genital tract locations.

C84.6 Anaplastic large cell lymphoma, ALK-positive

This is a rare lymphoma more common in young adults, affecting twice as many males as females. The lymphoma will usually be made of aberrant, cancerous T cell lymphocytes, but sometimes remains unclear as to cell type, designated as null (neither B or T) cell type. Specific 'hallmark' cells are present in ALCL with abundant cytoplasm, kidney-shaped nucleus, and an eosinophilic region located around the nucleus. The classic, systemic form is found most often in younger patients and is associated with a chromosomal abnormality resulting in production of anaplastic lymphoma kinase protein (ALK positive) in about 70% of cases. The first sign is often painless enlargement of lymph nodes in the neck, armpit, or groin, loss of weight, night sweats, and often presents when it is already advanced and displays symptoms of both systemic and extranodal, solid organ sites. This is a high-grade, aggressively growing cancer that needs prompt chemotherapy treatment. Newer therapies target the CD30 gene and ALK.

Note: ALCL can present in two ways: systemic, divided into two groups— either ALK positive or negative, and cutaneous, either in or on the skin. The primary cutaneous form is not reported here, but with C86.6-. ALK negative is reported with C84.7-.

C84.7 Anaplastic large cell lymphoma, ALK-negative

Anaplastic large cell lymphoma is a rare lymphoma more common in young adults, affecting twice as many males as females. The lymphoma will usually be made of aberrant, cancerous T cell lymphocytes, but sometimes remains unclear as to cell type, designated as null (neither B or T) cell type. Specific 'hallmark' cells are present in ALCL with abundant cytoplasm, kidney-shaped nucleus, and an eosinophilic region located around the nucleus. The ALK-negative systemic form; however is commonly found in patients over age 60 and does not have the usual chromosomal abnormality that causes anaplastic lymphoma kinase (ALK) protein to be expressed. ALK negative ALCL does respond to chemotherapy but mostly relapses within 5 years and these cases are often treated more aggressively with autologous stem cell transplantation. The first sign is often painless enlargement of lymph nodes in the neck, armpit, or groin, loss of weight, and night sweats. It often presents when it is already advanced and displays symptoms of both systemic and extranodal, solid organ sites.

Note: ALCL can present in two ways: systemic, divided into two groups— either ALK positive or negative, and cutaneous, either in or on the skin. The primary cutaneous form is not reported here, but with C86.6-. ALK positive is reported with C84.6-.

C86.6 Primary cutaneous CD30-positive T-cell proliferations

Use this code to report the primary cutaneous form of anaplastic large cell lymphoma limited to the skin. This is slow growing and may manifest as a solitary nodule or tumor or multiple, raised red lesions which do not go away. The lesions can appear on any part of the body, tend to itch and ulcerate. This is an indolent, or slow-growing lymphoma and the skin lesions may be present for a long term before being diagnosed. In almost all cases, it is confined to the skin. Spontaneous remission with relapses also confined to the skin often occur, and chemotherapy is used when cutaneous lesions are generalized.

C88 Malignant immunoproliferative diseases and certain other B-cell lymphomas

Disorders of the immune system involving abnormal proliferation of primary cells including B-cells, T-cells, Natural Killer (NK) cells and/or excessive production of immunoglobulins (antibodies).

C88.0 Waldenström macroglobulinemia

Macroglobulinemia is a malignant disease of the blood and lymphatic system. It manifests as the production of an excessive number of large antibodies called macroglobulins, which in turn cause the production of an excess amount of an antibody called IgM. IgM causes thickening of the blood, which in turn results in symptoms of fatigue, headache, weight loss, a tendency to bleed easily, vision problems, confusion, dizziness, and loss of coordination. Treatment of this disease is usually through a combination of medication (including blood-thinners) and chemotherapy.

C88.2 Heavy chain disease

Heavy chain diseases (HCDs) are rare lymphoplasmacytic proliferation disorders characterized by the overproduction of abnormal monoclonal proteins resulting in structurally incomplete immunoglobulin heavy chains that are unbounded by light chains. HCDs are recognized based on the class of immunoglobulin heavy chain produced, such as gamma HCD (IgG), also known as Franklin disease, and Mu HCD (IgM). Gamma HCD is usually associated with a systemic lymphoma, while Mu HCD resembles chronic lymphocytic leukemia. Nearly one third of all Franklin disease cases have an associated autoimmune disorder, such as lupus erythematosus or rheumatoid arthritis. Patients often report progressive weakness, malaise, fatigue, upper respiratory tract infections, dysphagia from soft palate edema, intermittent fevers, and lymphoma-like illness such as splenomegaly, hepatomegaly, and lymphadenopathy. The clinical course may be rapidly progressive or long and uneventful, but is still generally malignant with a survival time of months to 5 years. Most patients eventually succumb to bacterial infections.

C88.3   Immunoproliferative small intestinal disease

This reports alpha heavy chain disease, which is the most commonly reported heavy chain disease (HCD). HCDs are rare lymphoplasmacytic proliferation disorders caused by the overproduction of an abnormal monoclonal protein resulting in structurally incomplete immunoglobulin heavy chains unbounded by light chains. HCDs are recognized based on the class of immunoglobulin heavy chain that is produced. Alpha HCD (IgA) is actually a form of mucosa associated lymphoid tissue (MALT) lymphoma, also known as immunoproliferative small intestinal disease, IPSID, or Mediterranean lymphoma, recognized as the late stage of alpha HCD. This type of HCD tends to occur in younger patients in the Mediterranean area with a median age under 40 and presents with diarrhea, steatorrhea, abdominal pain, weight loss, and fever. It is often associated with a chronic *Campylobacter jejuni* infection and malabsorption syndrome. Lymphoplasmacytic infiltrate is present, forming lymphoepithelial lesions, usually involving the mucosa and submucosa, causing extensive villous atrophy of the small intestinal mucosa, that may form tumors. Prognosis is poor.

C88.8 Other malignant immunoproliferative diseases

Myelofibrosis with myeloid metaplasia is a progressive disorder in which bone marrow is initially overactive, and then slowly becomes replaced by scar tissue (fibrosis), which in turn reduces the patient's ability to produce new blood cells, resulting in chronic anemia. Signs and symptoms include fatigue, enlarged liver and spleen, bruising, bleeding, fever, pallor, and night sweats. This condition is also referred to as agnogenic myeloid metaplasia, idiopathic, chronic, or primary myelofibrosis and develops without known cause. This disease is accurately described as a type of chronic leukemia, that may develop into acute leukemia, occurring mainly in persons over the age of 50.

Note: Use this code for other lymphatic and hematopoietic tissue diseases such as unspecified chronic lymphoproliferative disease, megakaryocytic myelosclerosis, unspecified chronic myeloproliferative disease, and acute panmyelosis.

C90.0 Multiple myeloma

Multiple myeloma is the most common type of plasma cell tumor. Plasma cells are the white blood cells that make antibodies. This cancer begins in the blood cells and affects the bones, since plasma cells reside mainly in bone marrow, but it is not really considered a bone cancer. When plasma cells turn abnormal, they become myeloma cells. As they replicate out of control, they accumulate throughout the bone marrow to form tumors, called multiple myelomas, causing bone pain usually worse with movement. Normal blood cell formation and bone marrow function is affected, resulting in anemia and fatigue; a lack of normal white blood cells to fight off infections; and a shortage of platelets, causing excessive bleeding. Myeloma cells also secrete a substance that stimulates osteoclasts to dissolve bone, leading to weak and fractured bone tissue.

C90.1 Plasma cell leukemia

Plasma cell leukemia (PCL) is considered a variant of multiple myeloma that resembles a very late stage, and is very rare and aggressive. Survival rates are in the months. It is defined by an overabundant, significant number of circulating plasma cells in the peripheral blood. Primary types arise from a malignant plasma cell clone proliferation in peripheral blood. Secondary types arise from cloning in an underlying multiple myeloma. Patients have anemia, cytopenias, recurrent infections, pathologic fractures, renal failure, enlarged organs, lymphadenopathy, and more compromised bone marrow function. PCL exhibits some clinically distinct immunophenotypes and cytogenetic abnormalities that differentiate it from myeloma. Treatment is aimed at prolonging life with maximum quality.

C91 Lymphoid leukemia

Lymphoid leukemia is also called lymphocytic or lymphoblastic leukemia. Leukemias are cancers that affect the blood forming cells in the bone marrow and spread to the bloodstream and other parts of the body, such as the lymph nodes, liver, spleen, and brain. The main type of cell forming the lymphoid tissue of the immune system is the lymphocyte, which develops from immature lymphoblasts. These blasts normally constitute about 5 percent of healthy bone marrow, but in lymphoblastic leukemia, these cells remain abnormally immature and proliferate continuously, filling up the bone marrow, preventing the production of normal blood cells, and spilling out into the bloodstream and lymph system, traveling to the brain and other organs.

Neoplasms

C86.6 – C91

C91.0 Acute lymphoblastic leukemia [ALL]

Also known as acute lymphocytic or acute lymphoid leukemia (ALL), this is the most common type of leukemia affecting children, mainly those under 10 years of age. This type of leukemia occurs when immature lymphocytic white blood cells, called lymphoblasts, reproduce abnormally fast in the bone marrow without maturing properly. They crowd out healthy blood cell production and then spread into the bloodstream and other organs. ALL comes on suddenly and develops quickly. It can be fatal in a few months if not treated. Symptoms include fever, fatigue, aching bones and joints, swollen glands, bleeding gums, bruising or petechiae, slow healing cuts, and frequent infections.

C91.1 Chronic lymphocytic leukemia of B-cell type

Also known as chronic lymphoid or chronic lymphoblastic leukemia (CLL), this is the most common type of leukemia affecting adults and is rare in those under 30, with most cases occurring between the ages of 60 and 70. This type of leukemia is caused when immature lymphocytic white blood cells, called lymphoblasts, do not mature properly or mature only part of the way, and are unable to function normally. They continue to proliferate and live too long. The natural process of older cells dying off and being replaced by new cells that have matured properly is upset. Over time, these abnormal cells accumulate in large numbers and crowd out healthy blood cells, leading to life-threatening problems. Typical leukemic symptoms develop slowly because the cancer progresses at a slow rate.

C91.4 Hairy cell leukemia

Hairy cell leukemia, also called leukemic reticuloendotheliosis, is a rare cancer of the blood that comprises only about two percent of leukemias diagnosed each year. This type occurs 5 times more often in men than women, usually in those over 55. This leukemia is caused by abnormal growth of B cell lymphocytes that appear 'hairy' under the microscope because of fine filament projections on their surface. This leads to low blood counts of white blood cells, red blood cells, and platelets. Symptoms include weakness, fatigue, easy bruising, swollen lymph glands, weight loss, recurrent infections, fevers, and early feeling of fullness after eating only a little.

C91.9 Lymphoid leukemia, unspecified

Unspecified lymphoid, or lymphocytic, leukemia reports the subacute classification that simply refers to the disease duration and rate of progression not being quite as fast as the rapidly progressing, sudden onset of acute lymphoid leukemia. Subacute forms are known to have a few months' duration, but not last the 1-2 years found in chronic cases.

C91.Z Other lymphoid leukemia

This code is used to report aleukemic and subleukemic forms of lymphoid (lymphocytic or lymphoblastic) leukemia, in which the leukemia occurs without elevated levels of white blood cells in the blood. This type of classification is based on the leukocyte count found in the peripheral blood. In subleukemic cases, the total white blood cell count is normal at less than 15,000 WBC per cu mm, but immature or abnormal forms of lymphocytes are present in the peripheral blood. In aleukemic leukemia, the white blood cell count is also less than 15,000 WBC per cu mm with no immature or abnormal forms of lymphocytes in the peripheral blood. The difference between these forms depends on thorough searching for abnormal cells. This also reports T-cell large granular lymphocytic leukemia associated with rheumatoid arthritis.

C92 Myeloid leukemia

Myeloid leukemia is also called myelogenous, myelocytic, myeloblastic, granulocytic, and nonlymphocytic leukemia. Leukemias are cancers that affect the blood forming cells in the bone marrow and spread to the bloodstream and other parts of the body, such as the lymph nodes, liver, spleen, brain, and testes. The type of cell responsible for myeloid leukemia is the immature or primitive blood forming cell called the myeloblast. The myeloblast develops into granulocytes, other types of infection-fighting white blood cells besides lymphocytes, which include neutrophils, basophils, and eosinophils. These types of cells have granules of different sizes containing enzymes and other substances that destroy invading bacteria. Myeloblasts normally constitute a small percent of healthy bone marrow, but in myeloblastic leukemia, these cells remain abnormally immature and proliferate continuously, filling up the bone marrow, preventing the production of normal blood cells. They spill out into the bloodstream and lymph system and travel to other organs.

C92.0 Acute myeloblastic leukemia

Also known as acute myelogenous, myeloid, myelocytic, granulocytic, and nonlymphocytic leukemia (AML), this is the most common type of acute leukemia in adults and accounts for half of leukemias diagnosed in teenagers and people in their 20s. This type of leukemia occurs when immature granulocytic white blood cells, called myeloblasts, reproduce abnormally fast in the bone marrow without maturing properly, crowd out healthy blood cell production, and then spread into the bloodstream and other organs. AML gets worse very quickly if not treated and can be fatal in a few months. Symptoms include fever, weakness, fatigue, aching bones and joints, swollen glands, bleeding gums, bruising or petechiae, slow healing cuts, and frequent infections.

C92.1 Chronic myeloid leukemia, BCR/ABL-positive

Also known as chronic myelogenous, myeloblastic, myelocytic, granulocytic, and nonlymphocytic leukemia (CML), this is a relatively uncommon type of leukemia. Most cases occur in adults between 25 and 60 years old. BCR/ABL-positive CML has a cytogenetic code abnormality known as the Philadelphia (Ph) chromosome, resulting from reciprocal translocation that causes fusion of the BCR and ABL gene. This combined oncogene encodes a protein causing aberrant Abl tyrosine kinase activity that is causally related to CML, although this is not an inherited disorder. This leukemia develops when immature granulocytic white blood cells, called myeloblasts, or myeloid cells, do not mature properly or mature only part of the way, and are unable to function like mature basophils, neutrophils, and eosinophils. They continue to proliferate and live too long. The natural process of older cells dying off and being replaced by new cells that have matured properly is upset. Over time, these abnormal cells accumulate in large numbers and crowd out healthy blood cells, leading to life-threatening problems. Symptoms develop less dramatically than acute cases because the cancer progresses at a slower rate.

C92.2 Atypical chronic myeloid leukemia, BCR/ABL-negative

Atypical chronic myeloid leukemia (CML), BCR/ABL-negative is a relatively uncommon type of leukemia and more rare than BCR/ABL-positive or Philadelphia CML. Most cases occur with a median age of about 70 or 80 years old. This leukemia develops when immature granulocytic white blood cells, called myeloblasts, or myeloid cells, do not mature properly or mature only part of the way, and are unable to function like mature basophils, neutrophils, and eosinophils. This rare type of leukemia is characterized by increased numbers of both mature and immature neutrophils in the blood; neutrophil precursors in the blood constituting more than 10% of the white blood cells; monocytes less than 10%; and basophils less than 2%. The immature granulocytes proliferate with myelodysplasia associated with the bone marrow. The blood patterns are similar to typical CML, but without the Philadelphia chromosome or fused BCR/ABL gene. It presents with anemia, fatigue, thrombocytopenia, and splenomegaly.

C92.3 Myeloid sarcoma

This is a type of solid malignant tumor associated with myelogenous leukemia, in which immature leukemic white blood cells of the myeloid type form a solid, green-colored tumor, also called a granulocytic sarcoma or chloroma.

C92.4 Acute promyelocytic leukemia

Acute promyelocytic leukemia is an aggressive, specified subtype of AML, associated with a chromosomal abnormality.

C92.9 Myeloid leukemia, unspecified

Unspecified myeloid leukemia reports the subacute type classification which simply refers to the disease duration and rate of progression not being quite as fast as the rapidly progressing, sudden onset of acute myeloid leukemia. Subacute forms are known to have a few months' duration, but not to last the 1-2 years found in chronic cases.

C92.Z   Other myeloid leukemia

This code is used to report aleukemic and subleukemic forms of myeloid leukemia, in which the leukemia occurs without elevated levels of white blood cells in the blood. This type of classification is based on the leukocyte count found in the peripheral blood. In subleukemic cases, the total white blood cell count is normal at less than 15,000 WBC per cu mm, but immature or abnormal forms of myelocytes are present in the peripheral blood. In aleukemic leukemia, the white blood cell count is also less than 15,000 WBC per cu mm with no immature or abnormal forms of myelocytes in the peripheral blood. The difference between these forms depends on thorough searching for abnormal cells.

C93   Monocytic leukemia

Monocytic leukemia is also called monocytoid and monoblastic leukemia. Leukemias are cancers that affect the blood forming cells in the bone marrow and spread to the bloodstream and other parts of the body, such as the lymph nodes, liver, spleen, and central nervous system. The type of cell responsible for monocytic leukemia is the immature or primitive blood forming cell called the monoblast. The monoblast develops into a mature monocyte, another type of infection-fighting white blood cell related to granulocytes. Monocytes circulate in the bloodstream for about a day before entering tissues, where they become macrophages (histiocytes) that destroy invading germs by engulfing and ingesting them. Monoblasts normally constitute a small percent of healthy bone marrow, but in monoblastic leukemia, these cells remain abnormally immature and proliferate continuously, filling up the bone marrow, preventing the production of normal blood cells, spilling out into the bloodstream and lymph system, and traveling to other organs.

C93.0   Acute monoblastic/monocytic leukemia

Acute monoblastic, monocytic leukemia (AML M5) occurs when immature monocytic white blood cells, called monoblasts, reproduce abnormally fast in the bone marrow without maturing properly into monocytic macrophages (histiocytes). They crowd out healthy blood cell production and then spread into the bloodstream and other organs. AML M5 is a rare disease sometimes considered an uncommon type of acute myelogenous leukemia, in which the predominating cells are of the monocyte lineage. Acute monocytic leukemia gets worse very quickly if not treated and can be fatal in a few months. Symptoms include fever, weakness, fatigue, aching bones and joints, swollen glands, bleeding gums, bruising or petechiae, slow healing cuts, and frequent infections.

C93.1   Chronic myelomonocytic leukemia

This is a rare type of leukemia also known as chronic monocytic leukemia. This type of leukemia develops when immature monocytic white blood cells, called monoblasts, do not mature properly or mature only part of the way, and are unable to function like mature macrophages (histiocytes). They continue to proliferate and live too long. The natural process of older cells dying off and being replaced by new cells that have matured properly is upset. Over time, these abnormal cells accumulate in large numbers and crowd out healthy blood cells, leading to life-threatening problems. Symptoms develop less dramatically than acute cases because the cancer progresses at a slower rate.

C93.9   Monocytic leukemia, unspecified

Unspecified monocytic leukemia reports the subacute type of classification which simply refers to disease duration and rate of progression not being quite as fast as the rapidly progressing, sudden onset of acute leukemia. Subacute forms are known to have a few months' duration, but not to last the 1-2 years found in chronic cases.

C93.Z   Other monocytic leukemia

This code is used to report aleukemic and subleukemic forms of monocytic leukemia, in which the leukemia occurs without elevated levels of white blood cells in the blood. This type of classification is based on the leukocyte count found in the peripheral blood. In subleukemic cases, the total white blood cell count is normal at less than 15,000 WBC per cu mm, but immature or abnormal forms of monocytes are present in the peripheral blood. In aleukemic leukemia, the white blood cell count is also less than 15,000 WBC per cu mm with no immature or abnormal forms of monocytes in the peripheral blood. The difference between these forms depends on thorough searching for abnormal cells.

C94.0   Acute erythroid leukemia

Acute erythroid leukemia, also called erythroleukemia, is a malignant neoplasm of the bone marrow that results in an overproduction of red blood cells.

C94.2   Acute megakaryoblastic leukemia

Megakaryocytic leukemia is a form of leukemia which produces abnormally large-sized blood cells. These cells can impede blood flow or block smaller vessels and capillaries, in addition to causing the usual symptoms of leukemia.

C96.0   Multifocal and multisystemic (disseminated) Langerhans-cell histiocytosis

Disseminated, or multisystemic Langerhans cell histiocytosis is also known as Letterer-Siwe disease or progressive histiocytosis X. This disease occurs in very early childhood from autosomal recessive inheritance and is rapidly fatal when not treated. It presents with cutaneous lesions that look like seborrheic dermatitis; enlargement of the liver, spleen, and lymph nodes typical of lymphoma; hemorrhagic problems; and progressive anemia.

Note: The adult form of pulmonary Langerhans cell histiocytosis is coded to J84.82.

C96.2   Malignant mast cell tumor

Malignant mast cell tumors are also called malignant mastocytomas or malignant mast cell sarcomas. They are very rare in humans. The spectrum of disease may range from solitary or multiple cutaneous mastocytoma(s) to systemic mast cell disease and malignant mastocytosis, which is uniformly fatal. The disease is caused by overproliferation and excessive accumulation of mast cells in different tissue and the release of mast cell mediators, most often seen in the skin but also involving other tissues such as bone, bone marrow, and the nervous system.

C96.A   Histiocytic sarcoma

Histiocytic sarcoma, or malignant histiocytosis, is a rare disease caused by the malignant proliferation of histiocytes—immune cells called macrophages that eat foreign invaders. The histiocytes invade organs and tissues, attacking bones, skin, lung, liver, spleen, and other sites. Most cases affect young adults and children around age 10. Malignant histiocytosis has a poor prognosis and progresses very quickly. Symptoms include fever, weight loss, sweating, and enlarged lymph glands, liver, and spleen. Skin involvement appears as purple or skin-colored lumps that can ulcerate. Holes in bones may be seen on x-ray with increased calcium levels in the blood. Other blood cell counts decrease, causing anemia, lack of clotting, and low white cell counts.

D00   Carcinoma in situ of oral cavity, esophagus and stomach

Carcinoma in situ is a tumor that has the characteristics of malignancy and is undergoing aberrant growth changes but still remain contained and has not invaded other tissues. Many forms of cancer are initially carcinomas in situ, but are not detected early enough. If a neoplasm that was previously diagnosed and coded as carcinoma in situ is later found to have invaded the surrounding tissue, it must be recoded as a malignant tumor.

D01.3   Carcinoma in situ of anus and anal canal

The anal canal is the terminal part of the large intestine situated between the rectum and anus, below the level of the pelvic diaphragm. The anal canal is approximately 2.5 to 4 cm long, extending from the anorectal junction to the anus. It is directed downwards and backwards. It is differentiated from the rectum by the transition of the internal surface from endodermal to skinlike ectodermal tissue.

Neoplasms

C92.Z – D01.3

D01.5 Carcinoma in situ of liver, gallbladder and bile ducts

The liver is a large, flat organ positioned just above and in front of the stomach, which produces bile, a substance that aids the body in the digestion of fats. This code includes the whole biliary system, including the biliary passages that connect the liver to the small intestine and the gallbladder.

D02.0 Carcinoma in situ of larynx

The larynx, or voicebox, is an organ in the neck involved in protection of the trachea and sound production. The larynx houses the vocal cords, and is situated at the point where the upper tract splits into the trachea and the esophagus.

D07 Carcinoma in situ of other and unspecified genital organs

Carcinoma in situ in female genital organs has been linked to infection with the human papilloma virus. The malignancy develops over a period of time from dysplasia, the precancerous form of abnormal cell growth in tissues. As long as the cancer remains confined to its originating tissue and has not invaded other surrounding tissues, it is coded as 'in situ.'

D07.1 Carcinoma in situ of vulva

Vulvar carcinoma in situ is a rare disease of malignant cells in the female external genitalia, including the labia majora and minora, clitoris, the opening of the vagina, and its glands. The malignancy usually develops slowly over years from abnormal, dysplastic cells that grow on the surface of the skin. This abnormal growth of cells is a precancerous condition called dysplasia or vulvar intraepithelial neoplasia [VIN]. When the full thickness of epithelium has abnormal cells, particularly when the basement membrane has been invaded, then severe dysplasia, or VIN III, is diagnosed as vulvar carcinoma in situ. Chronic changes have usually been taking place in the skin for years, including itching, burning, and raised multifocal skin lesions that may be pink, white, gray, red, or hyperpigmented like a mole. The average age of VIN III diagnosis is 45-50 years old and has been associated with herpex simplex virus and granulomatous STDs in addition to the human papilloma virus. In those over 55, the cancer is usually unifocal, following years of itching and burning with lichen sclerosis changes, but no signs of viral DNA or VIN changes in neighboring tissue.

D07.2 Carcinoma in situ of vagina

A malignancy of vaginal cells that has developed from the continued abnormal growth of cells in a precancerous state, called dysplasia or vaginal intraepithelial neoplasia [VAIN]. This is similar to, though not as common as, what occurs in the cervix. When the level of dysplasia in individual cells has penetrated the epithelial layers deep enough, then severe dysplasia or VAIN III is diagnosed as vaginal carcinoma in situ. Vaginal carcinoma in situ may have no presenting symptoms and if the patient had been exposed to human papilloma virus as a causative agent, the virus could have incubated for up to 12 years before progressing to severe dysplasia. Pap smear tests that take cells from the vagina help to detect it.

D10 Benign neoplasm of mouth and pharynx

A benign neoplasm is one that is neither growing excessively nor causing destruction in the surrounding cells. Even so, it may cause dysfunction due to its size or its effect on adjacent tissue.

D14.0 Benign neoplasm of middle ear, nasal cavity and accessory sinuses

The sinuses are hollow chambers in the skull which serve to decrease the weight of the skull and serve as resonant chambers to affect the tone and quality of the person's voice. Though not a part of the respiratory system per se, the sinuses are connected to the nasal cavity by connecting tubes in order to equalize the air pressure within them to that of the outside, and are therefore usually classified with the upper respiratory system. This code includes the maxillary sinuses, the ethmoidal sinuses, the frontal sinus and the sphenoidal sinus in addition to the septum and cartilage of the nose, the eustachian tubes (which connect to the ears), and the nares, the openings that connect the nasal passages to the throat and the outside world.

D17 Benign lipomatous neoplasm

A lipoma is a benign neoplasm comprised of mature fat cells which can appear in any subcutaneous tissue. These tumors only require treatment if they are causing discomfort or are compressing an organ in such a way as to impede its function. They are the most common benign tumor in adults.

D18 Hemangioma and lymphangioma, any site

A hemangioma is a type of benign neoplasm that results in a mass of enlarged blood vessels, and is almost always either congenital or appears shortly after birth. When visible on the surface of the skin, this mass presents as a red to reddish-purple raised lesion of varying size. The principle complications from this disease are malformations due to the hemangioma pushing healthy tissue out of its way. Lymphangioma is a similar disorder, but affecting the lymph nodes instead of the blood vessels and is rarer than hemangioma.

D18.0 Hemangioma

Hemangioma typically begins in a rapid-growth phase, followed by a rest phase, and then an involutional phase in which it shrinks and, if small enough, disappears altogether. Smaller hemangiomas are generally left alone, while larger ones or those in areas where they may cause complications are generally either removed surgically or shrunk with a combination of steroid drugs and a special laser.

D21 Other benign neoplasms of connective and other soft tissue

A benign neoplasm is one that is neither growing excessively nor causing destruction in the surrounding cells. Even so, it may cause dysfunction due to its size or its effect on adjacent tissue. These connective tissues include the ligaments, tendons, muscle, fascia, blood vessels, bursa, synovia, cartilage, and fat.

D25 Leiomyoma of uterus

A leiomyoma is a benign neoplasm that appears in the smooth muscle of the uterus, and is also called a uterine fibroid or uterine myoma. The tumor may contain fatty, fibrous, or other tissue and is classified by its location in the tissue layers of the uterus. Symptoms are rare, and might include abdominal discomfort, frequent urination, and/or constipation.

D31 Benign neoplasm of eye and adnexa

A benign neoplasm is one that is neither growing excessively nor causing destruction in the surrounding cells. Even so, it may cause dysfunction due to its size or its effect on adjacent tissue. The adnexa for the eye includes extraocular muscles, connective and retrobulbar tissue of the eye and orbit, and peripheral nerves of the orbit. A benign tumor of the eye can have varying symptoms, including vision loss; floaters, spots, or squiggles in the field of vision, flashes of light, a dark spot on the iris, or a change in the position and/or shape of the eyeball.

D33 Benign neoplasm of brain and other parts of central nervous system

A benign neoplasm is one that is neither growing excessively nor causing destruction in the surrounding cells. It may cause dysfunction due to its size or its effect on adjacent tissue. A benign neoplasm of the brain and other parts of the nervous system may or may not present with symptoms, depending on the size and location of the tumor. The most common symptoms are headache, loss of coordination, weakness, and seizures. Other symptoms may include changes in concentration, memory, mental capacity, emotional state or alertness; nausea and/or vomiting; and vision and/or speech abnormalities.

D33.3 Benign neoplasm of cranial nerves

The cranial nerves are composed of twelve pairs of nerves that emanate directly from the brain (rather than the spinal cord, as all other nerves) and which control and receive information from the sensory organs and muscles in the head.

D35 Benign neoplasm of other and unspecified endocrine glands

The body's endocrine glands can also be afflicted by benign neoplasms, each causing its own set of symptoms. A tumor of a gland may be defined as functioning, by which it is meant that the tumor is causing an overproduction of one or more hormones, or nonfunctioning, in which case it is not. This distinction does not affect the coding of the neoplasm itself, but it may affect the coding of secondary complications.

D35.1 Benign neoplasm of parathyroid gland

The parathyroid glands are two pea-sized glands on either side of the thyroid in the neck. The parathyroid hormone controls the release of calcium into the bloodstream, which is obtained either from the bones, or from absorbing more calcium from food in the digestive tract. It may present with a small lump on the neck, kidney stones and/or failure, aching in the bones or osteoporosis, hoarseness, constipation, muscular weakness, and/or vomiting.

D35.2 Benign neoplasm of pituitary gland

The pituitary gland is a gland about the size of a pea that is in the center of the brain. In young people, a functioning pituitary tumor can cause abnormal growth in the hands and feet. In adults, it can cause what is known as Cushing's disease, which presents with an accumulation of fat in the face, high blood sugar, and muscular weakness. Other symptoms of either a functioning or non-functioning pituitary tumor include headaches, difficulty seeing, and nausea and vomiting due to pressure by the tumor on the surrounding nerves.

D35.4 Benign neoplasm of pineal gland

The pineal gland is a small organ set in the ventricles of the brain. Its function is not entirely understood, but one thing it is known to do is produce melatonin, which regulates how much and when we sleep. It may present with increased cerebrospinal fluid due to blocking the ventricles, causing headaches, vomiting, balance loss, and vision problems similar to those found in pituitary cancer. A functioning pineal tumor may also cause sleep disorders.

D35.5 Benign neoplasm of carotid body

The carotid body comprises the division of the carotid artery into numerous smaller arteries that supply blood to both the inside and outside of the cranium. Tumors in this site, called chemodectomas, are benign only about 10-15% of the time, and usually present with blockage and decreased blood flow to the brain, as well as increased blood pressure below the blockage.

D37 Neoplasm of uncertain behavior of oral cavity and digestive organs

A neoplasm of uncertain behavior is one in which a cellular examination proves unable to determine whether the neoplasm is malignant or not. This is not to be confused with a neoplasm of unspecified behavior, which is one for which the documentation does not state the nature of the neoplasm and the coder cannot assign anything more specific. As with most neoplasms, those of uncertain behavior are coded by system and location.

D3A Benign neuroendocrine tumors

Both benign and malignant neuroendocrine tumors are generally classified as carcinoid and pancreatic endocrine tumors, which are often histologically indistinguishable. These tumors arise from hormone-producing cells throughout the body and are characterized by functional activity that produces hormonal syndromes, such as carcinoid syndrome or medulloadrenal hyperfunction. Rarely, the occurrence of neuroendocrine tumors may also be associated as a part of multiple endocrine neoplasia [MEN] syndrome, type 1. Pancreatic tumors are usually restricted to the pancreas. Carcinoid tumors arise from three areas that are grouped according to the embyonic site of origin: the foregut = bronchi, lungs, stomach, proximal duodenum, thymus; the midgut = second portion of duodenum, jejunum, ileum, cecum, ascending colon, and appendix;

hindgut = transverse, descending, and sigmoid colon, rectum, and organs of the genitourinary tract, such as the ovaries and testes.

Many carcinoid tumors behave like benign tumors, particularly in early stages. The occurrence of a carcinoid tumor having malignant metastasis is directly related to the size of the primary tumor. Those under 1 cm rarely metastasize and behave more benignly, while those over 2 cm frequently metastasize. These tumors are slow growing, difficult to diagnose, and often produce no symptoms, especially in early, benign stages. The signs of tumor vary with the organ of origin and are usually found incidentally during other procedures, such as an appendectomy or colonoscopy. Symptoms that actually cause people to seek medical attention are uncommon and tend to be vague, such as abdominal discomfort, flushing, telangiectastia, or spider-like veins on the face, diarrhea, hypotension, tachycardia, and pellagra. Benign carcinoids can be treated and cured. Surgical resection is the standard for curative approach.

Note: When multiple endocrine neoplasia syndrome is associated with any carcinoid tumor, the MEN syndrome should also be coded. Other associated endocrine syndromes, such as carcinoid syndrome, should be listed as an additional code.

D44 Neoplasm of uncertain behavior of endocrine glands

A neoplasm of uncertain behavior is one in which a cellular examination proves unable to determine whether the neoplasm is malignant or not. As with most neoplasms, those of uncertain behavior are coded by system and location. Within the endocrine system, the most common sites for a neoplasm of uncertain behavior are the pituitary gland, which produces hormones responsible for regulating the body's growth; the craniopharyngeal duct, which controls the pressure of craniospinal fluid around the brain; and the pineal gland, another small organ set in the ventricles of the brain that produces melatonin, which regulates sleep patterns.

D45 Polycythemia vera

Polycythemia vera (PV) is a rare blood disease with an abnormally increased production of red blood cells by the bone marrow. The increased amount of RBCs makes the blood thicker than normal. The blood then flows more slowly, preventing organs and tissues from receiving enough oxygen, even though the blood contains more oxygen-carrying red cells. The thicker blood also creates a condition in which clots can form more easily, blocking the flow of blood and potentially causing stroke or heart attack. PV is a chronic, serious disease that develops slowly and remains asymptomatic for years, becoming fatal if it is not diagnosed and treated. It is often discovered through routine blood tests done for other purposes. Signs and symptoms result from the slow flow of the thickened blood and the lack of tissue perfusion, causing dizziness, itching, headaches, vision changes, and serious problems such as angina and heart failure. The main cause of PV appears to be a gene mutation that is not inherited. Treatment is aimed at reducing the number of RBCs and the level of hemogloblin, bringing the blood back to a normal thickness, and avoiding serious complications. Phlebotomy may be done on a regular schedule to reduce the cell count and bring blood thickness back to normal. Medicines used to help keep the bone marrow in check from producing too many RBCs include hydroxyurea and interferon-alpha, as well as radiation treatments.

D46 Myelodysplastic syndromes

Myelodysplastic syndrome (MDS) is not any one disease, but is actually a group of closely related diseases involving the bone marrow's production of abnormal hematopoietic stem cells, the immature cells from which all blood cells develop. These immature cells are called blasts and their number within the bone marrow is an indicator in the type of MDS. The blasts fail to mature, which causes low blood counts (cytopenia) of one or more cell types, such as anemia (red blood cells), neutropenia (white blood cells), thrombocytopenia (platelets), or pancytopenia (all blood cell types). The number and type of cytopenia(s) present is another important indicator of the type of MDS. Faulty hematopoiesis in MDS also causes dysplasia seen in one or more lines of blood cell production. Low grade myelodysplastic syndromes coded in this category include refractory anemia (RA); refractory anemia with excess blasts-1 (RAEB-1); and refractory anemia with ringed siteroblasts (RARS). Refractory anemia with excess blasts-2 (RAEB-2) is a high grade myelodysplastic syndrome treated as acute myeloid leukemia cancer on a less frequent basis. Dysplasias in cell lines may include oval erythrocytes and other misshapen cells, nucleated red blood cells, agranular neutrophils, and large platelets.

Risk factors for myelodysplastic syndromes, besides a cytogenetic basis, include any type of previous chemotherapy or radiation treatment; exposure to heavy metals, such as mercury and lead; and exposure to other chemicals such as fertilizers, pesticides, benzene, and tobacco smoke. Myelodysplastic syndromes do not manifest in specifically identifiable symptoms. They are most often detected by tests that examine the blood and bone marrow. Symptoms include weakness, fatigue, pale skin, shortness of breath, petechiae, and easy bruising. Treatment and prognosis depend on the health and age of the patient; the level of manifesting symptoms, such like anemia, bleeding, or infection; the patient's level of risk for leukemia; chromosomal changes; and the number of blast cells present in the bone marrow as well as how many types of blood cells are affected. High grade cases may be treated the same as acute myeloid leukemia on a less frequent basis.

D46.0 Refractory anemia without ring sideroblasts, so stated

Refractory anemia does not respond to treatment targeted at increasing hemoglobin and red blood cell counts. There are too few red blood cells in the patient's blood, while the number of white blood cells and platelets remains normal. In refractory anemia without an excess of blasts, the condition has less than 5% immature blast cells in the bone marrow.

D46.1 Refractory anemia with ring sideroblasts

Refractory anemia remains unresponsive to treatment that should increase hemoglobin counts and the number of red blood cells. There are too few red blood cells in the patient's blood, while the number of white blood cells and platelets remains normal. In refractory anemia with ring sideroblasts (RARS), the red blood cells that are present have too much iron contained within the cell. The developing red blood cells cannot use the iron needed to produce hemoglobin and the iron forms a visible dark ring.

D46.20   Refractory anemia with excess of blasts, unspecified

Refractory anemia remains unresponsive to treatment that should increase hemoglobin counts and the number of red blood cells. There are too few red blood cells in the patient's blood, while the number of white blood cells and platelets remains normal. In refractory anemia with an excess of blasts (RAEB), approximately 5-19% of cells in the bone marrow are blasts. There may also be accompanying changes in white blood cells and platelets. RAEB has the potential to develop into acute myeloid leukemia.

D46.22 Refractory anemia with excess of blasts 2

Refractory anemia with excess blasts-2 (RAEB-2) is a high grade myelodysplastic syndrome in which there is cytopenia of at least two types of blood cells; however, this myelodysplastic disease type is primarily determined by the percentage of immature blasts in the bone marrow which is between 5%-29%. These patients receive the same chemotherapy regimens delivered to patients with acute myeloid leukemia, but less frequently.

D46.4   Refractory anemia, unspecified

Refractory anemia, unspecified is any type of anemia that is not further identified that remains unresponsive to treatment which should increase hemoglobin counts and the number of red blood cells.

D46.9 Myelodysplastic syndrome, unspecified

Myelodysplastic syndrome, also called myelodysplasia, or preleukemia, is actually a group of closely related diseases involving the bone marrow's production of abnormal hematopoietic stem cells, the immature cells from which all blood cells develop. This causes low blood counts of one or more cell types, such as anemia, neutropenia, thrombocytopenia, or pancytopenia and precedes the development of acute myelogenous or myeloid leukemia.

D46.A Refractory cytopenia with multilineage dysplasia

Refractory cytopenia is low blood counts of one or more cell types such as red blood cells and platelets, that remains unresponsive to treatment aimed at increasing the numbers of deficient blood cells. Although anemia is the most common type of low blood cell count, refractory thrombocytopenia as the presenting cytopenia is reported here. In refractory cytopenia with multilineage dysplasia, less than 5% of cells in the bone marrow are immature blast cells, while less than 1% of cells in the blood are blasts. This condition can progress to acute myeloid leukemia.

D46.B Refractory cytopenia with multilineage dysplasia and ring sideroblasts

Refractory cytopenia is low blood counts of at least two or more cell types such as red blood cells and platelets, that remains unresponsive to treatment aimed at increasing the numbers of deficient blood cells. Although anemia is the most common type of low blood cell count, refractory thrombocytopenia as the presenting cytopenia is reported here. In refractory cytopenia with multilineage dysplasia, less than 5% of cells in the bone marrow are immature blast cells, while less than 1% of cells in the blood are blasts. In cases where red blood cells are affected, they may contain extra iron. The developing red blood cells cannot use the iron needed to produce hemoglobin and the iron forms a visible dark ring. This condition can progress to acute myeloid leukemia.

D46.C Myelodysplastic syndrome with isolated del(5q) chromosomal abnormality

Myelodysplastic syndromes are linked in half of cases to a cytogenetic basis, particularly the complex abnormality involving the deletion of all or part of a specific chromosome. A deletion involving a specific portion of the 5q chromosome, or 5q minus syndrome, represents a unique subset of myelodysplastic patients and may be involed in up to thirty percent of cases. The cytogenetic abnormality causal relationship is still unclear although it is thought to cause the loss of function of a tumor suppressor gene related to the chromosomal deletion.

D47.1 Chronic myeloproliferative disease

Note: Use this code for other lymphatic and hematopoietic tissue diseases such as unspecified chronic lymphoproliferative disease, and chronic neutrophilic leukemia.

D47.2 Monoclonal gammopathy

Select this code to report monoclonal paraproteinemia. Monoclonal paraproteinemia is likewise a symptom rather than a cause of disease. This code indicates elevated levels of macroglobulins, or heavy plasma globulins, in the bloodstream, which may serve as an indicator of a malignant tumor in one or more blood-forming organs (e.g., the bone marrow, the liver, the spleen, etc.). This disorder is often associated with fatigue and weakness, easy bruising, and vision problems.

D47.3 Essential (hemorrhagic) thrombocythemia

Essential thrombocythemia (ET) is one of the rare myeloproliferative disorders characterized by uncontrolled over-production of certain types of blood cells by the bone marrow. Specifically, ET is an overproduction of megakaryocytes, which are the precursors to blood platelets — the cells essential to clotting — leading to a hugely increased concentration of platelets in the blood. Signs and symptoms include splenomegaly, hemorrhaging from the intestines, gums, or nose, and other minor bleeding, as well as blood vessel thrombosis. Clots in the small arteries of the fingers and toes cause pain, redness, burning, and even gangrene. This disorder is known by many synonyms, including essential hemorrhagic thrombocythemia, essential thrombocytosis, idiopathic hemorrhagic thrombocythemia, and primary thrombocytosis. In rare cases, ET may progress into acute leukemia or myelofibrosis.

D47.4 Osteomyelofibrosis

This includes myelofibrosis (myelosclerosis) with myeloid metaplasia, which is a progressive disorder in which bone marrow is initially overactive, and then slowly becomes replaced by scar tissue, which in turn reduces the patient's ability to produce new blood cells, resulting in chronic anemia. Signs and symptoms include fatigue, enlarged liver and spleen, bruising, bleeding, fever, pallor, and night sweats. This condition is also referred to as idiopathic chronic myelofibrosis and develops without known cause. This disease is accurately described as a type of chronic leukemia, that may develop into acute leukemia, occurring mainly in persons over the age of 50.

D47.Z1 Post-transplant lymphoproliferative disorder (PTLD)

Transplant patients taking immunosuppressive drugs to prevent rejection are vulnerable to malignancy and at risk for contracting infectious diseases. Post-transplant lymphoproliferative disorder (PTLD) appears in transplant patients following Epstein-Barr virus infection. It is characterized by B cell lymphocytes proliferating without control. When the immunosuppressive medication is reduced or discontinued, PTLD may regress spontaneously or it may need to be treated with anti-viral therapy. This disease is classified as a neoplasm of uncertain behavior because the uncontrolled B cell growth can cause tumor masses and bowel obstruction and progress to non-Hodgkin's lymphoma if left untreated.

D48.1 Neoplasm of uncertain behavior of connective and other soft tissue

A giant cell tumor of the tendon sheath is a fairly uncommon condition. It occurs when oversized cells with multiple nuclei appear in the tendon sheath, crowding the tendon and possibly causing an inflammation. The tumor itself is almost always benign, but may require surgical removal to protect the tendon.

D50 **Iron deficiency anemia**

Anemia is a condition in which the blood fails to convey sufficient oxygen to the body due to a decreased number of red-blood cells, a decrease in the amount of hemoglobin (the protein that enables blood to carry oxygen) per blood cell, or an abnormality in the shape of the blood cells being produced. Symptoms common to all forms of anemia include chest pain as the heart tries to increase blood-flow while being oxygen-deprived itself, fatigue, and shortness of breath. In iron deficiency anemia, the body lacks sufficient stores of iron to form hemoglobin properly.

D50.0 **Iron deficiency anemia secondary to blood loss (chronic)**

Anemia may be due to long-term bleeding, often from an ulcer or other internal source rather than an external wound, which uses up the body's stores of iron as the bone marrow tries to produce new blood cells to keep up with the loss.

D50.8 **Other iron deficiency anemias**

Note: Use this code to report anemia due to an iron deficiency in the patient's diet.

D51.0 **Vitamin B12 deficiency anemia due to intrinsic factor deficiency**

Anemia due to underlying Vitamin B12 malabsorption caused by inadequate production of intrinsic factor in the gastric mucosa. This is a chronic, progressive type of anemia, also known as pernicious anemia.

D51.3 **Other dietary vitamin B12 deficiency anemia**

Anemia due to a deficiency of vitamin B12 intake in the patient's diet. Since meat, fish, dairy products, and eggs are the best source of vitamin B12, this type of anemia is common to those pursuing a strictly vegan diet, as well as in alcoholics. Symptoms of this form of anemia include loss of appetite, diarrhea, numbness and tingling in the hands and/or feet, pale skin color that may include jaundice (a yellow tinge), and a soreness in the mouth and/or tongue. In advanced cases, the patient may also suffer from mental confusion.

D52 **Folate deficiency anemia**

Another cause of anemia is folate deficiency. Folate, more commonly called folic acid, is found naturally in dark-green leafy vegetables, citrus fruits, beans, whole grains, and liver. This form of anemia may also be called megaloblastic anemia, because it presents with unusually large blood cells, which are called megalocytes, or megaloblasts while still in the bone marrow. Its symptoms include those common to all forms of anemia and pale skin color.

D52.0 **Dietary folate deficiency anemia**

Another cause of anemia is due to folate deficiency. Folate, more commonly called folic acid, is found naturally in dark-green leafy vegetables, citrus fruits, beans, whole grains, and liver. This form of anemia may also be called megaloblastic anemia, because it presents with unusually large blood cells, which are called megalocytes, or megaloblasts while still in the bone marrow. Its symptoms include those common to all forms of anemia and pale skin color.

D53.1 **Other megaloblastic anemias, not elsewhere classified**

Non-dietary megaloblastic anemia may also be caused by leukemia, diseases of the bone marrow, certain hereditary disorders, chemotherapy, and excessive alcohol consumption.

D55.1 **Anemia due to other disorders of glutathione metabolism**

Anemias can also occur due to a disorder of glutathione metabolism. Gluthathione is a tripeptide that is widely used by red blood cells to protect against oxidative damage. If the substance is not available in sufficient amounts, high numbers of red blood cells may be damaged or destroyed, resulting in anemia.

D56 **Thalassemia**

Thalassemia is a common inherited disorder across the globe. Thalassemias are actually a family of hemoglobinopathies that range in severity from silent carriers of the trait who are asymptomatic to those that have disease requiring treatment. This is due to the fact that there are multiple genotype combinations that produce a wide spectrum of disease manifestation. Some people may carry the trait without being affected. Mild cases may experience fatigue and weakness from anemia that can be overcome with nutrition and exercise, and severe cases require life-long blood transfusions and chelation therapy for iron overload.

D56.0 **Alpha thalassemia**

Normal hemoglobin A (Hb A) makes up about 95% of all hemoglobin and is composed of four protein chains--two alpha and two beta globin chains arranged in a specific shape. Alpha thalassemia patients have a deficiency of the alpha globin. The decreased alpha globin produces fewer alpha globin chains and results in excess beta globin chains, which form unstable Hemoglobin H that leads to red blood cell breakage. Since there are two genes from each parent involved in the production of the hemoglobin chain, a different number of mutations are possible. Three and four gene mutations manifest the disease reported here. Three gene mutations result in moderate to severe symptoms, also called Hemoglobin H disease, of which Hemoglobin H Constant Spring is more severe. Four gene mutations cause alpha thalassemia major (severe) or hydrops fetalis in the newborn that can be fatal. This type is most prevalent in Southeast Asia, Malaysia, and southern China.

Note: One gene mutation results in a silent carrier who has no symptoms. Two gene mutations result in mild signs and symptoms, often called alpha thalassemia trait or alpha thalassemia minor. These milder cases are not reported here, but with D56.3. An additional code is necessary when reporting hydrops fetalis due to alpha thalassemia.

D56.1 **Beta thalassemia**

Normal hemoglobin A (Hb A) makes up about 95% of all hemoglobin and is composed of four protein chains--two alpha and two beta globin chains arranged in a specific shape. Beta thalassemia is a deficiency of beta globin production affecting either some or all formation of beta chains, leaving a relative excess of alpha chains that form insoluble aggregates that concentrate in immature red blood cells (RBCs). They interfere with RBC production, maturation, and membrane function, causing anemia. There is one gene from each parent involved. Two gene mutations manifest with moderate to severe disease reported here, also called Cooley's anemia, beta thalassemia major, homozygous beta thalassemia, and thalassemia intermedia. Babies born with this will appear healthy but develop signs within 2 years. This type is most prevalent in the Mediterranean area and Africa.

Note: Thalassemia major not specified as either alpha or beta is coded as beta type for the default.

Note: One gene mutation results in a condition with mild signs and symptoms called beta thalassemia trait or beta thalassemia minor. These milder cases are not reported here, but with D56.3.

D56.2   Delta-beta thalassemia

Although alpha and beta globin chains make up most hemoglobin (A), a minor variant of hemoglobin, called Hb A2, makes up about 3% of hemoglobin in the normal adult and is composed of two alpha and two delta chains. Mutations occur when gene deletions on the beta chain extend to include the delta chain gene. One from each parent is involved and so mutations can occur at different levels of severity. Homozygous delta-beta thalassemia or delta-beta thalassemia major is reported here. It occurs when both gene loci for the beta and the delta chain are completely deleted or inactivated on both chromosomes. This means that normal hemoglobin A and hemoglobin A2 cannot be produced and only the fetal form of hemoglobin (F) is present. Delta beta thalassemia occurs most commonly in people of Greece and Italy.

Note: When a beta chain gene mutation on only one chromosome extends to include the locus for the delta chain, it results in a milder condition called delta-beta thalassemia trait or delta-beta thalassemia minor. These milder cases are not reported here, but with D56.3.

D56.3   Thalassemia minor

Thalassemia minor is coded for all minor cases of the alpha, beta, and delta-beta forms of thalassemia as well as the trait or silent carrier forms that remain asymptomatic. These minor cases are caused by the lesser forms or number of gene mutations for each type and have milder signs and symptoms of anemia.

D56.5   Hemoglobin E-beta thalassemia

Hemoglobin E (Hb E) is an autosomal recessive variant of normal hemoglobin A (Hb A) caused by a variation in the beta globin chain gene. The substitution of lysine for glutamic acid at a certain location causes the formation of Hb E, which is mildly unstable and denatures easily. Hemoglobin E-beta thalassemia causes a chronic form of hemolytic anemia. Patients with the more severe form produce no Hb A. This can be life-threatening. Symptoms include moderate to severe microcytic anemia, heart failure, splenomegaly, hepatomegaly, and poor growth. Patients that still produce some Hb A will have mild anemia and nonpalpable spleen. This is most prevalent in Southeast Asia, particularly Cambodia, Laos, and Thailand.

Note: Hemoglobin E disease occurs when an infant inherits two copies of the variant gene--one from each parent. This is not considered a thalassemia and is coded elsewhere to D58.2.

D56.8   Other thalassemias

Other thalassemias include Hemoglobin C (Hb C) thalassemia in which this variant type of normal hemoglobin A (Hb A) is formed because of a variation in the beta globin chain gene. When it occurs along with a nullifying deletion in the beta chain, hemoglobin C thalassemia results which causes a mild, chronic form of hemolytic anemia similar to Hb SC disease, but no need for early intervention.

Note: Hemoglobin C disease is not considered a thalassemia and is reported as a hemoglobinopathy with code D58.2.

D56.9   Thalassemia, unspecified

Thalassemia is an inherited blood disease that causes a disruption in the normal production of hemoglobin and a high rate of red blood cell destruction. The type of thalassemia depends on which chain of the hemoglobin molecule is affected and the severity of the condition depends on the number of gene mutations. Lower hemoglobin and fewer red blood cells cause anemia and symptoms of fatigue and weakness. Other symptoms include shortness of breath, pallor, jaundice, slow growth and delayed puberty, and dark urine. More severe cases have complications such as iron overload, bone deformities from bone marrow expansion, splenomegaly from the destruction of such a large number of red blood cells, and heart problems.

Note: Thalassemia is also sometimes called Mediterranean anemia as the genetic trait causing thalassemia is known to be prevalent in Mediterranean areas and it may or may not be documented as with other hemoglobinopathy.

D57   Sickle-cell disorders

Sickle-cell disorders, commonly known as sickle-cell anemias, are chronic, hereditary diseases occurring mainly in people of African descent. The patient's red blood cells are stiff and misshapen, being pointed like a crescent. These sickle-shaped cells inhibit the flow of blood through the body and have a shorter life span than normal red blood cells, which leads to anemia. Common symptoms of sickle cell disease include joint pains, fever, ulcers on the leg, jaundice, and a variety of other complications involving the spleen and weight-bearing bones. It is believed that the disease originated as a beneficial mutation in the tropical climates of Africa, as patients with sickle-cells seem to have enhanced protection from the malaria parasite. A determining factor in the selection of sickle cell codes is the type of hemoglobin and the presence of absence of crisis, in which the patient is at immediate risk of severe damage to bodily structures or even death.

D57.01   Hb-SS disease with acute chest syndrome

Sickle-cell thalassemia presenting with immediate life-threatening complications. Acute chest syndrome is a complication of sickle-cell disease in which blood clots form in the tiny blood vessels of the lungs. The repeated episodes of bleeding from the alveoli causes a buildup of hemosiderin in the lungs. Hemosiderin is a protein that stores iron until it is needed in the blood, but its buildup in the lungs causes difficulty breathing. This condition primarily effects children and young adults. Common symptoms include bleeding from the lungs, bloody mucous, and fluid accumulations in the lungs. Primary symptoms include chest pain, fever, coughing, anemia, and difficulty breathing.

Note: This does not include acute idiopathic pulmonary hemorrhage in infants.

D57.02   Hb-SS disease with splenic sequestration

Splenic sequestration occurs when blood vessels leading away from the spleen become blocked, trapping blood in the spleen.

D57.1   Sickle-cell disease without crisis

In this type of the disease, most or all of the patient's normal red blood cells have been replaced with sickle-shaped cells. The red blood cells are stiff and misshapen and contain abnormal hemoglobin S. The sickled red blood cells inhibit the flow of blood through vessels. This is the most severe type of the disease, producing chronic and severe anemia, as well as other disorders.

D57.20   Sickle-cell/Hb-C disease without crisis

Sickle-cell/Hb-C disease, or Hb-C sickle-cell anemia, is sometimes referred to as Hb-SC, without crisis. Patients with this condition have a higher ratio of normal red blood cells to sickle-cell red blood cells than patients with Hb-SS. Mild to moderate anemia may occur, and the patient may exhibit some of the symptoms listed above, but to a less severe degree than Hb-SS patients.

D57.3   Sickle-cell trait

A condition in which the patient carries genes for both normal and sickle-cell hemoglobin. This condition rarely produces adverse effects.

D57.411   Sickle-cell thalassemia with acute chest syndrome

Sickle-cell thalassemia presenting with immediate life-threatening complications. This condition is a complication of sickle-cell disease in which blood clots form in the tiny blood vessels of the lungs. Primary symptoms include chest pain, fever, coughing, anemia, and difficulty breathing.

Note: Code the sickle-cell disease in crisis first.

D58.0   Hereditary spherocytosis

Hereditary spherocytosis is a congenital condition in which the walls of red blood cells are thickened, making the cell more fragile. This condition causes chronic anemia, jaundice, fever, and abdominal pain.

D58.1   Hereditary elliptocytosis

Hereditary elliptocytosis is a genetic disorder in which the red blood cells are elliptical in shape. The disease can be mild, in which no more than 15% of red blood cells are deformed and the patient suffers no ill effects. In more severe cases the patient may experience anemia, jaundice, and gallstones as the affected red blood cells rupture, releasing their hemoglobin.

D59   Acquired hemolytic anemia

This category reports cases of hemolytic anemia from acquired conditions such as infections, poisonings, or exposure to dangerous physical agents that result in the premature destruction of red blood cells, as opposed to hereditary disorders causing anemia.

D59.3   Hemolytic-uremic syndrome

Hemolytic-uremic syndrome is a condition in which platelets become clogged in the narrow blood vessels within the kidneys, leading to the destruction of red blood cells and kidney failure. This condition can be caused by the *E. coli* bacteria, shigella bacteria, tumors, toxins, and other factors. Preliminary symptoms include severe abdominal pain, diarrhea, nausea, and vomiting.

D59.5   Paroxysmal nocturnal hemoglobinuria [Marchiafava-Micheli]

A condition in which the premature death of red blood cells leads to the presence of red blood cells in the urine, brought on by exertion, cold exposure, or other external forces.

D60   Acquired pure red cell aplasia [erythroblastopenia]

Acquired pure red cell aplasia (PRCA), also known as adult acquired red cell aplasia (with thymoma), is a rare disorder in which RBC precursor cells in the bone marrow decline severely and are nearly absent while WBC precursors are present at normal levels. The affected precursor cells have developed from stem cells and express erythropoietin receptors, so patients develop normochromic, normoblastic anemia with almost no reticulocytes. Acquired pure red cell aplasia can be idiopathic, occurring for unknown reasons. The chronic form is often associated with underlying disorders such as thymomas and autoimmune disease. The most common form is acute and self-limiting, secondary to drug- and viral-induced damage to erythrocyte precursor cells. Patients have typical anemia symptoms of fatigue, lethargy, and pale skin. Profound, transfusion-dependent anemia develops as a common morbidity.

D61   Other aplastic anemias and other bone marrow failure syndromes

Aplastic anemia is a condition in which bone marrow fails to produce sufficient numbers of red blood cells. The aplastic anemias are considered bone marrow disorders which also involve pancytopenia and not only anemia.

D61.01   Constitutional (pure) red blood cell aplasia

Constitutional red blood cell aplasia, also known as congenital or primary pure red cell aplasia, Diamond-Blackfan syndrome, or familial hypoplastic anemia, is a rare disorder of bone marrow that affects the production of precursors to red blood cells, while other blood cell types are produced normally. The disease develops in the neonatal period and presents as a severe form of anemia with isolated reduction of red blood cells, with almost half of affected individuals also having some type of congenital abnormality, such as cleft palate, cardiac defects, urogenital and craniofacial malformations, abnormalities in the upper limbs, and retarded growth.

D61.09   Other constitutional aplastic anemia

Other constitutional aplastic anemia, Fanconi's anemia, or congenital pancytopenia with malformations is characterized by a decreased number of all cellular elements in the blood accompanied by multiple congenital musculoskeletal and genitourinary anomalies with underdevelopment of the bone marrow.

D61.81   Pancytopenia

Pancytopenia is a decreased count of all elements in the blood; red blood cells, white blood cells, and platelets.

D61.810   Antineoplastic chemotherapy induced pancytopenia

Antineoplastic chemotherapy induced pancytopenia is a reduction in the numbers of red blood cells, white blood cells, and platelets. These are all short-lived, permanently differentiated cells that must be continually replenished through cycles of hematopoietic stem cell differentiation. All these cells become acutely depleted by the cytotoxic action of anticancer drugs, especially myelosuppressive types of antineoplastic therapy since blood cells are formed in the bone marrow and these drugs suppress bone marrow.

Note: Antineoplastic chemotherapy induced aplastic anemia is reported as drug-induced aplastic anemia with D61.1.

D61.811   Other drug-induced pancytopenia

Other drugs besides antineoplastic chemotherapy can induce pancytopenia, although rarely. These drugs include antibiotics, blood pressure medication, and heart medication.

D61.818   Other pancytopenia

Other pancytopenias can be induced by other diseases or conditions such as copper deficiency, severe folate deficiency, low dose arsenic poisoning, chronic radiation sickness, leishmaniasis, an overwhelming viral infection, hypersplenism, and systemic lupus erythematosus.

D61.82   Myelophthisis

Myelophthisis or myelopathic anemia, also called leukoerythroblastic anemia, is caused by abnormal foreign matter infiltrates, or lesions, occupying the bone marrow and suppressing bone marrow function. This type of anemia may be brought on by other neoplastic disease processes or tuberculosis. Myelophthisis is characterized by the presence of nucleated red blood cells and immature neutrophils (myeloid blast cells) circulating in the blood.

Note: The underlying disorder should also be coded.

D63   Anemia in chronic diseases classified elsewhere

Anemia is the low concentration of hemoglobin, a protein found on red blood cells (RBCs). Hemoglobin is necessary for the transport of oxygen molecules throughout the body. Anemia may result from different causes, such as bleeding, fragile blood cells that have a shorter life span, or improper production of cells by the bone marrow that are connected to other serious, chronic diseases classified elsewhere, such as a cancerous condition, or chronic kidney disease.

Note: The underlying condition or disease must be coded first when reporting anemia occurring with a chronic disease.

D64   Other anemias

This category includes sideroblastic anemia, which is a blood disorder in which the ability of bone marrow to produce normal red blood cells is impaired. The bone marrow produces red blood cells with insufficient iron to make hemoglobin. A patient suffering from this condition will have sideroblasts, which are deformed red blood cells, in their bloodstream. This disease is usually hereditary and sex linked (D64.0) but may be acquired through disease (D64.1), alcohol abuse, or from poisoning or adverse affects of certain toxins and drugs (D64.2).

D64.81   Anemia due to antineoplastic chemotherapy

This type of anemia is estimated to be one of the most common side effects of cancer treatment with antineoplastic chemotherapy, affecting up to 60% of cancer patients. The production of red blood cells is interrupted or inhibited by the cancer and its treatment, reducing the supply of red blood cells available to the body. This type of anemia is rarely destructive to the red blood cells themselves, nor truly aplastic in nature, (which causes the bone marrow to be wiped out). The anemia caused by antineoplastic chemotherapy is diagnosed with a blood test that measures the RBC volume in whole blood. The changes are usually short-lived, although the resulting fatigue affects the patient's quality of life by reducing the ability to perform everyday activities.

Note: Aplastic anemia due to antineoplastic chemotherapy is reported with D61.1.

D65   Disseminated intravascular coagulation [defibrination syndrome]

Defibrination syndrome is a bleeding disorder characterized by an abnormal reduction in the elements used in blood clotting. Many different diseases and conditions can cause this disorder. Profuse bleeding in the late stages is the most common symptom.

D66   Hereditary factor VIII deficiency

There are several factors in blood that are necessary for clotting, and a deficiency of one or more of these factors leads to hemophilia. Factor VIII deficiency is the most common form of hemophilia, and is sometimes referred to as classic hemophilia or hemophilia A. This condition is hereditary and occurs exclusively in men. The most common symptom is profuse bleeding from injuries, as well as bleeding from the joints, muscles, digestive tract, and brain.

D67   Hereditary factor IX deficiency

Congenital factor IX disorder is also known as Hemophilia B or Christmas disease. This condition presents identically to factor VIII disorder (D66). Unlike factor VIII disorder, however, hereditary factor IX deficiency can affect women.

D68.0   Von Willebrand's disease

Von Willebrand's disease is a hereditary defect in which von Willebrand protein, a substance that helps protect the walls of red blood cells, is deficient or defective. This disease is more common that hemophilia, and is usually mild. Most patients will only need treatment following surgery, trauma, or other instances that lead to blood loss.

D68.1   Hereditary factor XI deficiency

Hereditary factor XI deficiency, also known as hemophilia C, is the least common form of hemophilia, and is more mild than factor VIII or factor IX disorder. This condition rarely requires medical treatment, except in the case of operations where blood loss may be extensive.

D68.2   Hereditary deficiency of other clotting factors

Deficiencies of the other clotting factors: I (fibrinogen), II (prothrombin), V (labile), VII (stable), X (Stuart-Prower), XII (Hageman), and XIII (Fibrin stabilizing) are rare, and produce symptoms similar to other hemophilia disorders with varying degrees of severity.

D68.31   Hemorrhagic disorder due to intrinsic circulating anticoagulants, antibodies, or inhibitors

These type of hemorrhagic disorders occur shen the body begins to produce its own antibodies or anticoagulants against certain blood clotting factors or its own blood proteins.

D68.311   Acquired hemophilia

Acquired hemophilia is also known as autoimmune hemophilia and secondary hemophilia and occurs when the body develops antibodies against its own blood-clotting proteins, usually Factor VIII, but antibodies against other factor proteins have also been reported. This disorder is rare but dangerous and is hard to detect because it can occur in both men and women with normal hemostasis who have no personal or family history of bleeding episodes. It also presents differently from hereditary hemophilia. This disorder causes spontaneous, uncontrolled bleeding into the skin, muscles, soft tissues, and mucous membranes, as well as internal or cerebral bleeding. Muscle bleeding can cause compartment syndrome and tissue death. Many cases are not diagnosed until surgery, childbirth, or trauma causes excessive and dangerous bleeding. Even though secondary hemophilia does not cause joint bleeding as in classical hemophilia, the

bleeding episodes are more frequent and more severe. Acquired hemophilia is diagnosed with lab tests that measure clotting time and Factor VIII levels.

D68.312   Antiphospholipid antibody with hemorrhagic disorder

Antiphospholipid antibodies are a rare autoimmune occurrence. The body makes antibodies that react against its own blood proteins. Systemic lupus erythematosus (SLE) inhibitor, or lupus anticoagulant, is the main antibody directed against protein phospholipid complexes, although other kinds may be present. These antibodies can occur even without having SLE. Phospholipids are present in all cell membranes and living cells, including blood cells. When these antibodies attack phospholipids, it normally causes a hypercoagulable state in which clots form in the arteries and veins and block blood flow, causing organ damage; however, antiphospholipids may also cause thrombocytopenia that can lead to serious bleeding. Although the presence of these antiphospholipids does not normally cause hemorrhagic disease, there have been some cases where these antibodies seem to be related to bleeding when no other problems were found. This code is reported for the presence of these antibodies with hemorrhagic disorder.

Note: Other antiphospholipid antibodies causing hemorrhagic disorder reported with this code include anticardiolipin, antiphosphatidylinositol, antiphosphatidylglycerol, and antiphosphatidylserine.

Note: Antiphospholipid antibodies normally cause a hypercoagulable state (as opposed to a hemorrhagic disorder) known as antiphospholipid antibody syndrome. When this syndrome is the case, report D68.61.

Note: When the presence of antiphospholipid antibodies or SLE inhibitor is found, but without diagnosis, report R76.0.

D68.318   Other hemorrhagic disorder due to intrinsic circulating anticoagulants, antibodies, or inhibitors

Hemorrhagic disorder due to intrinsic circulating anticoagulants, antibodies, or inhibitors covers other bleeding disorders not specifically coded elsewhere caused by the body's production of these substances against its own blood proteins. This could be the production of antibodies against any of the coagulation factors, causing an increase in anti-VIIIa, -IXa, -Xa, or -XIa; the presence of anticoagulants in the blood such as antithrombin and antiprothrombin, causing antithrombinemia, antithromboplastinemia, or antithromboplastinogenemia.

D68.4   Acquired coagulation factor deficiency

Liver disease, vitamin K deficiency, drug abuse, and other conditions can also cause an acquired reduction in a clotting factor.

D68.5   Primary thrombophilia

Primary thrombophilia, or primary hypercoagulable state is a disorder causing the abnormal development of blood clots in arteries and veins that is not secondary to any medical intervention, or other identified disease process.

D69.0   Allergic purpura

Allergic purpuras occur when an allergic reaction produces hemorrhages of the skin and mucous membranes, producing purple discolorations on the skin surface.

D69.1   Qualitative platelet defects

Qualitative platelet defects are conditions in which the quality of platelets in the patient's bloodstream is substandard. This code can cover a wide range of conditions with a variety of symptoms, such as excessive hemorrhaging or clotting.

D69.2   Other nonthrombocytopenic purpura

Purpuras occur when bleeding in the skin and mucous membranes leads to purple spots on the skin, caused by something other than an abnormal decrease in the number of platelets in the blood stream.

D69.41   Evans syndrome

Evan's syndrome is a condition in which the patient suffers from low levels of iron in the body as well as low levels of platelets.

D69.5   Secondary thrombocytopenia

Secondary thrombocytopenia occurs when a patient has a low platelet count due to some other disease or condition, such as a viral infection, drug, or the receipt of a blood transfusion.

Note: Secondary thrombocytopenia does not include heparin-induced thrombocytopenia, which is reported with its own specific code, D75.82.

D69.51   Posttransfusion purpura

Posttransfusion purpura is sudden and severe thrombocytopenia with a platelet count less than 10,000/ L, usually appearing between 5 and 12 days after a transfusion of blood products containing any platelets, (i.e., RBCs, granulocytes, platelets, or whole blood). This occurs when the body has an adverse reaction to the transfusion and begins producing alloantibodies against the platelet-specific antigens introduced into the body. This happens in patients who have already been sensitized to platelets through transfusion or pregnancy. The exact mechanism is not known, but it is thought that recall of the previously formed alloantibodies also produces a transient kind of autoantibody that destroys the patient's own platelets, or the alloantibodies then begin destroying the patien's own platelets. This leads to a rapid decline in platelet count and severe thrombocytopenia.

D69.59   Other secondary thrombocytopenia

Secondary thrombocytopenia is a decreased platelet count brought about by another condition or circumstance such as drugs, dilution, extracorporeal circulation of blood, or platelet alloimmunization.

D70   Neutropenia

Neutropenia, also called agranulocytosis, is an acute disease featuring high fever and a steep drop in the number of neutrophils, a type of white blood cell, circulating in the bloodstream. Neutrophils typically make up 50-70% of circulating WBC and are the primary defense against infection. Causes of neutropenia can include autoimmune disorders (systemic lupus erythematosus), exposure to chemicals, toxins, or drugs (chemotherapy agents or other drugs), ionizing radiation, genetic disorders (Kostmann's syndrome) and infections (hepatitis, HIV, Lyme disease, malaria).

Note: Any associated conditions such as fever and mucositis need to be reported in addition to the specified type of neutropenia.

D70.0   Congenital agranulocytosis

Congenital neutropenia, also called infantile genetic agranulocytosis or Kostmann's syndrome, is caused by a gene defect that results in the absence of neutrophils in the blood. Neutrophil precursors are arrested in development and eosinophils and monocytes are present in high numbers. Without neutrophils, the type of white blood cell responsible for fighting infection, children are highly susceptible to recurring bacterial infections, especially of the skin and lungs, that can lead to early death. Children are also at risk for developing leukemia.

D70.1   Agranulocytosis secondary to cancer chemotherapy

This is a drop in circulating neutrophils as a side effect of the administration of cancer chemotherapy drugs. Chemotherapy affects bone marrow and attacks normal, rapidly growing cells at the same time it is killing abnormal cancer cells. A reduction in these infection-fighting white blood cells is a serious side effect that can lead to discontinuing therapeutic doses and life-threatening infections from a debilitated immune system.

Note: The underlying neoplasm must also be coded as well as an additional code to report the adverse effect of the specified drug.

D70.2   Other drug-induced agranulocytosis

Drug-induced neutropenia is a drop in circulating neutrophils as a side effect of medication. A reduction in these infection-fighting white blood cells is a serious side effect that can lead to discontinuing therapeutic doses

and increased infections from a debilitated immune system. Some cases of other drug-induced neutropenia can also present asymptomatically.

Note: An additional code must be assigned to report the adverse effect of a particular drug or class of drugs.

D70.3   Neutropenia due to infection

Neutropenia due to infection is an abnormally decreased count of circulating neutrophils as the direct result of an infection, most commonly a virus, such as infectious mononucleosis, but also seen with bacterial infections causing sepsis. The infection strains the immune system, removing many neutrophils from the circulating blood pool and depleting the reserve pool of neutrophils in the bone marrow.

D70.4   Cyclic neutropenia

Cyclic neutropenia is a rare pediatric blood disorder in which the neutrophilic number of white blood cells responsible for fighting infection drops from a normal level to an extremely low level in a repeating cyclical pattern about every three weeks. The extremely low level of neutrophils lasts about three days to a week and leaves the child open to serious infections. Symptoms present as fever without a cause, enlarged lymph nodes, sore throat, ulcers of the mouth, and skin and other serious infections.

D70.8   Other neutropenia

Other specified neutropenia or agranulocytosis may be caused by bone marrow or blood toxicity, or an autoimmune mechanism due to IgG or IgM antibodies seen in diseases like rheumatoid arthritis and systemic lupus erythematosus.

D70.9   Neutropenia, unspecified

Unspecified neutropenia is a decreased number of neutrophils circulating in the blood. Neutrophils are mature polymorphonuclear white blood cells responsible for fighting infection by moving in on the site of inflammatory reactions and engulfing invading organisms.

D71   Functional disorders of polymorphonuclear neutrophils

Polymorphonuclear neutrophils are the chief variety of white blood cells that attack microorganisms in the body. Diseases resulting from a functional disorder of this type of white blood cell are marked by recurrent infections and granulomatosis due to a lack of properly functioning white blood cells in the bloodstream that can fight off harmful microorganisms.

D72.1   Eosinophilia

Eosinophilia is a condition in which elevated levels of eosinophils are found in the bloodstream. Eosinophils are white blood cells that target parasites. High levels of these cells indicate a parasitic infection or an allergic reaction.

D72.810   Lymphocytopenia

Lymphocytopenia is a decrease in the usual number of lymphocytes, the type of white blood cells responsible for nonphagocytic cellular and humoral immunity.

D72.818   Other decreased white blood cell count

Other decreased white blood cell counts includes decreased counts for basophilic leukocytes, the cells that release histamine and seratonin; decreased eosinophil counts, a phagocytic leukocyte derived from the same progenitor cells as macrophages, neutrophils and basophils; decreased monocytes counts, phagocytic white blood cells with a nucleus that are formed in the bone marrow and mature into macrophages in the liver and lungs; and decreased counts of plasma cells in the blood.

D72.820   Lymphocytosis (symptomatic)

Lymphocytosis is an excessive amount of normal lymphocytes in the blood. Lymphocytes are the types of white blood cells responsible for nonphagocytic cellular and humoral immunity.

Diseases of the Blood/Blood-Forming

D69.41 – D72.820

D72.821 Monocytosis (symptomatic)

Monocytosis is an increased proportion of monocytes in the blood. Monocytes are phagocytic white blood cells with a nucleus that are formed in the bone marrow and mature into macrophages in the liver and lungs.

D72.822 Plasmacytosis

Plasmacytosis is an increased amount of plasma cells circulating in the blood. Plasma cells, also called plasmacytes, are a type of lymphocyte that evolves from B memory cells after they have been actived by contact with an antigen.

D72.823 Leukemoid reaction

Leukemoid reaction is a state of circulating blood presenting a clinical picture that resembles leukemia or is indistinguishable from leukemia based on the appearance of an abnormal increase in white blood cells and immature cells in the peripheral blood. This reaction occurs with infections such as tuberculosis, staphylococcal and streptococcal infections; with tumors and bone marrow compromise; liver failure, and inflammatory disorders like rheumatoid arthritis; and with toxic conditions like eclampsia or poisoning.

D72.824 Basophilia

Basophilia, also called basophilism and basophilic leukocytosis, is an abnormally increased number of basophils in the blood. Basophils are the cells that release histamine and seratonin upon stimulation.

D72.825 Bandemia

Band cells are immature white blood cells. They are often released from the bone marrow into the blood stream in their immature form when an infection is present. Bandemia is an elevated count of immature white blood cells in the blood that may occur when other white blood cell counts are normal. This is a nonspecific indicator of infection, particularly bacteremia that can help to predict bloodstream infection prior to visible symptoms and microbiology test results.

Note: Any confirmed infection or leukemia diagnosis should be coded to the infection or leukemia.

D73.1 Hypersplenism

Hypersplenism is a condition in which the spleen becomes markedly enlarged and increases the production of bone marrow cells. This leads to a deficiency of some components of blood.

D73.2 Chronic congestive splenomegaly

Chronic congestive splenomegaly occurs when the blood vessels of the spleen suffer from hypertension. This condition often presents along with cirrhosis.

D73.81 Neutropenic splenomegaly

Neutropenic splenomegaly, also called splenic or hypersplenic neutropenia, is a syndrome marked by an enlarged spleen, profound drops in neutrophil counts and other white blood cells, resulting in susceptibility to infections, with hypercellular bone marrow. Anemia is often found in combination with this syndrome.

D74 Methemoglobinemia

Methemoglobinemia is a condition in which levels of methemoglobin are elevated in the bloodstream. Methemoglobin is a non-functional from of hemoglobin created by the oxidation of iron contained in hemoglobin. While trace levels are normal, elevated levels can lead to cyanosis. Symptoms of this condition are bluish discolorations of the skin and mucous membranes, as well as headache, dizziness, and abnormal heartbeat. In severe cases, coma and death can occur.

D74.0 Congenital methemoglobinemia

Hereditary methemoglobinemia is caused by a recessive gene that results in the impaired production of a specific enzyme, NADH methemoglobin reductase. It can also appear in patients with abnormal hemoglobin variants, such as hemoglobin M or H (HbM or HbH), despite intact enzymes. Hemoglobin is converted to methemoglobin when iron is oxidized. This gives the blood a reduced oxygen carrying capacity and a reduced ability to release oxygen to the tissues. Increased levels of methemoglobin therefore cause hypoxia. Skin turns a bluish hue and the arterial blood is brown instead of the normal red color. Methemoglobin that is spontaneously formed in the body is normally reduced back to normal functioning hemoglobin by the protective enzyme NADH. The genetic deficiency of this enzyme does not allow for the normal reduction process back to functioning hemoglobin as does the presence of abnormal hemoglobin variants, even when the enzyme production is intact.

D75.1 Secondary polycythemia

Polycythemia is marked by an overgrowth of bone marrow, increased levels of red blood cell production, and enlargement of the spleen. In this case, the primary disease causing the polycythemia would be treated.

D75.81 Myelofibrosis

This code is used to report myelofibrosis that is not otherwise specified or secondary myelofibrosis. Myelofibrosis is a progressive disorder in which bone marrow is initially overactive, and then slowly becomes replaced by scar tissue (fibrosis). The normally fine structure of fibers in the bone marrow that support the blood forming tissues become thickened and coarse, which in turn reduces the patient's ability to produce new blood cells and results in chronic anemia. Secondary myelofibrosis differentiates itself from primary or idiopathic myelofibrosis (with myeloid metaplasia) by arising as a complication of other identified bone marrow diseases.

Note: Additional codes are needed to report the adverse effect when due to anti-neoplastic chemotherapy or for any associated therapy-related myelodysplastic syndrome (D46).

D75.82 Heparin induced thrombocytopenia (HIT)

Heparin is one of the most commonly prescribed medications. Its use can lead to a common but devastating adverse reaction, known as heparin-induced thrombocytopenia, or HIT. Without prompt recognition and treatment, half of those will develop devastating or fatal arterial or venous thrombotic complications resulting in limb amputation, pulmonary embolus, stroke, or acute MI. HIT is a distinct syndrome that appears in a totally different degree from other drug-induced thrombocytopenias. The timing, the diagnostic tests, the complications, and the treatment are all completely different. Whereas other iatrogenic thrombocytopenias occur with bleeding and platelet tranfusion is indicated, HIT presents with thrombosis and requires the initiation of an alternative anticoagulant or direct thrombin inhibitors. Even patients without a new blood clot at the time of HIT diagnosis must be given therapeutic alternative anticoagulants because the risk of blood clot stays very high for more than two weeks after heparin therapy is stopped and the platelet count has recovered.

D80 Immunodeficiency with predominantly antibody defects

Humoral immunity refers to the production of antibodies and the processes that it involves. This deficiency is a loss of immune response to infection due to a lack of immunoglobulins (antibodies) circulating in the bloodstream.

D80.0 Hereditary hypogammaglobulinemia

Congenital hypogammaglobulinemia is a genetic disorder in which the body does not produce enough of one or more classes, or isotypes, of antibodies.

D80.1 Nonfamilial hypogammaglobulinemia

An acquired loss of the body's ability to respond to infection because of a lack of immunoglobulins, or antibodies, produced by the body and circulating within the bloodstream.

D80.5 Immunodeficiency with increased immunoglobulin M [IgM]

An immunodeficiency in which several classes of antibodies are not produced in sufficient numbers but in which there is increased production of the IgM antibody.

D81   Combined immunodeficiencies

Combined immunodeficiencies affect both the humoral immunity and the cell-mediated immunity, and are usually genetic in nature. One type of this disorder, called agammaglobulinemia, results in either extremely low levels or a complete absence of antibodies. Another, called thymic alymphoplasia, results from a failure of the lymphatic system to form correctly.

D81.0   Severe combined immunodeficiency [SCID] with reticular dysgenesis

This type deficiency affects both the humoral immunity and the cell-mediated immunity, and is usually genetic in nature. One type of this disorder, called agammaglobulinemia, results in either extremely low levels or a complete absence of antibodies. Another, called thymic alymphoplasia, results from a failure of the lymphatic system to form correctly.

D81.4   Nezelof's syndrome

Nezelof's syndrome is an extremely rare immune deficiency disorder which primarily affects the cell-mediated immunity, which may affect the humoral immunity. Nezelof's syndrome is caused by an absence of the thymus gland.

D82.0   Wiskott-Aldrich syndrome

Wiskott-Aldrich syndrome is another rare, X-linked genetic immunodeficiency disorder in which not enough IgM antibodies are produced, causing infection. It also reduces the number of platelets produced, which prevents the blood from clotting properly and in fact can lead to internal hemorrhaging. It may also present with eczema, thrombocytopenia, and recurrent pyogenic infections.

D82.1   Di George's syndrome

DiGeorge's syndrome is a rare genetic disorder which results in a deficiency of the T-cells and abnormal growth of the thymus and parathyroid glands as well as deformities in other body structures: hypoplasia or aplasia of the thymus and parathryroid glands; associated congenital heart defects; anomalies in the great vessels; esophageal atresia; and abnormal facial structure.

D83.0   Common variable immunodeficiency with predominant abnormalities of B-cell numbers and function

Select this code to report common variable immunodeficiency, sometimes abbreviated as CVID. This is a disorder in which the body produces insufficient levels of most or all types of immunoglobulin (e.g., IgM, IgA, etc.) while also lacking B lymphocytes (white blood cells) or other plasma cells that are capable of producing other antibodies, resulting in frequent infections.

D86   Sarcoidosis

Sarcoidosis is a rare disease that occurs when tissues in the body, usually the lungs or lymph nodes, develop small nodules (lumps). The cause of the disease is unknown, and is often chronic. Common symptoms include persistent cough, skin rashes, and inflammation of the eyes. Weight loss, fatigue, fever, and night sweats are also common.

D89.0   Polyclonal hypergammaglobulinemia

Polyclonal hypergammaglobulinemia is a condition in which there is an elevated amount of a type of protein known as gammaglobulins in the bloodstream. It is less a disease or disorder in and of itself than an indicator of the presence of another chronic and infectious disease or disorder. It presents no specific symptoms and can only be detected by a blood test.

D89.81   Graft-versus-host disease

Graft-versus-host disease, GVHD, occurs when immunologically competent cells are transplanted into an immunocompromised host. The disease describes the immunologic shock to the organism and the consequences following hematopoietic cell transplantation. Histoincompatibility alone does not account for the development of GVHD, since autologous or syngeneic transplant recipients also develop GVHD. The residual number of T cells and other type of immune response cells in the graft also have an effect. The pathophysiology involves the competent cells recognizing epithelial target tissues as foreign and beginning the immune response. Treatment involves corticosteroids and immune supressants. Despite attempts at immune response manipulation, GVHD is a primary cause of morbidity and mortality in transplant patients.

Note: Graft versus host disease is most often a complication of bone marrow transplantation; however, it can also occur after blood transfusion or any solid organ transplant in which normal white blood cells are present in the organ being transplanted. Although the condition is classified with its own specific codes, the underlying complication should be listed first, while manifestations, such as diarrhea or hair loss, should be coded in addition.

D89.810 Acute graft-versus-host disease

Acute GVHD is normally observed within the first 100 days following transplant. Classic characterization affects the skin, gastrointestinal tract, and liver. The triad of symptoms consists of dermatitis with scattered macules or papules and desquamation over an increasing body surface area as GVHD progresses; enteritis with diarrhea; and hepatitis with increased bilirubin. The patient also has an increased susceptibility to infection. Acute GVHD patients are at risk for sepsis, electrolyte imbalances from diarrhea, bilirubinemia, and hepatorenal syndrome. Mortality is directly related to severity. Overpowering sepsis is the main cause of death in acute GVHD.

D89.811 Chronic graft-versus-host disease

Chronic GVHD usually begins more than three months after transplantation and may occur as a late phase in those who had acute GVHD, or it may present as a distinct entity. The skin is still the primary organ involved and can lead to lichen-planus type lesions, scleroderma, and complete epidermal necrosis. Liver damage and intestinal affects may also be present with chronic cases. Patients are additionally susceptible to hair loss, joint contractures from scleroderma, esophageal stricture, keratoconjunctivitis sicca, and lung disorders. Global immune impairment causes morbidity and mortality.

D89.82   Autoimmune lymphoproliferative syndrome [ALPS]

Autoimmune lymphoproliferative syndrome, also known as ALPS, is a rare, inherited immune system disorder in which unusually high numbers of white blood cells accumulate in specific areas of the body, such as the spleen, liver, and lymph nodes, causing organ enlargement. ALPS also causes additional problems from an imbalanced, low number of other types of blood cells in the body: anemia (low red blood cell count), neutropenia (low neutrophil count), and thrombocytopenia (low platelet count). Less often, autoimmune attacks can occur in any organ, like the skin, liver, nerves, and kidneys. The disease typically develops in early childhood and affects both children and adults and may range of mild to severe cases. Patients with ALPS do not become sicker over time but appear to have a lessening of symptoms in teenage and young adult years. There is no cure, but complications can be treated. Careful consideration of splenectomy may be necessary.

Endocrine, Nutritional and Metabolic Diseases | E00-E89

E00 Congenital iodine-deficiency syndrome

Congenital iodine-deficiency syndrome, or endemic cretinism, is a condition in which a child has low or no thyroid hormone produced from birth. It is usually caused by an absence of the thyroid, which sometimes is hereditary and sometimes occurs because the mother was taking anti-thyroid medication (e.g. for thyrotoxicosis) during pregnancy. If not caught and treated with hormone replacement medication right away, the condition can cause lasting damage to the central nervous system and cause both physical and mental developmental delay. Symptoms include poor eating, excessive sleeping, lack of crying or other activity, constipation, and below normal body temperature, heart rate, and blood count. The child may have a large head, belly, and/or tongue, and the soft spot of the skull may be abnormally large and take an unusually long time to close. Most will also present with an umbilical hernia that may seem to enlarge when the child is crying or straining and which usually disappears within 1-5 years.

Note: Assign another code to note any associated intellectual disabilities.

E02 Subclinical iodine-deficiency hypothyroidism

Subclinical hypothyroidism is an early stage of hypothyroidism that is usually detected by measuring the levels of serum TSH, or thyrotropin-stimulating hormone. This is generally considered the best screening test. Patients whose TSH levels are increased, while their free thyroxin T4 levels are normal are considered to be in a state of subclinical hypothyroidism in which the body is making enough thyroxine, but needs the additional stimulation from TSH in order to produce it. This condition can resolve, remain unchanged, or develop into overt hypothyroidism within a few years, in which case, low levels for free T4 will be present along with raised levels of TSH. The likelihood of progression to overt hypothyroidism is linked to greater levels of raised TSH with more consistency and the presence of detectable antithyroid antibodies. Symptoms are mild and nonspecific and include easy fatigability, dry skin, constipation, and an intolerance to cold, which are often attributed to other causes or normal aging. Mild abnormalities in cardiac function, serum lipoproteins, and cholesterol levels may also be present, in which case treatment may be initiated, particularly when higher levels of TSH are consistently detected. Worldwide, iodine deficiency is the number one cause of hypothyroidism because the body needs iodine to make thyroxine. Treatment normally consists of low daily doses of levothyroxine, which is partially converted to tri-iodothyronine (T3) in the body and helps maintain consistent blood levels of both T3 and T4.

E03.0 Congenital hypothyroidism with diffuse goiter

This includes nontoxic congenital goiter. Congenital goiter is a diffuse enlargement of the thyroid gland that is present from birth. It may be caused by genetic defects in thyroid hormone production, or maternal antibodies or goitrogens crossing the placenta. Genetic defects cause abnormal production of thyroid hormone levels which cause increased levels of thyroid stimulating hormone (TSH), resulting in the congenital goiter. Antibodies produced in mothers with autoimmune thyroid disorder can cross the placenta in the third trimester, which block TSH receptors, causing congenital hypothyroidism. In these cases, the related hormonal changes and the associated congenital goiter usually clear up within 6 months. Goitrogens such as antithyroid drugs and amiodarone can also cross the placenta and cause congenital hypothyroidism, with or without goiter. Diagnosis is confirmed by ultrasonic measurement of the size of the thyroid gland and testing for T4 and TSH levels. Signs and symptoms include firm, nontender enlargement of the thyroid that may or may not be noticeable at birth, compression of the trachea, difficulty breathing, and dysphagia. The hypothyroidism is treated with thyroid hormone and an unresolving goiter causing breathing or swallowing problems may be removed surgically.

E03.1 Congenital hypothyroidism without goiter

Congenital hypothyroidism is a condition in which a child has low or no thyroid hormone produced from birth. It is usually caused by an absence of the thyroid, either aplasia or atrophy from hereditary causes, or because the mother was taking anti-thyroid medication (e.g. for thyrotoxicosis) during pregnancy. If not caught and treated with hormone replacement medication right away, the condition can cause lasting damage to the central nervous system and both physical and mental developmental delay. Symptoms include poor eating, excessive sleeping, lack of crying or other activity, constipation, and below normal body temperature, heart rate, and blood count. The child may have a large head, belly, and/or tongue, and the soft spot of the skull may be abnormally large and take an unusually long time to close. Most will also present with an umbilical hernia that may seem to enlarge when the child is crying or straining and which usually disappears within 1-5 years.

E03.2 Hypothyroidism due to medicaments and other exogenous substances

Iodine is vital for thyroid function. Even though those who are exposed to high doses of radiation, whether medically or due to an environmental situation, are often given iodine supplements in order to protect the thyroid, it is also possible to take too much iodine (more than 300 mg per day) and damage the thyroid. Hypothyroidism then results in which the gland can no longer produce enough hormone to maintain the body's metabolism. Iatrogenic hypothyroidism may also occur due to taking certain other medications, such as lithium for mood disorders, and amiodarone. Symptoms include fatigue, weight gain, muscle aches and cramps, an intolerance to cold temperatures, decreased sex drive, memory loss, and depression and irritability. It may also present with hair loss or coarseness, dry and/or rough skin, constipation, or a disruption of the menstrual cycles in females.

E03.3 Postinfectious hypothyroidism

Hypothyroidism is a condition in which the thyroid is not producing enough thyroxine (T4). In postinfectious cases, a previous infection has affected the thyroid, causing it to become underactive and not able to produce enough thyroxine. This in turn triggers the pituitary gland to make thyroid stimulating hormone (TSH) and release it into the bloodstream to stimulate the thyroid gland to make more thyroxine. A raised level of TSH indicates an underactive thyroid gland, and hypothyroidism is confirmed by low levels of T4. Low levels of thyroxine cause many body functions to slow down. Signs and symptoms include tiredness, weight gain, constipation, cold intolerance, dry skin, lifeless hair, slowed mental function, and depression. Less common symptoms include hoarseness, heavy menstrual periods, loss of libido, and mental confusion.

E03.4 Atrophy of thyroid (acquired)

Atrophy of the thyroid is a state in which the thyroid gland has withered away and shriveled to an abnormally small size. The glandular tissue has degenerated and wasted away, becoming nonviable or severely reduced in effective functioning. Acquired thyroid atrophy has developed gradually over time, and is often the end result of years of inflammation, an autoimmune or infective disease process, or long-term under or overfunctioning of the gland. The remaining thyroid tissue may be surgically removed to prevent any further disease process and hormone replacement therapy is required.

E03.5 Myxedema coma

The full-blown expression of symptomatic hypothyroidism as a well-defined disease is known as myxedema. Coma is a rare and life-threatening complication of myxedema. Coma occurs in a state of decompensated hypothyroidism such as when a stressful event, like a myocardial infarction or serious infection, induces a myxedematous coma state. This is an extreme manifestation that usually occurs in the elderly. In addition to the altered state of consciousness, other symptoms include hypothermia, hypoventilation and hypoxia, hypotension, hyponatremia, hypercapnia, and bradycardia. Treatment consists of gradual warming with blankets, mechanical ventilation, intravenous doses of T3 and/ or T4, and levothyroxine, and prophylactic administration of antibiotics if infection is the precipitating cause.

E03.8 Other specified hypothyroidism

Hypothyroidism is a condition in which the thyroid is not producing enough thyroxine (T4). This in turn triggers the pituitary gland to make thyroid stimulating hormone (TSH) and release it into the bloodstream to stimulate the thyroid gland to make more thyroxine. A raised level of TSH indicates an underactive thyroid gland, and hypothyroidism is confirmed by low levels of T4. Low levels of thyroxine cause many body functions to slow down. Signs and symptoms include tiredness, weight gain, constipation, cold intolerance, dry skin, lifeless hair, slowed mental function, and depression. Less common symptoms include hoarseness, heavy menstrual periods, loss of libido, and mental confusion. All of these symptoms may be attributed to other causes or conditions and a diagnosis of hypothyroidism is not obvious. These conditions may gradually appear and worsen over years as the levels of T4 decrease. Other specified cases of hypothyroidism may be due to various rare conditions that affect the pituitary or cause other types of thyroid inflammation, resulting in hypothyroidism. Acquired hypothyroidism is also associated with certain genetic syndromes in which hypothyroidism develops later in life and is not present at birth, such as occurs with Down syndrome and Turner syndrome.

E03.9 Hypothyroidism, unspecified

This code reports acquired hypothyroidism that is not otherwise specified as to the causative reason. This is a condition in which the thyroid gland fails to produce enough thyroid hormone to maintain the body's metabolism. As a result, the person suffers with fatigue, weight gain, muscle aches and cramps, an intolerance to cold temperatures, decreased sex drive, memory loss, and depression and irritability. Hypothyroidism may also present with hair loss or coarseness, dry and/or rough skin, constipation, or a disruption of the menstrual cycles in females. Hypothyroidism affects more women then men, mostly in middle age. Many of the signs and symptoms of hypothyroidism are often attributed to aging and come on gradually. There is no obvious clinical picture pointing to hypothyroidism and diagnosis is confirmed by blood tests.

Note: The full-blown expression of hypothyroidism as a definitive disease is known as myxedema.

E04 Other nontoxic goiter

Goiter is an enlargement of the thyroid gland, which most often occurs due to an overload of thyroid-stimulating hormone (TSH) from the pituitary gland. Initially, goiter presents as a simple, painless swelling of the throat. In the early stages, the condition can be treated with thyroid-hormone supplements, which cause the pituitary to produce less TSH. This treatment usually stops the growth of the thyroid, but rarely causes it to decrease in size. If swelling continues, it can compress the larynx and esophagus, leading to difficulty in swallowing, coughing, and waking up at night with the sensation of being choked, as well as a compression of the blood vessels in the neck. At this stage, surgical removal of part or all of the thyroid is the only effective treatment. Biopsies and surgical intervention are also employed in any case where there is a suspicion of malignancy in the enlarged thyroid.

E04.0 Nontoxic diffuse goiter

A goiter is an enlargement of the thyroid gland, which most often occurs due to an overload of thyroid-stimulating hormone (TSH) from the pituitary gland and initially presents as a simple, painless swelling of the throat.

A nontoxic goiter is not impairing the function of the thyroid or causing thyroid disease or attributed to any specific inflammatory or neoplastic disease process. Nontoxic diffuse goiter is a generalized enlargement of the whole thyroid gland without the presence of individual hard nodules or cysts. They are also known as simple goiters. Nontoxic goiters usually grow very slowly over years without developing any symptoms. However if there is evidence of rapid growth, or the goiter presses on the esophagus or trachea causing cough, stridor, difficulty breathing or swallowing, the goiter may be removed surgically. Other treatments include radioactive iodine therapy to reduce the thyroid volume and medicaments such as levothyroxine or T4 to reduce the amount of TSH being produced by the pituitary and suppress thyroid hormone activity to shrink the goiter.

E04.1 Nontoxic single thyroid nodule

A single, non-toxic nodular or cystic goiter appears as a node or cyst on the thyroid that can be detected by palpating the neck with the fingers. As in the case of simple goiter, these knobs or cysts are not impairing the normal function of the thyroid or causing hyperthyroidism. Cysts may also contain infected material or bleed into the thyroid and the cyst may require drainage.

E04.2 Nontoxic multinodular goiter

Nontoxic multinodular (cystic) goiter has multiple hard knobs, or cysts appearing in the thyroid that can be detected by palpating the neck. These multiple nodules do not impair the function of the thyroid or cause thyroid disease; however, the cysts can bleed into the thyroid, and nodules may have the potential to become malignant. Biopsies may be done to analyze the tissue sample.

E04.9 Nontoxic goiter, unspecified

Unspecified goiter is an enlargement of the thyroid gland, which most often occurs due to an overload of thyroid-stimulating hormone (TSH) from the pituitary gland and initially presents as a simple, painless swelling of the throat. A nontoxic goiter is not impairing the function of the thyroid or causing thyroid disease. An unspecified nontoxic goiter may also be nodular, in which individual hard knobs or cysts are present in the thyroid that may be detected by palpating the neck. In the early stages, the condition can be treated with thyroid-hormone supplements, which usually stop the growth of the thyroid, but rarely cause it to decrease in size. If the goiter is large enough, it can compress the larynx and esophagus, causing dysphagia, coughing, and a sensation of being choked, as well as compressing blood vessels in the neck. In these cases, the thyroid may be surgically removed.

E05 Thyrotoxicosis [hyperthyroidism]

Thyrotoxicosis, also called hyperthyroidism, is a condition in which the thyroid produces too much of its hormone. Since the thyroid hormone controls the body's metabolism, this results in weight loss despite an increased appetite, a rapid heart rate (tachycardia), trembling, nervousness and emotional instability, overheating and profuse sweating, staring and/or bulging eyes, and goiter. Thyrotoxicosis can appear in several forms as with diffuse goiter, with a uninodular or multinodular goiter, or ectopic tissue and with or without thyrotixic crisis or storm. A thyrotoxic crisis is a sudden worsening of the toxic condition caused by excess thyroid hormone in the body, usually as a result of shock, injury, illness, stress, or removal of the thyroid gland.

E05.00 Thyrotoxicosis with diffuse goiter without thyrotoxic crisis or storm

Toxic diffuse goiter or Grave's disease is a condition in which the patient's immune system produces an antibody called thyrotropin receptor antibody, that mimics the action of the normal regulatory hormone produced by the pituitary gland, essentially overriding it and causing production of more thyroid hormone. Enlarged thyroid as a whole and bulging eyes are particularly notable in this disorder which causes anxiety, irritability, fatigue, tremor in the hands, sweating, sensitivity to heat, weight loss, and sometimes dermopathy as thick, red skin on the feet and shins. Grave's disease is usually treatable with medication that blocks the production of the excessive hormone.

E05.01 Thyrotoxicosis with diffuse goiter with thyrotoxic crisis or storm

Toxic diffuse goiter or Grave's disease is a condition in which the patient's immune system produces an antibody called thyrotropin receptor antibody, that mimics the action of the normal regulatory hormone produced by the pituitary gland, essentially overriding it and causing production of more thyroid hormone. Enlarged thyroid as a whole and bulging eyes are particularly notable in this disorder which causes anxiety, irritability, fatigue, tremor in the hands, sweating, sensitivity to heat, weight loss, and sometimes dermopathy as thick, red skin on the feet and shins. Grave's disease is usually treatable with medication that blocks the production of the excessive hormone. It may appear with thyrotoxic crisis or storm, which is a rare, but severe, sudden worsening of symptoms caused by injury, sickness, stress, or removal of the thyroid. Crisis causes fast heart rate, arrhythmia, vomiting, fever over 104 degrees F, diarrhea, and dehydration and can lead to coma and death.

E05.10 Thyrotoxicosis with toxic single thyroid nodule without thyrotoxic crisis or storm

Thyrotoxicosis, also called hyperthyroidism, is a condition in which the thyroid produces too much hormone. Since the thyroid hormone controls the body's metabolism, this results in weight loss despite an increased appetite, a rapid heart rate (tachycardia), trembling, nervousness and emotional instability, overheating and profuse sweating, changes in hair, rapid fingernail growth, thinning skin, shaky hands, muscle weakness, and goiter. Thyrotoxicosis that occurs with a toxic uninodular goiter appears with gland enlargement and a single, autonomously functioning nodule growing in the thyroid, increasing the gland's activity and causing hyperthyroidism. Diagnosis is made with blood tests, thyroid uptake tests with radioactive iodine, thyroid scans, and ultrasound. Treatment may depend on age, overall health, the severity of symptoms, and the specific cause of the hyperthyroidism. Medicaments are given to prevent the thyroid from making new hormone; radioactive doses of iodine can be taken orally to prevent hormone release and relieve symptoms; thyroidectomy may be done to remove part or all of the gland; and beta blockers may be given to slow the heart rate.

E05.11 Thyrotoxicosis with toxic single thyroid nodule with thyrotoxic crisis or storm

Thyrotoxicosis, also called hyperthyroidism, is a condition in which the thyroid produces too much hormone. Since the thyroid hormone controls the body's metabolism, this results in weight loss despite an increased appetite, a rapid heart rate (tachycardia), trembling, nervousness and emotional instability, overheating and profuse sweating, changes in hair, rapid fingernail growth, thinning skin, shaky hands, muscle weakness, and goiter. Thyrotoxicosis that occurs with a toxic uninodular goiter appears with gland enlargement and a single, autonomously functioning nodule growing in the thyroid, increasing the gland's activity and causing hyperthyroidism. This condition may present with thyrotoxic crisis or storm. A thyrotoxic crisis is a sudden worsening of the toxic condition caused by excess thyroid hormone in the body, usually as a result of shock, injury, illness, stress, or removal of the thyroid gland. Crisis causes symptoms of fast heart rate, arrhythmia, vomiting, fever over 104 degrees F, diarrhea, and dehydration and can lead to coma and death. Diagnosis is made with blood tests, thyroid uptake tests with radioactive iodine, thyroid scans, and ultrasound. Treatment may depend on age, overall health, the severity of symptoms, and the specific cause of the hyperthyroidism. Medicaments are given to prevent the thyroid from making new hormone; radioactive doses of iodine can be taken orally to prevent hormone release and relieve symptoms; thyroidectomy may be done to remove part or all of the gland; and beta blockers may be given to slow the heart rate.

E05.20 Thyrotoxicosis with toxic multinodular goiter without thyrotoxic crisis or storm

Thyrotoxicosis, also called hyperthyroidism, is a condition in which the thyroid produces too much hormone. Since the thyroid hormone controls the body's metabolism, this results in weight loss despite an increased appetite, a rapid heart rate (tachycardia), trembling, nervousness and emotional instability, overheating and profuse sweating, changes in hair, rapid fingernail growth, thinning skin, shaky hands, muscle weakness, and goiter. Thyrotoxicosis that occurs with a toxic multinodular goiter appears with gland enlargement and autonomously functioning nodules growing within the thyroid, increasing the gland's activity and causing hyperthyroidism. Diagnosis is made with blood tests, thyroid uptake tests with radioactive iodine, thyroid scans, and ultrasound. Treatment may depend on age, overall health, the severity of symptoms, and the specific cause of the hyperthyroidism. Medicaments are given to prevent the thyroid from making new hormone; radioactive doses of iodine can be taken orally to prevent hormone release and relieve symptoms; thyroidectomy may be done to remove part or all of the gland; and beta blockers may be given to slow the heart rate.

E05.21 Thyrotoxicosis with toxic multinodular goiter with thyrotoxic crisis or storm

Thyrotoxicosis, also called hyperthyroidism, is a condition in which the thyroid produces too much hormone. Since the thyroid hormone controls the body's metabolism, this results in weight loss despite an increased appetite, a rapid heart rate (tachycardia), trembling, nervousness and emotional instability, overheating and profuse sweating, changes in hair, rapid fingernail growth, thinning skin, shaky hands, muscle weakness, and goiter. Thyrotoxicosis that occurs with a toxic multinodular goiter appears with gland enlargement and autonomously functioning nodules growing within the thyroid, increasing the gland's activity and causing hyperthyroidism. This condition may present with thyrotoxic crisis or storm. A thyrotoxic crisis is a sudden worsening of the toxic condition caused by excess thyroid hormone in the body, usually as a result of shock, injury, illness, stress, or removal of the thyroid gland. Crisis causes symptoms of fast heart rate, arrhythmia, vomiting, fever over 104 degrees F, diarrhea, and dehydration and can lead to coma and death. Diagnosis is made with blood tests, thyroid uptake tests with radioactive iodine, thyroid scans, and ultrasound. Treatment may depend on age, overall health, the severity of symptoms, and the specific cause of the hyperthyroidism. Medicaments are given to prevent the thyroid from making new hormone; radioactive doses of iodine can be taken orally to prevent hormone release and relieve symptoms; thyroidectomy may be done to remove part or all of the gland; and beta blockers may be given to slow the heart rate.

E05.30 Thyrotoxicosis from ectopic thyroid tissue without thyrotoxic crisis or storm

Thyrotoxicosis, also called hyperthyroidism, is a condition in which the thyroid produces too much hormone. Since the thyroid hormone controls the body's metabolism, this results in weight loss despite an increased appetite, a rapid heart rate (tachycardia), trembling, nervousness and emotional instability, overheating and profuse sweating, changes in hair, rapid fingernail growth, thinning skin, shaky hands, muscle weakness, and goiter. Thyrotoxicosis can result from an ectopic thyroid nodule; that is, from a nodule forming in thyroid tissue that is not in its proper position in the neck. This usually results from a failure of the thyroid to descend. In gestation, the thyroid forms beneath the tongue and then slowly moves down the throat into its normal position. In some cases, it remains at the base of the tongue or high in the neck. In other cases, thyroid tissue remains along the path of the thyroid's descent that may produce extra thyroid hormone.

E05.31 Thyrotoxicosis from ectopic thyroid tissue with thyrotoxic crisis or storm

Thyrotoxicosis, also called hyperthyroidism, is a condition in which the thyroid produces too much hormone. Since the thyroid hormone controls the body's metabolism, this results in weight loss despite an increased appetite, a rapid heart rate (tachycardia), trembling, nervousness and emotional instability, overheating and profuse sweating, changes in hair, rapid fingernail growth, thinning skin, shaky hands, muscle weakness, and goiter. Thyrotoxicosis can result from an ectopic thyroid nodule; that is, from a nodule forming in thyroid tissue that is not in its proper position in the neck. This usually results from a failure of the thyroid to descend. In gestation, the thyroid forms beneath the tongue and then slowly moves down the throat into its normal position. In some cases, it remains at the base of the tongue or high in the neck. In other cases, thyroid tissue remains along the path of the thyroid's descent that may produce extra thyroid hormone. This condition may also appear with or without thyrotoxic crisis or storm, which is a rare, but severe worsening of symptoms caused by injury, sickness or stress, or removal of the thyroid. Crisis causes fast heart heart, arrhythmia, vomiting, fever over 104 degrees F, diarrhea and dehydration, and can lead to coma and death.

E05.90   Thyrotoxicosis, unspecified without thyrotoxic crisis or storm

Thyrotoxicosis, also called hyperthyroidism, is a condition in which the thyroid produces too much hormone. Since the thyroid hormone controls the body's metabolism, this results in weight loss despite an increased appetite, a rapid heart rate (tachycardia), trembling, nervousness and emotional instability, overheating and profuse sweating, changes in hair, rapid fingernail growth, thinning skin, shaky hands, muscle weakness, and goiter. Diagnosis is made with blood tests, thyroid uptake tests with radioactive iodine, thyroid scans, and ultrasound. Treatment may depend on age, overall health, the severity of symptoms, and the specific cause of the hyperthyroidism. Medicaments are given to prevent the thyroid from making new hormone; radioactive doses of iodine can be taken orally to prevent hormone release and relieve symptoms; thyroidectomy may be done to remove part or all of the gland; and beta blockers may be given to slow the heart rate.

E05.91   Thyrotoxicosis, unspecified with thyrotoxic crisis or storm

Thyrotoxicosis, also called hyperthyroidism, is a condition in which the thyroid produces too much hormone. Since the thyroid hormone controls the body's metabolism, this results in weight loss despite an increased appetite, a rapid heart rate (tachycardia), trembling, nervousness and emotional instability, overheating and profuse sweating, changes in hair, rapid fingernail growth, thinning skin, shaky hands, muscle weakness, and goiter. This condition may present with thyrotoxic crisis or storm. A thyrotoxic crisis is a sudden worsening of the toxic condition caused by excess thyroid hormone in the body, usually as a result of shock, injury, illness, stress, or removal of the thyroid gland. Crisis causes symptoms of fast heart rate, arrhythmia, vomiting, fever over 104 degrees F, diarrhea, and dehydration and can lead to coma and death. Diagnosis is made with blood tests, thyroid uptake tests with radioactive iodine, thyroid scans, and ultrasound. Treatment may depend on age, overall health, the severity of symptoms, and the specific cause of the hyperthyroidism. Medicaments are given to prevent the thyroid from making new hormone; radioactive doses of iodine can be taken orally to prevent hormone release and relieve symptoms; thyroidectomy may be done to remove part or all of the gland; and beta blockers may be given to slow the heart rate.

E06   Thyroiditis

Thyroiditis is an inflammation of the thyroid gland which can cause either hyper- or hypothyroidism. It can be caused by a bacterial or viral infection, a hormone production disorder in another gland (particularly the adrenal glands), a reaction to medication, or another problem altogether. In addition to a noticeably swollen thyroid (often on just one side), this disorder may present with the typical symptoms of hyper- or hypothyroidism. Thyroiditis is classified according to the acuteness and causation of the disorder.

E06.0   Acute thyroiditis

Acute thyroiditis can be life threatening and is considered a medical emergency. It presents with a high fever in which the neck is particularly hot, in addition to being red, swollen, and very tender to the touch. This condition accompanies an abscess, or infection, in the thyroid.

E06.1   Subacute thyroiditis

Subacute thyroiditis is less serious, and usually develops as a complication to another disease, such as mumps, flu, or an upper respiratory infection. It presents with fever and pain that radiates through the whole neck as well as with the symptoms of hyperthyroidism. It rarely becomes a chronic condition, though it can sometimes take several months for normal hormone production to resume.

E06.3   Autoimmune thyroiditis

Autoimmune thyroiditis is inflammation of the thyroid gland with lymphocyte infiltration that presents with painless thyoid enlargement and hypothyroid symptoms. Also known as lymphocytic thyroiditis, or Hashimoto's disease, this is an autoimmune disorder in which the bodyitself attacks the thyroid, causing the inflammation and enlargement.

E06.4   Drug-induced thyroiditis

Iatrogenic thyroiditis is an inflammation of the thyroid that can occur due to taking certain medications, such as taking lithium for mood disorders. It may also be due to an overdose of iodine in the body.

E06.5   Other chronic thyroiditis

Chronic fibrous thyroiditis, sometimes called Riedel's thyroiditis, is a rare disease in which tough and stringy (fibrous) tissue grows within the thyroid, usually resulting in a hard mass that can only be distinguished from a tumor by a biopsy. This mass decreases the amount of thyroid hormone produced in the affected area. This disease most often strikes women in their late forties, and is most often treated by surgical removal of the fibrous mass.

E07.0   Hypersecretion of calcitonin

Thyrocalcitonin, or calcitonin, is a hormone secreted by the thyroid that lowers calcium levels in the blood by preventing reabsorption of calcium from the bones; in this it acts as a counterbalance to the effect of parathyroid hormone. A disorder in the secretion of thyrocalcitonin results in too much or too little calcium being reabsorbed from the bone, which if left untreated, results in bones that are too brittle or too thick.

E07.1   Dyshormogenetic goiter

Dyshormonogenetic goiter is a condition that is often present at birth in which the thyroid is enlarged or swollen, but produces insufficient amonts of hormone for the body. It presents with the usual symptoms of hypothyroidism, and when congenital, causes dwarfism and delayed mental development unless the hormones are supplemented medically.

E07.81   Sick-euthyroid syndrome

Euthyroid sick syndrome is a condition in which thyroid hormone levels are off due to a non-thyroid related problem.

E08   Diabetes mellitus due to underlying condition

This category reports diabetes mellitus cases that develop from other known disease processes, or underlying conditions. Some of the diseases known to induce diabetes include pancreatic disorders (pancreatitis, hemochromatosis); endocrinopathies such as Cushing's disease, acromegaly, and hyperaldosteronism; malignancy; congenital disorders such as cystic fibrosis, and congenital rubella; and affective disorders like schizophrenia. Overt diabetes is caused secondarily by pancreatic disorders or endocrinopathies causing counter-regulatory hormone production. The end metabolic effect in secondary diabetes is dependent upon the impact the underlying disorder has on insulin secretion, insulin sensitivity, and the unmasking of genetic tendencies. The manifestations accompanying this classification of secondary diabetes parallel those occurring with type 1 and 2 diabetes.

Note: This category of diabetes excludes type 1, type 2, gestational, neonatal, drug or chemical induced, postpancreatectomy or other postprocedural diabetes, diabetes due to genetic defects, as well as secondary diabetes mellitus not classified elsewhere.

Note: Proper sequencing regarding diabetes caused by underlying conditions requires the coder to assign the code for the underlying condition first.

Note: Associated insulin use should also be coded additionally.

Note: Controlled or uncontrolled status is not considered an axis of coding for the selection of the diabetes code; however, out of control or poorly controlled cases that are so stated in the documentation are reported by using the appropriate code for the type of diabetes with hyperglycemia.

E08.0 Diabetes mellitus due to underlying condition with hyperosmolarity

Diabetes with hyperosmolarity is a medical emergency that involves extremely high blood glucose levels, dehydration, and decreased consciousness that can lead to coma, without the presence of ketones or acidosis. Hyperosmolarity occurs when high blood concentrations of glucose, sodium, and other molecules become even higher because the kidneys are conserving water. The kidneys normally help balance high blood glucose and ion levels by excreting extra amounts in the urine, but when the kidneys begin conserving water, the concentrations climb higher and there is a greater need for water. Signs include weakness, increased thirst, lethargy, confusion, speech impairment, loss of muscle function, and convulsions. These symptoms may progress over days or weeks and may occur with or without coma. Treatment aims to correct the dehydration with intravenous fluids and electrolytes to improve blood pressure, urine output, and circulation, and the administration of insulin to bring down high glucose levels.

E08.1 Diabetes mellitus due to underlying condition with ketoacidosis

Ketoacidosis is a dramatic, emergency complication that can develop quickly and can also lead to coma and death. Without insulin, sugar in the blood cannot be used for energy. Cells needing energy to survive switch to a back-up method in which fat cells break down, producing compounds called ketones that are used for some energy, but make the blood too acidic. This condition may first appear with excessive thirst, urination, nausea, vomiting, and abdominal pain. Breathing becomes deep and fast as the body attempts to balance the pH acidity level of the blood. Breath smells like acetone (nail polish remover) because of the escaping ketones. If left untreated, ketoacidosis progresses to coma and death within a few hours. Treatment consists of large amounts of fluids and electrolytes given intravenously with careful control of blood sugar back to normal levels in order to prevent sudden fluid shifts into the brain.

E08.2 Diabetes mellitus due to underlying condition with kidney complications

In diabetics, the renal blood vessels may thicken and leak protein into the urine, which cannot be filtered properly. An abnormally high level of protein in the urine is a sign of early kidney damage. Kidney malfunction or nephropathy can lead to chronic kidney disease and failure. Kidney complications are associated with long term diabetes.

E08.3 Diabetes mellitus due to underlying condition with ophthalmic complications

Diabetes affects both large and small blood vessels throughout the body, such as those in the eyes. Complex sugar-based substances adhere to vessel walls, causing them to thicken and leak, which makes them incapable of supplying as much blood and oxygen to the tissues as is needed. Leaking blood vessels of the eye cause retinal damage. Ophthalmic conditions such as retinopathy and cataracts occurring as long-term diabetic complications can lead to blindness.

E08.311 Diabetes mellitus due to underlying condition with unspecified diabetic retinopathy with macular edema

In diabetic retinopathy, the arteries supplying blood and nutrients to the retina become weakened and leak, causing hemorrhaging that damages parts of the retina and leaks blood into the inner eye, causing floaters and general vision loss. Diabetic macular edema is a swelling of the retina as an aspect of diabetes mellitus occurring when blood vessels leak and cause fluid and protein deposits to build up and collect within the macula, the yellowish central portion of the retina rich in the nerve endings and responsible for fine detailed, daytime vision.

E08.351 Diabetes mellitus due to underlying condition with proliferative diabetic retinopathy with macular edema

In background diabetic retinopathy, the arteries in the retina become weakened and leak, causing tiny hemorrhages, and decreasing the patient's vision. Proliferative diabetic retinopathy is the next stage when continued problems in the blood vessels cause parts of the retina to become oxygen- and nutrient-deprived. At the same time, hemorrhaging of the vessels continues to leak blood into the inner eye, causing the patient to experience floating black spots in their vision, called floaters, in addition to suffering from general vision loss. This can occur with macular edema, a swelling of the retina that occurs when fluid leaks from the blood vessels in the opaque spot on the cornea.

Note: In the final stage of this process, the patient frequently experiences retinal detachment and/or glaucoma, which should be classified with the appropriate codes for those disorders.

E08.4 Diabetes mellitus due to underlying condition with neurological complications

Diabetic nerve damage occurs because glucose is not being metabolized normally and blood supply is inadequate. Signs and symptoms of diabetic neuropathies differ depending on which nerve(s) are affected. In peripheral neuropathy, the patient may experience painful sensations, tingling, burning, or weakness in the limbs. Muscle weakness, pain, and difficulty with walking may occur. The patient may become hyerpsensitive to the slightest touch, which causes agony. Nerve damage in the skin also affects the ability to sense pain, pressure, and temperature changes, particularly in the feet and toes. Injuries can result that go unnoticed due to the neurological damage. Autonomic (poly)neuropathy affects the nerves that control functions such as heart rate, digestion, blood pressure, and body temperature regulation resulting in problems such as gastroparesis. Nerves other than peripheral nerves may also be affected, causing amyotrophy, or radiculoplexus neuropathy affecting the thighs, hips, abdomen, and buttocks.

E08.41 Diabetes mellitus due to underlying condition with diabetic mononeuropathy

Mononeuropathy involves damage to one specific nerve and can affect a limb, the face, or the trunk. It often comes on suddenly and can cause severe pain, although symptoms are not usually long-term problems and may diminish over time, unless considerably damage to the nerve has already occurred. Areas affected depend on which nerve is involved. Diabetic mononeuropathy can appear as pain in only one particular area of a limb, such as the front of the thigh or the shin, paralysis is one area of the face, abdominal pain, or aching behind one eye.

E08.43 Diabetes mellitus due to underlying condition with diabetic autonomic (poly)neuropathy

Autonomic neuropathy affects the nervous system that controls functions such as the heart, lungs, stomach and intestines, bladder, and body temperature and blood pressure regulation. Symptoms conditions of autonomic neuropathy in the diabetic include gastroparesis in which the stomach empties very slowly; constipation or uncontrolled diarrhea; incontinence and bladder problems; difficulty swallowing, inability to regulate heart rate when resting or moving; and sharp drops in blood pressure when rising.

E08.44 Diabetes mellitus due to underlying condition with diabetic amyotrophy

Amyotrophy can occur with any type of diabetes, although it is most common in type 2 diabetics. It is also called diabetic radiculoplexus neuropathy and affects nerves closer to the trunk, such as those of the thighs, hips, and buttocks, as opposed to affecting the nerve endings like in peripheral neuropathy. The patient experiences weakening and atrophying thigh muscles; sudden, extremely painful sensations in the hips, thighs, and buttocks; difficulty getting up from in the sitting position; and abdominal swelling, if the abdomen is affected.

E08.5 Diabetes mellitus due to underlying condition with circulatory complications

Diabetes has a big effect on blood vessels. Complex sugar-based substances adhere to vessel walls, causing them to thicken and leak, which makes them incapable of supplying as much blood and oxygen to the tissues as is needed. Poorly controlled blood sugar levels also cause an increase in fatty substances in the blood with the adherence of plaque material to the vessel walls. This atherosclerotic buildup also reduces blood flow and causes poor circulation. Poor circulation to the extremities causes slow-healing wounds prone to infection. Some wounds may never heal and lead to gangrene with the need for amputation.

E08.62 Diabetes mellitus due to underlying condition with skin complications

Because diabetes has such a big effect on blood vessels due to complex sugar-based substances adhering to vessel walls, making the arteries incapable of supplying as much blood and oxygen to the tissues as is needed, the skin may break down and not be able to heal, even without the occurrence of an external wound. This prevents healing and leads to skin problems such as dermatitis, the breakdown of collagen with build-up of fatty deposits, and ulcers, especially in the legs and feet. Diabetic skin ulcers, particularly of the foot and lower leg, often stem from vascular problems caused by poor circulation and poor oxygen supply to the extremities.

E08.620 Diabetes mellitus due to underlying condition with diabetic dermatitis

Diabetic dermatitis includes diabetic necrobiosis lipoidica, which is a necrotizing skin condition marked by collagen breakdown, deposits of fatty build-up, and the thickening of blood vessels. This is chronic condition that progresses slowly with flare-ups occurring. A reddish-brown rash appears at first, usually on the lower legs in most people, with well-defined borders on lesions that slowly grow larger, turning shiny and red with a yellowish center. Some people experience itching and burning with the rash, which may also appear on the trunk, arms, face, or scalp. The lesions eventually turn into a purple depression in the skin that may scar. During flare-ups, treatment may consist of topical creams with sterile dressings, cortizone injections or oral steroids, and ultrviolet light treatment for the lesions. If the lesions do not break open, treatment may not be required and rest and support stockings are used.

E08.64 Diabetes mellitus due to underlying condition with hypoglycemia

In hypoglycemia, the blood sugar falls abnormally low. This happens in diabetics when too much insulin or oral antidiabetic medication is taken, not enough food is ingested, or exercise is suddenly increased without a corresponding increase in food intake. Confusion, shaking, sweating, headache, aggression, heart palpitations, dizziness, and fainting are all symptoms. Small, sugar-laden snacks or fruit juice can reverse the low blood sugar, but if not treated promptly, severe hypoglycemia can progress to seizures and unconsciousness, called hypoglycemic or insulin shock. When the brain is deprived of glucose, neurons in the brain that process memory are destroyed and permanent memory loss can result.

E08.65 Diabetes mellitus due to underlying condition with hyperglycemia

This code is used to report diabetes mellitus due to an underlying condition when it is stated as "out of control", "poorly controlled", or 'inadequately controlled". Diabetes complications often require multiple coding. This code may be assigned with other appropriate diabetes codes to describe the complete clinical picture of the patient.

E09 Drug or chemical induced diabetes mellitus

This category reports diabetes mellitus cases that develop from poisoning due to exposure to toxic chemicals or medicinal drugs. The end metabolic effect in secondary diabetes due to drugs or chemicals is dependent upon the impact the substance has on insulin secretion, insulin sensitivity, and the unmasking of genetic tendencies. Sometimes, the effect of treatment for existing chronic conditions also increases diabetes risk in addition to the condition itself. Drugs and chemical agents known to be associated with secondary diabetes include diuretics, antihypertensives, hormones, psychoactive agents, anticonvulsants, antineoplastics, antiprotozoals, and antiretrovirals. The manifestations accompanying this classification of secondary diabetes parallel those occurring with type 1 and 2 diabetes.

Note: Secondary diabetes due to drugs or chemicals excludes type 1, type 2, gestational, neonatal, postpancreatectomy or other postprocedural diabetes, diabetes due to genetic defects, diabetes due to another underlying condition, as well as secondary diabetes mellitus not classified elsewhere.

Note: Proper sequencing requires the coder to assign the code for poisoning due to drug or toxin first and to use an additional code for the adverse effect of a drug, when applicable.

Note: Associated insulin use should also be coded additionally.

Note: Controlled or uncontrolled status is not considered an axis of coding for the selection of the diabetes code; however, out of control or poorly controlled cases that are so stated in the documentation are reported by using the appropriate code for the type of diabetes with hyperglycemia.

E09.0 Drug or chemical induced diabetes mellitus with hyperosmolarity

Diabetes with hyperosmolarity is a medical emergency that involves extremely high blood glucose levels, dehydration, and decreased consciousness that can lead to coma, without the presence of ketones or acidosis. Hyperosmolarity occurs when high blood concentrations of glucose, sodium, and other molecules become even higher because the kidneys are conserving water. The kidneys normally help balance high blood glucose and ion levels by excreting extra amounts in the urine, but when the kidneys begin conserving water, the concentrations climb higher and there is a greater need for water. Signs include weakness, increased thirst, lethargy, confusion, speech impairment, loss of muscle function, and convulsions. These symptoms may progress over days or weeks and may occur with or without coma. Treatment aims to correct the dehydration with intravenous fluids and electrolytes to improve blood pressure, urine output, and circulation, and the administration of insulin to bring down high glucose levels.

E09.1 Drug or chemical induced diabetes mellitus with ketoacidosis

Ketoacidosis is a dramatic, emergency complication that can develop quickly and can also lead to coma and death. Without insulin, sugar in the blood cannot be used for energy. Cells needing energy to survive switch to a back-up method in which fat cells break down, producing compounds called ketones that are used for some energy, but make the blood too acidic. This condition may first appear with excessive thirst, urination, nausea, vomiting, and abdominal pain. Breathing becomes deep and fast as the body attempts to balance the pH acidity level of the blood. Breath smells like acetone (nail polish remover) because of the escaping ketones. If left untreated, ketoacidosis progresses to coma and death within a few hours. Treatment consists of large amounts of fluids and electrolytes given intravenously with careful control of blood sugar back to normal levels in order to prevent sudden fluid shifts into the brain.

E09.2 Drug or chemical induced diabetes mellitus with kidney complications

In diabetics, the renal blood vessels may thicken and leak protein into the urine, which cannot be filtered properly. An abnormally high level of protein in the urine is a sign of early kidney damage. Kidney malfunction or nephropathy can lead to chronic kidney disease and failure. Kidney complications are associated with long term diabetes.

E09.3 Drug or chemical induced diabetes mellitus with ophthalmic complications

Diabetes affects both large and small blood vessels throughout the body, such as those in the eyes. Complex sugar-based substances adhere to vessel walls, causing them to thicken and leak, which makes them incapable of supplying as much blood and oxygen to the tissues as is needed. Leaking blood vessels of the eye cause retinal damage. Ophthalmic conditions such as retinopathy and cataracts occurring as long-term diabetic complications can lead to blindness.

E09.311 Drug or chemical induced diabetes mellitus with unspecified diabetic retinopathy with macular edema

In diabetic retinopathy, the arteries supplying blood and nutrients to the retina become weakened and leak, causing hemorrhaging that damages parts of the retina and leaks blood into the inner eye, causing floaters and general vision loss. Diabetic macular edema is a swelling of the retina as an aspect of diabetes mellitus occurring when blood vessels leak and cause fluid and protein deposits to build up and collect within the macula, the yellowish central portion of the retina rich in the nerve endings and responsible for fine detailed, daytime vision.

E09.351 Drug or chemical induced diabetes mellitus with proliferative diabetic retinopathy with macular edema

In background diabetic retinopathy, the arteries in the retina become weakened and leak, causing tiny hemorrhages, and decreasing the patient's vision. Proliferative diabetic retinopathy is the next stage when continued problems in the blood vessels cause parts of the retina to become oxygen- and nutrient-deprived. At the same time, hemorrhaging of the vessels continues to leak blood into the inner eye, causing the patient to experience floating black spots in their vision, called floaters, in addition to suffering from general vision loss. This can occur with macular edema, a swelling of the retina that occurs when fluid leaks from the blood vessels in the opaque spot on the cornea.

Note: In the final stage of this process, the patient frequently experiences retinal detachment and/or glaucoma, which should be classified with the appropriate codes for those disorders.

E09.4 Drug or chemical induced diabetes mellitus with neurological complications

Diabetic nerve damage occurs because glucose is not being metabolized normally and blood supply is inadequate. Signs and symptoms of diabetic neuropathies differ depending on which nerve(s) are affected. In peripheral neuropathy, the patient may experience painful sensations, tingling, burning, or weakness in the limbs. Muscle weakness, pain, and difficulty with walking may occur. The patient may become hyerpsensitive to the slightest touch, which causes agony. Nerve damage in the skin also affects the ability to sense pain, pressure, and temperature changes, particularly in the feet and toes. Injuries can result that go unnoticed due to the neurological damage. Autonomic (poly)neuropathy affects the nerves that control functions such as heart rate, digestion, blood pressure, and body temperature regulation resulting in problems such as gastroparesis. Nerves other than peripheral nerves may also be affected, causing amyotrophy, or radiculoplexus neuropathy affecting the thighs, hips, abdomen, and buttocks.

E09.41 Drug or chemical induced diabetes mellitus with neurological complications with diabetic mononeuropathy

Mononeuropathy involves damage to one specific nerve and can affect a limb, the face, or the trunk. It often comes on suddenly and can cause severe pain, although symptoms are not usually long-term problems and may diminish over time, unless considerably damage to the nerve has already occurred. Areas affected depend on which nerve is involved. Diabetic mononeuropathy can appear as pain in only one particular area of a limb, such as the front of the thigh or the shin, paralysis is one area of the face, abdominal pain, or aching behind one eye.

E09.43 Drug or chemical induced diabetes mellitus with neurological complications with diabetic autonomic (poly)neuropathy

Autonomic neuropathy affects the nervous system that controls functions such as the heart, lungs, stomach and intestines, bladder, and body temperature and blood pressure regulation. Symptoms conditions of autonomic neuropathy in the diabetic include gastroparesis in which the stomach empties very slowly; constipation or uncontrolled diarrhea; incontinence and bladder problems; difficulty swallowing, inability to regulate heart rate when resting or moving; and sharp drops in blood pressure when rising.

E09.44 Drug or chemical induced diabetes mellitus with neurological complications with diabetic amyotrophy

Amyotrophy can occur with any type of diabetes, although it is most common in type 2 diabetics. It is also called diabetic radiculoplexus neuropathy and affects nerves closer to the trunk, such as those of the thighs, hips, and buttocks, as opposed to affecting the nerve endings like in peripheral neuropathy. The patient experiences weakening and atrophying thigh muscles; sudden, extremely painful sensations in the hips, thighs, and buttocks; difficulty getting up from in the sitting position; and abdominal swelling, if the abdomen is affected.

E09.5 Drug or chemical induced diabetes mellitus with circulatory complications

Diabetes has a big effect on blood vessels. Complex sugar-based substances adhere to vessel walls, causing them to thicken and leak, which makes them incapable of supplying as much blood and oxygen to the tissues as is needed. Poorly controlled blood sugar levels also cause an increase in fatty substances in the blood with the adherence of plaque material to the vessel walls. This atherosclerotic buildup also reduces blood flow and causes poor circulation. Poor circulation to the extremities causes slow-healing wounds prone to infection. Some wounds may never heal and lead to gangrene with the need for amputation.

E09.62 Drug or chemical induced diabetes mellitus with skin complications

Because diabetes has such a big effect on blood vessels due to complex sugar-based substances adhering to vessel walls, making the arteries incapable of supplying as much blood and oxygen to the tissues as is needed, the skin may break down and not be able to heal, even without the occurrence of an external wound. This prevents healing and leads to skin problems such as dermatitis, the breakdown of collagen with build-up of fatty deposits, and ulcers, especially in the legs and feet. Diabetic skin ulcers, particularly of the foot and lower leg, often stem from vascular problems caused by poor circulation and poor oxygen supply to the extremities.

E09.620 Drug or chemical induced diabetes mellitus with diabetic dermatitis

Diabetic dermatitis includes diabetic necrobiosis lipoidica, which is a necrotizing skin condition marked by collagen breakdown, deposits of fatty build-up, and the thickening of blood vessels. This is chronic condition that progresses slowly with flare-ups occurring. A reddish-brown rash appears at first, usually on the lower legs in most people, with well-defined borders on lesions that slowly grow larger, turning shiny and red with a yellowish center. Some people experience itching and burning with the rash, which may also appear on the trunk, arms, face, or scalp. The lesions eventually turn into a purple depression in the skin that may scar. During flare-ups, treatment may consist of topical creams with sterile dressings, cortizone injections or oral steroids, and ultrviolet light treatment for the lesions. If the lesions do not break open, treatment may not be required and rest and support stockings are used.

E09.64 Drug or chemical induced diabetes mellitus with hypoglycemia

In hypoglycemia, the blood sugar falls abnormally low. This happens in diabetics when too much insulin or oral antidiabetic medication is taken, not enough food is ingested, or exercise is suddenly increased without a corresponding increase in food intake. Confusion, shaking, sweating, headache, aggression, heart palpitations, dizziness and fainting are all symptoms. Small, sugar-laden snacks or fruit juice can reverse the low blood sugar, but if not treated promptly, severe hypoglycemia can progress to seizures and unconsciousness, called hypoglycemic or insulin shock. When the brain is deprived of glucose, neurons in the brain that process memory are destroyed and permanent memory loss can result.

E09.65 Drug or chemical induced diabetes mellitus with hyperglycemia

This code is used to report diabetes mellitus due to an underlying condition when it is stated as "out of control", "poorly controlled", or "inadequately controlled". Diabetes complications often require multiple coding. This code may be assigned with other appropriate diabetes codes to describe the complete clinical picture of the patient.

E10 Type 1 diabetes mellitus

Diabetes mellitus is a systemic, metabolic disease arising from insulin-related problems. Insulin is a hormone made by the beta cells of the pancreas and secreted into the digestive system. Insulin regulates blood sugar levels as well as the transport, storage, and use of glucose and amino acids. Without effective insulin action, blood sugar levels are difficult to control and become dangerously high. This causes many different complications, especially over time, including poor circulation and blood vessel damage, kidney problems, nerve damage, ophthalmic degeneration, skin breakdown, atherosclerosis, heart disease, and stroke.

Diabetes mellitus has different types. Type 1, formerly referred to as juvenile onset or insulin dependent diabetes, occurs when more than 90% of the cells in the pancreas that produce insulin have been permanently damaged or destroyed. The body produces little or no insulin on its own. This type accounts for about 10% of diabetes cases and most people affected will be diagnosed before age 30. These patients require regular injections of insulin to survive. Type 1 diabetes is often linked backed to autoimmune processes, childhood or teenage viral infections, nutritional factors, drug overdoses-- particularly of antibiotics, and genetic predispositions.

Symptoms are related to the effects of high blood sugar. Too much sugar in the blood moves into the urine and then the kidneys excrete high amounts of water to dilute the large amount of sugar. People urinate frequently and are excessively thirsty. Excessive calories are also lost and weight loss occurs with a feeling of hunger. Blurred vision, nausea, sleepiness, and decreased physical endurance are also symptoms. These symptoms often develop abruptly and dramatically in type 1 patients.

Note: This category excludes diabetes due to an underlying condition or exposure to toxic chemicals or medicaments, any other types of secondary diabetes, gestational, neonatal, type 2, and postpancreatectomy or postprocedural diabetes.

Note: Diabetes is a pervasive, systemic disease that should be coded even when documentation does not reflect that current medical care was actively aimed at diabetic treatment or intervention.

Note: Report also the appropriate code to identify the use of insulin. Because the record states that a person is using or requiring insulin does not constitute type 1 diabetes. Type 2 patients may also depend on insulin for controlling blood sugar.

Note: Controlled or uncontrolled status is not considered an axis of coding for the selection of the diabetes code; however, out of control or poorly controlled cases that are so stated in the documentation are reported by using the appropriate code for the type of diabetes with hyperglycemia.

E10.1 Type 1 diabetes mellitus with ketoacidosis

Ketoacidosis is a dramatic, emergency complication that can develop quickly and can also lead to coma and death. Without insulin, sugar in the blood cannot be used for energy. Cells needing energy to survive switch to a back-up method in which fat cells break down, producing compounds called ketones that are used for some energy, but make the blood too acidic. This condition may first appear with excessive thirst, urination, nausea, vomiting, and abdominal pain. Breathing becomes deep and fast as the body attempts to balance the pH acidity level of the blood. Breath smells like acetone (nail polish remover) because of the escaping ketones. If left untreated, ketoacidosis progresses to coma and death within a few hours. Treatment consists of large amounts of fluids and electrolytes given intravenously with careful control of blood sugar back to normal levels in order to prevent sudden fluid shifts into the brain.

E10.2 Type 1 diabetes mellitus with kidney complications

In diabetics, the renal blood vessels may thicken and leak protein into the urine, which cannot be filtered properly. An abnormally high level of protein in the urine is a sign of early kidney damage. Kidney malfunction or nephropathy can lead to chronic kidney disease and failure. Kidney complications are associated with long term diabetes.

E10.3 Type 1 diabetes mellitus with ophthalmic complications

Diabetes affects both large and small blood vessels throughout the body, such as those in the eyes. Complex sugar-based substances adhere to vessel walls, causing them to thicken and leak, which makes them incapable of supplying as much blood and oxygen to the tissues as is needed. Leaking blood vessels of the eye cause retinal damage. Ophthalmic conditions such as retinopathy and cataracts occurring as long-term diabetic complications can lead to blindness.

E10.311 Type 1 diabetes mellitus with unspecified diabetic retinopathy with macular edema

In diabetic retinopathy, the arteries supplying blood and nutrients to the retina become weakened and leak, causing hemorrhaging that damages parts of the retina and leaks blood into the inner eye, causing floaters and general vision loss. Diabetic macular edema is a swelling of the retina as an aspect of diabetes mellitus occurring when blood vessels leak and cause fluid and protein deposits to build up and collect within the macula, the yellowish central portion of the retina rich in the nerve endings and responsible for fine detailed, daytime vision.

E10.351 Type 1 diabetes mellitus with proliferative diabetic retinopathy with macular edema

In background diabetic retinopathy, the arteries in the retina become weakened and leak, causing tiny hemorrhages, and decreasing the patient's vision. Proliferative diabetic retinopathy is the next stage when continued problems in the blood vessels cause parts of the retina to become oxygen- and nutrient-deprived. At the same time, hemorrhaging of the vessels continues to leak blood into the inner eye, causing the patient to experience floating black spots in their vision, called floaters, in addition to suffering from general vision loss. This can occur with macular edema, a swelling of the retina that occurs when fluid leaks from the blood vessels in the opaque spot on the cornea.

Note: In the final stage of this process, the patient frequently experiences retinal detachment and/or glaucoma, which should be classified with the appropriate codes for those disorders.

E10.4 Type 1 diabetes mellitus with neurological complications

Diabetic nerve damage occurs because glucose is not being metabolized normally and blood supply is inadequate. Signs and symptoms of diabetic neuropathies differ depending on which nerve(s) are affected. In peripheral neuropathy, the patient may experience painful sensations, tingling, burning, or weakness in the limbs. Muscle weakness, pain, and difficulty with walking may occur. The patient may become hyerpsensitive to the slightest touch, which causes agony. Nerve damage in the skin also affects the ability to sense pain, pressure, and temperature changes, particularly in the feet and toes. Injuries can result that go unnoticed due to the neurological damage. Autonomic (poly)neuropathy affects the nerves that control functions such as heart rate, digestion, blood pressure, and body temperature regulation resulting in problems such as gastroparesis. Nerves other than peripheral nerves may also be affected, causing amyotrophy, or radiculoplexus neuropathy affecting the thighs, hips, abdomen, and buttocks.

E10.41 Type 1 diabetes mellitus with diabetic mononeuropathy

Mononeuropathy involves damage to one specific nerve and can affect a limb, the face, or the trunk. It often comes on suddenly and can cause severe pain, although symptoms are not usually long-term problems and may diminish over time, unless considerably damage to the nerve has already occurred. Areas affected depend on which nerve is involved. Diabetic mononeuropathy can appear as pain in only one particular area of a limb, such as the front of the thigh or the shin, paralysis is one area of the face, abdominal pain, or aching behind one eye.

E10.43 Type 1 diabetes mellitus with diabetic autonomic (poly)neuropathy

Autonomic neuropathy affects the nervous system that controls functions such as the heart, lungs, stomach and intestines, bladder, and body temperature and blood pressure regulation. Symptoms conditions of autonomic neuropathy in the diabetic include gastroparesis in which the stomach empties very slowly; constipation or uncontrolled diarrhea; incontinence and bladder problems; difficulty swallowing, inability to regulate heart rate when resting or moving; and sharp drops in blood pressure when rising.

E10.44 Type 1 diabetes mellitus with diabetic amyotrophy

Amyotrophy can occur with any type of diabetes, although it is most common in type 2 diabetics. It is also called diabetic radiculoplexus neuropathy and affects nerves closer to the trunk, such as those of the thighs, hips, and buttocks, as opposed to affecting the nerve endings like in peripheral neuropathy. The patient experiences weakening and atrophying thigh muscles; sudden, extremely painful sensations in the hips, thighs, and buttocks; difficulty getting up from in the sitting position; and abdominal swelling, if the abdomen is affected.

E10.5 Type 1 diabetes mellitus with circulatory complications

Diabetes has a big effect on blood vessels. Complex sugar-based substances adhere to vessel walls, causing them to thicken and leak, which makes them incapable of supplying as much blood and oxygen to the tissues as is needed. Poorly controlled blood sugar levels also cause an increase in fatty substances in the blood with the adherence of plaque material to the vessel walls. This atherosclerotic buildup also reduces blood flow and causes poor circulation. Poor circulation to the extremities causes slow-healing wounds prone to infection. Some wounds may never heal and lead to gangrene with the need for amputation.

E10.62 Type 1 diabetes mellitus with skin complications

Because diabetes has such a big effect on blood vessels due to complex sugar-based substances adhering to vessel walls, making the arteries incapable of supplying as much blood and oxygen to the tissues as is needed, the skin may break down and not be able to heal, even without the occurrence of an external wound. This prevents healing and leads to skin problems such as dermatitis, the breakdown of collagen with build-up of fatty deposits, and ulcers, especially in the legs and feet. Diabetic skin ulcers, particularly of the foot and lower leg, often stem from vascular problems caused by poor circulation and poor oxygen supply to the extremities.

E10.620 Type 1 diabetes mellitus with diabetic dermatitis

Diabetic dermatitis includes diabetic necrobiosis lipoidica, which is a necrotizing skin condition marked by collagen breakdown, deposits of fatty build-up, and the thickening of blood vessels. This is chronic condition that progresses slowly with flare-ups occurring. A reddish-brown rash appears at first, usually on the lower legs in most people, with well-defined borders on lesions that slowly grow larger, turning shiny and red with a yellowish center. Some people experience itching and burning with the rash, which may also appear on the trunk, arms, face, or scalp. The lesions eventually turn into a purple depression in the skin that may scar. During flare-ups, treatment may consist of topical creams with sterile dressings, cortizone injections or oral steroids, and ultrviolet light treatment for the lesions. If the lesions do not break open, treatment may not be required and rest and support stockings are used.

E10.64 Type 1 diabetes mellitus with hypoglycemia

In hypoglycemia, the blood sugar falls abnormally low. This happens in diabetics when too much insulin or oral antidiabetic medication is taken, not enough food is ingested, or exercise is suddenly increased without a corresponding increase in food intake. Confusion, shaking, sweating, headache, aggression, heart palpitations, dizziness and fainting are all symptoms. Small, sugar-laden snacks or fruit juice can reverse the low blood sugar, but if not treated promptly, severe hypoglycemia can progress to seizures and unconsciousness, called hypoglycemic or insulin shock. When the brain is deprived of glucose, neurons in the brain that process memory are destroyed and permanent memory loss can result.

E10.65 Type 1 diabetes mellitus with hyperglycemia

This code is used to report diabetes mellitus due to an underlying condition when it is stated as "out of control", "poorly controlled", or "inadequately controlled". Diabetes complications often require multiple coding. This code may be assigned with other appropriate diabetes codes to describe the complete clinical picture of the patient.

E11 Type 2 diabetes mellitus

Diabetes mellitus is a systemic, metabolic disease arising from insulin-related problems. Insulin is a hormone made by the beta cells of the pancreas and secreted into the digestive system. Insulin regulates blood sugar levels as well as the transport, storage, and use of glucose and amino acids. Without effective insulin action, blood sugar levels are difficult to control and become dangerously high. This causes many different complications, especially over time, including poor circulation and blood vessel damage, kidney problems, nerve damage, ophthalmic degeneration, skin breakdown, atherosclerosis, heart disease, and stroke.

Diabetes mellitus has different types. Type 2, formerly referred to as adult onset or non-insulin dependent diabetes, occurs when the body develops a resistance to the action of insulin. Even though the pancreas is still producing insulin, sometimes even at higher levels in response to elevated blood sugars, the body's resistance results in not enough insulin to meet the body's needs. Most type 2 patients are diagnosed in adulthood at ages older than 30. With the increasing problems of obesity, sedentary lifestyle, and lack of exercise, type 2 diabetes is being diagnosed more and more often in children and adolescents. Type 2 diabetes can be controlled with oral medications, diet, and exercise, but sometimes also requires insulin injections.

Type 2 diabetes has several risk factors including obesity, age, some racial and cultural group risk factors, certain drugs such as corticosteroids, the presence of other diseases, and familial tendency. Of these risk factors, obesity is the major one for developing type 2 diabetes. Up to 90% of type 2 diabetics are overweight. Obese people require much larger amounts of insulin to maintain normal blood sugar.

Symptoms of diabetes are related to the effects of high blood sugar. Too much sugar in the blood moves into the urine and then the kidneys excrete high amounts of water to dilute the large amount of sugar. People urinate frequently and are excessively thirsty. Excessive calories are also lost and weight loss occurs with a feeling of hunger. Blurred vision, nausea, sleepiness, and decreased physical endurance are also symptoms. Those with type 2 diabetes may not have symptoms for years or even decades before diagnosis. Symptoms may be subtle and mild at first and gradually worsen. Laboratory tests confirm diagnosis by testing for glucose levels in urine and blood.

Note: This category excludes diabetes due to an underlying condition or exposure to toxic chemicals or medicaments, any other types of secondary diabetes, gestational, neonatal, type 1, and postpancreatectomy or postprocedural diabetes.

Note: Diabetes is a pervasive, systemic disease that should be coded even when documentation does not reflect that current medical care was actively aimed at diabetic treatment or intervention.

Note: Report also the appropriate code to identify the use of insulin.

Note: Controlled or uncontrolled status is not considered an axis of coding for the selection of the diabetes code; however, out of control or poorly controlled cases that are so stated in the documentation are reported by using the appropriate code for the type of diabetes with hyperglycemia.

E11.0 Type 2 diabetes mellitus with hyperosmolarity

Diabetes with hyperosmolarity is a medical emergency that involves extremely high blood glucose levels, dehydration, and decreased consciousness that can lead to coma, without the presence of ketones or acidosis. Hyperosmolarity occurs when high blood concentrations of glucose, sodium, and other molecules become even higher because the kidneys are conserving water. The kidneys normally help balance high blood glucose and ion levels by excreting extra amounts in the urine, but when the kidneys begin conserving water, the concentrations climb higher and there is a greater need for water. Signs include weakness, increased thirst, lethargy, confusion, speech impairment, loss of muscle function, and convulsions. These symptoms may progress over days or weeks and may occur with or without coma. Treatment aims to correct the dehydration with intravenous fluids and electrolytes to improve blood pressure, urine output, and circulation, and the administration of insulin to bring down high glucose levels.

E11.2 Type 2 diabetes mellitus with kidney complications

In diabetics, the renal blood vessels may thicken and leak protein into the urine, which cannot be filtered properly. An abnormally high level of protein in the urine is a sign of early kidney damage. Kidney malfunction or nephropathy can lead to chronic kidney disease and failure. Kidney complications are associated with long term diabetes.

E11.3 Type 2 diabetes mellitus with ophthalmic complications

Diabetes affects both large and small blood vessels throughout the body, such as those in the eyes. Complex sugar-based substances adhere to vessel walls, causing them to thicken and leak, which makes them incapable of supplying as much blood and oxygen to the tissues as is needed. Leaking blood vessels of the eye cause retinal damage. Ophthalmic conditions such as retinopathy and cataracts occurring as long-term diabetic complications can lead to blindness.

E11.311 Type 2 diabetes mellitus with unspecified diabetic retinopathy with macular edema

In diabetic retinopathy, the arteries supplying blood and nutrients to the retina become weakened and leak, causing hemorrhaging that damages parts of the retina and leaks blood into the inner eye, causing floaters and general vision loss. Diabetic macular edema is a swelling of the retina as an aspect of diabetes mellitus occurring when blood vessels leak and cause fluid and protein deposits to build up and collect within the macula, the yellowish central portion of the retina rich in the nerve endings and responsible for fine detailed, daytime vision.

E11.351 Type 2 diabetes mellitus with proliferative diabetic retinopathy with macular edema

In background diabetic retinopathy, the arteries in the retina become weakened and leak, causing tiny hemorrhages, and decreasing the patient's vision. Proliferative diabetic retinopathy is the next stage when continued problems in the blood vessels cause parts of the retina to become oxygen-

and nutrient-deprived. At the same time, hemorrhaging of the vessels continues to leak blood into the inner eye, causing the patient to experience floating black spots in their vision, called floaters, in addition to suffering from general vision loss. This can occur with macular edema, a swelling of the retina that occurs when fluid leaks from the blood vessels in the opaque spot on the cornea.

Note: In the final stage of this process, the patient frequently experiences retinal detachment and/or glaucoma, which should be classified with the appropriate codes for those disorders.

E11.4 Type 2 diabetes mellitus with neurological complications

Diabetic nerve damage occurs because glucose is not being metabolized normally and blood supply is inadequate. Signs and symptoms of diabetic neuropathies differ depending on which nerve(s) are affected. In peripheral neuropathy, the patient may experience painful sensations, tingling, burning, or weakness in the limbs. Muscle weakness, pain, and difficulty with walking may occur. The patient may become hyerpsensitive to the slightest touch, which causes agony. Nerve damage in the skin also affects the ability to sense pain, pressure, and temperature changes, particularly in the feet and toes. Injuries can result that go unnoticed due to the neurological damage. Autonomic (poly)neuropathy affects the nerves that control functions such as heart rate, digestion, blood pressure, and body temperature regulation resulting in problems such as gastroparesis. Nerves other than peripheral nerves may also be affected, causing amyotrophy, or radiculoplexus neuropathy affecting the thighs, hips, abdomen, and buttocks.

E11.41 Type 2 diabetes mellitus with diabetic mononeuropathy

Mononeuropathy involves damage to one specific nerve and can affect a limb, the face, or the trunk. It often comes on suddenly and can cause severe pain, although symptoms are not usually long-term problems and may diminish over time, unless considerably damage to the nerve has already occurred. Areas affected depend on which nerve is involved. Diabetic mononeuropathy can appear as pain in only one particular area of a limb, such as the front of the thigh or the shin, paralysis is one area of the face, abdominal pain, or aching behind one eye.

E11.43 Type 2 diabetes mellitus with diabetic autonomic (poly)neuropathy

Autonomic neuropathy affects the nervous system that controls functions such as the heart, lungs, stomach and intestines, bladder, and body temperature and blood pressure regulation. Symptoms conditions of autonomic neuropathy in the diabetic include gastroparesis in which the stomach empties very slowly; constipation or uncontrolled diarrhea; incontinence and bladder problems; difficulty swallowing, inability to regulate heart rate when resting or moving; and sharp drops in blood pressure when rising.

E11.44 Type 2 diabetes mellitus with diabetic amyotrophy

Amyotrophy can occur with any type of diabetes, although it is most common in type 2 diabetics. It is also called diabetic radiculoplexus neuropathy and affects nerves closer to the trunk, such as those of the thighs, hips, and buttocks, as opposed to affecting the nerve endings like in peripheral neuropathy. The patient experiences weakening and atrophying thigh muscles; sudden, extremely painful sensations in the hips, thighs, and buttocks; difficulty getting up from in the sitting position; and abdominal swelling, if the abdomen is affected.

E11.5 Type 2 diabetes mellitus with circulatory complications

Diabetes has a big effect on blood vessels. Complex sugar-based substances adhere to vessel walls, causing them to thicken and leak, which makes them incapable of supplying as much blood and oxygen to the tissues as is needed. Poorly controlled blood sugar levels also cause an increase in fatty substances in the blood with the adherence of plaque material to the vessel walls. This atherosclerotic buildup also reduces blood flow and causes poor circulation. Poor circulation to the extremities causes slow-healing wounds prone to infection. Some wounds may never heal and lead to gangrene with the need for amputation.

E11.62   Type 2 diabetes mellitus with skin complications

Because diabetes has such a big effect on blood vessels due to complex sugar-based substances adhering to vessel walls, making the arteries incapable of supplying as much blood and oxygen to the tissues as is needed, the skin may break down and not be able to heal, even without the occurrence of an external wound. This prevents healing and leads to skin problems such as dermatitis, the breakdown of collagen with build-up of fatty deposits, and ulcers, especially in the legs and feet. Diabetic skin ulcers, particularly of the foot and lower leg, often stem from vascular problems caused by poor circulation and poor oxygen supply to the extremities.

E11.620   Type 2 diabetes mellitus with diabetic dermatitis

Diabetic dermatitis includes diabetic necrobiosis lipoidica, which is a necrotizing skin condition marked by collagen breakdown, deposits of fatty build-up, and the thickening of blood vessels. This is chronic condition that progresses slowly with flare-ups occurring. A reddish-brown rash appears at first, usually on the lower legs in most people, with well-defined borders on lesions that slowly grow larger, turning shiny and red with a yellowish center. Some people experience itching and burning with the rash, which may also appear on the trunk, arms, face, or scalp. The lesions eventually turn into a purple depression in the skin that may scar. During flare-ups, treatment may consist of topical creams with sterile dressings, cortizone injections or oral steroids, and ultrviolet light treatment for the lesions. If the lesions do not break open, treatment may not be required and rest and support stockings are used.

E11.64   Type 2 diabetes mellitus with hypoglycemia

In hypoglycemia, the blood sugar falls abnormally low. This happens in diabetics when too much insulin or oral antidiabetic medication is taken, not enough food is ingested, or exercise is suddenly increased without a corresponding increase in food intake. Confusion, shaking, sweating, headache, aggression, heart palpitations, dizziness and fainting are all symptoms. Small, sugar-laden snacks or fruit juice can reverse the low blood sugar, but if not treated promptly, severe hypoglycemia can progress to seizures and unconsciousness, called hypoglycemic or insulin shock. When the brain is deprived of glucose, neurons in the brain that process memory are destroyed and permanent memory loss can result.

E11.65   Type 2 diabetes mellitus with hyperglycemia

This code is used to report diabetes mellitus due to an underlying condition when it is stated as "out of control", "poorly controlled", or "inadequately controlled". Diabetes complications often require multiple coding. This code may be assigned with other appropriate diabetes codes to describe the complete clinical picture of the patient.

E13   Other specified diabetes mellitus

This category reports other specified types of secondary diabetes mellitus that are due to genetic defects affecting either beta cell function or insulin action, and also cases of diabetes due to pancreatectomy or other procedures. Overt diabetes is caused secondarily by removal of the pancreas or interference with normal insulin action or functioning of the beta cells. The manifestations accompanying this classification of secondary diabetes parallel those occurring with type 1 and 2 diabetes.

Note: This category of diabetes excludes type 1, type 2, gestational, neonatal, drug or chemical induced diabetes, and diabetes due to another underlying disease or condition.

Note: Associated insulin use should be coded additionally.

Note: Controlled or uncontrolled status is not considered an axis of coding for the selection of the diabetes code; however, out of control or poorly controlled cases that are so stated in the documentation are reported by using the appropriate code for the type of diabetes with hyperglycemia.

E13.0   Other specified diabetes mellitus with hyperosmolarity

Diabetes with hyperosmolarity is a medical emergency that involves extremely high blood glucose levels, dehydration, and decreased consciousness that can lead to coma, without the presence of ketones or acidosis. Hyperosmolarity occurs when high blood concentrations of glucose, sodium, and other molecules become even higher because the kidneys are conserving water. The kidneys normally help balance high blood glucose and ion levels by excreting extra amounts in the urine, but when the kidneys begin conserving water, the concentrations climb higher and there is a greater need for water. Signs include weakness, increased thirst, lethargy, confusion, speech impairment, loss of muscle function, and convulsions. These symptoms may progress over days or weeks and may occur with or without coma. Treatment aims to correct the dehydration with intravenous fluids and electrolytes to improve blood pressure, urine output, and circulation, and the administration of insulin to bring down high glucose levels.

E13.1   Other specified diabetes mellitus with ketoacidosis

Ketoacidosis is a dramatic, emergency complication that can develop quickly and can also lead to coma and death. Without insulin, sugar in the blood cannot be used for energy. Cells needing energy to survive switch to a back-up method in which fat cells break down, producing compounds called ketones that are used for some energy, but make the blood too acidic. This condition may first appear with excessive thirst, urination, nausea, vomiting, and abdominal pain. Breathing becomes deep and fast as the body attempts to balance the pH acidity level of the blood. Breath smells like acetone (nail polish remover) because of the escaping ketones. If left untreated, ketoacidosis progresses to coma and death within a few hours. Treatment consists of large amounts of fluids and electrolytes given intravenously with careful control of blood sugar back to normal levels in order to prevent sudden fluid shifts into the brain.

E13.2   Other specified diabetes mellitus with kidney complications

In diabetics, the renal blood vessels may thicken and leak protein into the urine, which cannot be filtered properly. An abnormally high level of protein in the urine is a sign of early kidney damage. Kidney malfunction or nephropathy can lead to chronic kidney disease and failure. Kidney complications are associated with long term diabetes.

E13.3   Other specified diabetes mellitus with ophthalmic complications

Diabetes affects both large and small blood vessels throughout the body, such as those in the eyes. Complex sugar-based substances adhere to vessel walls, causing them to thicken and leak, which makes them incapable of supplying as much blood and oxygen to the tissues as is needed. Leaking blood vessels of the eye cause retinal damage. Ophthalmic conditions such as retinopathy and cataracts occurring as long-term diabetic complications can lead to blindness.

E13.311   Other specified diabetes mellitus with unspecified diabetic retinopathy with macular edema

In diabetic retinopathy, the arteries supplying blood and nutrients to the retina become weakened and leak, causing hemorrhaging that damages parts of the retina and leaks blood into the inner eye, causing floaters and general vision loss. Diabetic macular edema is a swelling of the retina as an aspect of diabetes mellitus occurring when blood vessels leak and cause fluid and protein deposits to build up and collect within the macula, the yellowish central portion of the retina rich in the nerve endings and responsible for fine detailed, daytime vision.

E13.351 Other specified diabetes mellitus with proliferative diabetic retinopathy with macular edema

In background diabetic retinopathy, the arteries in the retina become weakened and leak, causing tiny hemorrhages, and decreasing the patient's vision. Proliferative diabetic retinopathy is the next stage when continued problems in the blood vessels cause parts of the retina to become oxygen- and nutrient-deprived. At the same time, hemorrhaging of the vessels continues to leak blood into the inner eye, causing the patient to experience floating black spots in their vision, called floaters, in addition to suffering from general vision loss. This can occur with macular edema, a swelling of the retina that occurs when fluid leaks from the blood vessels in the opaque spot on the cornea.

Note: In the final stage of this process, the patient frequently experiences retinal detachment and/or glaucoma, which should be classified with the appropriate codes for those disorders.

E13.4 Other specified diabetes mellitus with neurological complications

Diabetic nerve damage occurs because glucose is not being metabolized normally and blood supply is inadequate. Signs and symptoms of diabetic neuropathies differ depending on which nerve(s) are affected. In peripheral neuropathy, the patient may experience painful sensations, tingling, burning, or weakness in the limbs. Muscle weakness, pain, and difficulty with walking may occur. The patient may become hyerpsensitive to the slightest touch, which causes agony. Nerve damage in the skin also affects the ability to sense pain, pressure, and temperature changes, particularly in the feet and toes. Injuries can result that go unnoticed due to the neurological damage. Autonomic (poly)neuropathy affects the nerves that control functions such as heart rate, digestion, blood pressure, and body temperature regulation resulting in problems such as gastroparesis. Nerves other than peripheral nerves may also be affected, causing amyotrophy, or radiculoplexus neuropathy affecting the thighs, hips, abdomen, and buttocks.

E13.41 Other specified diabetes mellitus with diabetic mononeuropathy

Mononeuropathy involves damage to one specific nerve and can affect a limb, the face, or the trunk. It often comes on suddenly and can cause severe pain, although symptoms are not usually long-term problems and may diminish over time, unless considerably damage to the nerve has already occurred. Areas affected depend on which nerve is involved. Diabetic mononeuropathy can appear as pain in only one particular area of a limb, such as the front of the thigh or the shin, paralysis is one area of the face, abdominal pain, or aching behind one eye.

E13.43 Other specified diabetes mellitus with diabetic autonomic (poly)neuropathy

Autonomic neuropathy affects the nervous system that controls functions such as the heart, lungs, stomach and intestines, bladder, and body temperature and blood pressure regulation. Symptoms conditions of autonomic neuropathy in the diabetic include gastroparesis in which the stomach empties very slowly; constipation or uncontrolled diarrhea; incontinence and bladder problems; difficulty swallowing, inability to regulate heart rate when resting or moving; and sharp drops in blood pressure when rising.

E13.44 Other specified diabetes mellitus with diabetic amyotrophy

Amyotrophy can occur with any type of diabetes, although it is most common in type 2 diabetics. It is also called diabetic radiculoplexus neuropathy and affects nerves closer to the trunk, such as those of the thighs, hips, and buttocks, as opposed to affecting the nerve endings like in peripheral neuropathy. The patient experiences weakening and atrophying thigh muscles; sudden, extremely painful sensations in the hips, thighs, and buttocks; difficulty getting up from the sitting position; and abdominal swelling, if the abdomen is affected.

E13.5 Other specified diabetes mellitus with circulatory complications

Diabetes has a big effect on blood vessels. Complex sugar-based substances adhere to vessel walls, causing them to thicken and leak, which makes them incapable of supplying as much blood and oxygen to the tissues as is needed. Poorly controlled blood sugar levels also cause an increase in fatty substances in the blood with the adherence of plaque material to the vessel walls. This atherosclerotic buildup also reduces blood flow and causes poor circulation. Poor circulation to the extremities causes slow-healing wounds prone to infection. Some wounds may never heal and lead to gangrene with the need for amputation.

E13.62 Other specified diabetes mellitus with skin complications

Because diabetes has such a big effect on blood vessels due to complex sugar-based substances adhering to vessel walls, making the arteries incapable of supplying as much blood and oxygen to the tissues as is needed, the skin may break down and not be able to heal, even without the occurrence of an external wound. This prevents healing and leads to skin problems such as dermatitis, the breakdown of collagen with build-up of fatty deposits, and ulcers, especially in the legs and feet. Diabetic skin ulcers, particularly of the foot and lower leg, often stem from vascular problems caused by poor circulation and poor oxygen supply to the extremities.

E13.620 Other specified diabetes mellitus with diabetic dermatitis

Diabetic dermatitis includes diabetic necrobiosis lipoidica, which is a necrotizing skin condition marked by collagen breakdown, deposits of fatty build-up, and the thickening of blood vessels. This is chronic condition that progresses slowly with flare-ups occurring. A reddish-brown rash appears at first, usually on the lower legs in most people, with well-defined borders on lesions that slowly grow larger, turning shiny and red with a yellowish center. Some people experience itching and burning with the rash, which may also appear on the trunk, arms, face, or scalp. The lesions eventually turn into a purple depression in the skin that may scar. During flare-ups, treatment may consist of topical creams with sterile dressings, cortizone injections or oral steroids, and ultrviolet light treatment for the lesions. If the lesions do not break open, treatment may not be required and rest and support stockings are used.

E13.64 Other specified diabetes mellitus with hypoglycemia

In hypoglycemia, the blood sugar falls abnormally low. This happens in diabetics when too much insulin or oral antidiabetic medication is taken, not enough food is ingested, or exercise is suddenly increased without a corresponding increase in food intake. Confusion, shaking, sweating, headache, aggression, heart palpitations, dizziness and fainting are all symptoms. Small, sugar-laden snacks or fruit juice can reverse the low blood sugar, but if not treated promptly, severe hypoglycemia can progress to seizures and unconsciousness, called hypoglycemic or insulin shock. When the brain is deprived of glucose, neurons in the brain that process memory are destroyed and permanent memory loss can result.

E13.65 Other specified diabetes mellitus with hyperglycemia

This code is used to report diabetes mellitus due to an underlying condition when it is stated as "out of control", "poorly controlled", or "inadequately controlled". Diabetes complications often require multiple coding. This code may be assigned with other appropriate diabetes codes to describe the complete clinical picture of the patient.

E16.2 Hypoglycemia, unspecified

Hypoglycemia is a condition in which the sugar levels in the blood are too low for the body to function normally. Symptoms of this condition include weakness, trembling, hunger, headache, irritability, a racing heartbeat, blurred vision, and in extreme cases, confusion, convulsions, and even coma. Hypoglycemia is caused by having too much insulin in the bloodstream (hyperinsulinism) usually due to an overproduction of insulin by the pancreas in nondiabetics.

E16.3   Increased secretion of glucagon

Glucagon is another hormone secreted by the pancreas which stimulates an increase in blood sugar and breaks down glucose in the liver, and serves to balance insulin. Abnormalities in its secretion are rare and usually present no symptoms, but are thought to contribute to diabetes in many cases. The most common cause of glucagon abnormalities is an unusual (but non-tumorous) increase in the number of a certain type of cell in the pancreas, called the alpha islet cells.

E16.4   Increased secretion of gastrin

Gastrin is another hormone secreted by the pancreas which stimulates the production of stomach acid and controls hunger. An abnormality in its secretion, like an abnormality of the secretion of glucagon, is rare and is often the result of an unusual (but non-tumorous) increase in the number of a certain type of cell in the pancreas, called the alpha islet cells. It may also be the result of Zollinger-Ellison syndrome, in which numerous small tumors appear on the pancreas and/or small intestine. Both of these can cause an increase in the amount of gastrin produced, causing wearing away of the stomach wall (ulcers).

E20   Hypoparathyroidism

Hypoparathyroidism is a disorder in which the parathyroid glands don't secrete enough hormone (PTH). The reduced production of PTH causes symptoms that range from mild tingling in the hands, fingers, and around the mouth to more severe muscle cramps. In rare cases, convulsions can result from this disorder. If left untreated over an extended period of time, this disorder can result in unusually thick bones. Hypoparathyroidism is rare, and most often results from surgical removal of one or more of the parathyroids.

Note: Postprocedural cases of hypoparathyroidism are coded to E89.2. Transitory neonatal cases are coded to P71.4.

E20.1   Pseudohypoparathyroidism

Pseudohypoparathyroidism is a condition in which the body exhibits the symptoms of hypoparathyroidism due to an inadequate response to the parathyroid hormone, rather than an insufficient amount of the hormone in the body.

E21   Hyperparathyroidism and other disorders of parathyroid gland

The parathyroid glands are four pea-sized glands located on the thyroid gland in the neck. They produce parathyroid hormone (PTH), which helps to balance the amount of calcium in the body by increasing absorption of calcium from the intestine and resorption from the bones. PTH is counter-balanced by thyrocalcitonin, which is sometimes called calcitonin.

E21.0   Primary hyperparathyroidism

A condition in which the parathyroid glands secrete too much hormone, causing calcium levels in the blood to rise and calcium deposits in the bone to decrease. The excessive resorption of calcium from the bones may cause them to become brittle, while excess calcium deposits in the blood may cause kidney stones to form. Primary hyperparathyroidism indicates that this disorder is not due to another underlying disease process, but caused by hyperplasia of the gland itself. This code also includes von Recklinghausen's disease of bone, or osteitis fibrosa cystica generalista.

E21.1   Secondary hyperparathyroidism, not elsewhere classified

A condition in which the parathyroid glands secrete too much hormone, causing calcium levels in the blood to rise and calcium deposits in the bone to decrease. The excessive resorption of calcium from the bones may cause them to become brittle, while excess calcium deposits in the blood may cause kidney stones to form. Secondary hyperparathyroidism indicates that this disorder is due to another underlying disease or disorder not of

the kidneys. If the underlying condition is addressed, parathyroid hormone levels will normalize.

Note: Secondary hyperparathyroidism that is caused by a disorder of renal origin is coded to N25.81.

E21.2   Other hyperparathyroidism

A condition in which the parathyroid glands secrete too much hormone, causing calcium levels in the blood to rise and calcium deposits in the bone to decrease. The excessive resorption of calcium from the bones may cause them to become brittle, while excess calcium deposits in the blood may cause kidney stones to form. Other forms include tertiary, or chronic types of secondary hyperparathyroidism in which abnormal parathyroid hormone levels remain irreversibly high.

E21.3   Hyperparathyroidism, unspecified

Hyperparathyroidism is a condition in which the parathyroid glands secrete too much PTH, causing calcium levels in the blood to rise and calcium deposits in the bone to decrease. The excessive resorption of calcium from the bones may cause them to become brittle, while excess calcium deposits in the blood may cause kidney stones to form. Hyperparathyroidism is often the result of a tumor or growth in one or more of the parathyroids.

E21.4   Other specified disorders of parathyroid gland

Note: Use this code for other specified disorders of the parathyroid glands such as a cyst or bleeding within one or more of the glands.

E22   Hyperfunction of pituitary gland

The pituitary is a small gland located at the base of the brain which secretes a number of important hormones. It is connected to the brain by the hypothalmus, and secretes releasing (RH) or release-inhibiting hormones (RIH) specific to each of the other glands of the endocrine system into the bloodstream. The hypothalmus and pituitary are the primary link between the nervous and endocrine systems. The pituitary is divided into three lobes, each of which secretes different hormones. The anterior (forward) lobe secretes the following: growth hormone; prolactin, which stimulates milk production after giving birth; ACTH (adrenocorticotropic hormone), which stimulates the adrenal glands; TSH (thyroid-stimulating hormone), which stimulates the thyroid gland; FSH (follicle-stimulating hormone), which stimulates the ovaries and testes; LH (luteinizing hormone), which stimulates the ovaries or testes. The intermediate lobe secretes melanocyte-stimulating hormone, which controls skin pigmentation. The posterior lobe, or neurohypophysis, secretes ADH (antidiuretic hormone), which increases absorption of water into the blood; and oxytocin, which contracts the uterus during childbirth and stimulates milk production.

E22.0   Acromegaly and pituitary gigantism

Acromegaly and gigantism are two related disorders caused by the overproduction of the growth hormone. Acromegaly strikes adults, usually in their forties, and typically presents with a swelling of the soft tissues and a corresponding enlargement of the hands, feet, and facial features. Gigantism appears during childhood and causes a more even growth of the body's features, including the long bones of the arms and legs, resulting in an extremely tall stature. In both cases, the excessive growth can cause dangerous complications (e.g., overloading the heart) and surgical intervention may be required.

E23   Hypofunction and other disorders of the pituitary gland

The pituitary is a small gland located at the base of the brain which secretes a number of important hormones. It is connected to the brain by the hypothalmus, and secretes releasing (RH) or release-inhibiting hormones (RIH) specific to each of the other glands of the endocrine system into the bloodstream. The hypothalmus and pituitary are the primary link between the nervous and endocrine systems. The pituitary is divided into three lobes, each of which secretes different hormones. The anterior (forward) lobe secretes the following: growth hormone; prolactin, which stimulates milk production after giving birth; ACTH (adrenocorticotropic hormone), which stimulates the adrenal glands; TSH (thyroid-stimulating hormone), which stimulates the thyroid gland; FSH (follicle-stimulating hormone), which stimulates the ovaries and testes; LH (luteinizing hormone), which stimulates the ovaries or testes. The intermediate lobe secretes melanocyte-stimulating hormone, which controls skin pigmentation. The posterior lobe, or neurohypophysis, secretes ADH (antidiuretic hormone), which increases absorption of water into the blood; and oxytocin, which contracts the uterus during childbirth and stimulates milk production.

E23.0 Hypopituitarism

Hypopituitarism is a type of dwarfism with retention of infantile characteristics, due to undersectrion of growth hormone and gonadotropin deficiency. Panhypopituitarism is included here and is a condition in which the pituitary fails to secrete sufficient amounts of any of its hormones. Since many of these hormones are specifically for the purpose of stimulating hormone production in other hormones (e.g., the thyroid), this results in a secondary failure of each of these other hormones to produce sufficient amounts to properly regulate the body as well. Thus, panhypopituitarism usually presents with the symptoms of low hormone production of one or more other glands, and may be misdiagnosed initially. In children, dwarfism occurs, though the limbs remain in proportion to the body, and patients do not go through puberty. This disorder is treated by hormone supplements as needed to maintain normal body function.
Pituitary dwarfism, or short stature, is also included here. This is a condition caused by a deficiency in the amount of growth hormone that is produced. Patients with this disorder are small, but perfectly proportioned and do mature sexually and are able to reproduce.

E23.2 Diabetes insipidus

Diabetes insipidus is a disorder in which the kidneys don't retain enough water from the urine due to a lack of antidiuretic hormone, ADH. It presents with frequent urination and pronounced thirst.

E24 Cushing's syndrome

Cushing's syndrome is a rare hormonal disorder caused by prolonged exposure of the body's tissues to high levels of the hormone cortisol, which is produced in the adrenals. It presents with obesity, especially in the upper body, a rounded face, increased fat around the neck, and thinning arms and legs. The skin becomes frail and easily bruised, the bones become brittle and easily broken even in everyday activities, and most patients also have severe fatigue and weakness, high blood pressure and blood sugar levels, and suffer from irritability and depression. Treatment of Cushing's syndrome depends on the cause. If a tumor is causing excess secretion of adrenal hormones into the bloodstream, for example, removing it surgically may correct the imbalance. Removing or treating one or both adrenals to reduce the flow of hormones may also be carried out.

E25 Adrenogenital disorders

Adrenogenital disorders result from defects in the regulation of cholesterol levels by the adrenal hormones, which in turn can affect sexual maturation. In infants and children, these disorders can impair development of sexual characteristics in puberty causing male virilization in females or feminizing characteristics in males as well as sexual precocity or precocious pseudopuberty. In post-menopausal women, it can present with diabetes and the acquiring of male traits, such as facial hair. If left untreated, adrenogenital disorders can also result in high blood pressure and heart disease. Treatment usually involves removal of part or all of one or both adrenal glands.

E26 Hyperaldosteronism

Hyperaldosteronism is a disease caused by an excess production of the aldosterone hormone, which is responsible for sodium and potassium balance, which then directly controls water balance to maintain appropriate blood pressure and blood volume. It results in a high amount of sodium and low potassium in the bloodstream, which in turn results in high blood pressure. While often showing no symptoms at all, it may also present with a headache, muscle weakness, and an intolerance for carbohydrates.

E26.01 Conn's syndrome

Conn's syndrome is a form of primary hyperaldosteronism with excess secretion of aldosterone due to an adrenocortical adenoma. It results in

hypokalemia, alkalosis, muscular weakness, polyuria, polydipsia, and hypertension.

Note: The adrenocortical adenoma should also be coded with D35.0-.

E26.02 Glucocorticoid-remediable aldosteronism

A rare form of primary hyperaldosteronism in which the secretion of aldosterone is solely under the control of the adrenocorticotropic hormone (ACTH), causing an imbalance in the body. Aldosterone is secreted in smaller excess amounts and is quickly remedied by taking glucosteroids.

E26.1 Secondary hyperaldosteronism

Secondary aldosteronism is an overproduction of aldosterone caused by another underlying disorder or disease.

E26.81 Bartter's syndrome

Bartter's syndrome is actually a group of symptoms caused by the inability of the kidneys to reabsorb potassium. Signs and symptoms include the enlargement of certain kidney cells, the accumulation of excess base in the body (alkalosis), hyperaldosteronism, cramping, constipation, urinary frequency, and weakness. This syndrome is also known as urinary potassium wasting.

E27 Other disorders of adrenal gland

The adrenal glands are set on top of the kidneys. The center of the gland (the medulla) produces adrenaline, while the exterior (the cortex) provides hormones that maintain the body's fluid and electrolyte (salt) balance as well as hormones used during sex.

E27.1 Primary adrenocortical insufficiency

The primary form of adrenocortical insufficiency, or ACTH-independent glucocorticoid insufficiency, is also known as Addison's disease. It results from disease or destruction of the adrenal cortex itself, often from autoimmune causes. Glucocorticoid insufficiency is low levels of cortisol secretion by the adrenal glands. Cortisol is the vital glucocorticoid hormone responsible for maintaining blood pressure and cardiovascular function; slowing the inflammatory response; balancing insulin effects; and regulating metabolism. Symptoms include weakness, anorexia, anemia, low blood pressure, nausea, vomiting, and electrolyte imbalances.

Secondary and tertiary forms are caused by the pituitary or hypothalamus not acting normally on the adrenal glands and present with clinical features similar to the primary form, with hypoglycemia common in children.

E27.2 Addisonian crisis

Acute adrenal insufficiency, called adrenal or Addisonian crisis, is precipitated by serious infection or stress, adrenal infarction, or hemorrhage. Combined mineralocorticoid (aldosterone) deficiency with glucocorticoid (cortisol) deficiency is a major factor in acute cases, causing hyperkalemia, metabolic acidosis, shock and hypotension, which can lead to coma and death if not treated.

E27.40 Unspecified adrenocortical insufficiency

Corticoadrenal insufficiency is related to impaired function of the adrenal cortex, causing decreased production of cortisol and/or aldosterone. The clinical manifestations depend on the extent to which hormone production is decreased, particularly whether or not aldosterone production is preserved. Corticoadrenal insufficiency may present as a lack of cortisol (a glucocorticoid) with or without concomitant aldosterone (a mineralocorticoid) insufficiency. Aldosterone levels alone may also be deficient. Symptoms of chronic adrenal insufficiency may go unnoticed until illness or other stress causes adrenal crisis or acute adrenal insufficiency.

Note: Primary adrenal insufficiency is caused by diseases or conditions that damage the adrenal cortex. Secondary adrenal insufficiency is related to the pituitary gland and the secretion of adrenocorticotropic hormone (ACTH); tertiary causes are related to the hypothalamus and secretion of corticotropic-releasing hormone.

E27.49 Other adrenocortical insufficiency

Other adrenocortical insufficiency includes mineralocorticoid deficiency, adrenal hemorrhage, and adrenal infarction. Mineralocorticoid deficiency is caused by a lack of aldosterone, produced by the adrenal cortex, and results in hyperkalemia, hyponatremia, dehydration, and metabolic acidosis and can lead to profound weakness and cardiac arrhythmias. Aldosterone helps maintain blood pressure and water and salt balance by helping the kidneys to retain sodium and excrete potassium. When aldosterone levels are deficient, the kidneys cannot regulate the body's salt and water balance and blood volume and blood pressure drop.

E27.5 Adrenomedullary hyperfunction

Overproduction of the adrenaline hormones by the medulla, which if left untreated can cause heart disease, high blood pressure, and related problems.

E28 Ovarian dysfunction

The ovaries are a pair of small, oval, whitish organs that sit to either side of the uterus. In addition to producing an egg each month (at about the midpoint between periods), they provide the female hormones estrogen and progesterone, which control the menstrual cycle, as well as play a key role in the development of the female sexual organs, breasts, and body shape during puberty.

E28.2 Polycystic ovarian syndrome

Polycystic ovaries, a condition also called polycystic ovary syndrome (PCOS) or Stein-Leventhal syndrome, the ovaries produce too many androgens, or male hormones. This can cause immature eggs to transform into cysts (small sacks filled with fluid) instead of mature eggs. Because these cysts can interfere with the menstrual cycle, missed or irregular periods are a common feature of this disorder. Other symptoms and problems caused by this disease are infertility, abdominal discomfort and/or heavy periods, excessive hair growth or thinning growth of the hair on the head, acne, weight gain, diabetes, heart disease, abnormal bleeding from the uterus, and cancer.

E28.310 Symptomatic premature menopause

The ovaries permanently fail to produce enough hormone before age 40 of unknown cause.

E29 Testicular dysfunction

The testes are two egg-shaped male reproductive organs located in the scrotum. They produce sperm and the male hormone, testosterone, which is responsible for sexual maturation and drive, increased skeletal and muscular growth, and other changes associated with puberty.

E29.0 Testicular hyperfunction

Testicular hyperfunction is the secretion of too much testosterone into the body. This is often due to an active tumor on the testicle, and most often presents with increased muscle and bone growth in children and increased growth of secondary sex characteristics; for example, growth of the breasts. Testicular hypofunction, the secretion of too little testosterone into the body, affects children and adults differently. In small children, it can cause the patient to exhibit the characteristics of both genders. In adults, it most often presents with obesity, muscle and hair loss, and a decreased sex drive.

E30.0 Delayed puberty

Delayed sexual development and/or delayed onset of puberty is generally defined as a condition in which testicular or breast enlargement has not begun by the age of 13, pubic hair has not appeared by age 14 (in girls) or 15 (in boys), and/or there is a time lapse of more than 5 years from the beginning of puberty to the completion of genital enlargement (in boys) or the first menstrual period (in girls).

E30.1 Precocious puberty

In precocious sexual development the signs of puberty appear before the age of 7 or 8 in girls or the age of 9 in boys.

E31.2 Multiple endocrine neoplasia [MEN] syndromes

This subcategory covers multiple endocrine neoplasia [MEN] syndromes, also called multiple or familial endocrine adenomatosis. These are geneticallly distinct groups of inherited conditions that involve hyperplasia and malignant tumor formation in several endocrine glands that can appear in infants to those in their 70s. The adenomatous growth causes glandular malfunction and myriads of concomitant disease conditions associated with glandular and hormonal malfunction. Three distinct forms have been identified with some overlapping similarities, but each syndrome is the sum of the effect of multiple tumors or adenomatous hyperplasia on various glands and organs occuring at the same time.

E31.21 Multiple endocrine neoplasia [MEN] type I

MEN type I, or Wermer's syndrome, is characterized by hyperplasia or tumors of the parathyroid, the islet cells of the pancreas, and the pituitary gland. The tumors are usually benign and cause the glands to secrete high levels of hormones, inducing multiple other medical problems. Kidney stones, infertility, and severe peptic ulcers from gastric hypersecretion are common. Patients also show an increased incidence of disease or tumors of the adrenal cortex and thyroid glands, along with the parathyroid. Tumors inside the pancreas may become cancerous. Multiple soft tissue lipomas and tumors of the bronchus, gastrointestinal tract, and mediastinum are also associated with MEN I.

E31.22 Multiple endocrine neoplasia [MEN] type IIA

MEN type IIA, also referred to as Sipple's syndrome, is characterized by a triad of medullary carcinoma of the thyroid, pheochromocytoma, and hyperplasia of the parathyroid gland. Pheochromocytoma is an adrenal gland tumor that causes epinephrine and norepinephrine to be released in excessive amounts, resulting in severely raised blood pressure, palpitations, and tachycardia. Calcitonin and catecholamine levels are also elevated and patients sometimes have glioblastomas and meningiomas. Hyperparathyroidism results due to increased secretion from the adenomatous parathyroid gland.

E31.23 Multiple endocrine neoplasia [MEN] type IIB

MEN type IIB is similar to Type IIA, or Sipple's syndrome, having medullary thryroid carcinoma with pheochromocytoma as the major characteristics, but with the additional distinguishing feature of mucosal neuromas. Type IIB does not have parathyroid involvement. The medullary thyroid cancers occurring with type IIB tend to develop at an earlier age and have been reported in infants at three months of age. The cancer tends to grow more rapidly and spread faster than in type IIA. MEN type IIB has also been found in people who had no known family history of MEN.

E32 Diseases of thymus

The thymus gland is a small gland in the upper chest. It weighs approximately an ounce at birth, grows to over a pound on average during puberty, but then ceases to grow and returns to its original mass by the time that the person is in his or herr forties. This organ plays an important role in developing the body's immune system. The hormones that the thymus secretes mature and differentiate the white blood cells. This role is principally carried out in childhood, and the thymus may be removed from an adult patient without any side effects.

E32.0 Persistent hyperplasia of thymus

Persistant hyerplasia of the thymus is a condition in which the thymus grows to an unusual size. In some cases, this may occur where drugs (especially steroids), surgery, stress, or infection caused the thymus to shrink, and it subsequently grew to a greater than normal size in what is known as rebound enlargement. This growth can cause difficulty in breathing as it pushes against the lungs, as well as complications from an overproduction of the thymus hormone.

E34.0 Carcinoid syndrome

Carcinoid syndrome is a condition in which cancerous cells secrete hormones into the bloodstream, causing chemical imbalances in the body. The chief symptom of carcinoid syndrome is a periodic flushing (reddening) of the face and other parts of the body. It may also present with diarrhea, abdominal pain, and high blood pressure. If left untreated, carcinoid syndrome can cause damage to the valves of the heart.

E34.2 Ectopic hormone secretion, not elsewhere classified

Ectopic hormone secretion occurs when a tumor beginning in a gland metastasizes and moves from its original location to another area of the body and continues to secrete hormones. Symptoms can vary widely depending on the gland affected, the location of the tumor, and how much and what type of hormone is secreted.

E34.5 Androgen insensitivity syndrome

Androgen insensitivity syndromes (AIS) are the most common reasons for pseudohermaphroditism. All cases born have an XY chromosome genotype, but appear in a range of phenotypes. AIS is typically characterized by feminization of external genitalia, abnormal sexual development, and infertility. The syndromes represent a spectrum of defects in androgen action that may be complete, partial, or mild.

E34.51 Complete androgen insensitivity syndrome

Complete androgen insensitivity syndrome is also called testicular feminization, or Goldberg-Maxwell syndrome. Those affected develop as normal females in adult appearance, generally with a vagina but no uterus, and without the onset of menses, which is sometimes the first sign of the disorder. Testicles may be present but undescended or detected in the inguinal area and must be surgically removed due to the risk of malignancy.

E34.52 Partial androgen insensitivity syndrome

Partial androgen insensitivity has a wide variety of presentations from predominantly female phenotype with extreme undervirilization and presence of clitoromegaly and labial fusion, to predominantly male phenotype with small phallus, testes and infertility, to severe hypospadias with bifid scrotum, or ambiguous genitalia. Reifenstein syndrome is one form of partial AIS that presents with hypospadias, gynecomastia, and hypogonadism combined with testicular atrophy and azoospermia occurring after puberty.

E40 Kwashiorkor

Kwashiorkor is a form of malnutrition due to inadequate protein intake which can occur even if overall calorie intake is good. The name is an African word meaning "first-child, second child," and refers to the nutritional deficit that can occur when the first child is weaned off of breast milk so that the second child can receive it instead. It is very rare in the United States, but is often seen in countries affected by famine and drought. Kwashiorkor initially presents with lethargy (tiredness) and irritability. As the protein deficiency continues, the child ceases to grow, loses muscle mass, and exhibits a general swelling of the body, especially in the abdomen. A loss of immunity to disease and skin conditions are also frequent, and coma and death can result if the child is not treated. Improving calorie and protein intake will correct the disorder if started early. However, the child may still fail to reach full height and growth and may exhibit a decreased IQ in cases of long-term kwashiorkor.

E41 Nutritional marasmus

Nutritional marasmus is malnutrition of both protein and caloric intake. It presents with a loss of body mass and general decline in health and immunity to disease, and may present with a reddish-orange tint to the hair, especially in tropical regions. This nutritional disorder is rarely seen in the United States, being more common in areas subject to drought and/or famine.

E44 Protein-calorie malnutrition of moderate and mild degree

Malnutrition can result from either inadequate intake of nutrients, or a disorder that prevents the body from properly digesting and/or using them. Malnutrition presents with a loss of body mass and general decline in health and immunity to disease, and in cases of inadequate protein intake, may present with a reddish-orange tint to the hair, especially in tropical regions. General malnutrition is categorized by degrees.

E44.0 Moderate protein-calorie malnutrition

In second degree, or moderate, malnutrition, the patient's weight is 25-40% below normal with biochemical changes in electrolytes, blood, and lipids present.

E44.1 Mild protein-calorie malnutrition

In first-degree, or mild, malnutrition, the patient's body weight is 10-25% below normal.

E45 Retarded development following protein-calorie malnutrition

Use this code to indicate arrested development in a patient following malnutrition in which the body did not receive enough protein; for example, a twelve-year-old patient that exhibits the appearance and development of a nine-year-old. Arrested development may include mental development as well as physical.

E50 Vitamin A deficiency

Vitamin A is a family of vitamins that includes retinol, and which plays an important role in vision, bone growth, reproduction, and cell division. It is found in animal foods such as whole eggs, whole milk, and liver, and is stored in the liver of humans. Vitamin A deficiency is rare in the United States, but remains a major health problem in much of the developing world, where it is a common companion of kwashiorkor.

Note: Vitamin A deficiency (VAD) is coded according to its primary manifestation. The most common manifestations involve the eyes.

E50.0 Vitamin A deficiency with conjunctival xerosis

Conjunctival xerosis is a dryness of the covering of the whites of the eyes.

E50.1 Vitamin A deficiency with Bitot's spot and conjunctival xerosis

Bitot's spots are greyish or white patches that appear on the surface of the conjunctiva. Patients manifesting Bitot's spots should avoid eyestrain, smoke-filled rooms, and sunlight.

E50.2 Vitamin A deficiency with corneal xerosis

Corneal xerosis, or dryness of the cornea, the dome shaped lens that protects the iris and true lens, is another common manifestation of vitamin A deficiency.

E50.4 Vitamin A deficiency with keratomalacia

Keratomalacia is a similar condition in which the cornea becomes not only dry, but infected and clouded due to vitamin A deficiency. It also affects the tear glands, resulting in inadequate tear production and even drier eyes. It is treated with antibiotic eye drops or ointments in addition to vitamin A supplements.

E50.6 Vitamin A deficiency with xerophthalmic scars of cornea

Xerophthalmic scars of the cornea result when corneal ulceration or keratomalacia do not receive adequate treatment early enough to prevent them. These scars result in long-term or permanent vision loss or even blindness.

E50.8 Other manifestations of vitamin A deficiency

Use this code for non eye-related manifestations of vitamin A deficiency. These may include respiratory, urinary, or other infections, and skin disorders marked by uneven pigmentation, dryness, and acne-like eruptions (e.g., follicular keratosis or phrynoderma) or extreme sensitivity to sunlight (xeroderma).

E51 Thiamine deficiency

Vitamin B is divided into many sub-groups. Thiamine, also called vitamin B1, is critical to the body for proper function of the nervous system.

E51.1 Beriberi

Beriberi is a disease caused by thiamine deficiency that has two major manifestations. "Wet beriberi" manifests as heart disease with swelling, increased heart rate, congestion of the lungs, and an increased heart size that can result in congestive heart failure. "Dry beriberi" manifests as a nervous disorder with pain, tingling, or loss of sensation in the hands and feet, and loss of function and/or wasting of the muscles, especially in the legs. In extreme cases, the patient can become paralyzed, develop brain damage, or even die.

E51.9   Thiamine deficiency, unspecified

Unspecified manifestations of thiamine deficiency may include depression, fatigue, headache, nausea, and loss of appetite.

E52   Niacin deficiency [pellagra]

Niacin, also called niacinamide, nicotinic acid, and vitamin B3, is essential for cell respiration; balancing the metabolism; digesting and utilizing carbohydrates, fats, and proteins; circulation of the blood; healthy skin; and normal function of the nervous and digestive systems. Pellagra is a disease that occurs due to a deficiency of niacin in a person's diet. It presents with scaly skin sores, diarrhea, inflamed mucous membranes (e.g., in the nose or throat), and mental confusion. It is sometimes seen in conjunction with alcoholism.

E53.0   Riboflavin deficiency

Riboflavin, or vitamin B2, supports the body's metabolism and aids in synthesizing a number of compounds that the body needs. Ariboflavinosis is a deficiency of riboflavin, and presents with dry throat and/or nasal passages, sores in the mouth, a magenta-colored tongue, and overproduction of oil on the skin.

E53.1   Pyridoxine deficiency

Vitamin B6, sometimes called pyridoxine, is essential to the growth of healthy blood cells and supports more body functions than any other vitamin. As a result, a deficiency of this vitamin can manifest in any number of ways. Common symptoms include nervousness, irritability, insomnia, muscles weakness, loss of balance or other difficulty walking, and cracking at the corners of the mouth (as if from dryness). In infants, it causes a failure to grow, irritability, and seizures.

E54   Ascorbic acid deficiency

Vitamin C, also called ascorbic acid, is essential for wound healing and healthy connective tissue. It has also been linked to preventing heart disease by preventing stiffening of the arteries and clotting by the platelets. Vitamin C is known to be an antioxidant, which blocks the damage done by certain waste byproducts (called free radicals) in the body's cells, and promotes the immune system. A deficiency of this vitamin is commonly called scurvy. Scurvy causes the capilaries (the smallest blood vessels) to break down, causing hemorrhaging (which appears as bruising and red spots on the skin), weakness, and joint pain. After about five months of the vitamin deficiency, the skin develops sores, and the gums bleed and become weak, causing the teeth to loosen.

E55   Vitamin D deficiency

Vitamin D, sometimes called calciferol, is a very unusual vitamin in that it is the only vitamin that the body produces naturally (in response to the sun's ultraviolet light when it strikes the skin). It is technically considered a hormone. Vitamin D aids the body in absorbing calcium from food and accumulating it in the bone, as well as supporting the immune system. It is sometimes used in the treatment of psoriasis.

E55.0   Rickets, active

Rickets is a childhood disease due to a lack of vitamin D and/or sunlight that results in soft, spongy bones. This causes pain in the bones, as well as several tell-tale skeletal deformities such as bowlegs, distortion of the rib cage, an oddly-shaped skull, and spinal and pelvic deformities (e.g., scoliosis), and a loss of growth. There is also a greater risk of bone fractures, delayed and/or defective formation of the teeth, and a loss of muscle strength.

E56.1   Deficiency of vitamin K

Deficiency of vitamin K can occur after prolonged treatment by antibiotics. This causes hemorrhaging within the body, which is most often noted by the appearance of bruises on the skin after light impacts.

E65   Localized adiposity

Localized adiposity are localized fat deposits, such as cellulite in the thighs or buttocks. By themselves, they do not present a medical concern, though they can be disfiguring or may cause complications in other medical conditions.

E66.0   Obesity due to excess calories

Obesity is the condition of having increased body weight due to excessive accumulation of fat from ingesting excessive amounts of calories.

E66.01   Morbid (severe) obesity due to excess calories

Morbid obesity is defined as having a body mass index, BMI, of 40 or over; or anyone who is greater than 100 lbs. over his or her ideal body weight. Morbid obesity is large amounts of excess fat in the body often associated with profound health risks including diabetes, respiratory compromise, and cardiac disease.

E66.09   Other obesity due to excess calories

Obesity due to excess calories is defined as having a body mass index (BMI) of 30 and above because of excessive accumulation of fat from overconsumption of too many calories, particularly low-nutrient empty calories. BMI is calculated by the following formula: (Weight in pounds times 703) divided by (height in inches squared) or (weight in kilograms) divided by (height in meters squared).

E66.2   Morbid (severe) obesity with alveolar hypoventilation

Morbid obesity hypoventilation syndrome is also called Pickwickian syndrome. It involves sleep induced breathing disorders related to both obesity and chronic hypoventilation. This syndrome is defined as having a BMI of 30 or greater with daytime arterial hypercapnia (elevated carbon dioxide levels) and accompanying hypoxemia (decreased blood oxygen levels) in the absence of other known causes of hypoventilation. Patients present with excessive daytime sleepiness or hypersomnolence, morning headaches, mood disorders, and fatigue. Sleep apneic or hypopneic symptoms include loud snoring, gagging, and choking. Untreated patients can develop erythrocytosis, right-sided congestive heart failure (cor pulmonale), and pulmonary hypertension.

E66.3   Overweight

Patients who are overweight without being obese have a BMI of 25-29.

E66.9   Obesity, unspecified

Obesity is defined as having a body mass index (BMI) of 30 and above. BMI is calculated by the following formula: (Weight in pounds times 703) divided by (height in inches squared) or (weight in kilograms) divided by (height in meters squared).

E67.0   Hypervitaminosis A

Vitamin A is a fat-soluble vitamin, and as such accumulates in the body's fat reserves instead of being removed by the kidneys (like, for example, vitamin C). This code describes hypervitaminosis A, or vitamin A poisoning. This poisoning occurs when the body takes in and stores too much vitamin A, causing swelling, aching and/or softened bones, nausea and vomiting, dizziness, and blurry vision. As this condition almost always occurs due to misuse of vitamin supplements, treatment generally involves simply stopping the excess intake of the vitamin.

E67.1   Hypercarotinemia

Hypercarotinemia is the condition of having a yellowish tint to the skin as a result of having too much carotene, or vitamin A, in one's system. Like hyperitaminosis A, the best treatment is simply to avoid excess sources of vitamin A until the condition fades.

E67.3 Hypervitaminosis D

Hypervitaminosis D presents with weight loss, fatigue, and weakness and can cause damage to the bones, soft tissues (e.g., the muscles), and kidneys. Choose this code to report hypervitaminosis D. Treatment likewise involves stopping the excess intake of the vitamin, though in severe cases, other treatment may also be necessary.

E70.0 Classical phenylketonuria

PKU is an inherited metabolic disorder caused by an enzyme deficiency in which the body does not properly regulate an amino acid called phenylalanine hydroxylase, a ring-shaped, or "aromatic," amino acid molecule. This results in the accumulation of phenylalanine and its metabolites in the blood with excess excretion in the urine. It most often manifests as a primary cause of mild mental retardation. It also presents with a mouse-like odor; light pigmentation of the skin; a peculiar walk, stance, or way of sitting; red, inflamed skin; and seizures. It is treated by a low-protein diet, which prevents the buildup of the amino acid in the bloodstream.

E70.20 Disorder of tyrosine metabolism, unspecified

Select this code for other disorders involving aromatic (ring-shaped) amino acids. These disorders include albinism, hypertyrosinemia, alkaptonuria, Oasthouse urine disease, Mende's syndrome, Smith-Strang disease, and van der Hoeve-Halbertsma-Waardenburg syndrome.

E70.4 Disorders of histidine metabolism

These disorders specifically involve the histidine amino acid, which is essential during childhood to promote both mental and physical growth. In both children and adults, it is used to produce histamine, which is important to gastric function; control of the bronchial muscles; and control of blood pressure. Overproduction of histamine can cause heightened allergic reactions.

E71.120 Methylmalonic acidemia

Branched-chain amino acid disorders are depicted by this code. These disorders are those involving amino acids whose atoms, instead of appearing ring-like, are arranged into chains (essentially straight lines) that branch at various points, such as forming into a Y-shape. There are three types of amino acids in this classification: leucine, isoleucine, and valine. These disorders include hypervalinemia, intermittent branched-chain ketonuria, leucine-induced hypoglycemia, and methylmalonic aciduria. These disorders are those in which the atoms of the amino acid molecules are laid out, as the name suggests, in a straight chain-like line. These disorders include glucoglycinuria; hyperglycinemia; hyper lysinemia; pepecolic acidemia; saccharopinuria; and other disorders of the metabolism of glycine, threonine, serine, glutamine, and lysine.

E71.2 Disorder of branched-chain amino-acid metabolism, unspecified

Branched-chain amino acid disorders are those involving amino acids whose atoms, instead of appearing ring-like, are arranged into chains (essentially straight lines) that branch at various points, such as forming into a Y-shape. There are three types of amino acids in this classification: leucine, isoleucine, and valine.

E71.31 Disorders of fatty-acid oxidation

Before they are able to be digested, fats in the intestinal tract go through a process of oxidation to be transformed into fatty acids. These fatty acids are able to be absorbed through the intestine into the bloodstream, where they are taken up into the cells with the aid of carnitines and other amino acids.

E71.43 Iatrogenic carnitine deficiency

Carnitine is an amino acid that the body uses to transport fatty acids into the cells. Use this code to depict a carnitine deficiency due to a reaction to medication or other medical treatment.

E71.44 Other secondary carnitine deficiency

Carnitine is an amino acid that the body uses to transport fatty acids into the cells. Use this code to depict a carnitine deficiency secondary to another medical condition that is, being caused by another, underlying disorder.

E71.5 Peroxisomal disorders

Peroxisomes are organelles (molecule-sized organ-like structures) within cells that contain enzymes critical for cellular function. There are several hundred types of peroxisomes per cell. Use this code to indicate peroxisomal disorders. These are genetic disorders in which one or more normal peroxisomes are missing. This can present with a wide variety of symptoms and disorders depending on the exact structures that are missing. In general, delays in normal growth and development, mental retardation, autism, and vision and hearing impairments are the most common complications, but lab tests are required to make the final determination. There is no treatment, but dietary changes and supplements can help to alleviate the worst of the complications.

E71.50 Peroxisomal disorder, unspecified

Peroxisomes are organelles (molecule-sized organ-like structures) within cells that contain enzymes critical for cellular function. There are several hundred types of peroxisomes per cell. Use this code to indicate peroxisomal disorders. These are genetic disorders in which one or more normal peroxisomes are missing. This can present with a wide variety of symptoms and disorders depending on the exact structures that are missing. In general, delays in normal growth and development, mental retardation, autism, and vision and hearing impairments are the most common complications, but lab tests are required to make the final determination. There is no treatment, but dietary changes and supplements can help to alleviate the worst of the complications.

E72 Other disorders of amino-acid metabolism

This category discusses disturbances of amino acid transport and metabolism. Amino acids are the building blocks of proteins, which in turn are the basic building blocks of the body's cells. Disorders in the absorption and use of amino acids result in chemical imbalances in the body and most often appear in infancy and can cause brain damage and mental retardation, seizures, coma, autism, and even death unless treated. Treatment depends on the specific disorder, but may include a special diet, vitamin and/or amino acid supplements, and close monitoring.

E72.0 Disorders of amino-acid transport

A disorder of the amino acid transport system affects the passage of amino acids in and out of the cells. Most such disorders are genetic, and are fairly common. Symptoms vary widely depending on the specific amino acid that is blocked from being properly transported. For example, cystinuria blocks the amino acid cystine, resulting in an excess amount of cystine in the urine. This causes the formation of cystine stones in the kidneys and bladder. These stones can cause permanent damage to the kidneys or even death if left untreated. Hartnup disease, which affects the amino acids that aid in the breaking down of proteins, causes a condition similar to pellegra. Other disorders of the amino acid transport system include renal gycinuria, cystinosis, and Fanconi syndrome (sometimes called Falconi-de Toni, Falconi-Debre, or Hart's syndrome). In all cases, the specific disorder must be determined by a blood or urine test.

E72.19 Other disorders of sulfur-bearing amino-acid metabolism

These disorders involve amino acids that, as the name implies, carry one or more sulfur atoms. Disorders of this type include cystathioninuria, methioninemia, and sulfite oxidase deficiency.

E72.2 Disorders of urea cycle metabolism

These disorders affect the production of urea, the main waste product in urine, which is hindered by an improper breakdown of amino acids (the chief components of urea). This can cause an accumulation of waste products in the bloodstream and cells. As with most amino-acid disorders, urea cyle disorders primarily develop in infancy due to a genetic disorder. They commonly present with vomiting, refusal to eat, lethargy that increases as time goes on, and then coma and death, if left untreated. Disorders of the urea cycle metabolism include argininosuccinic aciduria, citrullinemia, and hyperammonemia.

E73.9   Lactose intolerance, unspecified

This code is used to report disaccharidase deficiencies and disaccharide malabsoprtion. These deficiencies are actually a group of digestive problems in which the enzyme needed to properly digest a type of sugar called disaccharide is not produced in sufficient amounts, resulting in an inability to absorb it. This disorder presents as lactose intolerance, which causes abdominal bloating and cramping, excessive gas, nausea, and diarrhea when milk products are consumed.

E74   Other disorders of carbohydrate metabolism

Carbohydrates are the primary chemical compounds that biological systems, like the human body, use to store and consume energy. They are divided into sugars and starches. There are several disorders that can arise in the body's systems for transporting and metabolizing carbohydrates.

E74.00   Glycogen storage disease, unspecified

This disorder occurs when the body cannot convert its stores of glycogen into sugar due to a lack of the proper enzymes. In infants, it manifests as a failure to thrive and grow and is usually fatal within two years due to failure of the heart and lungs. In children, it usually appears in the first decade of life as weakness and respiratory difficulties. Most juvenile patients succumb to respiratory disease in their twenties and thirties. When it appears in adults, usually between age twenty and age sixty, it presents as a painless weakness in the limbs and respiratory muscles, and is sometimes, but not always, fatal as well.

E74.12   Hereditary fructose intolerance

This genetic disorder occurs when the body does not properly metabolize fructose, which is the type of sugar found in fruits and honey. This causes an accumulation of fructose-1-phosphate in the liver, kidney, and small intestine and severe hypoglycemia (low blood sugar) after ingesting a source of fructose. If the patient, particularly a young one, continues to ingest fructose, it can lead to kidney or liver failure and death. This condition is treated by a specialized, fructose- and sucrose (table sugar)-free diet.

E74.21   Galactosemia

Galactosemia is a rare genetic disorder in which the patient lacks the enzyme that converts lactose (contained in diary products) into both galactose and glucose (a form of sugar), resulting in too much of the former and not enough of the latter in the bloodstream. This disorder is usually picked up in the first week of life with standard blood-screening. However, though galactosemic children are started on a special diet from birth, a high number still suffer long-term disabilities in speech and language, delays in the development of their motor skills, and learning disabilities. In girls, the ovaries often fail to develop.

E75   Disorders of sphingolipid metabolism and other lipid storage disorders

Sphingolipid metabolic disorders are usually monogenetic inherited diseases caused by defects in lysosomal sphingolipid degradation. The defects cause an accumulation of lipids (fats) in one or more body organs. These diseases include Tay-Sachs, Sandhoff, Fabry-Anderson, Gaucher, Krabbe, and Niemann-Pick. Sphingolipid disorders may be treated with enzyme replacement therapy (ERT), cell medicated therapy (CMT) including bone marrow transplant (BMT), cell mediated cross correction and gene therapy.

E75.0   GM2 gangliosidosis

GM2 gangliosidoses are a group of inherited, related degenerative disorders in which an abnormal amount of lipids (fats) accumulate in the brain and/or spinal cord due to a deficiency of the enzyme beta-hexosaminidase. This enzyme catalyzes the breakdown of lipids--fatty acid derivatives known as gangliosides, which are made and degraded rapidly in early life as the brain is developing. Failure in the functioning of this enzyme causes the fats to accumulate in tissue of the brain and spinal cord, causing a rapid degeneration of the central nervous system that is almost ways fatal to the child, except in rare late-onset cases. When the disorder initially appears, development slows and there is a loss of peripheral vision. As it progresses, the child actually loses skills such as rolling over, crawling, sitting, and

so forth, and begins having difficulties in breathing. Eventually, the child becomes paralyzed and non-responsive and dies shortly thereafter. There is currently no cure or effective treatment for this condition.

Note: Tay-Sachs disease, Sandhoff disease, and AB variant GM2 gangliosidosis are all associated with a failure of the same metabolic pathyway, and all have the same clinical features and outcome. The three disorders are named for different points of failure, or chromosomal mutations, that affect activation of the enzyme.

E75.01   Sandhoff disease

Sandhoff disease is clinically indistinguishable from Tay-Sachs disease. It manifests in infancy and is usually fatal by early childhood. Sandhoff disease is named for a chromosome 5 mutation in the HEXB gene responsible for lysosomal enzymes beta-N-acetylhexosaminidase A and B. Without the functioning enzyme, fatty acids build up in the brain and spinal cord tissue and cause progressive destruction of the nerve cells.

E75.02   Tay-Sachs disease

Tay-Sachs disease is clinically indistinguishable from Sandhoff disease. It manifests in infancy and is usually fatal by early childhood. Tay-Sachs disease is named for a chromosome 15 mutation in the HEXA gene responsible for the lysosomal enzyme beta-N-acetylhexosaminidase A. Without the functioning enzyme, fatty acids build up in the brain and spinal cord tissue and cause progressive destruction of the nerve cells.

E75.29   Other sphingolipidosis

This code reports leukodystrophy, which is a genetic disorder that affects the brain, spinal cord, and peripheral nerves. It generally appears in early childhood and grows progressively worse. It causes degeneration of the white matter of the brain, which is responsible for communication between the various gray matter regions. Leukodystrophy presents with an increasing loss of muscle tone, loss of movement (especially walking), speech, the ability to eat and swallow, vision and hearing decreases, and personality and behavior changes. However, symptoms vary depending on which of the ten chemical compounds that make up the white matter are affected, so diagnosis may be difficult to obtain at first. There is no cure for leukodystrophy, and treatment focuses on improving quality of life through physical, occupational, and speech therapy.

E75.6   Lipid storage disorder, unspecified

Disorders that impair the body's ability to absorb and use fat from foods, resulting in lipids (fats and carbohydrates) accumulating in the body tissues. The symptoms, treatments, and long-term effects vary greatly. In most cases, these disorders are genetic, but lipidoses can also be caused by exposure to certain chemicals.

E76   Disorders of glycosaminoglycan metabolism

Glycosaminoglycan metabolic disorders are usually inherited genetic diseases that cause a failure in the breakdown of long chain sugar molecules causing them to accumulate and damage body organs. These diseases include Hurler's, Hurler-Scheie, Scheie's, Morquio, and Sanfilippo. Glycosaminoglycan disorders are most often treated with enzyme replacement therapy (ERT).

E76.3   Mucopolysaccharidosis, unspecified

Mucopolysaccharidosis may be any of a number of disorders that result in the deficiency of certain enzymes needed for the metabolism of complex carbohydrates in the bloodstream. Because these carbohydrates are major components of the body's connective tissue, mucopolysaccharidosis may present with a wide variety of muscular and skeletal malformations. There is no cure for the disorder itself, so treatment focuses on correcting the musculoskeletal deformities that the disorder presents instead.

E77   Disorders of glycoprotein metabolism

Glycoprotein metabolic disorders are rare inherited genetic diseases characterized by a failure to synthesize or degrade glycoprotein molecules causing them to accumulate in body organs and tissue.

E78 Disorders of lipoprotein metabolism and other lipidemias

Lipoprotein metabolic disorders are often inherited genetic diseases that cause elevated levels of remnant lipoproteins in the blood and deposits in body organs. These diseases include Fredrickson's hyperlipoproteinemia, hyperchylomicronemia, pure hypercholesterolemia, pure hyperglyceridemia, and mixed hyperlipidemia.

E78.0 Pure hypercholesterolemia

Pure hypercholesterolemia is more commonly called high cholesterol. In the average person, 80% of total cholesterol is produced by the liver, and 20% comes from what is eaten. When produced at its proper level, cholesterol serves to combine with protein and fat to transport them through the bloodstream. High cholesterol, however, can cause hardening and blockage of the blood vessels, leading to heart disease. This condition may be controlled by diet or medication and may be due to a hereditary condition that causes the liver to produce too much cholesterol.

E78.1 Pure hyperglyceridemia

Pure hyperglyceridemia is a condition in which there are too many glycerides (fats), usually triglycerides (saturated fat) in the blood. This can cause increased viscosity, or thickness, in the blood, which can raise blood pressure and lead to heart disease and other related problems (e.g., a stroke). This condition is treated with diet, exercise, and possibly medication.

E78.2 Mixed hyperlipidemia

Mixed hyperlipidemia is an elevation of lipids (fats and cholesterol) in the bloodstream. As with other disorders of lipoid metabolism, the most common complication of this disorder is heart disease, and it is usually treated with diet and exercise and sometimes with medication.

E78.3 Hyperchylomicronemia

Hyperchylomicronemia is a genetic disorder in which massive accumulation of fatty droplets, called chylomicrons, occurs in the bloodstream along with an increase in the amount of triglycerides (saturated fat) due to the absence or underproduction of a particular enzyme called lipoprotein lipase. Left untreated, this disorder can lead to severe heart disease, high blood pressure, and death. This disorder is treated with diet and medicine.

E78.4 Other hyperlipidemia

Other types of hyperlipidemia are diseases in which there is an accumulation of fats and cholesterol in the blood. Lipoproteins are formed when a particular type of protein, called an apolipoprotein, wraps around cholesterol and/or fat to transport them through the bloodstream.

E78.6 Lipoprotein deficiency

Lipoprotein deficiencies occur when there is an insufficient amount of lipoprotein to absorb fats and cholesterol adequately from the intestine and transport them to the rest of the body. These disorders are most often due to a genetic defect, and can cause failure to grow and develop in small children. They may be treated by a low-fat diet, large doses of fat-soluble vitamins (i.e., A, D, E, or K), or other dietary supplements and/or medications.

E79.8 Other disorders of purine and pyrimidine metabolism

Use this code for other disorders of the purine and pyrimidine metabolism, which, like porphyrins, are specialized molecules that combine with minerals and other nutrients to transport them through the body and change them to forms usable by the body's cells.

Note: Report gout conditions with M1A-,M10.-.

E80.2 Other and unspecified porphyria

Porphyrins are specialized molecules in the body which interact with minerals to aid in their metabolism. Porphyria is a disorder of the porphyrin metabolism which affects the nervous system and skin or both in a number of ways. A blood test is needed for diagnosis. Treatment focuses on the primary disease or disorder causing the porphyria, which may include exposure to certain types of toxic chemicals.

E80.4 Gilbert syndrome

A harmless, inborn error of bilirubin metabolism in which the liver enzyme that breaks down bilirubin is abnormal. This causes a mild elevation of unconjugated bilirubin in the blood, also known as familial nonhemolytic jaundice, appearing particularly after fasting or dehydration, but without liver damage or hematologic problems.

E80.6 Other disorders of bilirubin metabolism

Bilirubin is a waste product that is produced when red blood cells die and hemoglobin is broken down. It is broken down further in the liver and becomes part of the bile. This code is used to report a disorder of bilirubin metabolism that takes place when the bilirubin is not properly processed by the liver, often due to a genetic disorder (such as Dubin-Johnson syndrome) causing it to build up in the bloodstream. This can cause jaundice (yellowing of the skin and eyes).

E83.0 Disorders of copper metabolism

Disorders of copper metabolism involve either too much or too little copper being absorbed and utilized by the body, usually as a result of a genetic disorder (Wilson's disease). Too much copper can result in damage to the liver and/or brain, which will result in death if the disorder is not diagnosed via lab-test and treated. The disorder is treated by medication designed to reduce the absorption of copper.

E83.1 Disorders of iron metabolism

A disorder of iron metabolism causes too much iron to be absorbed into the bloodstream. This can cause a number of complications including chronic fatigue, loss of sexual drive, pain in the limbs or abdomen, a bronze-colored tint to the skin, and even failure of the kidneys (renal diabetes). These disorders may be treated with diet, or in some cases, by venesection (removing blood) so that the excess iron is reduced.

Note: Anemia due to iron deficiency should be coded to D50.-.

Note: An additional code may need to be assigned for the type of hemosiderosis caused by the underlying iron metabolism disorder, such as idiopathic pulmonary hemosiderosis.

E83.110 Hereditary hemochromatosis

Hereditary hemochromatosis is the build-up of too much iron in the body due to a genetic problem that interferes with the body's ability to break-down or metabolize iron. This condition causes the absorption of up to 4 times the normal amount of iron from the digestive tract and resuls in excess iron being stored within body organs. Hereditary hemochromatosis is the primary form of this disorder and the most common genetic disorder in the United States, seen in about 1 in every 200-300 people, affecting more men than women, particularly Caucasians. Too much iron builds up in the liver and spleen causing swelling and darkening or bronzing of skin color. Other symptoms include abdominal and joint pain; chronic fatigue; loss of sexual desire, body hair, and weight; and the development of diabetes, arthritis, testicular atrophy, and liver, heart, or kidney failure. Treatment aims to reduce excess iron and treat any organ damage.

Note: Report bronzed diabetes, pigmentary cirrhosis of the liver, and primary hereditary hemochromatosis with this code.

E83.111 Hemochromatosis due to repeated red blood cell transfusions

This is also known as exogenous hemochromatosis, or transfusion related iron overload, which causes progressive damage to the liver, heart, and endocrine glands, leading to debilitating or even life-threatening problems. Nonspecific initial symptoms of skin bronzing, abdominal pain, and fatigue may delay correct diagnosis until tissue damage is clinically evident. Excess iron deposits in the liver cause fibrosis, cirrhosis, and hepatocellular carcinoma. Iron deposits in myocardial tissue causes dilated cardiomegaly, pericarditis, conduction defects, angina, and heart failure. Iron overload can occur with as few as 10 RBC transfusions in a lifetime. When the serum ferritin is greater than 1000mcg/L, prognosis is worse.

E83.118 Other hemochromatosis

Other cases of hemochromatosis or iron overload may be caused by massive doses of iron from supplements and diet, such as taking iron pills for many years, or by secondary hemochromatosis brought on by other diseases such as thalassemia, certain kinds of anemia, chronic alcoholism, or liver disease.

E83.39 Other disorders of phosphorus metabolism

Phosphorus metabolism disorders more commonly result in inadequate amounts of phosphorus being absorbed (hypophosphatasia) than in the absorption of too much. Hypophosphatasia can strike while the patient is still in the womb, in infancy or childhood, or in an adult up to middle age. In a prenatal or infant patient, it presents with skin-covered spurs on the arms and legs, and causes skeletal deformities up through childhood. Adults may experience stress fractures. There is no current medical treatment for this disorder beyond orthopedic surgical correction of deformities and fractures, and it is often deadly to younger patients.

E83.41 Hypermagnesemia

Hypermagnesemia is the absorption of too much magnesium and presents with nausea and vomiting, flushed skin, weakness, lightheadedness, and in some cases may depress the patient's consciousness level. This disorder is treated with magnesium-blocking medications.

E83.42 Hypomagnesemia

Hypomagnesemia is the presence of too little an amount of magnesium in the body. It presents with irritability, decreased attention span, and mental confusion, and has been linked by some researchers to attention-deficit disorder. This disorder is treated with magnesium supplements.

E83.51 Hypocalcemia

Use this code to report low blood calcium. Hypocalcemia presents with a number of symptoms, including muscle and abdominal cramping, hyperactive reflexes, shortness of breath and coughing, numbness and tingling in the hands and feet, dry skin and coarse hair, cataracts, bad teeth, and in cases of severe or long-term hypocalcemia, psoriasis and heart-disease. Final diagnosis for this disorder is by blood test, and it is treated with calcium supplements.

E83.52 Hypercalcemia

Hypercalcemia is the condition of having too much calcium in the bloodstream. Mild elevations in calcium levels usually present with no problems, but larger elevations can result in nausea and vomiting, changes in mental status, abdominal pain, constipation, fatigue and weakness, depression, excessive urination, and headache. Severe elevations can lead to coma and death if left untreated. Hypercalcemia may be due to a genetic disorder that causes the absorption of excessive amounts of calcium in the intestine or be a side-effect of a malignant tumor in the bone or intestine. Treatment centers around stabilization and reduction of the calcium levels by medication and/or diet and treating the underlying cause of the excessive absorption, if possible.

E83.81 Hungry bone syndrome

Hungry bone syndrome is connected to treatment for thyrotoxicosis and to parathyroidectomy for primary or secondary hyperparathyroidism. The main characterization is a low level of calcium, sometimes with hypophosphatemia and hypomagnesemia. Hungry bone syndrome is connected to previously elevated levels of parathyroid hormone causing related bone demineralization and possibly osteoporosis. After treatment, as the levels of parathyroid hormone change to normal or low levels, the bones begin to sequester or hoarde calcium, causing an increased density in bone. The hypocalcemia may resolve in weeks or take years.

E84 Cystic fibrosis

Cystic fibrosis, often abbreviated as CF, is a genetic disease that causes the body to produce a thick, sticky mucus within the lungs that results in a steadily decreasing lung capacity and life-threatening lung infections. This mucus can also obstruct the pancreas and/or liver, causing digestive disorders and infections. There is no cure for CF, and treatment concentrates on clearing mucus from the lungs via physical therapy (e.g., chest tapping)

and medication on a daily basis. The average age of death for a person with CF is in the mid-30s. Cystic fibrosis is coded according to its manifestation. Meconium ileus is an obstruction of the intestinal tract due to the mucus produced by CF. It is most often initially noticed when the blockages causes the abdomen to distend.

E85 Amyloidosis

Amyloidosis is a classification of diseases in which one or more organ systems in the body accumulate deposits of abnormal proteins. Primary amyloidosis originates in the bone marrow and causes antibodies to be made that the body cannot break down; these eventually leave the bloodstream and accumulate in the organs. Secondary amyloidosis is caused by a chronic infection or inflammation such as rheumatoid arthritis and deposits a type of protein called the AA protein in the organs. Familial amyloidosis is a genetic disease which causes a build-up of the transthyretin protein, which is manufactured in the liver. Although amyloidosis is not a malignancy per se, it can be disabling or even life-threatening. There is no cure for this disease (except in the case of secondary amyloidosis, in which treating the underlying cause may cure the imbalance), so treatment focuses on management and slowing the production of the defective proteins.

E85.0 Non-neuropathic heredofamilial amyloidosis

Familial Mediterranean fever is an hereditary disease causing amyloidosis found in certain ethnic populations from the eastern Mediterranean region. The disease is caused by a gene mutation affecting the production of the specific protein, pyrin, found in white blood cells responsible for controlling the body's inflammatory response. The disease is characterized by recurrent attacks of fever; intense inflammatory response pain in the abdomen, joints, and chest; and red, swollen skin lesions. The misproduced protein deposits itself in organs and tissues throughout the body and often leads to kidney failure.

E85.3 Secondary systemic amyloidosis

Secondary amyloidosis is also known as reactive systemic amyloidosis, in which the deposited protein fibrils are of the AA type caused by a reaction to a chronic infection such as osteomyelitis, or a noninfectious inflammatory process, such as rheumatoid arthritis.

E85.8 Other amyloidosis

Other forms of amyloidosis include hereditary cardiac or systemic amyloidosis.

E86 Volume depletion

Volume depletion refers to the depletion of total body water (dehydration) or the volume of blood plasma (hypovolemia). Shock, coma, and death can occur when balanced fluids are not replaced.

Note: Postoperative hypovolemic shock is coded with T81.11; Traumatic hypovolemic shock is reported with T79.4; and hypovolemic shock, that is not otherwise specified is reported in the signs and symptoms chapter with R57.1.

E86.0 Dehydration

Dehydration is the excessive loss of free water without a corresponding loss of sodium and other solutes. The disproportionate loss of water to electrolytes causes a solute imbalance, particularly of increased serum sodium (hypernatremia) which is used as an indictor of dehydration. Dehydration can be caused by prolonged bouts of diarrhea or vomiting, polyuria, excessive sweating, and not drinking enough water. Other conditions that cause dehydration include painful infection or inflammation of the mouth or throat such as strep throat or stomatitis; disease of the kidneys or adrenal glands; and diabetes mellitus. Symptoms include pale skin, dry mucous membranes, thirst, constipation, lack of urination, rapid heart rate, low blood pressure, and confusion. A loss of body fluids greater than 10%-15% is an emergency and can lead to shock. Treatment involves the careful replacement of fluid volume gradually to restore correctly balanced plasma solutes and avoid sudden shifts in fluid. Treatment also requires addressing the underlying cause to resolve the reason for the dehydration.

Note: Since dehydration is usually the result of another underlying condition, either of which require medical management in itself, determining code sequencing can be difficult. Dehydration may be listed first when the physician documents that the dehydration is mainly responsible for the visit and treatment is directed at correcting it. If the patient was dehydrated as a result of another condition, such as severe burns, and the burns were the condition chiefly being treated, then the burns are sequenced first, followed by the dehydration as a secondary code.

E86.1 Hypovolemia

Hypovolemia is a decrease in the volume of blood plasma or a drop in the total intravascular blood volume. This is considered true volume depletion, referring to a state of combined loss of blood volume and corresponding amounts of sodium electrolytes. Hypovolemia is caused by traumatic blood loss; diuretics or vasodilators; and excessive renal excretion of sodium and water such as occurs in acute tubular necrosis and poorly controlled diabetes. Hypovolemia is also caused by the sequestering of blood and fluids in third-space compartments, seen in significant cases of edema and ascites. Signs and symptoms include tachycardia, change in mental status, pale skin, thirst, low blood pressure, and dizziness or fainting upon standing. Lab tests will show decreased hematocrit and hemoglobin levels, elevated BUN, and increased urine specific gravity. Sequestering or loss of more than a liter of blood constitutes severe hypovolemia, which can lead to shock and cardiovascular collapse. Treatment is to replace body fluids of the same concentration using saline solution, lactated Ringers, plasma protein or albumin infusions, and blood transfusions.

E86.9 Volume depletion, unspecified

Unspecified volume depletion is the loss of total body water and contraction of intravascular blood plasma volume.

E87 Other disorders of fluid, electrolyte and acid-base balance

In the body, fluids, electrolytes (molecules with either a positive or negative charge, such as salts), and pH levels must be carefully balanced for the body to maintain its proper functioning. If any of these three elements is out of balance, it can cause long-term damage to the body.

E87.0 Hyperosmolality and hypernatremia

Hyperosmolality and/or hypernatremia are two terms that refer to an excess of sodium in the bloodstream. This most often occurs in a patient whose thirst response is not functioning properly, causing a low-fluid to high-sodium ratio. It can also be caused temporarily due to excessive vomiting, diarrhea, and urination. Treatment focuses on rehydration and using medication to remove excess sodium from the bloodstream; in extreme cases or cases of kidney disease or failure, dialysis may be used.

E87.1 Hypo-osmolality and hyponatremia

Hypo-osmolality and/or hyponatremia is too little sodium in the bloodstream, often due to diet or a disorder of the intestinal tract that prevents proper absorption. It presents with weight loss and loss of appetite, nausea and vomiting, loss of concentration, confusion, fatigue, agitation, headache, and in some cases, seizures. It is treated by increasing the body's sodium intake, sometimes by IV.

E87.3 Alkalosis

The symptoms of alkalosis, a condition in which the acidity of the body's fluids is unusually low, having a pH of more than 7.45, vary depending on which acids are affected.

E87.4 Mixed disorder of acid-base balance

These disorders are those in which more than one acid or base in the body is out of balance at the same time. These can be very tricky to diagnose because they can vary so wildly in their symptoms, and must be discerned by careful examination of a blood test. For all three types of disorders, treatment concentrates on restoring a proper pH to the body, often by IV, and depending on the cause, may involve continuing medication and/or a special diet.

E87.5 Hyperkalemia

Report hyperpotassemia with this code. This is a condition in which the body retains an excessive amount of potassium. It can result in an irregular heartbeat, weakness, and partial paralysis in the arms and legs.

E87.6 Hypokalemia

Report hypopotassemia with this code. This is a condition in which the amount of potassium in the body is too low for normal function. It can present with an irregular heartbeat, muscles weakness or paralysis, constipation, nausea or vomiting, abdominal cramps, confusion, and depression.

E87.70 Fluid overload, unspecified

Fluid overload, also called fluid retention, is often caused by kidney disease, and results in swelling, fatigue, and shortness of breath. Left untreated, it can actually cause congestive heart failure due to increased resistance to the free flow of blood. As an emergency treatment, physicians may remove as much as half a liter of blood; continuing treatment depends on the original cause of the fluid overload.

E87.71 Transfusion associated circulatory overload

Transfusion associated circulatory overload, or TACO, occurs with high rates or volumes of infusion that cannot be processed effectively by the recipient. It also occurs with patients who have an underlying pathology affecting the heart or lungs, which causes the transfusion of blood or blood components to overload the patient's circulatory system, particularly in infants and the elderly. TACO is marked by acute respiratory distress, an overload of positive fluid balance, increased blood pressure, and pulmonary edema (secondary to congestive heart failure) that develops during the transfusion or within 6 hours of transfusion.

E88.01 Alpha-1-antitrypsin deficiency

Alpha-1-antitrypsin, or AAT, deficiency is a genetic disorder which can cause emphysema and liver disease; however, the exact mechanism that causes these diseases in some patients, while others have no symptoms at all, is not known. Treatment centers around medication to replace or augment the amount of AAT in the patient's body; however, it is not known how effective this treatment is once lung or liver disease has set in.

E88.1 Lipodystrophy, not elsewhere classified

Lipodystrophy is a disorder of fatty tissue (sometimes referred to as the adipose tissue) in which the body loses only certain kinds of fats. Patients with this disorder are prone to develop insulin resistance and diabetes, a high saturated fat level, and a fatty liver. This disease can be genetic or acquired, and is a known side-effect of certain medications used to treat HIV known as protease inhibitors.

E88.3 Tumor lysis syndrome

Tumor lysis syndrome is a life-threatening complication of cancer therapy. This syndrome is actually a group of metabolic complications known to occur after cancer treatment, or even without treatment, particularly for lymphomas and leukemias. The metabolic complications seen are hyperuricemia, hypocalcemia, hyperkalemia, hyperphosphatemia, and acute kidney failure. These are caused by the toxic byproducts produced when dying cancer cells break down.

Note: This code includes both post-chemotherapy syndrome and spontaneous tumor lysis syndrome. Spontaneous tumor lysis syndrome occurs prior to beginning chemotherapy and is associated with acute kidney failure due to uric acid nephropathy, but is not associated with hyperphosphatemia.

E88.4 Mitochondrial metabolism disorders

Mitochondria are best described as the power sources for the body's cells. They convert energy from nutrients into forms usable by the cell. A mitochondrial metabolism disorder can cause muscle weakness, heart disease, impaired mental function, and other symptoms. There is no cure, and treatment concentrates on managing the symptoms of the disorder.

E88.81   Metabolic syndrome

Dysmetabolic syndrome X comprises a related group of metabolic disorders that affect the bloodstream. They present with resistance to insulin, weight increase and obesity, thickening and clotting of the blood, and increased uric acid levels. These in turn can create further complications such as stroke or heart disease.

Note: Use an additional code to report the associated manifestations, such as obesity.

E89.0   Postprocedural hypothyroidism

Postsurgical hypothyroidism occurs when part of the thyroid is removed and the remaining tissue cannot produce enough hormone to maintain the body's metabolism. Postablative or postirradiation hypothyroidism occurs when thyroid damage is due to radiation therapy, or the administration of radioactive iodine. This condition causes symptoms of fatigue, weight gain, muscle aches and cramps, an intolerance to cold temperatures, decreased sex drive, memory loss, and depression and irritability. It may also present with hair loss or coarseness, dry and/or rough skin, constipation, or a disruption of the menstrual cycles.

E89.1   Postprocedural hypoinsulinemia

Postsurgical hypoinsulinemia is a condition where the pancreas no longer provides sufficient insulin for the body due to being partially or completely removed surgically.

E89.2   Postprocedural hypoparathyroidism

Hypoparathyroidism is a disorder in which the parathyroid glands don't secrete enough hormone (PTH) resulting from the surgical removal of one or more of the parathyroids. The reduced production of PTH causes symptoms that range from mild tingling in the hands, fingers, and around the mouth to more severe muscle cramps. In rare cases, convulsions can result from this disorder. If left untreated over an extended period of time, this disorder can result in unusually thick bones. Hypoparathyroidism is rare.

F01 Vascular dementia

Vascular dementia is a generalized condition describing problems with impaired memory, reasoning, judgment, planning, and other cognitive thought processes from brain damage due to reduced blood flow. Vascular dementia is similar to Alzheimer's disease, but is often stroke-related and usually occurs more suddenly. Changes may also appear in noticeable downward declines from the previous level of functioning. This is a common form of dementia estimated to account for about 40% of dementia cases, particularly in the elderly, and is related to certain risk factors such as hypertension, atherosclerosis, cerebrovascular disease, diabetes, and smoking.

F01.50 Vascular dementia without behavioral disturbance

Vascular dementia occurs when the brain is deprived of vital oxygen and nutrients whenever blood vessels are chronically damaged or stenosed and blood flow to the brain is reduced or blocked, such as in a stroke. Symptoms include memory loss, depression, restlessness, agitation, trouble focusing or paying attention, confusion, unsteady gait, a decline in the ability to reason and organize thoughts, or analyze a situation. Risk factors such as high blood pressure, atherosclerosis, diabetes, smoking, lupus, and atrial fibrillation puts a person at high risk. Treatment mainly consists of controlling the underlying conditions posing the greatest risk. Medication aimed at regulating or boosting levels of brain cell chemical messengers involved in memory, judgment, and information processing may be given to help with the dementia symptoms.

F01.51 Vascular dementia with behavioral disturbance

Patients with vascular dementia may have behavioral disturbances at some point, which includes wandering off, hoarding, aggressiveness, sexual disinhibitions, screaming or incessant vocalizations, perseveration on bathroom activities, attention seeking, and any combative or violent behavior that puts patients and others in danger. Behavioral disturbances cause additional comorbidity and mortality, and increase stress for caregivers. Treatment is pharmacological with environmental interventions, as well as addressing any other causes of behavioral issues, such as pain, other medical illnesses, personal emotional needs, and the current use of any inappropriate medications.

Note: When wandering in vascular dementia is noted as a behavioral disturbance, assign code Z91.83 in addition.

F02 Dementia in other diseases classified elsewhere

Dementia is a generalized condition reflecting a loss of cognitive and intellectual functions, such as impaired memory, reasoning, judgment, and other cognitive thought processes, without impaired perception or consciousness, due to some form of brain damage. Dementia occurs in many other diseases, such as with Alzheimer's, epilepsy, multiple sclerosis, Parkinson's, niacin and vitamin B deficiencies, systemic lupus erythematosus, acquired hypothyroidism, and poisoning and toxic reactions.

Note: The underlying disease, such as recurrent seizures, must be reported first. Although dementia in Parkinson's disease is reported here, dementia with Parkinsonism is reported with G31.83 as dementia with Lewy bodies. Dementia occurring with substance abuse disorders is coded elsewhere in chapter 5, and dementia that occurs dues to atherosclerosis or hypertensive cerebrovascular disease is reported at vascular dementia.

F02.80 Dementia in other diseases classified elsewhere without behavioral disturbance

Dementia is a generalized condition reflecting a loss of cognitive and intellectual functions, such as impaired memory, reasoning, judgment, and other cognitive thought processes, without impaired perception or consciousness, due to some form of brain damage. Dementia occurs in many other diseases, such as Alzheimer's or epilepsy, typically due to the changes in the brain that the disease process itself effects on that organ. This can stem from hormonal imbalances, nutritive deficiencies, brain tissue degeneration, or infection. Symptoms of dementia include memory loss, depression, restlessness, agitation, trouble focusing or paying attention, confusion, unsteady gait, a decline in the ability to reason and organize thoughts, analyze a situation, or plan out an action. Treatment is aimed at the underlying condition, attempting to halt further permanent brain damage, and alleviating dementia symptoms, possibly with medicaments that regulate brain cell chemistry.

F02.81 Dementia in other diseases classified elsewhere with behavioral disturbance

Most patients with dementia will have behavioral disturbances at some point, which includes wandering off, hoarding, aggressiveness, sexual disinhibitions, screaming or incessant vocalizations, perseveration on bathroom activities, attention seeking, and any combative or violent behavior that puts patients and others in danger. Behavioral disturbances cause additional comorbidity and mortality, and increase stress for caregivers. Treatment is pharmacological with environmental interventions, as well as addressing any other causes of behavioral issues, such as pain, other medical illnesses, personal emotional needs, and the current use of any inappropriate medications.

Note: When wandering in dementia with other diseases is noted as a behavioral disturbance, assign code Z91.83 in addition.

F03 Unspecified dementia

This category includes both senile and presenile dementia, NOS and senile and presenile psychoses, NOS. Primary degenerative dementia and senile dementia expressed as depressive or paranoid type is also reported here as unspecified dementia either with or without behavioral disturbance. This is a loss of cognitive and intellectual functions, such as impaired memory, judgment, reasoning, and other intellectual or cognitive thought processes, without impaired perception or consciousness, generally in patients older than 65, and brought on by atrophy of parts of the brain. In the uncomplicated state it is often mild in manifestation.

Note: Unspecified senility is not considered to be dementia, but a symptom coded R41.81.

F03.90 Unspecified dementia without behavioral disturbance

Dementia is a group of symptoms caused by changes in the brain resulting in intellectual and social disabilities that interfere with regular functioning. Different symptoms are experienced with dementia, which includes problems with at least 2 brain functions, such as memory loss and impaired judgment. Symptoms vary with the cause and the etiology is often unknown. Other signs and symptoms include inability to reason; difficulty communicating, planning, coordinating motor functions, or learning new information; as well as personality and mood changes.

F03.91 Unspecified dementia with behavioral disturbance

Most patients with dementia will have behavioral disturbances at some point, which includes wandering off, hoarding, aggressiveness, sexual disinhibitions, screaming or incessant vocalizations, perseveration on bathroom activities, attention seeking, and any combative or violent behavior that puts patients and others in danger. Behavioral disturbances cause additional comorbidity and mortality, and increase stress for caregivers. Treatment is pharmacological with environmental interventions,

Mental/Behavioral/Neuro Disorders

F01 – F03.91

and addressing causes such as pain, other medical illnesses, personal needs, and inappropriate medications.

Note: When wandering off is noted as a behavioral disturbance, assign code Z91.83 in addition.

F04 Amnestic disorder due to known physiological condition

Amnestic disorder involves the loss of previously established memories, the inability to create new memories, or to learn new information. Amnestic disorder often results from an underlying physiological condition that causes structural or chemical damage to parts of the brain that produces disturbances in memory.

Note: Amnestic disorder brought about by the use of alcohol or other psychoactive substance is coded elsewhere in chapter 5.

F05 Delirium due to known physiological condition

This category level code is used to report delirium resulting from other known physiological conditions that may be temporary, lasting for a brief period of time, or more permanent. Conditions known to produce delirium reported here include psycho-organic brain syndromes, confusional states not due to alcohol, infective psychoses, and dementia with delirium superimposed. Delirium can be defined as an acute state of confusion and agitation in which the patient will seem to be disoriented, and will overreact to emotional and physical stimuli.

Note: Delirium that is not otherwise specified is reported as a symptom with code R41.0.

F06 Other mental disorders due to known physiological condition

This category is used to report mental disorders that are the result of other medical conditions. These conditions are classified as due to another known physiological condition and may be temporary, lasting for a brief period of time, or more permanent. Conditions known to cause the mental disorders reported here include endocrine disorders, circulating exogenous hormones, other drugs and substances the body finds toxic, systemic diseases affecting the brain, and epilepsy. Some of the disorders classified here include hallucinations, catatonia, depression, anxiety, and other psychotic disorders.

Note: Delirium due to a known physiological factor is coded to F05 and can be defined as an acute state of confusion and agitation in which the patient will seem to be disoriented, and will overreact to emotional and physical stimuli.

F06.1 Catatonic disorder due to known physiological condition

Catatonia is defined as a state of apparent unresponsiveness in someone who is apparently awake to experience external stimuli. The patient usually will not be able to provide a coherent history, is withdrawn, and often mute. One group of symptoms relates to motor behavior disturbances such as slowed motor activity or immobility in which the same rigid body position is held for days, weeks, or even months. Catatonic patients may also display a waxy flexibility in which they hold a body position placed by someone else. Other signs and symptoms relate to behavioral responses to others and include negativistic halting against or going along with blindly; automatic obedience; echolalia in which the patient automatically repeats the vocalizations made by another; echokinesis, the involuntary imitation of another's actions; and the inappropriate repetition of stereotypical movements such as body rocking, tapping, abdomen patting, and moving the jaw, eyes, or mouth. There is also an alternative presentation of catatonia in an excited state with agitated, purposeless movements unrelated to the environment, possible combativeness, and autonomic instability. Underlying physiological causes include infectious, metabolic, and neurological conditions such as encephalitis, diffuse encephalopathy, poisoning by neuroleptics or other toxic substances, neuroleptic malignant syndrome, or nonconvulsive status epilepticus. Medications used in treatment include lithium carbonate, amobarbitol, benzodiazepines, carbamazepine, tricyclic antidepressants, thyroid hormone, zolpidem, and muscle relaxants. Electroconvulsive therapy may be indicated when

the patient is not responding to pharmacotherapy within 5 days, or is displaying signs of malignant catatonia.

Note: The underlying physiologic condition must be reported first. Schizophrenic catatonia is considered another type of catatonia and is reported with F20.2 as is depressive catatonia, reported with codes from categories F31-F33. Unspecified catatonia is reported as stupor with R40.1.

F06.4 Anxiety disorder due to known physiological condition

Anxiety disorder is marked by persistent, uncontrollable worry and fear about aspects of a person's life, usually lasting at least 6 months, that becomes too much for the person to control, negatively affecting their day to day life. Although there are many types of anxiety disorders with differing symptoms, such as generalized, obsessive-compulsive, post-traumatic, and panic disorders, similar psychological symptoms can also occur in anxiety disorder specifically due to a known underlying medical condition. The main set of symptoms clusters around uncontrollable, excessive, and irrational fear or dread that leaves the person filled with obsessive worry, fearfulness, and uncertainty. Medication may be used to control the symptoms of anxiety while treatment is aimed at the underlying medical condition, which may include pain disorders, metabolic disturbances, nutritional deficiencies, encephalopathy, or other nervous system disorders.

Note: Anxiety disorder due to alcohol or substance abuse is not considered an underlying physiological condition and is reported elsewhere in chapter 5.

F07.0 Personality change due to known physiological condition

A change in personality due to an injury or disease of the brain, resulting from damage to the frontal lobe. The effects of this injury vary, but typically result in the patient showing apathy, a lack of planning, emotional bluntness, and the absence of abstract thought.

F07.81 Postconcussional syndrome

Postconcussional syndrome is a condition in which the patient suffers symptoms such as headache, amnesia, and lack of concentration due to a severe blow to the skull.

F10 Alcohol related disorders

Alcohol related disorders usually occur along with heavy, prolonged bouts of drinking and normally occur mainly in patients with alcoholism. Alcohol produces a depressant effect, and over time it can seriously impair brain function, besides the effects on other body systems. Alcohol related disorders are classified based on whether the patient is abusing or dependent upon alcohol, intoxicated or in withdrawal, and whether the patient suffers from other related disorders, such as anxiety, sleep, or mood disorders, or psychotic disorders with delusions or hallucinations, or amnesia.

Note: Delirium can be defined as an acute state of confusion and agitation. The patient will seem to be disoriented, and will overreact to emotional and physical stimuli. Delusional patients exhibit false beliefs inconsistent with their own knowledge and experiences. Hallucinations, however, involve false sensory stimulation.

F10.2 Alcohol dependence

Alcohol dependence is a substance use disorder characterized by an individual's compulsive need to use alcohol.

F10.920 Alcohol use, unspecified with intoxication, uncomplicated

Idiosyncratic alcohol intoxication presents as a disorder unique to the individual that occurs after ingesting a small amount of alcohol, and is not caused by excessive drinking.

F19.930 Other psychoactive substance use, unspecified with withdrawal, uncomplicated

Drug withdrawal occurs when drug use is curtailed, resulting in physical or psychological symptoms that can vary widely depending on the drug(s) the patient was taking. Symptoms can last anywhere from hours to weeks, and commonly feature headache, anxiety, depression, chills, sweats, and tremors.

F20 Schizophrenia

Schizophrenia is a term for a group of chronic, severe mental disorders which affect behavior and thought patterns. The cause of these disorders is unknown, but is believed to be genetic. The onset of the disease usually happens in late adolescence or early adulthood, and affects males more often than females. While there are several variations of schizophrenia, symptoms such as hallucinations, delusions, and disorganized behavior are common among all of them.

F20.0 Paranoid schizophrenia

Paranoid schizophrenia is marked by displays of megalomania, delusions of persecution and/or grandeur, hallucinations, and aggressive behavior.

F20.1 Disorganized schizophrenia

Disorganized schizophrenia is characterized by inappropriate, disinhibited behavior. The patient may display strange emotional responses, and may appear agitated. Hallucinations and delusions may occur, but are not the prominent features of the disorder.

F20.2 Catatonic schizophrenia

Catatonic schizophrenia is marked by a state of rigid stupor in which the body's limbs can be posed, or the patient displays purposeless motion and refusal to follow commands or suggestions.

F20.5 Residual schizophrenia

Residual schizophrenia is observed in patients recovering from schizophrenia during which mild symptoms return.

F20.81 Schizophreniform disorder

Schizophreniform disorder is used as a preliminary diagnosis for schizophrenia. If the schizophreniform disorder cannot be cured in six months, then the diagnosis is changed to schizophrenia.

F20.89 Other schizophrenia

Simple type schizophrenia is often undiagnosed, and is the least severe type of the disease. Symptoms include a gradual withdrawal from contact with others, as well as mild hallucinations and delusions.

F21 Schizotypal disorder

Schizotypal disorder is a condition in which the patient is uncomfortable forming close relationships with others and suffers abnormal anxiety in social situations.

F23 Brief psychotic disorder

Brief psychotic disorder includes paranoid reaction and psychogenic paranoid psychosis. An acute paranoid reaction causes the patient to have severe delusions of persecution, believing that someone or something is conspiring to do them harm. Psychogenic paranoid psychosis is a type of disorder in which the patient's paranoid state is in response to an external stimulus, and has a longer duration than an acute paranoid reaction.

F24 Shared psychotic disorder

A shared psychotic disorder occurs when a delusional person convinces another person that their delusions are real. The person convinced to accept the delusions as real typically shares a close relationship with the delusional person.

F30 Manic episode

Mood disorders reports dramatic, recurrent, or severe forms of mood disturbances that are accompanied by extreme changes in energy and behavior, either very low depressive type or the high manic type. Psychoses may also be present in bipolar and major depressive disorder

with hallucinations of things that are not there or delusions of false ideas or beliefs. These disorders may occur in singular episodes, may be cylic or recurring in nature, and may also appear mixed at the same time.

Note: *The Diagnostic and Statistical Manual of Mental Disorders* (DSM-IV) criteria require that when coding bipolar disorders, the episode(s) cannot be better accounted for by any kind of schizophrenic-related type of disorder, delusional disorder, or psychotic disorder.

This category codes bipolar disorder, single manic episode. Bipolar disorder is one of the most common mental disorders, also referred to as manic depressive disorder. A single manic episode is the presence of only one manic period when it is not a recurrence, and with no past major depressive episodes. Approximately 90% of those with a single manic episode will go on to have recurrent episodes. The manic mood is characterized by unusually high levels of energy; a lack of need for very much sleep; racing thoughts or fast speech; a euphoric mood; difficulty concentrating; unrealistic beliefs in one's own abilities; excessive spending; and intrusive or aggressive behavior. Up to 70% of all manic episodes occur immediately preceding or following a major depressive episode, so caution should be used when reporting this category.

F31.0 Bipolar disorder, current episode hypomanic

Current hypomanic episode is a mild to moderate level of mania associated by patients with good feelings that increase functioning and productivity. It can turn into severe mania or depression and the mood symptoms, although perceived as good, can actually cause distress or impairment in social and occupational functioning. A hypomanic episode that turns into a more severe manic episode later is still considered hypomanic in the current episode.

F31.1 Bipolar disorder, current episode manic without psychotic features

Bipolar disorder is one of the most common mental disorders, also referred to as manic depressive disorder. The occurrence of a cyclical manic episode is coded here in which there has previously been at least one major depressive episode. The current manic mood is characterized by unusually high levels of energy; a lack of need for very much sleep; racing thoughts or fast speech; a euphoric mood; difficulty concentrating; unrealistic beliefs in one's own abilities; excessive spending; and intrusive or aggressive behavior.

Note: If "recurrent manic episode" is stated, but not otherwise specified, report code F31.89.

Note: When the current manic episode is severe and occurs with psychotic symptoms report F31.2.

F31.3 Bipolar disorder, current episode depressed, mild or moderate severity

Bipolar disorder is one of the most common mental disorders, also referred to as manic depressive disorder. The occurrence of a cyclical depressed episode is coded here in which there has previously been at least one major manic episode. A current depressive episode is characterized by feelings of hopelessness, worthlessness, guilt, or helplessness; decreased energy and fatigue; difficulty remembering or making decisions; a lasting sad, empty, or anxious mood; pervasive pessimism; sleeping too much or not being able to sleep; weight loss or gain; and suicidal thoughts or attempts.

Note: When a current depressed episode is severe, occurring with psychotic symptoms, report F31.5.

Note: A recurrent episode of major (reactive) (psychogenic) (endogenous) (seasonal affective) depression is coded to category F33.

F31.6 Bipolar disorder, current episode mixed

Use this subcategory to report a current episode of bipolar disorder stated to be a mixed episode. In a mixed episode, symptoms of both mania and depression are present together, but neither one dominates. For instance, a person may feel sad on one hand, but also very energetic at the same time. Patients often present as agitated with trouble sleeping or lack of need for much sleep. They may have suicidal thoughts or even display psychosis.

F31.81   Bipolar II disorder

This code reports bipolar II disorder, which is defined as a history of one or more major depressive episodes, accompanied by at least one hypomanic episode, and without history of a manic or mixed episode. The major difference between bipolar I and bipolar II relies on bipolar II having hypomania, but no manic episodes. Bipolar II cannot have psychotic features such as hallucinations and delusions that may occur in bipolar I. Symptoms do cause distress or impair functioning, but not markedly enough to require hospitalization.

F31.9   Bipolar disorder, unspecified

This code is used to report the circular type of bipolar disorder, or manic depressive psychosis, in which the current state or most recent episode is not specified as either manic, depressive, or mixed. This code also reports atypical bipolar affective disorder not otherwise specified.

F32   Major depressive disorder, single episode

A single major depressive episode is the presence of only one depressive period with no past manic episodes and no recurrence of a previous depressive episode-defined as a shift in polarity from mania, or an interval of less than two months without depressive symptoms. The depressive episode is characterized by feelings of hopelessness, worthlessness, guilt, or helplessness; decreased energy and fatigue; difficulty remembering or making decisions; a lasting sad, empty, or anxious mood; pervasive pessimism; sleeping too much or not being able to sleep; weight loss or gain; and suicidal thoughts or attempts.

Note: Single episodes of major depressive disorder are only coded when there has been no previous major manic episode. If the depressive episode follows a previous manic episode, it should be coded as bipolar disorder with most recent (or current) episode depressed.

Note: This category also includes singles episodes of severe depression with psychotic symptoms, reactive depressive psychosis, or psychotic depression.

F34.0   Cyclothymic disorder

Cyclothymic disorder is characterized by mild mood swings between elevated mood and mild depression. Be careful not to confuse this condition with bipolar disorder, a similar condition in which the mood swings are much more severe.

F34.1   Dysthymic disorder

Dysthymic disorder is also described as chronic depressive personality disorder, or neurotic depression. Dysthymia is a serious, chronic, depressive state that persists for at least 2 years and is accompanied by symptoms such as fatigue, insomnia, anxiety, low self-esteem, and disruption of appetite. Dysthymia is a mood disorder that is less severe than a psychosis, lasting longer than major depressive disorder. Sufferers may have symptoms for a long time before being diagnosed and many believe that depression is simply part of their character.

F40.01   Agoraphobia with panic disorder

Agoraphobia is a fear of open spaces or crowds, traveling, or leaving a safe place. The patient will suffer panic attacks when forced into these situations.

F40.1   Social phobias

Patients suffering from social functioning have an intense fear of appearing in public, especially in situations where they are the center of attention.

F40.10   Social phobia, unspecified

Patients suffering from this condition have an intense fear of appearing in public, especially in situations where they are the center of attention.

F40.2   Specific (isolated) phobias

Phobias are an intense fear or loathing of an object or situation.

F41.0   Panic disorder [episodic paroxysmal anxiety] without agoraphobia

Panic disorder without agoraphobia, or a fear of crowds, is thought to be a malfunction of the patient's flight or fight response. The patient suffers unexplained bouts of intense fear or anxiety, accompanied by symptoms such as elevated heart rate, sweating, trembling, dizziness, and/or shortness of breath. Fear of dying is also a hallmark of panic disorder.

F41.1   Generalized anxiety disorder

This condition is marked by persistent, uncontrollable worry about aspects of a person's life. This disorder is diagnosed when the anxiety symptoms last longer than six months, with anxiety present on the majority of days in that time.

F42   Obsessive-compulsive disorder

Obsessive-compulsive disorders occur when a person suffers from recurrent obsessions of thought or action that are time-consuming or disruptive to daily life. These obsessions can be ideas, thoughts, images, or impulses which produce anxiety or distress.

F43.0   Acute stress reaction

This condition occurs when an extremely high stress level causes a patient to experience intense anxiety and panic.

F43.1   Post-traumatic stress disorder (PTSD)

This condition, once thought to occur mostly in combat veterans, occurs commonly in all levels of society as a response to traumatic events such as rape, physical assault, and natural disasters. A patient afflicted with PTSD will often suffer sudden, powerful memories (flashbacks) of the event that triggered the condition, causing anxiety and panic. They may also withdraw from family and friends, and avoid situations which resemble aspects of the original traumatic event. The patient's emotions may swing wildly, and they may turn to drugs or alcohol as a way of coping.

F43.2   Adjustment disorders

Adjustment reactions and disorders occur when the patient has difficulty adjusting to a new environment or situation. They could be a reaction to grief, moving away from home to a different culture, being hospitalized, or other such situations.

F43.25   Adjustment disorder with mixed disturbance of emotions and conduct

An adjustment disorder with mixed disturbances of different emotions, as well as a disturbance in conduct that causes the patient to act out in ways that are not socially acceptable.

F43.29   Adjustment disorder with other symptoms

Adjustment disorder with withdrawal occurs when the patient abnormally isolates themselves to avoid dealing with a new situation. The condition commonly occurs in young children, who become sullen and withdrawn.

F44   Dissociative and conversion disorders

Dissociative disorders are a type of alternate, or multiple personality disorders that occur when an individual is incapable of remembering or maintaining his or her own true identity. An alternate, or two or more different distinct personalities, each with its own thoughts, emotions, and behaviors is created. These disorders are very rare. A conversion disorder occurs when impaired physical function occurs due to a psychological problem instead of a physical problem. The patient may suffer seizures, paralysis, loss of the voice, or temporary blindness or deafness, also known as hysterical blindness or hysterical deafness. It is thought that this condition is a response to stress.

F44.0   Dissociative amnesia

Dissociative amnesia is the result of psychological trauma which causes the patient to temporarily forget personal information and renders him or her unable to perform complex tasks, such as driving or cooking.

F44.1   Dissociative fugue

Dissociative fugue is a disorder occurring in response to a severe, recent stressor, in which the patient invents a new personality and becomes unable to remember his or her previous identity, lasting from days to months.

F44.4 Conversion disorder with motor symptom or deficit

A conversion disorder occurs when symptoms impairing physical function occur due to a psychological problem instead of a physical problem. The patient may suffer seizures, paralysis, voice loss, or temporary blindness. It is thought that this condition is a response to stress.

F44.81 Dissociative identity disorder

Dissociative identity disorder is commonly known as multiple personality disorder. This condition arises due to severe emotional and mental stress or trauma in childhood. The patient creates one or more distinct personalities separate from their own as a protective device, each with its own memory, behaviors, thoughts, and motivations. Any of the different personalities may be dominant, lived by the person, with suppression of the true identity.

F44.89 Other dissociative and conversion disorders

This code includes reactive or psychogenic confusion, also called psychogenic twilight state. A patient with this disorder will seem severely disoriented and results from a severe emotional reaction.

F44.9 Dissociative and conversion disorder, unspecified

An unspecified dissociative disorder or reaction is a temporary state of hysteria in which the patient will lapse into an alternate personality in response to a stressor.

F45 Somatoform disorders

Somatoform disorders are psychological problems which manifest themselves with physical symptoms.

F45.0 Somatization disorder

This condition is marked by physical symptoms that are a manifestation of psychological conflicts. The patient will present with symptoms of illness affecting multiple organ systems, for which the physician will find no physical source.

F45.1 Undifferentiated somatoform disorder

An undifferentiated somatoform disorder is a condition in which the patient has symptoms of a specific physical disease, but does not actually suffer from that disease.

F45.2 Hypochondriacal disorders

Hypochondriasis is also called health fear or health phobia. This is a somatoform disorder marked by an overwhelming fear that one has a serious disease, or by excessive preoccupation with serious illness, even though medical practiotioners cannot find any evidence of the disease(s) being present.

F48.1 Depersonalization-derealization syndrome

Depersonalization disorder is a condition in which the patient recurrently looks at themselves from an outsider's point of view, to the point of feeling that they are not in control of themselves. Symptoms of this disorder are similar to those of panic disorder and other anxiety problems.

F48.2 Pseudobulbar affect

Pseudobulbar affect (PBA) is a condition that occurs secondary to underlying neurological conditions, disease, or injury. The structural damage to the brain causes involuntary, frequent, disruptive outbursts of crying or laughing that is incongruent or magnified out of proportion with the patient's emotional state and situation. It is often mistaken for psychiatric disorders such as bipolar disorder, schizophrenia, and depression. PBA has been reported in patients with amyotrophic lateral sclerosis, multiple sclerosis, those who have had traumatic brain injury, and patients one year after suffering stroke.

Note: The underlying neurologic disease or sequelae cause must be reported first, if known, as pseudobulbar affect is a secondary neurologic condition.

F48.8 Other specified nonpsychotic mental disorders

Other specified nonpsychotic mental disorders includes other specified types of neurosis, such as occupational, or psychasthenic neurasthenia, and psychogenic syncope. The patient suffers physical weakness, fatigue, or collapse due to mental exertion and inadequate rest.

F50.0 Anorexia nervosa

Anorexia nervosa is an eating disorder caused by an extreme, irrational fear of becoming overweight that leads to radical restriction of food intake. Patients may exercise excessively or binge eat and induce self vomiting. Sufferers also have a distorted self image of their body and diet to the point of starvation and malnutrition, causing serious ill health and even death.

F50.2 Bulimia nervosa

Bulimia nervosa is a serious eating disorder than mainly affects young women, characterized by binge eating, secretive episodes of consuming a large amount of food in a short time, followed by an attempt to purge the calories eaten, often by self-induced vomiting or with the use of strong laxatives or diuretics, or excessive exercise. A patient with this disease will typically eat compulsively and see themselves as being overweight, even if their weight is normal. The cycles of insatiable appetite and purging are often set apart by long periods of food restriction. Binge eating and purging can cause stomach rupture, acidic erosion of tooth enamel, an inflamed esophagus, irregular menstrual periods, and even irregular heart rhythms due to the lack of necessary vitamins and minerals, such as potassium.

F50.8 Other eating disorders

This code includes pica in adults, which is the urge to eat nonfood substances, such as dirt, paper, paint, and rocks. It also includes the psycogenic loss of appetite, which is characterized by an aversion to eating or food without a pathologic/physiologic explanation for the condition. It may occur after an illness when the brain, as a conditioned response, sends signals to the body to avoid a food that was eaten just previous to the illness as a protection against becoming ill again.

Avoidant/Restrictive Food Intake Disorder (ARFID) is a complex eating disorder characterized by decreased interest in food/eating, avoidance of certain foods due to sensory characteristics and/or an increased concern with the consequences or disadvantages of food/eating. The disorder occurs in the absence of psychological or physiological disease or conditions and ultimately results in a failure to meet nutritional needs. ARFID is often associated with a fear of eating and may be triggered by an episode of choking or vomiting or unpleasant memories associated with certain places (work, school, home, restaurant).

F50.9 Eating disorder, unspecified

Atypical types of anorexia and bulimia nervosa are included here. One type of atypical anorexic disorder, sometimes called orthorexia nervosa, is characterized by an obsession with avoiding "unhealthy" foods that eventually leads to restrictive eating and can cause malnutrition. The disorder does not usually involve body dysmorphia but does cause anxiety and distress that negatively interfers with everyday life.

Binge Eating Disorder (BED) is a complex eating disorder characterized by recurrent episodes of overeating not followed by purging, exercise, or fasting. Individuals who engage in this behavior are usually overweight or obese and experience guilt, shame, and distress which perpetuates the cycle.

F51.03 Paradoxical insomnia

A disorder marked by violent, vigorous behavior perceived in a dream, such as running, jumping, punching, or kicking. During normal REM sleep, the muscles are deactivated so that this type of activity cannot take place. Patients suffering from this condition risk injuring themselves or their bedmates.

Mental/Behavioral/Neuro Disorders F44.4 – F51.03

F51.11   **Primary hypersomnia**

Primary hypersomnia is a condition in which the patient is chronically unable to wake up from sleep and maintain wakefulness throughout a normal day.

F51.4   **Sleep terrors [night terrors]**

Patients with this sleep arousal disorder, commonly known as night terrors, will become active during sleep, and may experience terror, panic, and episodes of screaming. The patient will be unable to recall these episodes upon waking.

F52.4   **Premature ejaculation**

Premature ejaculation occurs when a male chronically ejaculates almost immediately during sexual intercourse.

F52.5   **Vaginismus not due to a substance or known physiological condition**

Psychogenic vaginismus is a condition in which psychological factors cause a female to suffer painful contractions of the muscles in the vagina.

F52.6   **Dyspareunia not due to a substance or known physiological condition**

A condition in which a female feels psychosomatic pain during sexual activity.

F60   **Specific personality disorders**

This class of mental disorders is characterized by inflexible, pervasive thought patterns that interfere with a person's daily life.

F60.0   **Paranoid personality disorder**

A patient with paranoid personality disorder mistakenly believes that others are exploiting, harming, or deceiving them. They may hold grudges for little or no reason, and are constantly suspicious of their friends and loved ones.

F60.1   **Schizoid personality disorder**

Schizoid personality disorders are characterized by weak social skills, difficulty expressing anger, and a desire to be alone.

F60.2   **Antisocial personality disorder**

Antisocial personality disorder is a condition in which the sufferer shows a total disregard for the rule of law and the rights of other people, and will violently resist living by the accepted norms of a society.

F60.3   **Borderline personality disorder**

Borderline personality disorder is characterized by mood swings, unstable interpersonal relationships, fear of abandonment, suicidal thoughts, and other symptoms. This also includes an explosive or aggressive personality in which the sufferer is quick to anger, aggressive, abnormally emotional, and argumentative.

F60.4   **Histrionic personality disorder**

Histrionic personality disorder manifests as excessive emotional behavior, theatrics, and an extreme need for attention. Sufferers of this disorder will often make inappropriate sexual advances.

F60.5   **Obsessive-compulsive personality disorder**

A patient with obsessive-compulsive personality disorder will place undue attention on nearly every task they are given to perform, and will attempt it compulsively until they feel it is perfect. These people tend to be rigid in thought and action and show an aversion to delegate responsibility.

F60.6   **Avoidant personality disorder**

Avoidant personality disorder occurs when the patient avoids social contact out of a fear of rejection or humiliation.

F60.7   **Dependent personality disorder**

Dependent personality disorder manifests as helplessness, an inability to make independent decisions, and low self-esteem.

F60.81   **Narcissistic personality disorder**

Symptoms of narcissistic personality disorder are an exaggerated sense of self-importance and a focus on self wants, lack of social inhibition, lying, lack of empathy for others, and a sense of entitlement.

F60.89   **Other specific personality disorders**

This includes eccentric, immature, and self-defeating personality disorders as well as passive-aggressive personality disorder in which a person's aggressive feelings are manifested as procrastination and passive resistance to demands.

F63.1   **Pyromania**

The impulse to set fires.

F63.2   **Kleptomania**

An irresistible impulse to steal; pathological stealing. This condition usually manifests as shoplifting.

F63.3   **Trichotillomania**

Hair plucking or pulling out hair.

F63.81   **Intermittent explosive disorder**

Intermittent explosive disorder causes the patient to experience periods where he or she is unable to control his or her anger.

F64.1   **Gender identity disorder in adolescence and adulthood**

Patients with this disorder express an overwhelming desire to anatomically change their sex. These patients feel that they were born as the wrong gender.

Note: Use an additional code, Z87.890, to report surgical status for sex change or sex reassignment.

F64.2   **Gender identity disorder of childhood**

This condition occurs when a child becomes confused about the role and behavior that is appropriate for their gender.

F65.0   **Fetishism**

The term fetishism describes a sexual fixation on a particular item, fantasy, or situation that is exploited for sexual purposes.

F65.1   **Transvestic fetishism**

Transvestic fetishism is a disorder in which the patient desires to wear clothing associated with the opposite sex.

F65.2   **Exhibitionism**

Exhibitionism causes the individual to feel a compulsion to expose their genitals while in public.

F65.3   **Voyeurism**

Voyeurism is a disorder in which the patient suffers from a compulsion to covertly observe others who are nude or engaged in sexual activity.

F65.4   **Pedophilia**

A condition in which an adult engages in sexual activity with a child or children.

F65.51   **Sexual masochism**

A patient with this disorder feels the need to be humiliated or hurt to achieve sexual gratification.

F65.52   **Sexual sadism**

Sexual sadism occurs when the patient must humiliate or injure others to achieve sexual gratification.

F68.1   **Factitious disorder**

In factitious disorders, the patient purposely assumes psychological symptoms, or physical illnesses for psychological reasons in the presence of others, especially physicians and other health care workers.

F68.10 Factitious disorder, unspecified

Factitious disorder consists of the patient purposely assuming psychological symptoms in the presence of others, especially physicians and other health care workers. Sufferers of this disease seek attention by pretending to have medical problems, and frequently seek treatment, even surgery, at the hands of medical professionals. Some people who suffer this disease are quite adept at tricking health care providers into believing that they are physically ill.

F70 Mild intellectual disabilities

Patients with mild intellectual disabilities will be high-functioning, but will be of below average intelligence. Those afflicted will have problems learning complex tasks and comprehending language, and often have difficulty in an academic environment. Use other codes to identify psychiatric or physical conditions associated with the intellectual disability.

F71 Moderate intellectual disabilities

Moderate intellectual disability is usually noticeable in the first year of a child's life, as the child will be delayed in crawling, sitting upright, walking, and other normal landmarks of early development. A patient with this condition will have lifelong problems developing and learning on pace with their peers, but can typically become a fully functional and independent member of society.

F72 Severe intellectual disabilities

A condition in which the patient has trouble performing basic self-care tasks, such as hygiene and food preparation. Patients suffering from this level of retardation will need constant support and supervision throughout their lives.

F73 Profound intellectual disabilities

Patients afflicted with profound intellectual disabilities will never progress past the mental levels of a toddler, and will need constant support and supervision throughout their lives.

F80.0 Phonological disorder

Phonological disorder is a problem with the proper pronunciation of words.

F80.1 Expressive language disorder

An impairment is which an individual has difficulty expressing him or herself using spoken and written language. Persons with expressive language disorder will understand language better than they are able to communicate themselves. In children, this may be a developmental problem that occurs with normal intelligence, or part of a condition that does affect mental function. Adults may acquire it as a result of brain damage or injury. Patients will have trouble accessing and organizing their words into sentences to describe or define the idea they wish to convey. They may also have trouble with spelling, using words correctly, and forming sentences when writing.

F80.2 Mixed receptive-expressive language disorder

This is a communication disorder in which the patient has difficulty both in expressing him or herself, particularly with spoken language, and with understanding what others are saying. This is generally a childhood disorder and may be developmental or acquired. The child has trouble constructing his or her own coherent sentences as well as understanding some types of terms that others are using, such as abstract nouns and spatial terms, and well as complex sentences.

F80.4 Speech and language development delay due to hearing loss

Children who are born with hearing loss or deafness, and those that acquire it before language and speech skills are developed have a greater risk for not acquiring those skills normally at appropriate ages. Without the ability to hear language being spoken, the ability to learn by mimicking is reduced.

F80.81 Childhood onset fluency disorder

Childhood onset fluency disorder is the preferred terminology for childhood 'stuttering.' This is a disruption in the flow of speech production usually occurring between 2 and 5 years of age marked by sound and syllable repetitions, articulatory blocks that prevent the speaker from moving forward with speech, and incorrect prolongations of speech sounds. These disruptions in speech are accompanied by noticeable signs of self-awareness, tension, and struggle. Fluency disorders are a potentially disabling and handicapping condition that can have significant educational and social consequences for the child.

Note: For adult onset fluency disorder, see code F98.5.

F81.0 Specific reading disorder

Specific reading disorder includes reading retardation and developmental dyslexia. Developmental dyslexia is a disorder in which the patient has great difficulty understanding written language, and this difficulty can not be traced to a deficit of inherent intelligence, proper instruction, or a neurological injury or condition.

F84.0 Autistic disorder

Autistic disorder, or autism, usually appears around 30 months of age. This neurological disorder results in the abnormal development or impairment of social interaction, communication skills, and behavior. Patients with autism will seem cold and aloof, and will not respond to typical emotional stimulus. The degree of severity of autism varies greatly, with some sufferers able to function normally, and others unable to function at all.

F84.3 Other childhood disintegrative disorder

Children with this disintegrative psychosis or dementia infantalis will develop normally until about age two, and then begin to deteriorate in language, social, and intellectual functioning. This condition is often mistaken for autism.

F90 Attention-deficit hyperactivity disorders

This is one of the most common disorders of childhood with symptoms of difficulty staying focused, paying attention, and controlling behavior, with overactivity of physical movement. To be diagnosed with this disorder, a child must have symptoms of inattention, hyperactivity, and impulsivity to a degree that is more severe than children of the same age for at least 6 months.

F90.0 Attention-deficit hyperactivity disorder, predominantly inattentive type

The predominantly inattentive type of ADHD has most of its manifesting symptoms in the inattention category and less symptoms in the hyperactive-impulsive category. These children may sit quietly and even though they are not acting out or moving around impulsively, they are still not paying attention to what they are doing. This subtype is diagnosed when 6 or more of the following inattentive symptoms are present: be easily distracted and frequently switch from one project to another; become bored with any one task after a few minutes; have difficulty focusing on organizing and completing a task or learning something new; loses things necessary to completing tasks or assignment, such as homework; daydreaming; not appearing to listen when spoken to; struggles to follow instructions; or has trouble processing accurately or at the speed others can.

F90.1 Attention-deficit hyperactivity disorder, predominantly hyperactive type

The predominantly hyperactive type of ADHD present with the majority of symptoms in the overactive-impulsive category, with less of the inattentive symptoms. This subtype is diagnosed when 6 or more of the following hyperactive-impulsive symptoms are present: fidget and squirm when seated; dash around touching everything; being constantly in motion; talking incessantly; difficulty sitting still for meals, story time, etc; having trouble with quiet tasks; being very impatient; blurting out comments or answers; showing emotion without restraint; have difficult waiting their turn or for things they want.

F90.2 **Attention-deficit hyperactivity disorder, combined type**

The combined type of ADHD is diagnosed the most and occurs when at least 6 symptoms in both the inattentive category and the hyperactive-impulsive category are present together.

F91.1 **Conduct disorder, childhood-onset type**

This refers to unsocialized aggressive or solitary aggressive conduct disorder. Children with this condition have never learned age-appropriate behavior, commonly due to excessive isolation. Anger issues are the most common symptom, and the patient may lie, cheat, steal, and aggressively bully other children in their peer group.

F91.2 **Conduct disorder, adolescent-onset type**

This condition refers to socialized conduct disorder, or group type conduct disorder found among groups of adolescents who show anti-social tendencies. Members of the group may skip school, commit petty (occasionally serious) crime, and abuse drugs or alcohol. The common feature of this particular diagnosis is that the misbehavior takes place in the context of a group or gang.

F91.3 **Oppositional defiant disorder**

A condition in which the child stubbornly resists all authority, especially that exerted by parents.

F93.0 **Separation anxiety disorder of childhood**

A condition in which a child suffers abnormal anxiety when separated from their parent, guardian, or usual environment.

F94.0 **Selective mutism**

Children with this disorder will go long periods without speaking, remaining mute even to family members.

F95.2 **Tourette's disorder**

Tourette's disorder is a condition in which the patient experiences multiple muscular and motor tics, often occurring in episodes one or more times a day. To qualify as Tourette's, the episodes must occur for at least 12 months.

F98.0 **Enuresis not due to a substance or known physiological condition**

Bedwetting, or the lack of control of urination, particlarly during sleep, due to psychogenic reasons and not of organic origin.

F98.1 **Encopresis not due to a substance or known physiological condition**

The voluntary or involuntary bowel movements in places other than the toilet occurring in children past the age when fecal control is normally expected, due to a psychogenic reason.

F98.21 **Rumination disorder of infancy**

Rumination disorder is a condition in which the patient habitually regurgitates food and reswallows it.

F98.3 **Pica of infancy and childhood**

A disorder in which a child feels the compulsion to eat inedible substances, such as dirt or rocks.

Note: Pica occurring in adulthood is coded to F50.8.

F98.4 **Stereotyped movement disorders**

Stereotyped movement disorders cause the patient to make deliberate, repeated movements, such as rocking back and forth, or banging the head against a surface for no discernible reason.

F98.5 **Adult onset fluency disorder**

Adult onset fluency disorder is the terminology replacing 'stuttering.' This is a disruption in the flow of speech production with onset after puberty marked by sound and syllable repetitions, articulatory blocks that prevent the speaker from moving forward with speech, and incorrect prolongations of speech sounds. These disruptions in speech are accompanied by noticeable signs of self-awareness, tension, and struggle. Fluency disorders are a potentially disabling and handicapping condition that can have significant educational, social, and vocational consequences for adults.

Note: For childhood onset fluency disorder, see code F80.81.

G00 Bacterial meningitis, not elsewhere classified

Meningitis is an infection of the protective tissues lining the brain and spinal cord, called the meninges. This condition presents with a number of symptoms, including fever and chills, loss of appetite, severe headache, sensitivity to light, altered consciousness or changes in mental status, vomiting, stiffness in the neck, lethargy and/or drowsiness, irritability and/or confusion. The patient may also lose consciousness and go into convulsions. Bacteria are the more common cause of meningitis, which is usually severe and can cause serious complications. In some cases, the patient may suffer long-term conditions, such as deafness and brain damage.

G00.0 Hemophilus meningitis

Hemophilus meningitis is a bacterial infection of the protective tissues surrounding the brain and spinal cord caused by *Hemophilus influenzae* bacteria that have migrated to the central nervous system. This was the number one cause of bacterial meningitis in children under 5 before the advent of the Hib vaccine. The infection usually occurs when bacteria spread into the bloodstream, and then into the meninges. Upper respiratory infections, otitis media, pharyngitis, and sinusitis are all risk factors, as is exposure to another family member with an *H. influenzae* infection, attending school or daycare, older age, and a weakened immune system. Symptoms come on quickly, resulting in fever and chills, severe headache, vomiting, stiff neck, malaise, mental status changes, and photophobia. In very young children, symptoms may also present as agitation, irritability, feeding difficulties, high pitched cry, bulging fontanelle, rapid breathing, and arching the head and neck backwards. Diagnostic exams usually consist of physical examination, cultures of the blood and cerebrospinal fluid, chest x-rays, and cranial CT scan. Antibiotics are given as soon as possible, sometimes with corticosteroids to reduce inflammation. This is a very dangerous infection with a risk of mortality, especially in the very young and old. Other morbidity outcomes include brain damage, hearing loss, hydrocephalus, and seizures.

G00.1 Pneumococcal meningitis

Pneumococcal meningitis is a bacterial infection of the protective tissues surrounding the brain and spinal cord caused by *Streptococcus pneumoniae* bacteria that have migrated into the central nervous system, usually from another infection elsewhere in the body, particularly a respiratory infection. This is the number one cause of bacterial meningitis in adults and second most common type of meningitis in children over age 2. Ear and heart valve infections are also risk factors, as is removal of the spleen, trauma to the head--particularly with open wound, diabetes, alcohol use, and any previous history of meningitis. Symptoms come on quickly resulting in fever and chills, severe headache, vomiting, stiff neck, fast heart rate, mental status changes, and photophobia. In very young children, symptoms may also present as agitation, irritability, decreased consciousness, feeding difficulties, bulging fontanelle, rapid breathing, and arching the head and neck backwards (opisthotonos). Diagnostic exams usually consist of physical examination, blood cultures, gram stain or other special cultures on cerebrospinal fluid, chest x-rays, cranial CT scan, and lumbar puncture. Antibiotics are given as soon as possible, sometimes with corticosteroids to reduce inflammation. This is a very dangerous infection with a high risk of mortality. Recovery depends on how quickly treatment is received and how well the patient responds. About 1 in 5 of those with pneumococcal meningitis will die from it. Many others experience long term complications such as brain damage, hearing loss, hydrocephalus, and seizures.

G00.2 Streptococcal meningitis

Streptococcal meningitis is a bacterial infection of the protective tissues surrounding the brain and spinal cord caused by other streptococcal bacteria, such as Group A, Group B, or Enterococcus, that have migrated to the central nervous system, usually from another infection or from tissue where the bacteria is normally found. Meningitis caused by *Streptococcus agalactiae* (Group B) is the highest cause of neonatal meningitis. The bacteria normally live in the bowels and vagina, as well as the back of the nose and throat, and are passed to the neonate either during birth or afterwards by contaminated contact. Symptoms usually occur in the first few days of life and present as fever, breathing and feeding difficulties, and fits. Antibiotics can be given to the mother in labor or to the baby after birth. Most babies survive with no serious problems. Fatalities are higher among premature babies. Others may suffer sequelae such as brain damage, deafness, and problems with motor coordination.

Group A streptococcal meningitis is rare but does occur if the bacteria, which normally live on the surface of the skin and in the throat, manage to gain access to the sterile protective coverings around the brain and spinal cord. Once there, the bacteria replicate rapidly in the cerebrospinal fluid, releasing toxins that cause inflammation, swelling, and increased pressure on the brain. Symptoms appear as fever and chills, severe headache, vomiting, stiff neck, and photophobia and can rapidly progress to drowsiness, confusion, delirium, seizures, and loss of consciousness. This is a very dangerous infection with a high risk of mortality. Long term complications include neurological damage, deafness, motor coordination problems, and learning difficulties.

Note: The causative organism must be coded in addition.

G00.3 Staphylococcal meningitis

Staphylococcal meningitis is a bacterial infection of the protective tissues surrounding the brain and spinal cord caused by *Staphylococcus aureus* bacteria that have migrated to the central nervous system. This is a rare, but deadly cause of bacterial meningitis and has a high mortality rate. The cause is often a complication of surgical procedures, particularly on neurological structures. The bacteria may also invade from another localized infection, during trauma, in weakened immunologic states, and with conditions such as alcoholism, cellulitis, osteomyelitis, and decubitus ulcers. Classic symptoms appear as fever and severe headache; lethargy; stiff neck in forced flexion; sudden altered consciousness as confusion or drowsiness, even stupor or coma; generalized or focal seizures; hypotension; the inability to extend the legs completely, known as Kernig sign; and flexed hips and knees in response to the forced flexion occurring in the neck (Brudzinski sign). Antibiotics are given as soon as possible with effective penetration into the central nervous system along with maintaining adequate blood pressure. This is a medical emergency with a high risk of mortality. Delayed treatment is associated with adverse outcomes and complications such as brain damage, hearing loss, hydrocephalus, and seizures.

Note: Staphylococcal meningitis may also be caused by *Staphylococcus epidermis*.

G00.8 Other bacterial meningitis

This is a bacterial infection of the protective tissues surrounding the brain and spinal cord caused by other strains of specified bacteria that have migrated to the central nervous system, usually from an infection elsewhere in the body or sites where the bacteria normally reside. Symptoms of bacterial meningitis come on quickly, resulting in fever and chills, severe headache, vomiting, stiff neck, malaise, mental status changes, and photophobia. In very young children, symptoms may also present as agitation, irritability, feeding difficulties, high pitched cry, bulging fontanelle, rapid breathing, and arching the head and neck backwards. Diagnostic exams usually consist of physical examination, cultures of the blood and cerebrospinal fluid, chest x-rays, and cranial CT scan. Antibiotics are given as soon as possible, sometimes with corticosteroids to reduce inflammation. This is a very dangerous infection with a risk of mortality, especially in the very young and old. Other morbidity outcomes include brain damage, hearing loss, hydrocephalus, and seizures.

Note: Other bacteria reported here as causing meningitis include *Mycoplasma pneumonia, Klebsiella pneumonia, Escherichia coli, Friedlaender's bacillus,* and *Bacteroides fragilis.*

G00.9 Bacterial meningitis, unspecified

This code includes meningitis due to gram-negative bacteria, and unspecified purulent, pyogenic, or suppurative meningitis cases (producing pus). Symptoms of bacterial meningitis come on quickly, resulting in fever and chills, severe headache, vomiting, stiff neck, malaise, mental status changes, and photophobia. In very young children, symptoms may also present as agitation, irritability, feeding difficulties, high pitched cry, bulging fontanelle, rapid breathing, and arching the head and neck backwards. Gram-negative bacteria are far more likely to cause disease than are gram-positive bacteria.

G03 Meningitis due to other and unspecified causes

Meningitis is an infection of the lining of the brain and spinal cord (called the meninges). This condition presents with a number of symptoms, including fever, a purplish rash, loss of appetite, headache, sensitivity to light, vomiting, stiffness in the neck, lethargy and/or drowsiness, irritability and/or confusion. The patient may also lose consciousness and go into convulsions. In some cases, the patient may suffer long-term conditions, such as deafness.

Note: This category reports meningitis caused by an unspecified organism, or an organism other than a bacterium, or a parasitic or infectious disease classified elsewhere.

G03.0 Nonpyogenic meningitis

Meningitis is an infection or inflammation of the protective tissues covering the brain and spinal cord. Nonpyogenic meningitis is not caused by a pus-producing bacterial source of infection, although it does cause serious inflammation around the brain. This is also known as aseptic or sterile meningitis and can range from mild and self-limiting, to severe and life-threatening. The main symptoms are fever, headache, stiff neck, photophobia, nausea and vomiting, and malaise, or drowsiness. Extreme lethargy, seizures, and mental confusion are not usually signs of aseptic meningitis, although patients can display signs of altered consciousness. Other meningeal signs may also be present upon physical examination, such as Kernig sign, when extension of the knee from a supine position with the hip flexed illicits pain; Brudzinski sign with flexion of the knees and hips in a supine position in response to neck flexion; and Amoss sign in which the patient assumes the tripod position. Causative factors can be many. Diagnosing aseptic meningitis and determining appropriate treatment is dependent upon the source of infection or inflammation and intensity of symptoms.

Note: Although viral meningitis and aseptic meningitis are sometimes meant interchangeably, viral meningitis is coded to category A87.

G03.1 Chronic meningitis

Chronic meningitis is present for an extended period of time, causing symptoms to develop over weeks or months instead of days. This type of meningitis is usually due to infection instead of injury, and is often associated with a depressed immune system.

G03.2 Benign recurrent meningitis [Mollaret]

Mollaret meningitis is a kind of recurring meningitis characterized by episodes of severe headache, fever, and meningismus that resolve spontaneously, followed by weeks or month without a relapse. Meningismus is a state of meningeal irritation when symptoms of meningitis are present without actual infection of inflammation. The causative factor is unknown. Patients also experience transient neurological signs and symptoms in half of cases, such as double vision, seizures, pathologic reflexes, paresthesia along cranial nerves, hallucinations, and even coma. Some patients show increased gamma globulins in cerebrospinal fluid without fever. Recent studies show data suggesting that herpes simplex virus 1 and 2 may be connected.

G04 Encephalitis, myelitis and encephalomyelitis

Encephalitis is an inflammation of the brain itself, which can present with fever, headache, confusion, and in extreme cases, can cause brain damage, stroke, seizures, or even death. Myelitis is an inflammation of the spinal cord, and presents with fever, headaches, tingling, pain, or loss of feeling and strength, and can cause paralysis. Encephalomyelitis is an inflammation of both the brain and spinal cord. Encephalitis, myelitis, and encephalomyelitis are conditions identified by the affected area of inflammation. The condition may affect the brain and not the spinal cord or vice versa, or both sites together. There are many possible underlying causes, including acute infection, post infectious processes, immunizations, and toxic substances.

G04.0 Acute disseminated encephalitis and encephalomyelitis (ADEM)

Acute disseminated encephalitis and encephalomyelitis (ADEM) is a serious neurological disease with inflammation of the brain and/or spinal cord occurring as a result of damage to the myelin sheath. The myelin sheath is the protective, insulating covering of nerve fibers. Infectious ADEM occurs in connection with a viral or bacterial infection. The onset is sudden, appearing more often in children than adults, with different symptoms among affected individuals. Symptoms include headache, fever, stiff neck, inflammation of the optical nerves, vomiting, delirium, seizures, coma, myelitis, and paralysis of one limb or one side of the body. Some cases may occur as postinfectious ADEM following measles or chicken pox, and other cases may occur as a complication or allergic reaction following immunization.

G05.3 Encephalitis and encephalomyelitis in diseases classified elsewhere

Use this code to report cases of encephalitis or encephalomyelitis that occur in diseases classified elsewhere. Encephalitis is an inflammation of the brain itself and encephalomyelitis is an inflammation of both the brain and the spinal cord. There are several diseases in which encephalitis appears, or may appear, as an intrinsic part of the disease process, such as West Nile and mumps. These types of root causes of encephalitis are excluded.

G06.0 Intracranial abscess and granuloma

An intracranial abscess is an infected pocket or cavity filled with pus within the cranium, or skull. The abscess can cause infection and pressure on the brain, presenting with fever, a persistent and usually localized headache, drowsiness, confusion, seizures, nausea and vomiting, and movement or sensory impairments. An untreated abscess can spread the infection beyond the pocket in which it is contained and cause permanent brain damage or death.

G06.1 Intraspinal abscess and granuloma

An intraspinal abscess is an infected pocket or cavity filled with pus within the spine. The abscess can cause infection and pressure on the spinal cord's nervous tissue, presenting with fever, back pain, fatigue, muscle weakness, and even paralysis. An untreated abscess can spread the infection beyond the pocket in which it is contained and cause permanent paralysis or death.

G08 Intracranial and intraspinal phlebitis and thrombophlebitis

Phlebitis is an inflammation of a vein which presents with pain, swelling, redness, and warmth around the affected area. Thrombophlebitis is an inflammation due to blood clot formation within the vein. Inflammation and blood clot formation of the veins and venous sinuses (open areas) within the skull or spine is a serious medical emergency. This code includes septic cases of intracranial or intraspinal phlebitis and thrombophlebitis.

G10 Huntington's disease

Huntington's disease, also called Huntington's chorea, is a genetic disorder that causes degeneration of the neurons of the brain. This initially presents with mood swings, depression, and irritability; trouble driving; difficulty in learning and remembering things; and difficulty in making decisions. As the disease progresses, it becomes increasingly difficult to concentrate on intellectual tasks, even to the point of the patient being unable to feed him or herself and swallow. Dementia and death occur within 15 years of onset. This disease is genetic in origin, and there is a 50% chance of it passing to the child of a parent who has the gene. The age at which symptoms appear and the rate of progression vary from person to person. There is no cure, and treatment concentrates on maintaining quality of life for as long as possible via medication and exercise.

G11 Hereditary ataxia

Hereditary ataxias are a group of genetic disorders that display a characteristic uncoordinated gait that is slowly progressive, wide in its stance, and unsteady. The unbalanced, uncoordinated gait is usually associated with poor coordination of the fingers and hands, eyes, and speech. Patients often demonstrate nystagmus and dysarthria. In many cases, atrophy of the cerebellum with dysfunction of its associated systems is a causative factor. Spinal cord lesions as well as peripheral sensory loss are also known to result in hereditary ataxia. The genetic forms are diagnosed by finding a positive family history of ataxia, detection of typical clinical signs and symptoms with physical examination, neuroimaging, and the use of molecular genetic testing. These ataxias may be inherited in an autosomal dominant, autosomal recessive, or X-linked manner and are categorized by the mode of inheritance and the gene in which the causative mutations occur. There is no specific treatment, except when vitamin E deficiency is present. The use of canes, walkers, and wheelchairs is appropriate for the ataxic gait. The use of special devices to help with writing, eating, and buttoning may be employed as well as speech therapy or computerized aids in cases of severe impairment.

G11.1 Early-onset cerebellar ataxia

Early-onset cerebellar ataxia includes Friedreich's ataxia, a genetic disorder that slowly progresses over several years after symptoms first appear, usually between the ages of five and fifteen. It presents with weakness and an inability to coordinate muscle activity (ataxia) in the limbs, head, and neck, though without loss of sensation. It does not affect mental capacity, though within 8-10 years it results in an inability to walk and causes speech difficulties. Scoliosis, a curvature of the spine, abnormalities of the heartbeat, and diabetes mellitus also often accompany this disease. In the late stages of the disease, there is little if any movement capability left. Remissions (pauses in the progress of the disease) are rare, but can last 5-10 years or longer in some cases. There is no cure, though medication and orthopedic intervention (braces, surgery, etc.) can help to alleviate symptoms and improve quality of life.

G11.4 Hereditary spastic paraplegia

Hereditary spastic paraplegia, sometimes abbreviated HSP, is not a single disease, but a group of disorders characterized by lower-limb spasticity, a condition in which the joints lose flexibility until they become virtually immobile, while the upper limbs remain unaffected. In some instances, called complicated HSP, additional symptoms may include epilepsy, loss of coordination of the muscles (ataxia), optic or hearing problems, mental retardation, dementia, problems with speech, and difficulty swallowing and/or breathing. Fortunately, complicated HSP is rare. While there is no cure, medications can reduce symptoms and assistive devices (canes, wheelchairs, etc.) can improve quality of life.

G12.0 Infantile spinal muscular atrophy, type I [Werdnig-Hoffman]

Werdnig-Hoffman disease is a genetic disorder which appears in infancy which causes the degeneration of spinal and brain nerve cells leading to atrophy (wasting away) of the skeletal muscles and paralysis. There is no cure or effective treatment for this disease, and death typically occurs in early childhood.

G12.1 Other inherited spinal muscular atrophy

This code includes Kugelberg-Welander disease, also called Type III spinal muscular atrophy (SMA), juvenile type. It most often appears in children before the age of 3-6 months. A child with Type III SMA usually never accomplishes even the most basic of motor skills such as lifting the head, though they are not completely without movement.

G12.2 Motor neuron disease

Motor neuron disease (MND) is actually a group of related diseases that affect the motor neurons in the brain and spinal cord. Unlike Werdnig-Hoffman disease and SMA, it is far more common in adults over the age of 40 than in children. It presents with weakness and wasting away of the muscles, usually starting in the arms and legs. In some patients, the weakness extends to the face and throat, making speech and swallowing difficult. It does not affect sensation. MND is a progressive disease, but the rate of progression varies from person to person. There is no cure, and treatment concentrates on bettering quality of life.

G12.21 Amyotrophic lateral sclerosis

Amyotrophic lateral sclerosis (LAS) is also called motor neuron disease but is better known as Lou Gehrig's Disease. The cause is unknown, although some cases are known to be inherited. This is a serious disease that affects the nerve cells of the brain and spinal cord that control voluntary muscle movement causing weakness and progressing to death. Early symptoms include weakness in the legs, feet, and ankles with difficulty lifting the front of the foot; hand weakness and clumsiness; slurring speech; and muscle cramps in the arms, shoulder, and tongue. It usually begins in the hands and feet, progresses to other parts of the body, and weakens muscles until they become paralyzed and the patient can no longer chew, swallow, speak, or breathe.

G12.22 Progressive bulbar palsy

Progressive bulbar palsy (PBP) affects primarily the face, jaw, tongue, and throat, and is so known because the area of the brain that controls these muscles, the lower brainstem, was once known as the bulb. Pure PBP, which has no affect on the limbs, is very rare, and is usually the result of surgery or radiation therapy. PBP is often initially misdiagnosed as Parkinson's.

G12.29 Other motor neuron disease

Primary lateral sclerosis (PLS) is an extremely rare disease that usually begins in the legs, but may occasionally begin in the hands or tongue; in the latter case, the first symptom is the slurring of words. Diagnosing PLS is difficult, as there is no one test that can be used to identify it. Instead, a battery of tests must be run to eliminate all other possible conditions. There is no cure for PLS, and treatment focuses on assisting the patient's quality of life. PLS is not life-threatening.

G20 Parkinson's disease

Parkinson's disease is a type of brain disease that occurs when 80% or more of a certain type of nerve cells in a part of the brain called the substantia die or otherwise become impaired. These cells produce a chemical called dopamine, which allows the body's muscles to move smoothly and in a coordinated fashion. It presents with uncontrollable shaking, slowness of movement, stiffness in the muscles and facial expression, loss of balance, a shuffling walk, muffled speech, and depression. It mostly affects patients over the age of 60.

G21 Secondary parkinsonism

The symptoms of secondary Parkinsonism are similar to Primary Parkinson's disease but are caused by an identifiable underlying illness, injury, or disease process. Nerve cells in the brain that produce dopamine are slowly destroyed. Without dopamine, the transmission of messages in the brain slows down ultimately affecting the movement of muscles throughout the body. Causes may include chemical or environmental toxins, drugs, encephalitis or meningitis, and cerebral vascular disease.

G21.0 Malignant neuroleptic syndrome

Neuroleptic malignant syndrome is a rare but life-threatening reaction to certain types of medication called neuroleptics. It occurs in reaction to any medication affecting nerve cells that produce dopamine in up to 1% of patients. Most patients develop symptoms within two weeks after initial exposure to the medication. Symptoms include severe fever, change in mental status, muscle rigidity and/or tremors, seizures, and rapid heart beat (tachycardia), as well as changes in the autonomic nervous system that regulates organ activity such as breathing. Once symptoms appear, their progression is very rapid, reaching peak intensity within 72 hours and remaining at their peak anywhere from 45 minutes to 65 days. This disease is life-threatening unless it receives immediate treatment to maintain the body's fluid balance, discontinuing the medication that caused the disease in the first place, and starting medication to shorten the course of the disease via both IV and orally.

G23 Other degenerative diseases of basal ganglia

Other degenerative diseases of the basal ganglia may result in symptoms similar to Parkinson's disease, or may result in increased stimulation resulting in stronger but uncontrolled movement. Other symptoms include muscle and/or facial tics, tremors, or uncontrolled muscle contractions which force the body into abnormal and sometimes painful movements or postures (dystonia). Treatment of these disorders centers around replacing the chemicals the body is not producing naturally with medication or medication that acts to slow the degenerative process.

G24.01 Drug induced subacute dyskinesia

Subacute dyskinesia due to drugs is mostly reversible movement disorders associated with the direct or indirect affect of dopamine transmission. Subacute movement disorders may manifest in spasm of the eylid or mouth and face, and are credited as being an idiosyncratic extension of the intended action of the medicinal compound that was taken. This code also includes tardive dyskinesia, which is a more delayed movement disorder caused by long term exposure to drugs such as central dopamine blockers. The cranial musculature, trunk and limbs are affected with choreatic, meaning rapid and jerky, movements. In some cases of tardive dyskinesia, the muscles of the diaphragm may be affected causing respiratory distress.

G24.02 Drug induced acute dystonia

Acute dystonia due to drugs, including neuroleptic-induced acute dytonia, is characterized by stiff muscles causing dyskinetic movements, altered mental status, such as paranoid behavior, and autonomic nervous system dysfunction that leads to excessive sweating, saliva secretion, and abnormal swings in blood pressure. This acute disorder of muscle tone is brought on specifically as a reaction to drugs. The most common groups of drugs inducing this condition are the antipsychotics and major tranquilizers (called neuroleptic), such as thioridazine, chlorpromazine, haloperidol, and fluphenazine.

G24.1 Genetic torsion dystonia

Genetic torsion dystonia is a condition in which the patient suffers from debilitating muscular contractions which prevent normal muscle control. These contractions typically start at around the age of 12 in one part of the body, such as an arm or a leg, and then spread to the rest of the body within five years. This disease is not fatal, and its cause is not currently known. Treatment may involve medications such as dopamine replacements or sedatives, or in some cases may extend to brain surgery.

G24.3 Spasmodic torticollis

Spasmodic torticollis is a type of dystonia in which the muscular contractions contort the neck muscles and cause pain in the neck and/or arm and an abnormal posture of the head (e.g., being pulled forward or backwards) that usually disappears during sleep. Touching the opposite side of the face may reduce the pain and control the spasms. There is currently no cure for this disorder, though the symptoms may be treated with medication (e.g., botulinum toxin to paralyze the affected muscles), physical therapy, or cutting the affected nerves to stop the spasms.

G24.5 Blepharospasm

Blepharospasm is a dystonia, or involuntary muscular contraction, of the eyelids and surrounding facial muscles. This can cause the patient to blink for extended and variable lengths of time, preventing them from being able to see.

G24.8 Other dystonia

Note: Use this code for other acquired torsion dystonia, NOS in which the patient suffers debilitating muscle contractions that prevent normal muscle control.

G25.0 Essential tremor

An essential tremor produces uncontrollable shaking, the precise cause os which is not completely understood, but research shows that the cerebellum of the brain does not function properly in patients with an essential tremor. The shaking normally is concentrated in the hands, but can spread to other body parts, including the facial muscles. Stress, fatigue, anger and/or fear, caffeine, and nicotine can all temporarily worsen the tremors. For the most part, these tremors are not debilitating or life-threatening. These conditions may run in families (familial) or be due to a reaction to medication.

G25.1 Drug-induced tremor

Tremor is the involuntary, often rhythmic contraction and relaxation of one or more muscles. Commonly affecting the hands, tremors may also be observed in the arms, eyes, head, vocal cords, trunk, and legs. They can be occasional, temporary, or intermittent.

Note: An additional code must be assigend to identify the circumstances and specific drug as the cause.

G25.2 Other specified forms of tremor

Other specified forms of tremor are various disorders in which a person shakes uncontrollably. This code also reports intentional tremor. The shaking normally is concentrated in the hands, but can spread to other body parts, including the facial muscles. Stress, fatigue, anger and/or fear, caffeine, and nicotine can all temporarily worsen the tremors. For the most part, these tremors are not debilitating or life-threatening.

G25.3 Myoclonus

Myoclonus, which literally means muscle ("myo-") jerking ("clonus"), is a condition that results from damage to the central nervous system which causes sudden, uncontrolled electrical discharges through the nervous system and a corresponding sudden muscle contraction elsewhere in the body. These jerking motions may be continual in the affected body part, making it impossible to use it normally. In severe cases, the entire body may be affected, preventing the patient from being able to stand, walk, pick up objects, feed or dress themselves, speak, or even control the direction of their gaze because of the constant involuntary muscle spasms. Often, patients will show no signs of myoclonus when at rest or asleep. A number of medications are used to reduce the severity of myoclonus, usually in combination with each other. However, there is no cure for this disorder at this time.

G25.4 Drug-induced chorea

Chorea is an abnormal, involuntary, hyperkinetic muscle movement disorder. It is characterized by irregular, repetitive, dance-like rhythmic muscle movements which seem to flow from one muscle (or group of muscles) to another. The movements may also include twisting or writhing into odd postures that make walking difficult.

Note: This code reports chorea as an adverse affect of drugs or medications, which must be specifically identified by an additional code.

G25.5 Other chorea

Other choreas, or involuntary movement disorders, are characterized by brief, involuntary muscle contractions that follow no regular pattern or rhythm, but appear to flow from one muscle to the next. Hemiballism (or hemiballismus) and paroxysmal choreoathetosis both fall under this category. These disorders may or may not be debilitating, but are rarely life-threatening. Treatment generally involves using medication to control the muscle spasms.

G25.6 Drug induced tics and other tics of organic origin

Tics or tic disorders involve a discrete group of muscles and are characterized by sudden, repetitive motor movement or phonic utterances. Tics can be simple (eye blinking, throat clearing) or complex (hand clapping/touching, word repetition/uttering inappropriate words/phrases). Tics can be transient (lasting >1 month but <1 year) or chronic (lasting >1 year and appearing before age 18).

G25.61 Drug induced tics

Muscle and/or facial tics of organic origin, as opposed to those due to a psychological problem, are due to a biological or chemical disorder in the nervous system. In some cases, they result as a side-effect of medication, which is reported here. Tics are irritating, but rarely debilitating, and may be brought under control with proper medication.

Note: An additional code must be used to identify the adverse effect, if applicable, of the specific drug.

G25.71 Drug induced akathisia

Akathisia is a syndrome characterized by a feeling of inner restlessness. Symptoms can range from a sense of disquiet or anxiety to severe discomfort especially in the knees/legs that may make it impossible to sit still or be motionless. The condition usually results from increased levels of the (brain) neurotransmitter norepinephrine which regulates aggression, alertness, and arousal. Medications such as propranolol and clonazepam may be helpful in relieving the symptoms of akathisia.

Note: This code reports akathisia as an adverse effect of medication, which should be identified with an additional code to specify the drug.

G25.81 Restless legs syndrome

Restless legs syndrome (RLS) is a strong, almost irresistable urge to move the legs, particularly while at rest or when lying down. The longer one rests, the more probable the chance that the symptoms will occur and the more severe they become. The affected person feels sensations in the legs such as creeping, crawling, itching, tugging, or pulling. The symptoms get better upon movement of the legs. Complete or partial relief lasts as long as the motor activity continues. Many people with RLS also suffer from insomnia.

G25.82 Stiff-man syndrome

Stiff-man disease is a rare autoimmune neurologic disease that presents with progressive rigidity or stiffness of the muscles of the neck, shoulders, and trunk, that progresses to the arms, and legs, and may include painful muscle spasms. It affects approximately twice as many men as women. Characteristics of the disorder include an exaggerated upright posture with back discomfort, sleep disturbances (spasms are triggered when transitioning from REM sleep to Stage 1 or 2 sleep), and generally slowed physical movement because rapid muscle movement will trigger spasms. The condition has been identified in infancy through adulthood and there are subtle differences in its manifestations at different ages. There is also demonstrated comorbity to diabetes associated with positive GAD antibodies.

G25.83 Benign shuddering attacks

Benign shuddering attacks are an uncommon occurance in older infants and young children. They present while the child is awake with sudden flexion of the neck, adduction of the arms and shivering of the trunk. The movements last 5-10 seconds with no loss of consciousness. While benign shuddering attacks may mimic a seizure (motor and/or absence) an EEG, MRI or CT will be entirely normal. The etiology is unknown and no treatment is necessary.

G30 Alzheimer's disease

Alzheimer's disease is a common progressive degeneration of the cerebrum that destroys a person's memory, reason, judgment, communication, and ability to carry out day-to-day activities over a period of several years. It most commonly progresses over a period of three to twenty years before leading to death. There is presently no cure or effective treatment for Alzheimer's.

G31.01 Pick's disease

Pick's disease is the most common form of frontotemporal dementia, which presents with memory loss, difficulty in thinking, and disturbances in speech. The symptoms progress during a period of two to ten years before causing death. There is no cure or effective treatment for Pick's disease.

G31.1 Senile degeneration of brain, not elsewhere classified

Senile degeneration of the brain causes loss of memory and reason, and personality changes, though it is rarely a direct cause of death. In addition, it may be caused by depression, poor nutrition, thyroid dysfunction, or drug or alcohol abuse, in which case treatment focuses on correcting the contributing problem.

G31.83 Dementia with Lewy bodies

Lewy bodies are microscopic protein deposits sometimes found in deteriorating nerve cells in the brain. The symptoms and complications are very much like Alzheimer's disease, and in fact, one is often misdiagnosed as the other. This disease progresses fairly rapidly, typically lasting about five to seven years before ending in the death of the patient. There is no effective treatment currently available.

G31.84 Mild cognitive impairment, so stated

Mild cognitive impairment is defined as an impairment in memory or other specific cognitive function, beyond what is normally seen at that age, but with function remaining relatively intact in the other cognitive domains. Mild cognitive impairment is a slowly progressing precursor to dementia in 80 percent of cases and is diagnosed by a usual or standard set of criteria as follows: corroborated complaints of memory function, objective memory impairment for age, preserved general cognitive function for age, intact activities of daily life, and not demented.

G31.85 Corticobasal degeneration

Corticobasal degeneration is a rare, progressive neurodegenerative disease with a dual manifestation of cognitive impairment like that occurring in frontotemporal dementia, and movement disorders. Corticobasal degeneration is a degenerative disease not only of the basal ganglia, but also atrophy of the frontal and parietal cortical regions of the brain. Symptoms first appear around age 60 with asymmetrical movement disorders that do not affect both sides the same. Movement dysfunction can include myoclonus, dystonia, rigidity, poor coordination, akinesia, disequilibrium, and limb dystonia. Cognitive dysfunction includes visuospatial and number processing impairment, loss of executive function, hesitant and halting speech or other language impairment. It progresses slowly and is resistant to drug therapy. There is no treatment available and death usually occurs within eight years.

G35 Multiple sclerosis

Multiple sclerosis (MS) is not fully understood, but is thought to be an autoimmune disorder in which the body's immune system attacks its own nervous system. Myelin, a fatty tissue that helps nerve cells conduct electrical impulses, is lost in multiple areas, causing scar tissue and sclerosis. Symptoms of MS vary wildly between patients, but often include bladder and bowel problems, loss of memory, attention, and problem-solving capabilities, emotional problems, dizziness and vertigo, fatigue, pain, loss of flexibility in the joints (spasticity), and vision problems. There is no cure for MS, and treatment centers on managing symptoms and making the patient comfortable.

G36.0 Neuromyelitis optica [Devic]

Neuromyelitis optica, sometimes called Devic's syndrome, affects the nerves that carry information from the eyes, causing a corresponding vision loss. It can also present with numbness, loss of coordination, and weakness in the muscles, loss of flexibility (spasticity), and other loss of muscle function.

G37 Other demyelinating diseases of central nervous system

Other diseases that destroy myelin damage the protective tissue that helps nerve cells to conduct electrical impulses. In all cases, there is no cure, but medications and physical therapy can slow down the progression of the disorder and better the patient's quality of life.

G37.0 Diffuse sclerosis of central nervous system

Schilder's disease is a rare, progressive disorder that usually begins in childhood. It may present with dementia and personality changes, loss of speech (aphasia), seizures and tremors, loss of balance, muscle weakness, headache, and vomiting.

G37.3 Acute transverse myelitis in demyelinating disease of central nervous system

Acute transverse myelitis is a neurologic disorder of the spinal cord causing inflammatory lesions across both sides, or the entire width, of one level or segment of the spinal cord. These lesions are in areas where the myelin sheath that protects and encases the spinal cord is lost. The lesions can appear anywhere in the spinal cord, although they usually appear in one portion. Symptoms are related to the level affected. Acute transverse myelitis has a sudden onset and rapid progression within hours and days. Signs and symptoms may begin as weakness, numbness, severe back pain, sensory loss, and motor and sphincter deficits and progress to paraplegia, and paralysis of bladder or respiratory function. A prognosis for complete recovery is rare and many patients are left with considerable disabilities or gain no signs of recovery whatsoever.

G40 Epilepsy and recurrent seizures

Epilepsy is a disorder that causes the electrical signals in the brain to be disrupted, causing the person to go into a seizure or convulsive state. Since other conditions can cause seizures, diagnostic tests such as CT scans and lumbar punctures must be used to rule them out and come to a diagnosis of epilepsy.

G40.A Absence epileptic syndrome

Absence epileptic syndrome is sometimes known as childhood absence epilepsy, as this syndrome starts in early childhood, usually between the ages of four to nine. It occurs slightly more often in girls than boys. The typical seizures of this syndrome consist of a sudden absence, or loss of awareness in which the child drops their current activity and stares blankly into space, remaining unresponsive to voice prompts. This type of seizure usually lasts between 5 and 20 seconds and occurs many times a day, even hundred of times in a day. The absence seizure ends as suddenly as it began and the child resumes activity. Sometimes the seizure is accompanied by repetitive, purposeless facial movements such as eyelid fluttering or lip smacking. The seizures are far less likely to occur when the child is actively engaged in something he or she finds fun and enjoyable in contrast to being bored, tired, or just sitting. Diagnosis is made with a history of this seizure behavior and by asking the child to breathe quickly while counting out loud in a physical exam. This triggers an absence seizure 90% of the time in children with this syndrome. An EEG is also used to confirm the diagnosis. Treatment consists of antiepileptic drugs. Prognosis is excellent as most children develop normally. Only a small percentage of children with this syndrome will develop other types of seizures later in adolescence, such as tonic clonic type seizures.

G43 Migraine

A migraine is actually a neurological disorder involving various nerve pathways and chemicals in the brain, whose changes affect the flow of blood, although the exact causative events are not known. The migraine may have certain triggers like stress or food that induce abnormal brain activity. Status migrainosus is severe migraine lasting three days or more, despite treatment, and often requiring hospitalization. Intractable or refractory migraines are sustained migraines that do not respond to standard treatment or intervention.

Note: Unspecified headaches may mimic migraine, but are not coded as migraine until so diagnosed.

G43.0 Migraine without aura

Migraine without aura is also known as common migraine. This is a severe and debilitating migraine headache that occurs without warning signs of visual disturbances or other sensations.

G43.1 Migraine with aura

Migraine with aura is also known as classical migraine, basilar migraine, migraine equivalent, or migraine with transient neurological phenomena, and retinal migrane. This is a severe and debilitating migraine headache that occurs with certain visual sensation warnings that come before or with

the pain of a migraine attack. Characteristic visual disturbances include flashes of light, blindness in one eye, zigzag patterns in the field of vision, blind spots, and heat shimmering appearance of objects. Other sensations may also occur such as numbness, tingling, dizziness, and speech difficulty.

Note: When migraine aura occurs without the pain of the headache, it is known as migraine equivalent and is also coded here.

G43.4 Hemiplegic migraine

Hemiplegic migraine is a rare form of migraine disease with two variations--familial and sporadic, both of which are coded here. These headaches begin in childhood and cease in adulthood. Symptoms of both are similar and include: prolonged aura lasting several days or weeks; paralysis on one side of the body that may be sudden and mimic stroke; headache which may begin before the hemiplegia, or even remain absent; fever; impaired consciousness of differing degrees from confusion to coma; meningismus--symptoms without actual meningitis illness or inflammation; nausea and/or vomiting; photophobia and/or phonophobia. The difference is that familial hemiplegic migraines may be traced back in family history and are connected to mutuations of specific genes on chromosomes 1 and 19.

G43.5 Persistent migraine aura without cerebral infarction

A migraine attack similar to previous migraines with aura, except that the aura symptoms persist for longer than a week with no radiological evidence of infarction. The persisting aura symptoms are rare, often bilateral, and may last for months.

G43.6 Persistent migraine aura with cerebral infarction

A migraine attack similar to previous migraines with aura, except that the aura symptoms persist for longer than a week and a neuroimaging procedure shows an ischemic infarction or stroke in a relevant area.

G43.82 Menstrual migraine, not intractable

Also known as premenstrual migraine, these migraines affect women and are hormonally related to the changes that occur around menstruation. When compared to migraines occurring at other times, menstrual migraines have been reported as more severe, lasting longer--up to 72 hours, and occurring more often with nausea and vomiting. Some menstrual related headaches may be exaggerated by certain phytoestrogens, or naturally occurring plant estrogens, found in sunflower seeds, hops (beer), coffee, chamomille, and other spices.

G44.00 Cluster headache syndrome, unspecified

Note: This includes headaches described as ciliary neuralgia, histamine cephalgia, lower half migraine, and migrainous neuralgia.

G44.01 Episodic cluster headache

Cluster headaches are a distinctive kind of headache marked by excruciating pain that occurs in frequent attacks lasting from 15 min to 3 hrs in cyclical patterns, or cluster periods of up to 12 weeks, followed by remission periods. The pain develops quickly without warning and is described as a searing hot poker through the eye. Lying down increases the pain. Another identifying trait is that the pain develops only on one side or hemisphere, typically affecting the same side throughout a cluster period. The autonomic nervous system is also triggered and causes other symptoms like excessive tearing, nasal congestion, swelling, redness, and reduced pupil size of the eye on the affected side. Cluster periods typically last in episodes of 2-12 weeks. Chronic ones may continue for more than a year. The start date and duration of cluster periods are often amazingly consistent and may begin seasonally, right after the solstices in the spring and fall. During the cluster period, attacks usually occur every day, lasting from 15 min to 3 hrs. The majority of attacks occur between 9pm and 9am, during REM sleep. The pain recedes as quickly as it came, leaving the person free of pain but exhausted. Cluster type headaches occur more often in men between ages 20 and 40.

G44.03 Episodic paroxysmal hemicrania

Paroxysmal hemicrania is a rare kind of headache of adulthood causing severe throbbing or boring pain on one side of the face in or near the eye or temple, sometimes reaching to the back of the neck. Redness and tearing of the eyes, a drooping or swollen eyelid, and nasal congestion on the affected side also occur. In between attacks, persons affected may feel dull pain, soreness, or tenderness. In the episodic type, the headaches may occur in bouts of freqent, daily attacks, separated by relatively long periods lasting months or years without headache.

G44.04 Chronic paroxysmal hemicrania

Paroxysmal hemicrania is a rare kind of headache of adulthood causing severe throbbing or boring pain on one side of the face in or near the eye or temple, sometimes reaching to the back of the neck. Redness and tearing of the eyes, a drooping or swollen eyelid and nasal congestion on the affected side also occur. In between attacks, persons may feel dull pain, soreness, or tenderness. In the chronic form, also called Sjaastad syndrome, the attacks of one-sided severe pain localized in the eye or temple occur up to 40 times a day, lasting from 2-45 minutes and do not occur in recognizable patterns.

G44.05 Short lasting unilateral neuralgiform headache with conjunctival injection and tearing (SUNCT)

This rare type of headache, also known as SUNCT, occurs most often in men over 50. Attacks come in the daytime, lasting from a few seconds to a few minutes, and are characterized by moderate to severe throbbing or stabbing pain near the eye or temple. Attacks come about 6 times an hour. Autonomic nervous system responses accompany the headaches, including nasal congestion with runny nose, watery bloodshot eyes due to blood vessel dilation (conjunctival injection), and increased systolic blood pressure. SUNCT may be a form of trigeminal neuralgia and is considered a type of trigeminal autonomic cephalgia.

G44.2 Tension-type headache

Tension type headaches, also known as muscular contraction headaches, are the most common type of headache, but the causes are unclear. This kind of headache produces a mild to moderate, dull, achy tightening pain over the forehead and sides or pain like a band encircling the head. The pain can become severe and may also occur at the back of the neck or base of the skull. Tension headaches may happen only occasionally or nearly all the time. Generally, when the headache occurs more than 15 days a month for several months, it is considered chronic.

Note: This excludes tension headache due to psychological factors.

G44.3 Post-traumatic headache

Post-traumatic headache is a common result of head trauma, even mild head injury. The severity of the headache does not appear to be related to severity of head injury. Other symptoms often accompany the headache, such as insomnia, concentration problems, mood swings, personality changes, and dizziness. Frequency and severity of headaches diminish with time and are usually gone within 6-12 months. Some of these headaches result from vascular changes causing pulsating pain that takes on the characteristics of migraine pain. The other common cause is muscle contraction, particularly sustained muscle contraction in the scalp and neck in chronic cases.

G44.4 Drug-induced headache, not elsewhere classified

Also called medication overuse headache and rebound headache, this is the most common kind of chronic daily headache caused by overuse of migraine abortive ergot alkaloids and analgesic drugs. The International Headache Society defines it as a chronic headache (more than 15 days a month for at least three months), occurring after the intake of analgesics or ergots, which disappears after withdrawal therapy. Clinical features include daily headache varying in type and severity, frequently in early morning; headaches accompanied by other symptoms such as dizziness, parasthesias, nausea, irritability, tachycardia, and diminished pulse; overuse of analgesics with increased tolerance or multiple drugs used concomitantly; ineffective prophylactic medications; withdrawal symptoms with discontinuation of analgesics; spontaneous headache improvement with slow detoxification.

G44.51 Hemicrania continua

Hemicrania continua occurs in both sexes of all ages and appears with an underlying unilateral dull ache. Severe unilateral pain lasting up to an hour with pulsation or throbbing occurs in more than half of patients. Intermittent icepick type stabbing pains or focal, intense pain occurs throughout the day for a few minutes. Sensitivity to light and accompanying nausea may be present. Alcohol and physical exertion exacerbate the pain. Attacks may come up to five times a day. Autonomic features like watery, bloodshot eyes and nasal congestion may accompany flareups.

G44.52 New daily persistent headache (NDPH)

New daily persistent headache has no known underlying secondary cause. The mild to moderate pain is bilateral, consists of a pressing or tightening type, but non-throbbing quality, and must last more than three months and occur daily from within three days of onset to be diagnosed. Patients must also have symptoms of sensitivity to light and sound with mild nausea, but not severe nausea or vomiting. This headache can mimic other conditions that need to be ruled out before diagnosis, such as cerebrospinal fluid leak, and cerebral venous sinus thrombosis.

G44.53 Primary thunderclap headache

Thunderclap headaches are dramatic, sudden, severe headaches that come on without warning and peak within 60 seconds, then fade over several hours. Even though they may appear for no apparent reason, there may be cases in which the headache is a sign of a potentially life-threatening condition, such as a ruptured cerebral aneurysm, subarachnoid hemorrhage, a cerebral sinus thombosis, or carotid artery dissection. Medical evaluation should be sought immediately with such headaches.

G44.81 Hypnic headache

Hypnic headache is also known as alarm clock headache. It is a relatively rare type of headache marked by being awakened between 1 and 3 am with an intense throbbing or dull type pain through the whole head, accompanied by nausea. The attack will usually last about an hour. Episodes may sometimes strike in the daytime, but the headache is connected to REM sleep. Hypnic headaches almost always affect those over 65.

G44.83 Primary cough headache

Primary cough headache typically affects males over 40. The headache is triggered by bouts of coughing or other straining movements such as crying, laughing, sneezing, nose blowing, or bending over. The pain is often described as sharp, stabbing, or splitting on both sides of the head and around the back of the skull. The cause is unknown and a dull, aching type pain may last for hours.

G44.84 Primary exertional headache

Primary exertional headache occurs after strenuous, sustained exercise, particularly running, tennis, weightlifting, swimming, and rowing. Primary exercise headaches are not connected to any underlying problems, are harmless, and can be prevented with medication.

G44.85 Primary stabbing headache

Primary stabbing headache is commonly called ice pick headache as it is so descriptive of the pain, which occurs as intense, short, sharp, stabbing that comes with no warning anywhere on the head, but usually localized in the temple, orbit, or parietal region. The attack may last up to 30 seconds and can disappear before the affected person knows what has happened. Sometimes the pain may occur as a single stab. It is considered a primary headache since there is no deeper underlying cause.

G45.0 Vertebro-basilar artery syndrome

The basilar artery is in front of the brainstem and provides blood to many vital structures of the brain. A blockage of this artery can lead to severe disruption of vision, speech, and behavior. In vertebrobasilar artery syndrome, the blood flow to the brainstem is temporarily blocked. A myriad of neurological symptoms can occur in the afflicted patient, many of which are similar to the symptoms of a stroke and can include vertigo, visual disturbances such as double or blurred vision, and weakness of the quadricep muscles.

G45.1 Carotid artery syndrome (hemispheric)

Carotid artery syndrome involves the elongation of the styloid process, a slender, cylindrical bone that arises from the temporal bone in front of the stylomastoid foramen. Symptoms of the disorder can include neck and/or throat discomfort, facial pain, and difficulty swallowing.

G45.3 Amaurosis fugax

Amaurosis fugax is the transient loss of vision in one eye. The condition is not permanent and usually results from decreased blood flow to the retina causing retinal hypoxia. The condition is often a sign of carotid artery disease and may indicate impending stroke.

G45.4 Transient global amnesia

Transient global amnesia is a sudden, temporary loss of short-term memory due to interrupted blood flow to certain areas of the brain. This interrupted blood flow often has no apparent cause. Self identity is intact as is recognition of people that are known well to the individual. Perceptial skills are also retained along with deeply encoded facts and complex learned behavior. There is often an elevated emotional state and perseverance characterized by repeated questions or statements. A history of migraines is common with the disorder and triggers can include strenuous exercise, immersion in very hot or cold water, and certain medical procedures such as angiography and endoscopy.

G45.9 Transient cerebral ischemic attack, unspecified

Transient cerebral ischemia is the temporary disruption of cerebral blood flow without acute infarction or tissue death. Symptoms of the disorder can include sudden numbness, weakness or paralysis on one side of the body, difficulty with speech, and mental confusion.

G47.10 Hypersomnia, unspecified

Sleeping for an excessive amount of time.

G47.11 Idiopathic hypersomnia with long sleep time

Hypersomnia of an unknown origin, in which the patient sleeps for an abnormally long time in one sleep period.

G47.12 Idiopathic hypersomnia without long sleep time

Hypersomnia of an unknown origin, in which the patient sleeps too often without any one sleep period being abnormally long.

G47.13 Recurrent hypersomnia

Recurrent hypersomnia is diagnosed when the patient sleeps for more than 18 hours a day, lasting several consecutive days or weeks.

G47.2 Circadian rhythm sleep disorders

The circadian rhythm refers to events that typically occur at 24 hour intervals, especially the sleep wake cycle or schedule. When the sleep schedule is disrupted, the patient commonly experiences fatigue and sleepiness.

G47.20 Circadian rhythm sleep disorder, unspecified type

This code is used to report unspecified disruptions of the normal 24-hour sleep cycle. This typically occurs due to irregular working hours, stress, or other psychological disturbances.

G47.21 Circadian rhythm sleep disorder, delayed sleep phase type

Delayed sleep phase type circadian rhythm disorder, in which the patient has trouble falling to sleep, and consequently has trouble waking up on time.

G47.22 Circadian rhythm sleep disorder, advanced sleep phase type

A disorder in which the patient falls asleep too early, and wakes too early.

G47.23 Circadian rhythm sleep disorder, irregular sleep wake type

An irregular sleep-wake type disorder, in which the patient sleeps and wakes in an abnormal pattern without regard to time.

G47.24 Circadian rhythm sleep disorder, free running type

Free-running type circadian rhythm sleep disorder is a condition in which the patient is unable to maintain a normal sleep schedule without the use of an alarm clock or other aid to wake up.

G47.25 Circadian rhythm sleep disorder, jet lag type

A disorder in which rapidly crossing time zones temporarily disrupts the patient's sleep schedule.

G47.26 Circadian rhythm sleep disorder, shift work type

This sleep disorder occurs when the patient has trouble maintaining a normal sleep schedule due to a work schedule that forces them to be awake at odd hours.

G47.3 Sleep apnea

A condition in which the patient suffers recurring, temporary interruptions in breathing during sleep. Sleep apnea most often occurs in overweight patients or those who have an airway obstruction.

G47.31 Primary central sleep apnea

Primary central sleep apnea typically occurs in patients with lesions of the lower brain stem. This disorder is caused by defects in the part of the brain that regulates bodily functions during sleep, and is not caused by problems such as obesity or airway obstructions.

G47.32 High altitude periodic breathing

This disorder occurs when the breathing patterns during sleep consist of a few shallow breaths, followed by deep, sighing breaths, a few seconds of no respiratory activity, and then the cycle begins again. The patient may wake up and feel as though they were suffocating. This type of breathing is not considered abnormal if it occurs at high altitude, but at low altitude is a sign of illness or brain injury.

G47.33 Obstructive sleep apnea (adult) (pediatric)

This disorder affects people who are overweight, have an airway obstruction, or have an abnormally narrow airway.

G47.34 Idiopathic sleep related nonobstructive alveolar hypoventilation

A condition in which the body is deprived of oxygen during sleep although there is no recognized obstruction that causes the lack of ventilation.

G47.35 Congenital central alveolar hypoventilation syndrome

This congenital condition of the nervous system causes abnormally slow and shallow respiration, leading to an abnormal increase the amount of carbon dioxide in the blood. The patient may complain of waking up and feeling suffocated, and may have a tingling sensation in the hands, arms, and face.

G47.36 Sleep related hypoventilation in conditions classified elsewhere

The lack of oxygen and/or slow, shallow breathing during sleep as an aspect of a condition classified elsewhere.

G47.4 Narcolepsy and cataplexy

Narcolepsy is a neurological disorder in which the patient experiences bouts of excessive sleepiness. It may present with or without cataplexy, which is a sudden loss of muscle tone and deep tendon reflexes that leads to muscle weakness, temporary paralysis, or collapsing on the floor. Other symptoms of narcolepsy include sleep paralysis, in which the patient cannot move during the transition from sleep to wakefulness; waking dreams; automatic behaviors such as driving home and not remembering how they arrived there; and disruption of normal REM sleep on a daily basis.

G47.51 Confusional arousals

Confusional arousal is a condition that usually occurs in young children that involves partially waking up and thrashing about, muttering, moaning, or crying. These episodes typically last from 5 minutes to just short of an hour, after which the patient falls back asleep, remembering nothing of the episode upon waking.

G47.52 REM sleep behavior disorder

REM sleep behavior disorder is marked by violent, vigorous behavior that is perceived in a dream, such as running, jumping, punching, or kicking. During normal REM sleep, the muscles are deactivated so that this type of activity cannot take place. Patients suffering from this condition risk injuring themselves or their bedmates.

G47.53 Recurrent isolated sleep paralysis

This condition involves the patient experiencing episodes of being unable to move or speak just before falling asleep, or just after waking up. These episodes can be accompanied by intense feelings of dread or panic.

G47.6 Sleep related movement disorders

This code is used to report sleep related movement disorders, in which the patient experiences painful or random movements that disrupt sleep.

G47.61 Periodic limb movement disorder

Periodic limb movement disorder occurs when a limb moves or jerks involuntarily during or just before sleep.

G47.63 Sleep related bruxism

Grinding the teeth during sleep.

G50.0 Trigeminal neuralgia

Trigeminal neuralgia, sometimes called tic douloureux, is a condition that is usually caused by blood vessels compressing the trigeminal nerve root, causing pain in the face and particularly in the hinges of the jaw. It is usually treated with medication and painkillers, but in some cases surgery may be necessary.

G50.1 Atypical facial pain

Atypical face pain is similar to trigeminal neuralgia, but the pattern and quality of the pain is different. It is usually treated with medication and painkillers, but in some cases surgery may be necessary.

G51.0 Bell's palsy

Bell's palsy is a condition that causes the facial muscles to weaken or become paralyzed due to trauma to the 7th cranial nerve. The paralysis almost always affects only one side of the face and is rarely permanent, usually vanishing on its own after a few weeks to a few months without treatment. It is most common in diabetic patients, those with depressed immune systems, and pregnant women in their last trimester.

G51.1 Geniculate ganglionitis

Geniculate ganglionitis is a term that refers to any of a number of diseases that affect the facial nerves. These may manifest as facial muscle weakness, loss of the sense of taste or hearing, or decreased tear production. Treatment depends on the exact nature and extent of the disorder.

G51.2 Melkersson's syndrome

In Melkersson's syndrome, the patient experiences repeated bouts of Bell's palsy and facial swelling.

G51.4 Facial myokymia

Facial myokymia is a facial nerve disorder that manifests as a continual rippling motion in the facial muscles.

G52.0 Disorders of olfactory nerve

The olfactory nerve, or the 1st cranial nerve, relays the sense of smell to the brain. Disorders of this nerve may manifest either as a lack of smell or as strong, unexplained odors that others cannot detect.

G52.1 Disorders of glossopharyngeal nerve

Disorders of the glossopharyngeal nerve includes glossopharyngeal neuralgia. This presents as a sharp, jabbing, electric, or shock-like pain on one side of the throat, usually near the tonsil or deep inside the ear due to a disorder of the glossopharyngeal (9th) nerve. This pain may be triggered by chewing or swallowing.

G52.2 Disorders of vagus nerve

Disorders of the pneumogastric (10th) nerve may affect the ear, tongue, swallowing, and vocal cords, causing either weakness or paralysis with loss of sensation, or causing pain.

G52.3 Disorders of hypoglossal nerve

The hypoglossal (12th cranial) nerve innervates the tongue and is responsible for its ability to move. Disorders of this nerve cause weakness of the tongue on the affected side and eventually atrophy, or wasting away

G52.7 Disorders of multiple cranial nerves

This code should be used to report a disorder that affects more than one cranial nerve, causing muscle weakness or paralysis. Vernet's syndrome, which affects the 9th-11th nerves simultaneously, Collet-Sicard syndrome, which affects the 9th-12th nerves simultaneously, and polyneuritis cranialis are three such disorders.

G52.8 Disorders of other specified cranial nerves

Disorders of the accessory (11th) nerve affect the shoulders and neck, causing muscle weakness and/or pain.

G54 Nerve root and plexus disorders

A nerve root connects the peripheral nerves (those that extend throughout the body) to the spinal cord. A plexus is a bundle of nerves that exists outside of the spinal cord. An injury, or lesion, to either can have far-reaching consequences to the body.

G54.0 Brachial plexus disorders

The brachial plexus is located at the joining of the neck and shoulder and provides access between the arm and spinal cord. A lesion, or injury, to this bundle results in a corresponding loss of function and numbness or pain in the shoulder, arm, and/or hand. As a general rule patients will regain voluntary muscle control over a period of 12-18 months, after which any remaining numbness or muscle weakness is generally considered permanent. In some cases, surgical grafting of the nerves may be attempted.

G54.1 Lumbosacral plexus disorders

The lumbosacral plexus is the bundle of nerve fibers from which the nerves spread to the abdomen and pelvis. A lesion of the lumbosacral plexus causes a corresponding weakness of the voluntary muscles in those areas, along with pain or numbness.

G54.2 Cervical root disorders, not elsewhere classified

An injury to the nerve root, a connection between the spinal cord and the peripheral nerves which supply the rest of the body, in the cervical spine (neck). Injuries to the nerve root cause a corresponding weakness or paralysis in the area of the body that the nerve root innervates. While some patients may regain full function with physical therapy, these injuries often result in permanent impairment.

G54.3 Thoracic root disorders, not elsewhere classified

An injury to the nerve root, a connection between the spinal cord and the peripheral nerves which supply the rest of the body, in the thoracic (chest-level) spine. Injuries to the nerve root cause a corresponding weakness or paralysis in the area of the body that the nerve root innervates. While some patients may regain full function with physical therapy, these injuries often result in permanent impairment.

G54.4 Lumbosacral root disorders, not elsewhere classified

An injury to the nerve root, a connection between the spinal cord and the peripheral nerves which supply the rest of the body, in the lumbar (lower) spine. Injuries to the nerve root cause a corresponding weakness or paralysis in the area of the body that the nerve root innervates. While some patients may regain full function with physical therapy, these injuries often result in permanent impairment.

G54.5 Neuralgic amyotrophy

Neuralgic amyotrophy, sometimes called Parsonage-Turner syndrome or brachial plexus neuritis (not to be confused with a lesion of the brachial plexus), is a common disorder in which the patient experiences sudden, intense shoulder pain and weakness and in rare cases paralysis. Often, the site of the injury to the nerve that is causing the pain is unknown. While the condition may continue for months, or years in rare cases, the patient usually recovers completely without intervention.

G54.6 Phantom limb syndrome with pain

Phantom limb is a very common sensation in which an amputee continues to feel sensation in the absent limb as if it were still there. In some cases, this sensation comes in the form of pain, which may come and go or be constant. This is not a psychological disorder, but results from the severed nerve endings continuing to send information to the brain which is misinterpreted. Treatment for this disorder is varied and is often unsuccessful.

G56.3 Lesion of radial nerve

A lesion of the radial nerve causes muscle weakness, tingling, pain or numbness in the index and middle finger part of the hand.

G56.4 Causalgia of upper limb

Causalgia of the upper limb is a condition in which the patient experiences burning pain in a limb which has previously suffered injury. This pain is similar to the initial pain and swelling that an injured limb experiences as a normal reaction to cause the person to protect it while it is healing, but it appears long after the initial wound has healed. This pain can be bad enough to disrupt the patient's life, and is made worse by touching or moving the affected limb.

Note: This condition is often called complex regional pain syndrome (CRPS) type II.

G57.0 Lesion of sciatic nerve

A nerve lesion is a damaged or injured area of a nerve affecting its function. Nerve lesions can be caused by any number of conditions and manifest in a multitude of ways. Symptoms depend on the lesion's location, the extent of nerve signal interruption, and how much of the thick myelin sheath protecting the nerve is eroded or stripped away. Some causes include tumors, misplaced injections, chronic abrasion against bony structures, degenerative diseases, and prolonged pressure. The sciatic nerve is the longest and largest nerve in the body, beginning in the lower back and running down through the gluteal region into the lower leg. The sciatic nerve innervates all the skin of the leg and the muscles in back of the thigh, as well as those of the lower leg and foot. A lesion of the sciatic nerve affects the hamstrings and the muscles of the leg and foot, causing muscle weakness or paralysis, and pain or numbness that radiates down the leg. Imaging, electromyography, or nerve conduction tests are done to locate the lesion and the extent to which the nerve signals are being scrambled or blocked. It may be possible to repair the nerve lesion with surgery while others may eventually heal themselves. Medication along with physical therapy is also used in treating nerve lesions.

G57.1 Meralgia paresthetica

Maralgia paresthetica is a condition in which trauma to the femoral nerve results in pain, burning, and tingling sensations high on the outside curve of the thigh. It often results from obesity or in patients who wear tight corsets, undergarments, or tool belts.

G57.2 Lesion of femoral nerve

A nerve lesion is a damaged or injured area of a nerve affecting its function. Nerve lesions can be caused by any number of conditions and manifest in a multitude of ways. Symptoms depend on the lesion's location, the extent of nerve signal interruption, and how much of the thick myelin sheath protecting the nerve is eroded or stripped away. The femoral nerve is located in the leg and innervates the muscles of the hip, the front of the thigh, and part of the lower leg. A femoral nerve lesion results in numbness, tingling, burning, and decreased sensation in the front of the thigh, knee, or leg; weakness straightening the knee or bending at the hip with a sensation of knee buckling; difficulty in ambulation or going down stairs. Causes include prolonged lying in the lithotomy position (on the back with thighs and legs flexed and turned), and wearing tight belts. Imaging, electromyography, or nerve conduction tests are done to locate the lesion and the extent to which the nerve signals are being scrambled or blocked. It may be possible to repair the nerve lesion with surgery while others may eventually heal themselves. Medication along with physical therapy is also used in treating nerve lesions.

G57.3 Lesion of lateral popliteal nerve

A nerve lesion is a damaged or injured area of a nerve affecting its function. Nerve lesions can be caused by any number of conditions and manifest in a multitude of ways. Symptoms depend on the lesion's location, the extent of nerve signal interruption, and how much of the thick myelin sheath protecting the nerve is eroded or stripped away. The lateral popliteal nerve is located in the lower leg and is the most commonly damaged nerve in the lower limb due to its position traveling around the outside of the head of the fibula leaving it relatively unprotected. It innervates the muscles of the anterior and lateral compartments of the lower leg. A lesion affects the ability to flex the foot upward at the ankle, causing foot drop. Other symptoms include numbness, pain, and tingling in the lower lateral part of the leg and dorsum of the foot, and wasting of anterior tibial and peroneal muscles. Causes of lesions include stretching after prolonged kneeling and long term pressure over the back of the fibula, such as from bedrest or plaster casts. Imaging, electromyography, or nerve conduction tests are done to locate the lesion and the extent to which the nerve signals are being scrambled or blocked. Surgical exploration may be needed if it does not resolve or an obvious lesion is located.

G57.4 Lesion of medial popliteal nerve

A nerve lesion is a damaged or injured area of a nerve affecting its function. Nerve lesions can be caused by any number of conditions and manifest in a multitude of ways. Symptoms of nerve lesions depend on the location of the lesion, the extent to which the nerve signal is interrupted, and how much of the thick myelin sheath protecting the nerve is eroded or stripped away. The medial popliteal nerve is located in the lower limb and travels around the inner aspect of the fibular head. A lesion of the medial popliteal nerve will cause loss of muscle control and numbness, pain, and sensory loss in the sole of the foot and part of the calf as well as wasting of the calf muscle, claw toes from intrinsic paralysis, heel valgus, and when a complete lesion is present, the inability to plantar flex the foot. Imaging, electromyography, or nerve conduction tests are done to locate the lesion and the extent to which the nerve signals are being scrambled or blocked. Management often includes wearing a splint to prevent any over dorsiflexion and managing the source of any pressure causing the lesion.

G57.5 Tarsal tunnel syndrome

Tarsal tunnel syndrome is very similar to the better-known carpal tunnel syndrome, and results from a compression of the tibial nerve in the leg, causing pain and weakness in the ankle and foot. This disorder is treated by resting the ankle and applying ice and medication to reduce swelling. In some cases surgery may be employed to sever the tissue putting pressure on the nerve.

G57.6 Lesion of plantar nerve

A nerve lesion is a damaged or injured area of a nerve affecting its function. Nerve lesions can be caused by any number of conditions and manifest in a multitude of ways. Symptoms of nerve lesions depend on the location of the lesion, the extent to which the nerve signal is interrupted, and how much of the thick myelin sheath protecting the nerve is eroded or stripped away. A lesion of the plantar nerve in the sole of the foot leading to the toes is most often caused by excessive or long-term pressure and results in a localized, sharp, burning type pain in the ball of the foot. A lesion involving the digital nerves leading to the toes is known as Morton's neuroma or Morton's metatarsalgia. This results from thickening of the tissue surrounding the digital nerve leading to the toes and causes pain and burning in the ball of the foot with stinging or burning pain and numbness in the neighboring halves of the toes affected, most commonly between the third and fourth toes. This lesion occurs in response to long term irritation, trauma, or excessive pressure from wearing high-heeled shoes. Imaging, electromyography, or nerve conduction tests are done to locate the lesion and the extent to which the nerve signals are being scrambled or blocked. Wearing lower heeled shoes with wider toe space is recommended. Corticosteroid injections or surgery may needed.

G57.7 Causalgia of lower limb

Causalgia of the lower limb is a condition in which the patient experiences burning pain in a limb which has previously suffered injury. This pain is similar to the initial pain and swelling that an injured limb experiences as a normal reaction to cause the person to protect it while it is healing, but it appears long after the initial wound has healed. This pain can be bad enough to disrupt the patient's life, and is made worse by touching or moving the affected limb.

Note: This condition is often called complex regional pain syndrome (CRPS) type II.

G60.0 Hereditary motor and sensory neuropathy

Hereditary sensory neuropathy is a condition in which the patient suffers from four to six similar but distinct inherited degenerative disorders of the nervous system. These disorders cause sensory loss in various parts of the body, from the eyes and ears to the extremities, as well as loss of motor, reflex, or blood vessel function. Peroneal muscular atrophy, also known as Charcot-Marie-Tooth disease or CMT, is another inherited neurological disorder in which patients slowly lose sensation and the use of their arms, hands, legs, and feet as the nerves innervating the arms and legs degenerate. The loss of neural input to and from the legs usually precedes that in the arms by several years. Due to the loss of sensation, CMT patients may injure themselves and be unaware of it. There is no cure for CMT, so treatment concentrates on improving quality of life through orthopedic devices (e.g., braces) and physical therapy. Hereditary peripheral atrophy, sometimes called Dejerine-Sottas disease, is another genetic neuropathy that damages the peripheral nerves, resulting in muscle wasting and weakness, loss of sensation (particularly in the lower legs and arms), loss of coordination and balance (ataxia), curvature of the spine (scoliosis), and stiffened joints. The severity and rate of progression varies per patient.

G60.1 Refsum's disease

Refsum's disease is a genetic, progressive disease which, due to a disorder of the metabolism of lipids (fats), causes physical weakness, vision loss, and painful inflammation of the nerves. The progression is often marked by periods of remission, after which the disease progresses again. Treatment is primarily centered around providing a diet low in phytanic acid, which is found in dairy products and animal fat, which is believed to be connected to this disease.

G60.3 Idiopathic progressive neuropathy

Idiopathic progressive polyneuropathy refers to any progressive disorder of the nervous system that affects the limbs and for which the cause is not known.

G61.0 Guillain-Barre syndrome

Acute infective polyneuritis, also known as Guillain-Barre syndrome or GBS, is a neural disorder that begins with numbness, tingling, and burning sensations in the feet, followed by weakness and sometimes paralysis of the legs. This muscle weakness progresses upwards through the torso to the arms and face. This disease is the result of a viral or bacterial infection which causes the body's immune system to attack the nerves. Progression of the disease can take anywhere from less than ten days to up to two months, and paralysis can continue for six months to two years. This paralysis can

cause life-threatening respiratory distress, requiring the patient to be put on a ventilator.

G61.81 Chronic inflammatory demyelinating polyneuritis

Chronic inflammatory demyelinating polyneuritis is a progressive disorder in which the body's immune system attacks its own nervous system, causing numbness, weakness, and/or paralysis. This is different from Guillain-Barre syndrome in that no preceding infection is linked to the autoimmune disorder.

G62.0 Drug-induced polyneuropathy

polyneuropathy is a condition in which the patient loses nervous function due to damage caused by taking drugs that the body finds toxic. It most commonly presents with numbness, a burning sensation in the extremities, and/or muscle weakness. In severe cases, the autonomic nerves that control unconscious body functions like digestion, may also be affected. Polyneuropathy due to drugs presents much the same as that due to alcohol.

Note: This code includes more than elicit drugs; cancer medication may also cause some form of polyneuropathy as drug complications or adverse reactions occur.

G62.1 Alcoholic polyneuropathy

Alcoholic polyneuropathy is a condition in which the patient loses nervous function due to damage caused by excessive alcohol consumption over the course of many years. It most commonly presents with numbness, a burning sensation in the feet, and/or muscle weakness. In severe cases, the autonomic nerves, those that control internal body functions like the heartbeat, may become involved. The damage done is usually permanent.

G62.2 Polyneuropathy due to other toxic agents

Toxic polyneuropathies are disorders caused by damage to several different nerves after exposure to a toxic or poisonous substance.

G62.81 Critical illness polyneuropathy

Critical illness polyneuropathy is a frequent complication in critically ill patients as a result of sepsis (blood-poisoning by the infection or toxic agent) and multiple organ failure. It is thought to be a common factor in the difficulty many patients have in being weaned from dependence on a ventilator.

G70 Myasthenia gravis and other myoneural disorders

A myoneural disorder is one that affects both the nerves and the muscles that they connect to. Note that other neural disorders can indirectly cause muscle weakness and wasting, but this is due to signals from the brain not reaching all of the muscles in the affected area, resulting in the muscle not being exercised. In a myoneural disorder, the muscle is directly affected.

G70.0 Myasthenia gravis

In myasthenia gravis the immune system mistakenly attacks the connections between the nerve fibers and the muscles, preventing the muscles from receiving signals from the brain. It normally presents with muscle weakness in specific locations rather than general fatigue, and in two-thirds of patients, the first muscles affected are those controlling the eyes. This weakness usually spreads during the first two years before slowly improving over several more years.

G70.00 Myasthenia gravis without (acute) exacerbation

Use this code to indicate myasthenia gravis that is not life threatening. This is a muscle weakness that increases during periods of activity and improves after periods of rest.

G70.01 Myasthenia gravis with (acute) exacerbation

Myasthenia gravis may suddenly reach a state of acute exacerbation, in which the patient's life is threatened by the inability to use the respiratory muscles, requiring immediate emergency care.

Diseases of the Nervous System

G57.7 – G70.01

G70.1 Toxic myoneural disorders

Toxic myoneural disorders have the same range of symptoms, but are due to foreign and toxic substances that have entered the patient's body. This can include certain prescribed medications.

G70.80 Lambert-Eaton syndrome, unspecified

Lambert-Eaton syndrome (LEMS) is a rare autoimmune disorder that affects the neuromuscular junction where nerve cells and muscle cells meet and muscle activation occurs. LEMS is caused by the production of antibodies that interfere with the communication between the nerves and muscles. The presynaptic voltage-gated calcium channels of the motor nerve terminal are attacked and the nerve cells do not release enough acetylcholine to transmit electrical impulses across the junction. This causes muscle weakness and depressed tendon reflexes. The proximal muscles of the lower limbs are predominantly affected. Patients have difficult standing, walking, or climbing stairs. Symptoms may develop slowly over years. Oropharyngeal and ocular muscles are also affected causing eyelid ptosis, diplopia, and difficulty chewing or swallowing. Autonomic dysfunction may occur as constipation, urinary retention, sweating, and abnormal tearing and salivation. Dry mouth may be one of the first presenting symptoms. Some strength improvement does occur with activity. Electromyography and nerve conduction velocity tests help diagnose LEMS.

G70.81 Lambert-Eaton syndrome in disease classified elsewhere

Lambert-Eaton syndrome also occurs in the presence of other autoimmune diseases, such as vitiligo, and not always with cancer. Treatment aims to suppress the autoimmune response using steroids, immunoglobulin injections, and plasmapheresis to separate plasma from the blood as it is removed from the body, filter out harmful antibodies that are interfering with nerve function, and return the plasma to the body.

Note: The underlying disease classified elsewhere must be listed first, followed by Lambert-Eaton syndrome.

G71.0 Muscular dystrophy

Muscular dystrophy is a genetic myopathy which causes progressive weakness and wasting of the muscles. This weakness progresses at different rates for different patients. Some experience only minor muscle weakness over the course of their normal lifespan, while others are unable to walk within a matter of years or, in the late stages, even breathe without assistance. There is no cure for muscular dystrophy, so treatment focuses on enhancing the patient's quality of life.

G71.11 Myotonic muscular dystrophy

Myotonic muscular dystrophy, also known as dystrophia myotonica, proximal myotonic myopathy (PROMM), or Steinert's disease, is the most common form of adult-onset muscular dystophy. One form of the disease severely affects babies because the disease has an effect called 'anticipation,' in which it gets progressively worse with each generation. The earlier the disease appears, the more severe the symptoms. Symptoms vary and can appear at birth or in the first few years. The disease begins to show by age 20 for half of those with it, but it is not uncommon for some to live to 40 or 50 before definite symptoms begin to show, which are milder. Those affected as babies tend to have disabling weakness in the extremities and cognitive problems with developmental delays and/or learning disabilities. Their pattern of myotonic weakness is generally noted in the head and neck muscles, and in the hands and lower legs. Muscle weakness in the older-onset, milder form of the disease is more evident closer to the trunk in the neck, shoulders, hips, and upper legs. Cognitive manifestations include problems with organization or concentration. The disease also tends to cause other unusual problems like lack of energy and hypersomnia, insulin resistance, digestive problems, hair loss, and heart blocks and cataracts. The disease is diagnosed by genetic tests for the mutated gene; muscle biopsy to look for changes in muscle cell structure; blood tests for creatine kinase, even before symptoms appear; and electromyography.

G71.12 Myotonia congenita

This condition, also known as myotonia levior, presents in early childhood with a lack of ability to quickly relax muscles after voluntary contraction.

Symptoms are usually noticed around 2 or 3 years of age with muscle stiffness, especially in the legs, from sudden activity after rest. The myotonia is not painful. Patients may stumble and fall and have difficulty relaxing the grip of a handshake or opening the eyes after squinting. This type of myotonic disorder is also known as Thomsen's disease. It is not degenerative and does not cause muscle wasting, but in fact causes muscle enlargement with increased muscle strength. The disease is caused by gene mutations that shut off the electrical excitation in muscle. There are two forms of myotonia congenita--Thomsen's disease, the dominant form, which is milder, and the recessive Becker's disease type, which manifests in adolescence or later and is more severe.

G71.13 Myotonic chondrodystrophy

Myotonic chondrodystrophy (congenital), also known as Schwartz-Jampel syndrome, manifests in late infancy and has distinctive features of a mask-like face, abnormally short stature or dwarfism, blepharophimosis, small, fixed facial features like microstomia, limited mobility of major joints or joint contracture in fixed positions, and generalized myotonia. Abnormal bone development is also seen, especially in a prominent sternum and hip dysplasia. Death usually occurs because of respiratory compromise. The muscles of the diaphragm, tongue, and larynx are hypertrophied and repeated aspiration and laryngeospasm occur. IgA deficiency is also thought to contribute to respiratory compromise.

G71.14 Drug induced myotonia

This is muscle weakness and stiffness that is usually short-lived, brought on by the use of beta-blockers, diuretics, muscle relaxants or anesthetic drugs, and statins.

G71.19 Other specified myotonic disorders

This includes paramyotonia congenita of von Eulenburg, a sodium ion channel type of myotonia, in which muscle weakness and stiffness is brought on by exposure to cold or temperature changes and the weakness can persis for hours, even after the body is warmed. Periodic paralysis and myotonia is especially prominent in the eyelids. Potassium sensitivity is involved in some cases.

G71.2 Congenital myopathies

A congenital myopathy is a disorder or disease that causes direct damage to the muscles of the body that is present from birth. This is distinct from a neuropathy or myoneural disorder that results in muscle weakness; in such disorders, the muscles initially lose strength due to signals from the brain not reaching them, and waste over time from disuse. In a myopathy, muscle weakness, damage, and even paralysis is present from a problem within the muscle tissue itself. Loss of sensation is a common symptom in a neuropathy or myoneural disorder as a result of the nervous damage, while in a myopathy, the patient continues to feel sensation normally.

G72.3 Periodic paralysis

Familial periodic paralysis, also called hypokalemic periodic paralysis, is a genetic disorder which causes occasional episodes of muscle weakness which is greatest in the shoulders and hips, but which can also affect the respiratory and heart muscles. Unlike most other forms of periodic paralysis, people with this disorder have normal thyroid function, but very low levels of potassium in the blood during an episode as the muscles absorb the potassium from the blood. Although muscle strength is initially normal between attacks, repeated attacks can lead to permanent weakness. Potassium supplements given during an episode often ends the episode.

G72.41 Inclusion body myositis [IBM]

Inclusion body myositis (IBM) is considered a disease from the group of muscle diseases called the inflammatory myopathies, which are characterized by chronic muscle inflammation and weakness. The muscle weakness may affect both proximal trunk muscles and distal extremity muscles. The onset is generally gradual over years and may affect only one side of the body. Symptoms include falling or tipping over; difficulty swallowing; weakness that begins at the wrists causing difficulty gripping, pinching, or buttoning; and atrophic loss of muscle in the forearms and quadriceps of the leg. The disease usually affects more men than women and occurs after the age of 50. There is no cure or standard course of treatment and the disease has shown to be unresponsive to corticosteroids and immunosuppressants. Therapy is supportive for symptoms and may include physical therapy to help maintain mobility.

G72.81   Critical illness myopathy
Critical illness myopathy is a frequent complication in critically ill patients as a result of sepsis (blood-poisoning by the infection or toxic agent) and multiple organ failure, which result in widespread damage to the muscles. It is thought to be a common factor in the difficulty many patients have in being weaned from dependence on a ventilator.

G73.1   Lambert-Eaton syndrome in neoplastic disease
Lambert-Eaton syndrome (LEMS) (G70.80) is a rare disorder that affects the neuromuscular junction where nerve cells and muscle cells meet and muscle activation occurs. LEMS is caused by the production of antibodies that interfere with the communication between the nerves and muscles. The presynaptic voltage-gated calcium channels of the motor nerve terminal are attacked and the nerve cells do not release enough acetylcholine to transmit electrical impulses across the junction. This causes muscle weakness and depressed tendon reflexes. LEMS is also closely linked to cancer diagnoses and is considered a paraneoplastic syndrome, although it can occur alone, or in the presence of other autoimmune diseases. It is estimated that 50%-70% of those diagnosed with LEMS have an identified cancer, the majority of which is small cell lung cancer. Over half of those with LEMS will develop small cell lung cancer later. LEMS can also appear up to 3 years before any cancer manifests and is diagnosed. Other associated cancers include lymphomas, T cell leukemia, thymoma, prostate cancer, and neuroendocrine tumors. For those with cancer and LEMS, treatment is aimed at the underlying cancer first and help improve muscle strength.

Note: The underlying cancer must be coded first.

G80   Cerebral palsy
Cerebral palsy is a condition in which the cerebrum becomes damaged in the womb, during delivery, or in the first few weeks of life due to lack of oxygen (e.g., when the child becomes tangled in the umbilical cord) or a congenital malformation in the brain. It presents with an inability to fully control motor function, and is classified according to the affected area. There is no cure for cerebral palsy.

G80.0   Spastic quadriplegic cerebral palsy
Palsy presenting with paralysis of all four limbs.

G80.1   Spastic diplegic cerebral palsy
Diplegic cerebral palsy affects one set of limbs on both sides of the body (e.g., both arms or both legs).

G80.2   Spastic hemiplegic cerebral palsy
Hemiplegic cerebral palsy affects either the left or right side, e.g., the right arm and right leg.

G80.3   Athetoid cerebral palsy
Cerebral palsy is one of any number of permanent, but nonprogressive, motor disorders caused by intrauterine pathology in brain development and/or brain damage occurring from birth trauma. The brain's ability to effect movement and hold posture is disrupted. Muscle coordination may be stiff and spastic or floppy and loose, uncontrolled movements or tremors may be present, as well as difficulty swallowing, speaking, and walking. Other medical disorders such as mental retardation and seizures may or may not be present, depending on the location of the brain damage. Cerebral palsy is classified according to the different types of movement disorders that are manifested. Athetoid means that the palsy is characterized by uncontrolled, writhing movements of the hands, feet, arms, or legs.

G81.0   Flaccid hemiplegia
Flaccid hemiplegia indicates that while the patient cannot move the affected side, the limbs can be positioned by another or by the patient's good arm without difficulty.

G82.2   Paraplegia
Paraplegia is the paralysis of both lower limbs and possibly of the lower portion of the trunk of the body as well.

G82.5   Quadriplegia
Quadraplegia is paralyzation that affects all four limbs, typically caused by damage to the spinal cord in the area of the neck. These conditions are coded according to the level of vertebrae where the injury occurred in the cervical (neck) portion of the spine and how complete the severing of the spinal cord is.

G82.51   Quadriplegia, C1-C4 complete
The injury occurs in the top four vertebrae (C1-C4) and the spinal cord is completely severed.

G82.52   Quadriplegia, C1-C4 incomplete
The injury occurs in the top four vertebrae (C1-C4) and the spinal cord is only partially severed.

G82.53   Quadriplegia, C5-C7 complete
The injury occurs in the lower three cervical vertebrae (C5-C7) and the spinal cord is completely severed.

G82.54   Quadriplegia, C5-C7 incomplete
The injury occurs in the lower three cervical vertebrae (C5-C7) and the spinal cord is only partially severed.

G83.0   Diplegia of upper limbs
Diplegia is a condition in which both upper limbs are paralyzed and the use of the arms is lost, but the patient retains use of his or her legs and trunk.

G83.1   Monoplegia of lower limb
Monoplegia of the lower limb indicates that only one leg--either the right or the left is paralyzed. Codes are classified by whether the right or left leg was the dominant side or the patient's nondominant side.

G83.11   Monoplegia of lower limb affecting right dominant side
Paralysis affecting the right leg of a right-handed person.

G83.12   Monoplegia of lower limb affecting left dominant side
Paralysis affecting the left leg of a left-handed person.

G83.13   Monoplegia of lower limb affecting right nondominant side
Paralysis affecting the right leg of a left-handed person.

G83.14   Monoplegia of lower limb affecting left nondominant side
Paralysis affecting the left leg of a right-handed person.

G83.2   Monoplegia of upper limb
Monoplegia of the upper limb indicates that only one arm--either the right or the left is paralyzed. Codes are classified by whether the right or left arm was the dominant side or the patient's nondominant side.

Note: The right side is considered the dominant side as the default when not further specified.

G83.21   Monoplegia of upper limb affecting right dominant side
Paralysis affecting the right arm of a right-handed person.

G83.22   Monoplegia of upper limb affecting left dominant side
Paralysis affecting the left arm of a left-handed person.

G83.23 Monoplegia of upper limb affecting right nondominant side

Paralysis affecting the right arm of a left-handed person.

G83.24 Monoplegia of upper limb affecting left nondominant side

Paralysis affecting the left arm of a right-handed person.

G83.3 Monoplegia, unspecified

Monoplegia is paralysis of a single limb, muscle, or muscle group.

G83.4 Cauda equina syndrome

Cauda equina syndrome, sometimes abbreviated as CES, is a rare disorder in which the bundle of nerves at the lower end of the spinal cord are compressed and paralyzed, cutting off sensation and movement. It may present with bladder or bowel dysfunction which either prevents the patient from releasing waste or else from holding it; severe and/or progressive numbing of the area between the legs, over the buttocks, in the inner thighs or the back of the legs and feet; and pain and spreading numbness in one or both legs. This disorder may be caused by a ruptured disc, tumor, infection, or fracture and requires immediate emergency medical treatment to relieve the pressure and prevent paralysis.

G83.5 Locked-in state

Locked-in state is a condition in which the patient remains conscious and retains their normal cognitive function, but in which they lose all power of movement, except perhaps for their eyes, making it very difficult or impossible for them to communicate. Lou Gehrig's disease is a common cause of this condition. Diagnostic tests such as CT scans and MRIs may be required to distinguish between this condition and a permanent vegetative state.

G89 Pain, not elsewhere classified

The character and extent of pain can present in vastly different ways depending upon the cause, other contributing factors, and areas affected. Encounters for pain management consume a large part of health care resources and rightly necessitate codes that identify the type and/or cause of pain beyond the ability to classify pain only to the site or as a generalized symptom.

G89.0 Central pain syndrome

Central pain syndrome is caused by damage to the central nervous system, whether through trauma or conditions and diseases that affect the brain, such as cerebrovascular accident or stroke, multiple sclerosis, Parkinson's, and epilepsy. The type of pain described in central pain syndrome varies widely due to the many different varieties of causes. Patients sometimes require antidepressants and anticonvulsive medications in addition to pain medication.

G89.1 Acute pain, not elsewhere classified

Acute pain is moderate to relatively severe or intense, sudden in appearance, and mostly self-limiting to the causative period of injury before healing has occurred.

G89.11 Acute pain due to trauma

Acute pain due to trauma presents as relatively severe or intense pain, stemming from a specific traumatic, causal incident, but does not continue for a long course of time. Acute pain occurs in direct response to injury or trauma and subsides as the injury heals.

G89.12 Acute post-thoracotomy pain

Post-thoracotomy pain is an aching, burning, or sharp sensation that occurs in the chest wall around the surgical incision. Because a thoracotomy involves cutting, excising, and suturing skin, muscle, nerves, and other structures in the chest wall, pain can result from entrapment or fibrosis of nerve fibers in the scar tissue. Pain can also stem from disrupted muscles in the shoulders and chest. Acute post-thoracotomy pain may present in short duration, but relatively severe.

G89.18 Other acute postprocedural pain

The incidence and severity of acute postoperative pain occasions return trips to health care facilities, delays recovery, and can lead to other health problems when it remains unrelieved, driving up health care costs.

G89.2 Chronic pain, not elsewhere classified

Chronic pain is present for months or years and often does not respond to typical treatment models. It may be related to a causative injury or surgical procedure or may stem from a completely unidentifiable etiology. Chronic pain usually requires a multidisciplinary treatment approach using different kinds of therapy in addition to long-term pain medication management and treatment focused on related psychosocial factors.

G89.21 Chronic pain due to trauma

Chronic pain due to trauma persists for months, possibly years, even after the body has healed from the obvious injuries stemming from a particular traumatic incident.

Note: Pain that is not specified as to cause should be coded to pain by site.

G89.22 Chronic post-thoracotomy pain

Chronic post-thoracotomy pain is an aching, burning, or sharp sensation in the chest wall around the surgical incision that continues over a long period of time following the healing period. Because a thoracotomy involves cutting, excising, and suturing skin, muscle, nerves, and other structures in the chest wall, pain can result from entrapment or fibrosis of nerve fibers in the scar tissue. Pain can also stem from disrupted muscles in the shoulders and chest.

G89.28 Other chronic postprocedural pain

Chronic pain lasts for months, even after the body has healed from the surgical procedure, and may go on for years.

G89.3 Neoplasm related pain (acute) (chronic)

Neoplasm related pain includes both acute and chronic types. Use this code when the pain being treated is identified as being related to any type of malignancy, tumor, cancer, or neoplastic disease.

G89.4 Chronic pain syndrome

Chronic pain syndrome (CPS) is usually defined as pain lasting longer than six months, although some diagnosticians may use three months as the criterion and some consider it to be pain that persists beyond the reasonably expected healing time for the tissues involved. CPS is a challenging problem that can have a very complex natural history, an unidentified etiology, and a poor response to the model of care. It requires a multidisciplinary approach. Patients often require long-term pain management, including long-acting pain medications, antidepressants, physical therapy for muscle stretching and strengthening, and occupational therapy to help change habits in performing ordinary tasks. CPS has a significant psychosocial dysfunction component that arises from decreasing function and ability, emotional stress, isolation affecting relationships, financial strain and unemployment, legal issues, chemical dependency, and sleep problems.

G90 Disorders of autonomic nervous system

The autonomic nervous system controls body functions over which humans do not have conscious control, such as heartbeat, breathing, digestion, and unconscious reflexes.

G90.0 Idiopathic peripheral autonomic neuropathy

Idiopathic peripheral autonomic neuropathy is a condition in which there is damage to one or more non-spinal, autonomic nerves with no identified cause. Symptoms and treatments vary depending on which nerves (and connected systems) are affected.

G90.01 Carotid sinus syncope

Carotid sinus syndrome is also called carotid sinus syncope or tight-collar syndrome. The carotid sinus is a widened portion of the carotid artery containing nerve endings that are sensitive to pressure. When these nerve fibers are stimulated, or sense increased blood pressure within the carotid sinus, they send impulses to the brain that slow the heart rate and reduce arterial pressure. This reflex results in bradycardia and hypotension, causing syncope or brief unconsciousness from transient cerebral perfusion. This is an exaggerated response to carotid sinus baroreceptor stimulation and predominantly affects older males.

G90.4 Autonomic dysreflexia

Autonomic dysreflexia, also called hyperreflexia, is a condition that can occur in patients with a spinal cord injury to the fifth thoracic vertebrae (T-5) and above. It may occur when pain or another irritating stimulus (such as an overfull bladder) affects the body below the affected vertebrae. This sends nerve impulses to the spine, but it is stopped at the place where the spinal cord is severed and causes a reflex reaction that can cause an increase in blood pressure and spasms that can lead to seizures, stroke, and even death if not treated.

G90.5 Complex regional pain syndrome I (CRPS I)

Complex regional pain syndrome I (CRPS I) is also known as reflex sympathetic dystrophy. CRPS I is a chronic neurological disorder caused by nerve damage that presents with severe burning pain, changes in bone and skin, excessive sweating, swelling, and extreme sensitivity to the touch. There is currently no cure, and treatment focuses on managing the pain and maintaining the patient's quality of life.

G91.0 Communicating hydrocephalus

Communicating hydrocephalus is a degenerative disorder caused by an obstruction in the flow of cerebrospinal fluid (CSF). The blockage may be caused by a bout of meningitis, a hemorrhage within the ventricles (passages) of the brain, a congenital malformation, or other infection. In order to prevent swelling and permanent brain damage and degeneration, an artificial drainage tube must be surgically inserted into the ventricles of the brain.

Note: Communicating hydrocephalus includes secondary normal pressure hydrocephalus.

G91.1 Obstructive hydrocephalus

An obstructive hydrocephalus prevents the flow of CSF into the spinal canal. These blockages may be caused by a bout of meningitis, a hemorrhage within the ventricles (passages) of the brain, a congenital malformation, or other infection. In order to prevent swelling and permanent brain damage and degeneration, an artificial drainage tube must be surgically inserted into the ventricles of the brain.

G91.2 (Idiopathic) normal pressure hydrocephalus

This is a treatable condition that results from a disruption of normal cerebrospinal fluid (CSF) circulation with gradual enlargement of the ventricles in the brain. The triad of symptoms that emerge includes gait impairment, cognitive impairment or dementia, and urinary incontinence with urgency. This syndrome often occurs secondary to a disease process or brain injury, such as meningitis or traumatic subarachnoid hemorrhage. When this syndrome occurs without any known etiology, it is called idiopathic normal pressure hydrocephalus. INPH is treated with surgical diversion of CSF by implanting a shunt to drain the fluid, either from the ventricles in the brain or from the lumbar subarachnoid space in the spine, to a distal site where it can be reabsorbed by the body, such as the pleural or peritoneal cavity, or the venous system. Patients usually undergo tests of short-term removal of excess CSF through lumbar puncture or several days of drainage via a spinal catheter prior to shunt placement to see how they respond.

Note: This code includes normal pressure hydrocephalus that is not otherwise clarified, but excludes secondary normal pressure hydrocephalus, which is coded as communicating hydrocephalus.

G92 Toxic encephalopathy

Toxic encephalopathy is brain damage due to poison or other toxic substance. Toxic encephalitis and encephalomyelitis develop as a result of poisoning by one or more toxic substances, such as carbon tetrachloride, lead, or mercury, and can also occur as toxic levels of by-products from intrinsic metabolic processes build up. The symptoms can vary depending on the nature of the toxin and the location of the brain affected, but loss of memory and reasoning ability and weakness or paralysis are common. In mild cases the patient is administered oxygen and an anti-toxin (if available). In more severe cases, extensive physical and educational therapy may be needed to restore all or part of the patient's mental and physical function.

G93.0 Cerebral cysts

A cerebral cyst is a pocket in brain tissue filled with fluid, which is usually infected. As it expands, this can put pressure on the surrounding tissue, causing complications such as tremors, muscle weakness, and paralysis in one or more parts of the body. Treatment involves draining the cyst, which requires delicate and dangerous surgery to the brain.

G93.1 Anoxic brain damage, not elsewhere classified

Anoxic brain damage indicates a brain injury caused by a lack of oxygen (e.g., due to drowning). Symptoms can vary widely depending on which area of the brain is damaged and to what extent, but can include loss of memory, reasoning abilities, and paralysis.

Note: This code does not include brain damage that occurred during childbirth.

G93.2 Benign intracranial hypertension

Benign intracranial hypertension is a very rare condition that is also known as pseudotumor cerebri, in which high cerebrospinal fluid pressure in the brain can cause all the symptoms of a brain tumor. This can present with constant headaches, nausea and vomiting, problems with balance and memory, disturbances of vision, ringing in the ears (tinnitus), and neck and back pain. This disorder is most common in women between the ages of 20 and 50, and has been linked in some studies to hormonal changes. Treatment includes medication to reduce the blood pressure and exercise to encourage weight loss. In rare cases, a tube called a shunt may be surgically implanted to drain the excess fluid from the cranium.

G93.4 Other and unspecified encephalopathy

Encephalopathy is a general term that refers to a disease or disorder of the brain when another more specific diagnosis is not available.

G93.5 Compression of brain

Compression of the brain is caused by elevated pressure in the cranium due to a blood clot, tumor, fracture, abscess (infected pocket), or other condition. This condition presents with drowsiness, difficulty in breathing, a weak pulse, and paralysis on one side of the body (hemiplegia). If not treated, it can lead to coma and death. Treatment involves lowering the pressure and repairing the defect or injury that caused the blockage in the first place, usually by emergency surgery.

G93.6 Cerebral edema

Cerebral edema is the accumulation of excessive fluid in the body of the brain. Because the brain has no room to expand, this can cause severe injury. This condition presents with drowsiness, difficulty in breathing, a weak pulse, and paralysis on one side of the body (hemiplegia). If not treated, it can lead to coma and death. Treatment involves lowering the pressure and, if possible, repairing the defect or injury that caused the accumulation of fluid in the first place.

G93.7 Reye's syndrome

Reye's syndrome is a rare disease that usually appears in childhood. The cause of Reye's syndrome is unknown, but it is not contagious. It most often appears in the winter months in patients recovering from a viral infection, such as an upper respiratory infection. Abnormal accumulations of fat begin to develop in all of the organs, but most dangerously in the liver and brain. This causes a build-up of pressure within the brain that manifests in the usual signs of cerebral degeneration. Reye's syndrome initially presents with persistent vomiting and signs of dysfunction in the brain, such as loss of energy and drowsiness. In the second stage, the patient begins to exhibit personality changes, irritability and aggressiveness, confusion, irrationality, and delirium. In the final stages, the patient has convulsions and lapses into a coma, which leads to death. This disease is extremely dangerous and can lead to death within days. It can also be difficult to diagnose, especially in infants (who may not show the same pattern of symptoms as adults), and is often misdiagnosed as encephalitis, meningitis, diabetes, drug overdose, poisoning, sudden infant death syndrome, or a psychiatric illness. Final diagnosis of the disease is made by testing the liver function. Treatment concentrates on protecting the brain from permanent damage due to the swelling.

G93.81   Temporal sclerosis

Temporal lobe sclerosis, also called hippocampal or mesial temporal sclerosis, is scarring and loss of neurons in the deepest portion of the temporal lobe associated with damage from brain injuries such as trauma, infection, tumors, hypoxia, or uncontrolled seizures. The region begins to atrophy; neurons die and scar tissue forms, particularly in the hippocampal region of the temporal lobe. Temporal sclerosis usually results in partial, focal, temporal lobe epilepsy, where the seizure initiation is located. Other symptoms occur such as strange sensations, convulsions, muscle spasms, emotional changes, and alterations in behavior. Temporal lobectomy of the portion of the brain containing the focal point of the seizures is often done to remove the section of sclerotic temporal structures completely and relieve medically refractory epilepsy.

G93.82   Brain death

Brain death is the irreversible complete loss of all brain function, including the brain stem, resulting in the end of all brain activity and cessation of vital bodily functions required to sustain life. In brain death, the pupils are fixed and dilated; there is no eye movement; respiratory reflexes are absent; and there is no response to painful stimuli. Brain death requires that a flat EEG remain for a specific duration of time. A total lack of electrical activity in the brain is demonstrated by taking two different EEGs 12 hours apart. In some cases, the heart may continue to beat and there may be spinal reflexes that cause the limbs to move. Hypothermia and drug toxicities can mimic brain death and these must be ruled out. There is usually evidence of some trauma or disease that has caused brain injury.

G95.0   Syringomyelia and syringobulbia

Syringomyelia and syringobulbia are a pair of related disorders in which a cyst, a fluid-filled pocket or cavity, forms in the spinal cord (syringomyelia) or in the spinal cord where it connects to the brain stem (syringobulbia). This cyst is often referred to as a syrinx. These disorders present with back pain, headaches, weakness in the back, shoulders, arms, or legs, and the loss of the ability to feel extremes of hot and cold, especially in the hands. Treatment usually involves surgery to either enlarge the space around the syrix to relieve the pressure, or in some cases to drain the syrix. Both risk the possibility of paralysis.

G95.1   Vascular myelopathies

Vascular myelopathies are conditions in which the spine is damaged due to a malfunction in the blood vessels that feed it. Such malfunctions can include edema (swelling) of the spinal cord due to blood accumulation, clots that form in the veins (thrombosis) and/or break away and travel through the veins to become lodged in another location (embolism), and so on.

G96.0   Cerebrospinal fluid leak

Cerebrospinal rhinorrhea is a condition in which cerebrospinal fluid, which normally cushions the brain, flows from the nose, usually due to a fracture of the frontal bone of the skull and tearing of the membrane. This condition may be treated with bed rest, giving the body a chance to repair the damage itself, or by surgical intervention. Cerebrospinal fluid otorrhea is a condition in which the fluid which surrounds and protects both the brain and the spinal cord discharges from the ear.

G96.11   Dural tear

The dura mater is the tough, protective, outermost layer of the meninges that surround the spinal cord and the brain. Dural tears that are not a result of surgical procedures may be caused by trauma, such as a skull fracture.

G97.1   Other reaction to spinal and lumbar puncture

A lumbar puncture is a standard diagnostic procedure that enables the physician to collect a sample of cerebrospinal fluid for testing. However, in some cases, the patient may exhibit a bad reaction. A headache is the most common side-effect, but damage to the spinal cord and a corresponding weakness or even paralysis are also possible.

G97.41   Accidental puncture or laceration of dura during a procedure

The dura mater is the tough, protective, outermost layer of the meninges that surround the spinal cord and the brain. This protective layer can be breached inadvertently during brain and spinal cord procedures such as transphenoidal surgery for pituitary tumors, craniofacial surgery, laminectomy for spinal stenosis, or diskectomy for spinal decompression. Iatrogenic dural tears or inadvertent durotomies also occur during anterior spinal surgery with vertebrectomy, resection of calcified ligament, or adherent disc. The hole or tear allows cerebrospinal fluid to leak and must be sutured or repaired with a suitable material, such as dura graft matrix, to keep the brain or spinal cord protected.

G99.0   Autonomic neuropathy in diseases classified elsewhere

Autonomic neuropathy is a condition that manifests as a group of symptoms when there is damage to one or more of the nerves or nerve bundles that regulate unconscious body functions, such as heartrate, blood pressure, digestion, and bowel and bladder emptying. Symptoms and treatments vary depending on which nerves (and connected systems) are affected. The autonomic nerves send signals from the brain and spinal cord out to many different tissues, including the stomach, bladder, intestines, blood vessels, heart, and pupils. Symptoms could include urinary problems, dizziness or fainting when standing from a drop in blood pressure, sweating abnormally, delayed pupillary reaction, and gastric problems. Autonomic neuropathy often occurs in the presence of other conditions, such as hyperthyroidism and amyloidosis.

Note: Use this code if the disorder is due to a another disease classified elsewhere, in which case the underlying disease should be coded first, unless it is identified as diabetic autonomic neuropathy, which is coded within categories E09-E13.

H00.01 Hordeolum externum

A hordeolum externum is an infection of the sebaceous (oil) glands of Zeis at the base of the eyelashes, most often due to *Staphylococcus aureus bacteria*. Also known as a stye, the infected gland appears as a swollen, red bump on the outer edge of the eyelid that is sore and tender to touch. Other symptoms include watery eye, sensitivity to light, and a gritty or scratchy sensation within the eye. Styes appear with acute onset after the bacteria have entered the gland and last about 7-10 days. They are normally self-limiting and resolve on their own with basic care at home. Applying warm compresses several times a day is done to help drain the stye gently and loosen any blockages. The stye contains watery fluid, pus, and bacteria that can spread through the eye if the stye is ruptured. Excessive watering, pain even in low light, trouble seeing, or any stye that becomes very large or eyelids with crusting, scaling, or blistering requires medical attention.

H00.02 Hordeolum internum

A hordeolum internum is an infection of the Meibomian oil gland lining the inside of the eyelid most often due to *Staphylococcus aureus bacteria*. Upper eyelids are more commonly affected with internal styes than lower eyelids. The infection is located more within the tarsal plate, has less skin involvement, and often presents abruptly with a reaction to the bacterial infiltration that is more severe than an external stye. They appear as painful swelling and redness of the eyelid externally. Other symptoms include watery eye, sensitivity to light, and a gritty or scratchy sensation. A red, bumpy area with a central yellowish spot forms on the surface of the conjunctiva. Pus eventually drains through this area, either towards the skin or the conjunctival surface. These styes usually last about 7-10 days, during which most lesions will enlarge and drain spontaneously on the conjunctival, inner side of the eyelid. Applying warm compresses several times a day is done to help facilitate drainage and keep the gland open. Topical antibiotic eye drops may be used to treat the infection, and oral antibiotic treatment may be required in severe cases. Glands that become blocked and swell can cause a Meibomian cyst or chronic chalazion.

H00.03 Abscess of eyelid

An abscess of the eyelid is a pocket of infection producing pus, surrounded by inflamed tissue. The abscess must usually be drained to heal and prevent the spread of infection into the eye itself.

H00.1 Chalazion

Chalazion is a cyst-like lump, or swelling, in the eyelid caused by chronic inflammation or infection of a blocked meibomian gland, which secretes fluid to keep the eye moist. This swelling is usually tender and painful, although not always, and may cause excessive tearing and sensitivity to light. Obstruction of one of the ducts which drains the meibomian gland leads to chalazion, which often occurs after an internal hordeolum (stye) becomes chronic and turns into a cyst. This condition usually resolves itself after a few months without treatment, though if it continues to enlarge, surgical removal may be necessary. Surgical treatment is done by incision of the tarsal gland and curettage of the material blocked within the gland.

H01.0 Blepharitis

Blepharitis is an inflammation of the eyelids, a common condition which presents with burning, itching, irritation, and crusty, flaky skin on the eyelids. In severe cases, it can spread to cause inflammation of the conjunctiva as well.

H01.01 Ulcerative blepharitis

Ulcerative blepharitis is characterized by hard, matted crusts around the eyelashes which result in small sores that may ooze or bleed, as well as loss of eyelashes, changes in the shape of the edges of the eyelids, and excessive tearing.

H01.02 Squamous blepharitis

Squamous blepharitis does not form ulcers, though greasy flaking of the skin may occur at the margins of the lids and around the lashes, sometimes accompanied by excessive sweating from the scalp, brows, and skin behind the ears.

H01.11 Allergic dermatitis of eyelid

Allergic contact dermatitis of the eyelid is inflammation of the skin of the lid with redness, swelling, and itching that may include blisters with fluid drainage or oozing. This occurs at any point on the eyelid, particularly the upper eyelid, where contact is made with an allergenic agent, such as make-up, certain cosmetic ingredients, metals, adhesive glue, latex, dyes, and plants or animals, due to hypersensitization to that particular allergen.

H01.12 Discoid lupus erythematosus of eyelid

Discoid lupus erythematosus (DLE) is a benign, autoimmune disorder of the skin. The face, scalp, and ears are frequently affected. Development of DLE involving the eyelids is not very common and palpebral lesions as the first or sole manifestation of DLE without other cutaneous lesions are very rare and easily lead to misdiagnosis. This is a chronic skin condition that causes inflammation and skin lesions, wounds, discolorations, and other abnormalities which can result in scarring. DLE of the eyelid causes changes in the skin around the lids with thickened, erythematous, scaly, well-defined raised lesions or plaques that may scar, resulting in deformities along the edges of the eyelids. There appears to be a predilection of lesions to affect the lower eyelids. Permanent scarring, atrophy, and eye impairment is often attributed to long-term presence of the disease without proper diagnosis or treatment. The cause of this condition is unknown, but it appears to run in families and affects more women than men. The clinical course of the disease is not constant, but is unpredictable and occurs in repeating periods of remission and flare ups over time. Antimalarial drugs have shown to be quite effective in treating DLE of the eyelid.

H01.13 Eczematous dermatitis of eyelid

Eczematous dermatitis of the eyelid is generally a chronic, inflammatory, non-contagious skin condition appearing on the eyelids. It is characterized by pruritis, or itching, and sometimes a burning sensation that accompanies or precedes redness and rash, with flaking and cracking of the top layer of skin, making it susceptible to infection. The rash may actually arise from scratching in response to the itch. Oily discharge may also accompany a flare-up of the condition, which will then crust over. It may result from some kind of irritant contact, but the exact cause is often unknown.

H01.14 Xeroderma of eyelid

Xeroderma of the eyelids is disorder in which the skin of the eyelids is unable to repair DNA damage done by sunlight. This causes the cells to stop reproducing properly, resulting in thinning of the skin, splotchy pigmentation, visible blood vessels, and leading to cancer. There is no cure for this condition. Treatment centers on trying to protect the skin from further damage.

H02.0 Entropion and trichiasis of eyelid

Entropion and trichiasis of the eyelid are a pair of related conditions. In entropion, the eyelid, usually the bottom one, curls inward towards the eye, so that the margin is pressed against the orb. In trichiasis, the eyelashes curl inward so that they touch the orb. In both cases, irritation of the eye and possible damage to the patient's vision may result.

H02.01 Cicatricial entropion of eyelid

Entropion is an inward rotation of the eyelid margin towards the globe. Cicatricial entropion occurs due to scarring on or around the eyelid as a result of contracture of the tarsoconjunctival tissue with internal rotation of the eyelid. The chronic irritation of the globe comes from the inward-turned eyelashes and/or the margin of the lid when it has become keratinized. Causes of cicatricial entropion are many and include chronic conjunctivitis, ocular herpes zoster, infectious trachoma, surgical correction of lid ptosis, traumatic burns, and other sequelae causing scarring and contraction. Even the long-term use of glaucoma medications applied topically can result in eventual conjunctival contracture and cicatricial entropion. In cicatricial entropion, the abnormal lid margin position will not correct, and there is some degree of tarsoconjunctival scarring. Surgical removal is usually required to stop the lashes and the keratinized lid margin from coming into contact with the globe. Cases caused by utoimmune or inflammatory processes may be treated with lubricating drops and ointments, eyelash ablation, and prevention of symblepharon formation.

H02.02 Mechanical entropion of eyelid

Entropion is an inward rotation of the eyelid margin towards the globe. Mechanical entropion indicates that the inward curvature of the eyelid is occurring as a result of some another condition that is altering the shape or structure of the eye. Many conditions can cause mechanical entropion, particularly of the lower lid, such as abnormalities in the size or position of the globe itself as with enophthalmos or microphthalmos. A tumor beneath the eye can cause lid malformation. There have also been cases of mechanical entropion as a complication of morbid obesity. In many cases, surgery is done to correct the entropion itself, if not the causative condition.

H02.03 Senile entropion of eyelid

Entropion is an inward rotation of the eyelid margin towards the globe. Aging, or the related conditions affecting the skin due to aging, is the cause of senile entropion. As a person ages, the skin loses collagen and produces much less than in younger years. Muscles become more slack and skin loosens. When this loose tone of skin and muscles affects the skin of the eyelid, it causes it to turn inward and the eyelashes rub continually against the eye, causing redness, soreness, and chronic irritation that can lead to corneal abrasions. Senile entropion develops slowly and is not noticed in early stages. The lower eyelid is most often affected, and in most cases, surgery is needed to tighten the muscle and skin around the eye and place stitches that hold the lid back outward.

H02.04 Spastic entropion of eyelid

Entropion is an inward rotation of the eyelid margin towards the globe. In spastic entropion, the lid turns inward as a result of muscle spasms occurring in the lid. The eyelashes then rub continually against the eye, causing redness, soreness, and chronic irritation that can lead to corneal abrasions. Spastic entropion may be caused by other conditions such as dry eye syndrome and blepharitis. The treatment may be different based on the cause. Spastic cases of entropion have not proven to respond well to surgical treatment. Routine lubrication and the use of tear preparations not only help to protect the ocular surface, but sometimes also break the cycle causing spastic entropion in cases caused by dry eye. Blepharitis cases may be treated with extra care for eyelid cleansing with the use of antibiotics and corticosteroids to calm the inflammatory response, clear any infection, and break the cycle causing spastic entropion. In other types of cases, a small amount of injected botox is effective in weakening the orbicularis oculi muscle and calming the spasms.

H02.05 Trichiasis without entropian

Trichiasis without entropion indicates that though the lid itself has not turned inward towards the eye, some or all of the lashes have turned to face the eye, possibly due to the eyelash follicles forming on the wrong side of the lid margin. This condition usually needs to be treated by permanent removal of the afflicting lashes.

H02.1 Ectropion of eyelid

Ectropion is a disorder in which the eyelid, usually the bottom, curls outward away from the eye, often causing dryness and irritation, and possible damage to the patient's vision.

H02.11 Cicatricial ectropion of eyelid

Cicatricial ectropion occurs due to scarring on or around the eyelid that causes it to turn outward away from the eye.

H02.12 Mechanical ectropion of eyelid

Mechanical ectropion indicates that the outward curvature of the eyelid away from the eye is a side-effect of another condition which is altering the shape of the eye, or the condition of the eyelid. For example, a tumor of the skin beneath the eye could cause the lid to malform and curl outward away from the eye.

H02.13 Senile ectropion of eyelid

Senile ectropion occurs in older age, caused by a weakening of the muscles and decreased skin elasticity that causes the eyelid to turn outward away from the eye.

H02.14 Spastic ectropion of eyelid

Spastic ectropion is an outward turning of the eyelid away from the eye due to muscle spasms in the eyelid.

H02.2 Lagophthalmos

Lagophthalmos is a condition in which the patient has difficulty completely closing the eyelid. This can cause dryness of the eye, particularly at night, which can in turn result in inflammation and ulceration of the cornea. In general, this condition is treated by artificial lubrication of the eyes through the use of eye drops.

H02.21 Cicatricial lagophthalmos

Cicatrical lagophthalmos is due to scar tissue hampering the normal closure of the lids.

H02.22 Mechanical lagophthalmos

Mechanical lagophthalmos is due to another condition which alters the normal shape of the lid or eye, making it difficult to close the lids. For example, a patient with protruding corneas might suffer this condition due to the extended area that the lids must cover in order to close completely.

H02.23 Paralytic lagophthalmos

Paralytic lagophthalmos is an inability to close the lids completely due to muscle weakness or paralysis, whether caused by damage to the muscles themselves or to the nerves supplying the muscles of the lids.

H02.3 Blepharochalasis

Blepharochalasis, sometimes called pseudoptosis, is a drooping of the eyelids due to repeated edema (swelling), which causes the lids to lose their normal elasticity. This condition is often confused with actual ptosis, and can only be distinguished by careful examination.

H02.4 Ptosis of eyelid

Drooping or sagging of the upper eyelids. The excess amount of sagging is often caused by nerve damage, weakness in the muscles that raise the eyelid, and loss of elasticity in the skin. In extreme cases, surgery may be done to correct the sagging lid when it is interfering with vision.

H02.41 Mechanical ptosis of eyelid

Mechanical ptosis is drooping or sagging of the eyelid due to another condition which mechanically alters the normal shape, condition, and/or movement of the lid.

H02.42 Myogenic ptosis of eyelid

Myogenic ptosis occurs due to a disorder causing weakness in the muscles of the eyelids themselves.

H02.51 Abnormal innervation syndrome

Abnormal Innervation syndrome is a nervous disorder characterized by an unusual formation in the bundle of nerves which supply the lids, resulting in symptoms ranging from muscle weakness to tics.

H02.52 Blepharophimosis

Blepharophimosis is a hereditary disorder in which the palpebral fissures, the eye slits, or space between the eyelids, become narrowed, giving the patient the appearance of continually squinting. In extreme cases, this can block the patient's normal vision.

H02.53 Eyelid retraction

Lid retraction or lid lag is a condition in which the lower lid droops below the cornea, exposing the white of the eye. This is a common condition due to age, thyroid disease, or botched plastic surgery. It rarely presents with serious side-effects, but is unpleasant cosmetically and may cause some dryness of the eye.

H02.59 Other disorders affecting eyelid function

Sensorimotor disorders are those which affect the sensitivity of the eyelid and the motion of the eyelid. For example, a disorder preventing the brain from recognizing when the eyes are too dry and it is time to blink will affect the normal blink reflex so that the patient does not blink often enough to moisten the eye.

H02.60 Xanthelasma of unspecified eye, unspecified eyelid

Xanthelasma is a common skin disorder in which deposits of fatty materials build up under the skin, creating a yellowish patch of skin that is often impregnated with red or white nodules. While not dangerous, these deposits are cosmetically unattractive and may be removed surgically.

H02.7 Other and unspecified degenerative disorders of eyelid and periocular area

Disorders and disease processes which cause deterioration of the eyelid or area of the face around the eyes.

H02.71 Chloasma of eyelid and periocular area

Chloasma indicates hyperpigmentation of the eyelid in which excess coloration on the eyelid may or may not spread to the skin surrounding the eye. This pigmentation is not dangerous, but can give the eyes a sunken or tired look.

H02.72 Madarosis of eyelid and periocular area

Madarosis is the absence or excessive loss of the eyelashes and even the eyebrows in some cases. This can be caused by infection, autoimmune disease, or mechanical means. Hypotrichosis can cause complications and damage to the eye, insofar as the eyelashes help to protect the eye from foreign material.

H02.73 Vitiligo of eyelid and periocular area

Vitiligo is a condition of loss of skin pigmentation (hypo- or depigmentation) in the eyelid. This condition may occur in segments or patches of skin that gives the eyes a pale, ghostly appearance in comparison to the surrounding skin. The lack of functioning melanocytes also leaves the skin highly susceptible to radiation damage from sun exposure. The condition may be treated with an epithelial skin graft containing melanocytes.

H02.81 Retained foreign body in eyelid

A retained foreign body in the eyelid is an object, such as a splinter, which has become buried beneath the skin of the eye. Such an object can cause infection and blindness if not removed.

H02.82 Cysts of eyelid

A cyst of the eyelid is a pocket of fluid surrounded by inflamed tissue, which must often be surgically drained to heal.

H02.83 Dermatochalasis of eyelid

Dermatochalasis is a disorder in which excess, lax skin and muscle grow on and around the eyelids. This excess skin can obstruct the patient's peripheral vision. This is a common condition in the elderly.

H02.84 Edema of eyelid

Edema of the eyelid indicates swelling due to fluid retention. This condition will usually resolve itself without treatment.

H02.85 Elephantiasis of eyelid

Elephantiasis of the eyelid is a disorder in which the eyelid becomes permanently swollen, usually due to chronic blockage of the lymphatic system, which causes a continual build-up of fluid and tissue. This condition must be surgically corrected.

H02.86 Hypertrichosis of eyelid

Hypertrichosis of the eyelid is excessive eyelash growth.

H02.87 Vascular anomalies of eyelid

Vascular anomalies of the eyelid may include a number of disorders, ranging from insufficient blood flow through the vessels to enlarged, visible blood vessels.

H04.0 Dacryoadenitis

Dacryoadenitis is an inflammation of the lacrimal gland. It presents with pain and swelling of the gland, which is seen as a swelling of the skin over the gland, excessive tearing, and a swelling of the lymph nodes just in front of the ear. This disorder may be caused by an infection, in which case warm compresses and/or antobiotics may be all the treatment required, or by another cause such as blockage of the lacrimal ducts, in which case other treatments may be needed.

H04.01 Acute dacryoadenitis

Acute dacryodenitis is a sudden, severe inflammation of the lacrimal gland, usually due to infection. This type of inflammation will normally resolve itself as the infection is dealt cleared.

H04.02 Chronic dacryoadenitis

Ongoing inflammation of the lacrimal gland is less severe than an acute case and may last for months or even years. This type of inflammation is often associated with a blockage of the lacrimal ducts that backs up tear production within the gland.

H04.03 Chronic enlargement of lacrimal gland

Chronic enlargement of the lacrimal gland is not necessarily painful and may be due to a systemic disease or neoplastic growth.

H04.11 Dacryops

The lacrimal system is comprised of two lacrimal glands which produce lacrimal fluid, or tears, that are secreted onto the surface of the eye from the gland through its many tiny excretory ducts. The lacrimal sac in the corner of the eye at the distal end of the nasolacrimal duct receives the tears through the lacrimal canaliculi, the tube-shaped passages, or ducts beginning at the tiny openings, called punctum, in the upper and lower lids. The fluid is then drained into the cavity of the nose through the nasolacrimal duct. A fluid-filled pocket or cyst with possible infection that develops in these tear-producing glands is called dacryops. Dacryops may be painless or it may present with ongoing pain and discomfort, and a visible white or bluish cyst in the eye often at the outer canthus below the upper eyelid. The cyst usually requires surgical removal.

H04.12 Dry eye syndrome

Tear-film insufficiency, called dry-eye syndrome, in which the eye is unable to maintain a sufficient amount of tearing and moisture in order for the surface of the eye to be properly lubricated and prevent becoming dry. This causes anything from subtle irritation to inflammation of the tissues in the front of the eye. The patient experiences persistent dryness, scratchiness, redness, and a burning sensation in the eye.

H04.13 Lacrimal cyst

The lacrimal system is comprised of two lacrimal glands which produce lacrimal fluid, or tears, that are secreted onto the surface of the eye from the gland through its many tiny excretory ducts. The lacrimal sac in the corner of the eye at the distal end of the nasolacrimal duct receives the tears through the lacrimal canaliculi, the tube-shaped passages, or ducts beginning at the tiny openings, called punctum, in the upper and lower lids. The fluid is then drained into the cavity of the nose through the nasolacrimal duct. A fluid-filled pocket or cyst with possible infection may develop in any location of the system where lacrimal gland tissue is present, such as the (naso)lacrimal ducts or sacs. Treatment may range from local area massage, to antibiotics, to lacrimal duct probing, or nasal endoscopy with cyst marsupialization.

H04.14 Primary lacrimal gland atrophy

Lacrimal atrophy is wasting away of the lacrimal glands, which can cause severe dryness of the eyes as tear production decreases. Primary atrophy is not caused by another systemic disease or disorder.

H04.15 Secondary lacrimal gland atrophy

Lacrimal atrophy is wasting away of the lacrimal glands, which can cause severe dryness of the eyes as tear production decreases. This type of atrophy is secondary to another disease process.

H04.16 Lacrimal gland dislocation

A lacrimal gland that becomes separated from the excretory tear ducts, preventing the tears produced in the gland from passing normally into the eye.

H04.2 Epiphora

Epiphora is excessive tearing of the eye. This can be caused by an overproduction of tears from an enlargement of the glands, or distention (widening) of the ducts. Excessive tearing may also be the result of an inability of the eye to drain the tears away normally. The causative reason may require surgical correction to prevent the epiphora.

H04.21 Epiphora due to excess lacrimation

Excessive tearing caused by the overproduction of tears in the lacrimal gland coming through the excretory ducts into the eyes.

H04.22 Epiphora due to insufficient drainage

Excessive tearing due to insufficient drainage of tears from the eye through the lacrimal canaliculi that may be due to malformation, blockage, foreign body, or inflammation of the tear ducts.

H04.30 Unspecified dacryocystitis

Inflammation of the lacrimal sac, the dilated upper portion of the nasolacrimal duct in the corner of the eye that receives the tears drained through the punctum in the eyelids via the lacrimal ducts.

H04.31 Phlegmonous dacryocystitis

Phlegmonous dacryocystitis is an inflammation of the tear sac in which there is a build-up of pus, similar to an abscess. Surgical drainage of the pus is usually necessary.

H04.32 Acute dacryocystitis

Acute dacryocystitis is a sudden, severe, suppurative inflammation of the lacrimal sac, often following chronic blockage of the nasolacrimal duct or exudative rhinitis. The causative infecting organism may be staphylococcus, streptococcus, or pneumococcus. The patient experiences pain in the affected eye; a red, hot, diffuse swelling at the margin of the eyelids; infected discharge (pus); excessive watering of the eye; and fever and malaise.

H04.33 Acute lacrimal canaliculitis

Acute lacrimal canaliculitis is a severe, sudden inflammation of the passages or ducts which drain tears from the eyes into the lacrimal sac through the tiny punctum in the eyelids. It presents with reddening of the eye, pain and swelling of the eyelid, and a watery discharge back out of the tear ducts.

H04.41 Chronic dacryocystitis

Chronic dacryocystitis is a long-term, ongoing inflammation of the lacrimal sac in the corner of the eye, often due to blockage of the nasolacrimal duct that drains the tears received in the sac down into the cavity of the nose. This is the most common disorder affecting the lacrimal sac.

H04.42 Chronic lacrimal canaliculitis

Chronic lacrimal canaliculitis is an on going inflammation of the passages or ducts that drain tears from the eyes into the lacrimal sac through the tiny punctum in the eyelids. It presents with reddening of the eye that may be painful, swelling of the eyelid, and a watery discharge back out of the tear ducts.

H04.51 Dacryolith

A dacryolith is a lacrimal stone. It forms via excess mineral deposits in the lacrimal system, and can cause severe pain and inflammation. As it forms in one of the canals (most often the nasolacrimal duct), it can also cause blockage and other complications. Depending on the location and size of the stone, surgery may be necessary to remove it.

H04.52 Eversion of lacrimal punctum

Eversion of the lacrimal punctum is a condition in which the tiny exit in the margin of the eyelid that opens into the tear duct for drainage is turned away from the eye, so that natural tears flow directly onto the face instead of draining into the nasal cavity through the lacrimal ducts.

H04.53 Neonatal obstruction of nasolacrimal duct

Neonatal obstruction of the nasolacrimal duct is a condition found in infancy in which the duct that carries tears received in the lacrimal sac away to drain into the nasal cavity becomes blocked, causing swelling and excessive wateriness of the eyes. The obstruction often must be surgically removed.

H04.54 Stenosis of lacrimal canaliculi

Stenosis of the lacrimal canaliculi is an abnormal narrowing of the ducts that drain tears away from the eye through the tiny punctum of the eyelids into the lacrimal sac. The narrowed lumen of the tear ducts decreases the amount of natural tears that are effectively drained away from the eye, causing some flow directly onto the face instead of into the nasal cavity through the lacrimal ducts.

H04.55 Acquired stenosis of nasolacrimal duct

Acquired stenosis of the nasolacrimal duct is a condition in which the tear duct that carries tears drained from the eye away to the nasal cavity becomes narrowed, causing swelling and excessive wateriness of the eyes.

H04.56 Stenosis of lacrimal punctum

Stenosis of the lacrimal punctum is an abnormal narrowing of the tiny exits, or orifices in the corner of the eyelids where the lacrimal duct begin that drain normal tears from the eyes into the lacrimal sac and away into the nasal cavity. These openings into the lacrimal ducts are already very minute and any narrowing causes insufficient drainage with excessive watering of the eyes.

H04.61 Lacrimal fistula

A lacrimal fistula is an abnormal channel that forms between some part of the lacrimal system and another open space, often the outer skin. This connection usually results from a severe infection which pits the inner surface of the lacrimal gland or ducts, and must usually be drained of any pus or other discharge and surgically closed.

H04.81 Granuloma of lacrimal passages

A granuloma of the lacrimal passages is a nodular, inflamed lesion within the canaliculi or ducts of the lacrimal system. It usually appears as a result of a bacterial infection, and may partially or completely block one of the tear ducts. In some cases, surgical drainage of the granuloma may be necessary.

H05 Disorders of orbit

This category is used to report disorders of the eye orbit, the bony structure that contains the eye, and its external structures. The eye cavity, which is part of the orbit, is also known as the eye socket.

H05.01 Cellulitis of orbit

Orbital cellulitis is a condition which occurs when the fatty tissue around the eyeball, usually between the eye socket and the eyeball, becomes infected.

H05.02 Osteomyelitis of orbit

Orbital osteomyelitis is an inflammation of the bone of the eye socket.

H05.03   Periostitis of orbit

Orbital periostitis is an inflammation of the fibrous membrane that lines the orbital bone.

H05.04   Tenonitis of orbit

Tenonitis is an inflammation of the episcleral space, the gap between the outer sheath of the eye and the fibrous membrane of the sclera.

H05.12   Orbital myositis

Orbital myositis is an inflammation of the muscles that move the eyeball.

H05.2   Exophthalmic conditions

Exophthalmic conditions are those that cause the eyball to protrude outward in the eye socket, giving the eye a bulging appearance.

H05.20   Unspecified exophthalmos

An abnormal protrusion of the eyeball.

H05.21   Displacement (lateral) of globe

Lateral displacement of the globe is a condition in which the eyeball is situated towards the side of the head, away from the nose.

H05.22   Edema of orbit

Orbital edema is swelling of the orbit from an abnormal build-up of fluid (other than blood) behind the eye, causing it to protrude forward.

H05.23   Hemorrhage of orbit

Bleeding from the orbit of the eye. The accumulated blood creates pressure which causes the eyeball to protrude from the eye socket.

H05.24   Constant exophthalmos

A chronic state in which the eyeball continuously protrudes from its socket.

H05.25   Intermittent exophthalmos

Intermittent exophthalmos is a condition in which the eyeball alternately protrudes out of the eye socket, and then returns to its proper position for a time before protruding again.

H05.26   Pulsating exophthalmos

Pulsating exophthalmos is a condition in which the bulging of the eyeball is caused by either a fistula, or abnormal passage, located at the back of the eyeball, or an abnormality of the blood vessels. In both cases, the result is a regular pulsing of the eye in time with the heartbeat.

H05.31   Atrophy of orbit

In atrophy of the eye orbit, the bones of the eye socket waste away, causing deformity in the shape of the socket and putting the eye in jeopardy with its loss of bony protection.

H05.35   Exostosis of orbit

Exostosis of the eye orbit is a condition in which there is abnormal bone growth of the eye socket. The increased thickness of bone may occur in patchy areas and the condition can push on the globe, impair vision, and prevent the eye from moving properly in its orbit.

H05.4   Enophthalmos

Enophthalmos is a condition in which the eye is recessed abnormally deep within the eye socket.

H05.5   Retained (old) foreign body following penetrating wound of orbit

A foreign body left in the eye socket from an old injury or trauma in which the foreign body was allowed to remain due to the risks of removing it, or one which escaped detection during care of the original injury and remained in place.

Note: Use an additional code to identify the particular type of retained foreign body.

H05.82   Myopathy of extraocular muscles

Myopathy of extraocular muscles is a disease process that affects the muscles that control the movement of the eye, causing pain, twitching, and/or paralysis of the eye globe.

H10   Conjunctivitis

The conjunctiva is a thin, transparent membrane which covers and protects the sclera, the white of the eye, as well as the inside of the eyelids. It also secretes oils and fluids which moisten and lubricate the eye. One of the most common disorders of this membrane is conjunctivitis, sometimes called pink-eye, an inflammation that presents with the tell-tale pink coloration of the white of the eye, swelling and irritation, and excessive tearing. Conjunctivitis caused by an infection typically begins in one eye and spreads to the other and is highly contagious for other people, while conjunctivitis caused by an allergic reaction usually affects both eyes at the same time.

H10.0   Mucopurulent conjunctivitis

Mucopurulent conjunctivitis is associated with the production of mucus and pus.

H10.01   Acute follicular conjunctivitis

Acute follicular conjunctivitis presents with follicles in the pinkened conjunctiva. These follicles appear as gray-white, round, elevated patches of tissue, caused by infiltration of the lymphatic system by the infection. These symptoms are usually associated with viral conjunctivitis.

H10.1   Acute atopic conjunctivitis

Acute atopic conjunctivitis is a sudden, severe case of conjunctivitis caused by allergies.

H10.21   Acute toxic conjunctivitis

Acute toxic conjunctivitis or acute chemical conjunctivitis is known as pink eye and occurs as the result of any irritating substance entering the eye. The most common types of irritants include household cleaning products, sprays, smoke, smog, industrial strength pollutants, and chlorine in swimming pools. Even though chemically induced pink eye is not as serious as an alkali or acid burn, the condition can still endanger a patient's eyesight.

Note: The code to identify the specific chemical and intent must be assigned first. This code is not to be confused with a chemically-induced corrosive injury to the eye, nor does it include burns of the eye and adnexa

H10.22   Pseudomembranous conjunctivitis

Pseudomembranous conjunctivitis presents with an additional thin membrane which forms over the conjunctiva of the eye and eyelid. This membrane can be removed without causing damage to the conjunctiva. It is most common in bacterial infections, but can also be caused by viral, toxic, or allergic conjunctivitis.

H10.23   Serous conjunctivitis, except viral

Serous conjunctivitis indicates that the conjunctivitis presents with a thin, watery discharge in addition to the usual symptoms.

H10.3   Unspecified acute conjunctivitis

Acute conjunctivitis is a sudden, severe occurrence of the disease which will usually resolve itself relatively quickly.

H10.4   Chronic conjunctivitis

Chronic conjunctivitis is usually less severe than acute conjunctivitis, but occurs in repeating episodes over a period of months or years. Most cases are due to the staphylococcus or streptococcus viruses.

H10.43   Chronic follicular conjunctivitis

Chronic follicular conjunctivitis presents with follicles in the pinkened conjunctiva. These follicles appear as gray-white, round, elevated patches of tissue, caused by infiltration of the lymphatic system by the infection. These symptoms are usually associated with viral conjunctivitis.

Diseases of the Eye and Adnexa

H10.44 – H11.82

H10.44   Vernal conjunctivitis

Vernal conjunctivitis is a seasonal inflammation of the conjunctiva, almost always due to an allergic reaction to pollen, mold, or other seasonal factor.

H10.5   Blepharoconjunctivitis

Blepharoconjunctivitis is conjunctivitis combined with blepharitis, an inflammation of the eyelids.

H10.52   Angular blepharoconjunctivitis

Angular blepharoconjunctivitis is most severe at the juncture between the upper and lower eyelids, presenting as a scaly patch on the outside corner of the eye.

H10.53   Contact blepharoconjunctivitis

Contact blepharoconjunctivitis is an inflammation of the conjunctiva and eyelid due to wearing contact lenses.

H10.81   Pingueculitis

Pingueculae are yellowish, raised areas of limbal conjunctival tissue, usually seen in middle-aged patients with a history of chronic sun exposure. Normally, they remain asymptomatic, but can become acutely vascularized, irritated, and inflamed. Pingueculitis may then cause corneal thinning or corneal punctate epitheliopathy.

H11.0   Pterygium of eye

A pterygium is a raised, wedge-shaped overgrowth of the conjunctiva onto the cornea of the eye. In addition to the visible overgrowth, this condition may also cause irritation, redness, and excessive tearing. As the pterygium develops, it may distort the shape of the cornea, causing astigmatism, or may grow into the patient's vision, requiring surgery to remove it.

H11.02   Central pterygium of eye

A central pterygium is one which has grown into the center of the cornea, entering the patient's visual field.

H11.03   Double pterygium of eye

A double pterygium indicates that the overgrowth of the conjunctiva is taking place in two separate points around the cornea, often at opposite sides from each other.

H11.04   Peripheral pterygium of eye, stationary

A stationary pterygium is one which is not progressing, but is instead remaining on the periphery of the cornea.

H11.05   Peripheral pterygium of eye, progressive

A progressive pterygium has marked growth over time.

H11.06   Recurrent pterygium of eye

A recurrent pterygium is one which, following surgery to remove it from overgrowing the cornea, has regrown.

H11.1   Conjunctival degenerations and deposits

Deterioration of the conjunctiva due to a disease process, or mineral deposits within it.

H11.11   Conjunctival deposits

Mineral deposits which form in the conjunctiva.

H11.12   Conjunctival concretions

Conjunctival concretions are yellow-white granules or cysts which form just beneath the conjunctiva. As they wear away the surface of the conjunctiva above, they can present with the sensation of having a foreign body in the eye. They are easily removed.

H11.13   Conjunctival pigmentations

Conjunctival pigmentations can occur as a result of mineral deposits forming in the conjunctiva that alter its color.

H11.14   Conjunctival xerosis, unspecified

Conjunctival xerosis is a disorder in which the conjunctiva becomes dry, usually due to a vitamin A deficiency. If left untreated, this condition can lead to the formation of an ulcer in the cornea, xerophthalmia (dry eyes, extending to the layers below the conjunctiva), and keratomalacia (dryness and damage to the cornea). In some cases, Bitot's spots, small, greyish-white raised spots, may form and should be coded separately.

H11.15   Pinguecula

Pingueculae are yellowish, raised areas of limbal conjunctival tissue, usually seen in middle-aged patients with a history of chronic sun exposure. Normally, they remain asymptomatic and require no treatment, but they can become acutely vascularized and cause irritation.

H11.21   Conjunctival adhesions and strands (localized)

Localized adhesions and strands of the conjunctiva most often form between the membrane of the lids and the globe of the eye, forming a fiber-like connection between the two.

H11.22   Conjunctival granuloma

A granuloma of the conjunctiva is a nodular, inflamed lesion on the conjunctiva of the eye. It usually forms as a result of bacterial infection in a scratch in the conjunctiva.

H11.23   Symblepharon

Symblepharon is a condition in which the conjunctiva of one or both lids adheres to the eye, often partially or completely over the cornea. This overgrowth must typically be surgically removed.

H11.3   Conjunctival hemorrhage

Conjunctival hemorrhage is not in and of itself a serious condition, and may occur spontaneously as a result of straining, sneezing, or coughing. When a blood vessel supplying the conjunctiva bursts, the blood becomes trapped beneath it, pooling in a manner similar to a bruise and giving part or all of the white of the eye a red appearance. This normally resolves on its own after one to two weeks.

H11.41   Vascular abnormalities of conjunctiva

Vascular abnormalities of the conjunctiva can include a wide variety of syndromes, including aneurysms, dilated or constricted blood vessels, blood clots, etc.

H11.42   Conjunctival edema

Swelling of the conjunctiva due to fluid retention.

H11.43   Conjunctival hyperemia

Hyperemia of the conjunctiva is a redness of the eyes due to an increased blood flow into and congestion of the vessels supplying the conjunctiva rather than due to infection.

H11.44   Conjunctival cysts

A conjunctival cyst is a pocket of (possibly infected) fluid surrounded by inflamed tissue within the conjunctiva of the eye. A cyst may require drainage to prevent damage to the eye.

H11.81   Pseudopterygium of conjunctiva

A pseudopterygium is a small overgrowth of the conjunctiva over the cornea. Unlike a pterygium, it lacks firm adhesion to the cornea, and usually develops as the eye heals from an injury, such as a burn, in order to protect a thinned or scarred portion of the cornea. This disorder usually requires no treatment.

H11.82   Conjunctivochalasis

Conjunctivochalasis is a degenerative condition in which the conjunctiva's attachment to the eye loosens, causing a wrinkled appearance. It presents with dryness of the eyes and a tendency to trap particles in the folds, causing a chronic inflammatory state.

H15.0 Scleritis

Scleritis is an inflammation of the sclera, which is the fibrous outer covering of the eye (i.e., the white of the eye).

H15.01 Anterior scleritis

Anterior scleritis is an inflammation occurring in the front of the white of the eye above and below the cornea.

H15.02 Brawny scleritis

Brawny scleritis is a severe inflammation of the sclera that also affects the border between the sclera and the cornea.

H15.03 Posterior scleritis

Posterior sclerosis is an inflammation of the white of the eye at the rear of the eyeball.

H15.05 Scleromalacia perforans

Scleromalacia perforans is a condition that often occurs with severe rheumatoid arthritis or in patients with recurrent cases of scleritis. Also known as necrotizing scleritis, this is a serious condition and the most severe form of scleritis. It results in dangerous thinning of the sclera, either with or without inflammation, that can lead to loss of the eye.

H15.1 Episcleritis

Episcleritis is an irritation, inflammation, or infection of the episclera, the thin, protective membrane covering the white of the eye that connects the sclera to the conjunctiva.

H15.11 Episcleritis periodica fugax

Episcleritis periodica fugax is an often chronic condition in which the patient suffers from periodic attacks of inflammation of the sclera. These attacks typically have a rapid onset and a short duration.

H15.12 Nodular episcleritis

Nodular episcleritis is an inflammation of the outermost protective membrane overlying the sclera, with the formation of small nodules on the surface of the eye.

H15.81 Equatorial staphyloma

Equatorial staphyloma is a condition in which the sclera bulges outwards around the middle of the eye due to softening caused by inflammation.

H15.82 Localized anterior staphyloma

Anterior staphyloma is a localized spot on the front of the eye where the sclera bulges outward due to abnormal softening, usually caused by an inflammation.

H15.83 Staphyloma posticum

Staphyloma posticum is a condition in which the sclera bulges outwards at the back of the eye due to abnormal softening, often caused by inflammation.

H15.84 Scleral ectasia

Scleral ectasia is a condition in which the contents of the eyeball protrude through an abnormally thin section of the sclera.

H15.85 Ring staphyloma

In ring staphyloma, a ring-shaped area of the white of the eye bulges outwards around the center of the eye, usually due to abnormal softening caused by an inflammation.

H16 Keratitis

Keratitis is a term used to indicate a wide variety of infections and inflammations of the cornea. The cornea is the transparent part of the eye in front that covers the iris, the pupil, and the anterior chamber. The cornea also refracts light and is responsible for about two thirds of the eye's focusing power, even though it is fixed, and not adjustable like the lens.

H16.0 Corneal ulcer

A corneal ulcer is commonly caused by a bacterial or fungal infection after an otherwise superficial abrasion (scrape) of the cornea. In some cases, it may be linked to a vitamin A deficiency. Corneal ulcers present with redness of the eye; severe pain; the feeling that there is something in the eye; tears, pus, or other thick liquid draining from the eye; blurred vision; photophobia (pain caused by bright lights); and swollen eyelids. The ulcer itself may be visible as a white patch.

H16.01 Central corneal ulcer

A central corneal ulcer appears within the patient's field of vision and may directly interfere with sight.

H16.02 Ring corneal ulcer

A ring corneal ulcer encircles the entire edge of the cornea.

H16.03 Corneal ulcer with hypopyon

A hypopyon ulcer results in the accumulation of pus or other thick liquid discharge on the inside surface of the cornea.

H16.04 Marginal corneal ulcer

A marginal corneal ulcer appears as a patch towards one side of the cornea.

H16.05 Mooren's corneal ulcer

Mooren's ulcer appears at the juncture between the cornea and the sclera, the white of the eye, though if left untreated can spread across the surface of the cornea, resulting in blindness. This is an autoimmune disorder, in which the body's own immune system attacks the cornea, and is seen more often in men than in women, and is most common in the elderly.

H16.06 Mycotic corneal ulcer

A mycotic corneal ulcer is caused by a fungal infection.

H16.07 Perforated corneal ulcer

A perforated corneal ulcer is one in which the tissue damage and loss has passed through all layers of the cornea, resulting in a hole that directly connects the anterior chamber of the eye (the space between the iris and lens and the cornea) with the outside. This will often result in the leakage of ocular fluid, which can cause the eye to lose pressure, as well as become infected.

H16.1 Other and unspecified superficial keratitis without conjunctivitis

Superficial keratitis which does not present with conjunctivitis (inflammation of the protective membrane that covers the white of the eye) usually presents with painful, bloodshot, watery eyes sensitive to bright light, blurred vision, and a sensation of having something in the eye.

H16.11 Macular keratitis

Macular keratitis, also called areolar or nummular keratosis, is an inflammation of the cornea which appears as a circular film on the cornea that obscures the patient's vision, in addition to presenting with the common symptoms of keratitis.

H16.12 Filamentary keratitis

Filamentary keratitis is an inflammation of the cornea characterized by the development of tiny hair-like structures.

H16.13 Photokeratitis

Photokeratitis is a painful, inflamed cornea that develops due to over-exposure to ultraviolet light. Snow-blindness (due to the glare of the sun off the snow) and welders' keratitis both fall under this category. It can also afflict patients who have been over-exposed to sunglare off the water.

H16.14 Punctate keratitis

Punctate keratitis is an inflammatory condition caused by the death of cells on the surface of the cornea, which causes fiber-like deposits to form. It may be caused by a viral or bacterial infection, dry eyes, exposure to chemicals, over-exposure to ultraviolet light (e.g., from the sun), overuse of contact lenses, or from an allergy to eye-drops.

H16.2 Keratoconjunctivitis

Keratoconjunctivitis is an inflammation of both the cornea and the conjunctiva, the protective membrane that surrounds the white of the eye. It presents with (burning) painful, bloodshot, watery eyes, sensitivity to bright light, blurred vision, and a sensation of having something in the eye.

H16.21 Exposure keratoconjunctivitis

Exposure keratoconjunctivitis is a dryness and inflammation of the cornea and conjunctiva caused by the failure of the eyelid to close completely during sleep and/or with blinking.

H16.22 Keratoconjunctivitis sicca, not specified as Sjögren's

Keratoconjunctivitis sicca, sometimes called dry-eye syndrome, is a condition in which decreased production by the tear glands or increased evaporation of the tears has led to a dry, thickened cornea and conjunctiva. This disorder is common in older patients.

Note: This disorder excludes Sjögren syndrome.

H16.23 Neurotrophic keratoconjunctivitis

Neurotrophic keratoconjunctivitis is a rare, degenerative disease of the cornea and conjunctiva caused by impairment of the trigeminal nerve. This loss of corneal innervation causes significantly decreased or absent corneal sensation. The resulting anesthesia develops into inflammation and corneal epithelial defects without spontaneous healing. The dystrophic defects progress to ulceration and perforation. The most common cause of neurotrophic corneal anesthesia is herpes viral infection. Lesions that compress the trigeminal nerve are also possible causes, as are systemic diseases affecting the nervous system, such as diabetes and multiple sclerosis.

H16.24 Ophthalmia nodosa

Ophthalmia nodosa indicates the presence of nodules arising on the conjunctiva, the thin membrane that protects the white of the eye, due to the hairs of a caterpillar, tarantula, or similar organism penetrating the tissues of the eye.

H16.25 Phlyctenular keratoconjunctivitis

Phlyctenular keratoconjunctivitis is an inflammation of both the cornea and the conjunctiva caused by an allergic hypersensitivity response to microbial antigens, such as staphylococcus, mycobacteria, tuberculosis, and chlamydia. It is more common in children and presents with small, yellow-gray, discrete nodules called phlyctenules along the corneal limbus, the cornea, or the conjunctiva. These nodules persist up to two weeks. On the conjunctiva, ulceration that heals without a scar occurs. When the cornea is affected, it results in blurred vision, copious lacrimation, light sensitivity, aching, and the sensation of a foreign body. Subsequent recurrences with infection can lead to corneal opacity and loss of visual acuity.

H16.26 Vernal keratoconjunctivitis, with limbar and corneal involvement

Vernal keratoconjunctivitis is a recurring, bilateral, ocular inflammation that occurs with seasonal incidence. This self-limiting, allergic inflammation is known as springtime keratoconjunctivitis and affects young boys in particular causing itching, burning, and tearing in the eyes, along with photophobia. Swift diagnosis and treatment is necessary to help prevent possible secondary corneal damage, glaucoma, or cataract. The pathogenesis is thought to have multiple factors involving the immune system and mast cells, lymphocytes, and eosinophils; the nervous system and neural substances; and the endocrine system and sex hormones.

H16.31 Corneal abscess

A corneal abscess is a pocket of infected material surrounded by infected and inflamed tissue within the layers of the cornea. Such a pocket usually has to be surgically drained to heal, and will usually result in significant loss of vision.

H16.32 Diffuse interstitial keratitis

Diffuse interstitial keratitis is an inflammation of the middle layers of the cornea which may cause deposits to form that can obscure the patient's vision. This type of inflammation is called Cogan's syndrome if the inflammation spreads to the inner ears, where it can cause permanent hearing loss.

H16.33 Sclerosing keratitis

Sclerosing keratitis is an inflammation characterized by thickening and hardening of the cornea. This is usually a chronic disorder, and over time causes the cornea to become scarred and opaque, leading to blindness.

H16.4 Corneal neovascularization

Neovascularization is a process in which the body produces new, abnormal growth of blood vessels. Neovascularization of the cornea can result in loss of visual acuity as the new vessels interfere with light passing through the cornea.

H16.41 Ghost vessels (corneal)

Ghost vessels occur when the oxygen demands which set off neovascularization in the first place are met. Blood then ceases to flow through the new vessels, leaving them with a pale, translucent appearance which can obscure the vision when occurring in the cornea.

H16.42 Pannus (corneal)

Pannus indicates neovascularization just beneath the epithelium, the outer membrane, of the cornea. This growth of new vessels may be accompanied by the appearance of granulated (small and hard) tissue, and may be either very thick, causing the cornea to become opaque (pannus crassus); very dry (pannus siccus); or very thin, causing little visual disruption (pannus tenuis).

H16.43 Localized vascularization of cornea

Localized vascularization of the cornea indicates that there has only been partial or limited new vessel growth into the cornea. At this stage, the patient's visual acuity is usually not affected noticeably.

H16.44 Deep vascularization of cornea

Deep vascularization of the cornea indicates that the new vessel growth is very thick, obscuring the patient's vision and giving the cornea an opaque appearance.

H17 Corneal scars and opacities

While scratches to the surface of the cornea are painful, they usually resolve without any permanent scarring. However, injuries or diseases that penetrate to the inner layers of the cornea more often result in scarring, which can cause part or all of the cornea to become whitish and opaque, obscuring the patient's vision.

H17.0 Adherent leukoma

An adherent leukoma is a thick, opaque overgrowth of the cornea onto the iris. In addition to blocking peripheral vision in the area of the overgrowth, this can interfere with the iris' ability to dilate and contract properly.

H17.1 Central corneal opacity

Central opacity of the cornea is a whitish, clouded over area that forms in the center of the cornea, blocking the central vision.

H17.81 Minor opacity of cornea

Minor opacity of the cornea does not cover the whole cornea, but appears as a cloud in one part of it; for this reason, it may be called a corneal nebula.

H17.82 Peripheral opacity of cornea

Peripheral opacity of the cornea forms in a ring-shape around part or all of the edge of the cornea, while not interfering with central vision.

H18.0 Corneal pigmentations and deposits

Corneal pigmentation is caused by mineral deposits (often granular copper deposits) on or within the cornea, which can obscure vision as they build up over time. Pigmentation is distinguished from scarring by the fact that little or no actual physical damage to the eye results, although vision can still be affected since the cornea does refract light and provides a lot of the eye's focusing power.

H18.01 Anterior corneal pigmentations

Anterior pigmentations appear on the exterior (or forward) surface of the cornea, and are usually identified by a particular pattern of streaking called Stahli's lines. This particular form of pigmentation usually results from blood staining the cornea.

H18.02 Argentous corneal deposits

Argentous deposits are silver deposits that appear in the cornea.

H18.04 Kayser-Fleischer ring

A Kayser-Fleischer ring is a gray-green or brownish ring of copper deposits which appear on the exterior of the cornea first, slowly growing inward. This type of corneal pigmentation is often seen in liver disorders.

H18.05 Posterior corneal pigmentations

Posterior pigmentation appears on the inner layer of the cornea, closest to the iris.

H18.06 Stromal corneal pigmentations

Stromal pigmentations are those in which the deposits appear in the internal layers of the cornea which affects the focusing power that the cornea provides.

H18.1 Bullous keratopathy

Bullous keratopathy is a pathological condition of permanent edema, or swelling, of the cornea with the formation of fluid-filled, blister-like vesicles, or bullae, in the corneal epithelium. The blisters cause pain and can rupture and decrease visual acuity. Bullous keratopathy occurs when the corneal endothelial cells are damaged and can no longer keep the cornea from absorbing excess fluid by pumping it back into the aqueous. The cause of this damage has changed over the years and used to be common due to cataract surgery and certain intraocular lens implants. Surgery techniques and lens designs was improved so much in the last twenty years, that bullous keratopathy is seen more as trauma resulting from acute angle-closure glaucoma surgery when the cornea is directly damaged or decompensates after laser treatment.

H18.2 Other and unspecified corneal edema

Corneal edema is a swelling of the cornea due to an excessive amount of fluid in its cells. This swelling is almost always accompanied by clouding of the cornea, obscuring the patient's vision.

H18.3 Changes of corneal membranes

Changes of the corneal membranes include both folds and ruptures, either of which will result in lost visual acuity and distorted vision. These are often due to an underlying disease or other cause.

H18.31 Folds and rupture in Bowman's membrane

Folds and/or ruptures of Bowman's membrane affect the membrane just beneath the epithelium, the outermost layer of cells on the cornea. This membrane is comprised of strong fibers which help the cornea to maintain its shape.

H18.32 Folds in Descemet's membrane

Descemet's membrane lies between the endothelium, the innermost layer of cells in the cornea, and the stroma, a strong supportive layer. When the cornea becomes distended, such as in cases of corneal edema, particularly following phacoemulsification surgery or other intraocular procedures such as for glaucoma or corneal transplant, folds may appear in this membrane that can affect vision, as well as prevent the flow of nutrients to the rest of the cornea. The folds appear as deep, dark, criss-cross lines in the membrane and posterior stroma with loss of transparency from the edema, that may or may not be reversible after the edema has resolved.

H18.33 Rupture in Descemet's membrane

Descemet's membrane lies between the endothelium, the innermost layer of cells in the cornea, and the stroma, a strong supportive layer. When the cornea becomes distended, such as in cases of corneal edema, postoperative inflammation, or congenital glaucoma, the stroma and the epithelium can tolerate the change in shape from the distention better than the Descemet's membrane, which may tear or suffer a complete break from the increased pressure. This can affect vision, as well as prevent the flow of nutrients to the rest of the cornea. Ruptures can also occur from the use of surgical instruments.

H18.4 Corneal degeneration

Corneal degeneration is a gradual deterioration of the cornea due to age, disease, or another process, which occurs with a corresponding loss of visual acuity.

H18.41 Arcus senilis

Arcus senilis is a white, gray, or bluish appearing opaque ring in the periphery or margin of the cornea seen in older adults. It is caused by cholesterol deposits in the cornea or by hyaline degeneration of the corneal stroma associated with ocular defects or hyperlipidemia. Although it may appear even from birth or in childhood, it is most commonly seen in those over 50 years of age.

H18.42 Band keratopathy

Band-shaped keratopathy is a type of degeneration of the cornea in which calcium deposits are laid in horizontal band-like layers, obscuring the patient's vision.

H18.44 Keratomalacia

Keratomalacia is a degenerative condition which is normally seen in both eyes at once. It presents with poor night vision and extreme dryness of the eyes, followed by wrinkling of the corneal tissues, progressive cloudiness, and softening of the corneas. Dry, gray spots may also appear on the sclera, the white of the eye. Without effective treatment, permanent blindness may result.

Note: This condition is most often caused by a severe vitamin A deficiency, but keratomalacia from this cause is reported with E50.4.

H18.45 Nodular corneal degeneration

Nodular degeneration of the cornea, which includes Salzmann's nodular dystrophy, is a type of progressive deterioration which presents with small, white or grayish nodules within the area of the cornea. This condition usually presents with no discomfort in its initial stages, though it may present with dry eye or excessive tearing, sensitivity to bright light (photophobia), and loss of visual acuity as it progresses.

H18.46 Peripheral corneal degeneration

Peripheral degenerations of the cornea begin at the margins of the cornea, where it connects to the sclera, the white of the eye. In extreme cases, such degeneration can cause the cornea to fall partially or completely away from the rest of the eye.

H18.5 Hereditary corneal dystrophies

Hereditary corneal dystrophies are genetic conditions which cause the cornea to weaken and degenerate so as to become opaque, retain fluid, or develop other lesions. Several different types of hereditary corneal dystrophies result in the body errantly depositing bits of matter into the stroma of the cornea, the interior layer which gives the cornea its shape, eventually obscuring the patient's vision. These are classified according to the pattern of the deposits.

H18.51 Endothelial corneal dystrophy

Endothelial corneal dystrophy is a hereditary disorder which ordinarily does not appear until adulthood. It causes the endothelial (innermost) layer of the cornea to deteriorate, which in turn causes it to become less effective at removing excess fluid from the interior of the cornea, resulting in pain and swelling that distorts the patient's vision. Medication and other therapies designed to dry the eyes are commonly used to treat this disorder.

H18.52 Epithelial (juvenile) corneal dystrophy

Juvenile epithelial corneal dystrophy presents during the first two years of life as a slight irritation affecting both eyes, followed by multiple lesions on the epithelium, the outermost layer of the cornea, which gradually grow together and obscure vision.

H18.53 Granular corneal dystrophy

Granular corneal dystrophy is a condition in which the body deposits opaque granules, or specks, of matter into the cornea randomly.

H18.54 Lattice corneal dystrophy

In lattice corneal dystropy, deposits take on a streaked and latticework-like pattern.

H18.55 Macular corneal dystrophy

In macular corneal dystrophy, deposits form primarily in the center area of the cornea, obscuring the patient's vision.

H18.6 Keratoconus

Keratoconus is a condition in which the cornea of the eye protrudes in an abnormal fashion; (e.g., it may protrude abnormally far in the center or bulge to one side). This protrusion results in the patient having a distorted field of vision, much as an uneven pane of glass will result in a distortion of the light passing through it. In the early stages, the patient's vision is usually correctable by glasses or contact lenses, but in the later stages, a corneal transplant may be necessary in order to restore the patient's vision.

H18.61 Keratoconus, stable

This code should be used to report keratoconus where the corneas are not distorting or otherwise changing rapidly.

H18.62 Keratoconus, unstable

Use this code to report keratoconus with acute hydrops, meaning the corneas are changing shape rapidly due to thinning and the pressure of the ocular fluid behind them.

H18.71 Corneal ectasia

Corneal ectasia is a condition similar to keratoconus, but in which the cornea is bulging due to having become thin and scarred from trauma or surgery. This condition is a common complication of laser surgery.

H18.72 Corneal staphyloma

Corneal staphyloma is a bulging of the cornea in which the bulge contains uveal tissue, the tissue that supplies the eye with blood. This condition is sometimes seen as a secondary effect of glaucoma.

H18.73 Descemetocele

Descemetocele is a condition in which the Descemet's membrane, the inner layer of the cornea, separates from the rest of the cornea and bulges inward into the anterior chamber of the eye. It may form as a side-effect to a corneal ulcer. If left unchecked, this condition can cause permanent blindness and even loss of the eye.

H18.81 Anesthesia and hypoesthesia of cornea

Corneal anesthesia and hypoesthesia indicate that the cornea has a decreased or complete loss of sensitivity to pain and irritation, respectively. Lack of sensitivity in the cornea can result in damage from foreign particles which would normally be blinked out of the eye, or injuries which would normally result in favoring that eye while the cornea heals.

H18.83 Recurrent erosion of cornea

Recurrent erosion of the cornea is a condition which affects the outermost layer of the cornea, called the epithelium. It occurs when the epithelium is bonded poorly to the next layer of cells, causing them to shed easily. In particular, this shedding often occurs when the patient awakes from sleep and first opens the eyes. This presents with pain similar to that caused by a normal corneal abrasion, as well as blurred vision and pain in bright light. This recurs as new cells, also poorly bonded, regrow and are likewise shed.

H20 Iridocyclitis

The iris is the colored portion of the eye which dilates and constricts in order to regulate the amount of light entering the eye. The ciliary body is a ring of muscle just behind the iris which connects to the lens by numerous, hair-like ligaments to hold the lens suspended in the center of the iris. The ciliary body, like the iris, can dilate or contract, adjusting the tension on the lens to focus vision. Iridocyclitis is an inflammation of the iris and ciliary body.

H20.0 Acute and subacute iridocyclitis

Iridocyclitis is an inflammation of both the iris and the ciliary body. It presents with redness and watering of the eyes, pain, light sensitivity that can produce pain even when the light is shined in the unaffected eye, and vision loss.

H20.01 Primary iridocyclitis

Primary iridocyclitis is an inflammation of the iris and/or ciliary body which is not caused by another disease.

H20.02 Recurrent acute iridocyclitis

Recurrent iridocyclitis indicates that acute infection and inflammation of the iris and ciliary body continues to return after periods of remission, which are free of symptoms.

H20.03 Secondary infectious iridocyclitis

Secondary infectious iridocyclitis is a condition in which inflammation of the eye affecting the iris and ciliary body is caused by another underlying systemic disease or infection that is passed from one person to another.

H20.05 Hypopyon

Hypopyon is an accumulation of white blood cells, in the form of pus, between the cornea and the iris and lens. This is a common complication of trauma to the eye, especially where an infection occurred. Permanent damage and even blindness can result to the eye unless there is immediate medical intervention.

H20.1 Chronic iridocyclitis

Chronic iridocyclitis presents with few symptoms, but can severely damage the eye over the long period of time which it lasts. It is especially common in children with juvenile rheumatoid arthritis, particularly girls ages two to six.

H20.2 Lens-induced iridocyclitis

Lens-induced iridocyclitis is an inflammation of the iris and ciliary body due to an abnormality of the lens, usually caused by an immune reaction due to an overabundance of proteins in the lens.

H20.81 Fuchs' heterochromic cyclitis

Fuchs' heterochromic cyclitis is a congenital disorder of the eye which presents with inflammation, cataracts, and heterochromia--a condition in which the affected iris is either a different color than the unaffected one, or in which parts of the affected iris are different colors. This disorder usually first begins to affect the patient's vision in their twenties or thirties.

H20.82 Vogt-Koyanagi syndrome

Vogt-Koyanagi syndrome is an autoimmune disorder in which the body's immune system attacks healthy systems by mistake, usually after a viral infection. In this multisystemic syndrome, the immune system targets the cells that produce melanin, the chemical that causes the skin to tan in order to protect it from the sun. This syndrome presents with a loss of color in the hair and skin and hearing problems, as well as inflammation in the irises (the colored parts of the eyes) that causes the formation of pus. Retinal detachment is a frequent complication.

H21 Other disorders of iris and ciliary body

The iris is the colored portion of the eye which dilates and constricts in order to regulate the amount of light entering the eye. The ciliary body is a ring of muscle just behind the iris which connects to the lens by numerous, hair-like ligaments to hold the lens suspended in the center of the iris. The ciliary body, like the iris, can dilate or contract, adjusting the tension on the lens to focus vision.

H21.0 Hyphema

Hyphema is a condition where bleeding occurs in the iris, usually as a result of blunt trauma to the eye, and pools in the bottom of the cornea. This causes vision to become extremely blurred. Hyphema will usually resolve itself over the course of a few weeks, provided that the patient avoids re-bleeding.

H21.1 Other vascular disorders of iris and ciliary body

Other vascular disorders of iris and ciliary body includes rubeosis iridis, a condition in which the iris grows new and abnormal blood vessels (neovascularisation) that are visible from the surface as the growth continues. These can compress the iris, causing vision problems such as light sensitivity.

H21.21 Degeneration of chamber angle

The chamber angle is the rim at which the iris meets the cornea. It is at this angle that the aqueous fluid, which fills the cornea and protects the iris and lens, flows out from the eye in order to maintain its proper pressure. Degenerative changes of the chamber angle may cause the fluid to drain too slowly or too quickly, altering the pressure of the eye, and can also result in separation of the cornea from the rest of the eye.

H21.22 Degeneration of ciliary body

Degenerative changes of the ciliary body affect the eye's ability to focus the lens. The patient may experience completely blurred vision, an inability to focus on written text, or vision that is only clear at certain distances.

H21.23 Degeneration of iris (pigmentary)

Pigmentary iris degeneration is a condition in which the color of the iris fades, allowing light to seep in rather than be blocked by it. This condition presents with light-sensitivity and blurred vision.

H21.24 Degeneration of pupillary margin

In degeneration of the pupillary margin, the iris disintegrates into thin fibers that float freely in the anterior chamber, between the cornea and the lens of the eye. In many cases, this condition is associated with glaucoma. The free-floating fibers may obscure vision and in some cases can scratch the cornea.

H21.25 Iridoschisis

Iridoschisis is a rare condition that usually occurs late in life in which the iris becomes split into two layers: an anterior (forward) layer and a posterior (rear) layer. The posterior layer remains attached to the muscles that control the dilation of the iris, while the anterior layer disintegrates into thin fibers that float freely in the anterior chamber, between the cornea and the lens of the eye. In many cases, this condition is associated with glaucoma. The free-floating fibers may obscure vision or even scratch the cornea.

H21.26 Iris atrophy (essential) (progressive)

Essential, or progressive, iris atrophy is a very rare disorder that presents with a pupil that appears out of place and/or distorted, as well as areas of degeneration or holes in the iris which develop slowly over time. It usually affects only one eye. These degenerations cause a corresponding loss of vision, and are sometimes accompanied by glaucoma, a build-up of fluid pressure within the cornea.

H21.27 Miotic pupillary cyst

A miotic cyst of the pupillary margin is a fluid-filled pocket that forms in the iris at the edge of the pupil that causes the iris to contract. This in turn interferes with vision where light is less than optimal; e.g., in a dimly-lit room, or at night.

H21.3 Cyst of iris, ciliary body and anterior chamber

A cyst is an abnormal fluid-filled pocket or cavity, which is prone to infection and can cause structural changes in the iris, ciliary body, or anterior chamber (the area between the iris and the cornea) when it is present, which may effect vision to different degrees.

H21.31 Exudative cysts of iris or anterior chamber

An exudative cyst is one that forms due to serum or other fluid material, usually pus, produced by the body in response to injury or disease, collecting in a pocket of tissue rather than draining properly. An exudative cyst in the anterior chamber forms between the iris and cornea.

H21.32 Implantation cysts of iris, ciliary body or anterior chamber

An implantation cyst forms in response to trauma and/or surgery to the eye.

H21.34 Primary cyst of pars plana

A primary cyst of the pars plana is one that forms in the ring-shaped area of the interior of the eye between the edge of the retina and the ciliary body, but is not appearing because of another known disorder or disease process.

H21.35 Exudative cyst of pars plana

An exudative cyst forms due to serum or other fluid material, usually pus, produced by the body in response to injury or disease, collecting in a pocket of tissue rather than draining properly. An exudative cyst that forms in the pars plana appears in the ring-shaped area of the interior of the eye between the edge of the retina and the ciliary body.

H21.40 Pupillary membranes, unspecified eye

Pupillary membranes occur when the iris does not completely part over the pupil during formation of the eyes during fetal development, leaving thin strands of tissue over the lens. These strands may or may not interfere with normal vision, depending on their thickness.

H21.51 Anterior synechiae (iris)

An anterior synechiae involves the iris and the cornea growing together, causing distortion in the shape of the iris.

H21.52 Goniosynechiae

Goniosynechiae involves adhesion of the iris to the posterior surface of the cornea in the angle of the anterior chamber. The anterior chamber angle is the rim at which the iris meets the cornea. It is at this angle that the aqueous fluid, which fills the cornea and protects the iris and lens, flows out from the eye in order to maintain its proper pressure. Goniosynechiae can interfere with the proper flow of aqueous humor.

H21.53 Iridodialysis

Iridodialysis is a condition in which the iris becomes torn away from the edge of the cornea, usually as a result of an injury to the eye. This allows light to enter the eye without passing through the lens, obscuring vision.

H21.54 Posterior synechiae (iris)

A posterior synechiae is an adhesion where the lens and the iris grow together, preventing the iris from dilating and contracting properly.

H21.55 Recession of chamber angle

The chamber angle is the rim at which the iris meets the cornea. It is at this angle that the aqueous fluid, which fills the cornea and protects the iris and lens, flows out from the eye in order to maintain its proper pressure. Recession of the chamber angle can occur due to injury to the eye, usually blunt trauma. As the angle recedes, the flow of aqueous liquid is impaired, possibly resulting in glaucoma, or build-up of fluid pressure within the eye.

H21.56 Pupillary abnormalities

Use this code to report other abnormalities of the pupil, such as a deformed pupil that is not circular or a rupture of the sphincter (circular) muscle that controls the opening and closing of the iris.

H21.81 Floppy iris syndrome

Intraoperative floppy iris syndrome occurs when a person who has taken alpha-blockers, often for urine retention in prostatic hypertrophy, undergoes surgery for cataracts. During cataract surgery, the iris is dilated with medication, but in patients who have previously taken alpha blockers, the iris does not stay properly dilated. It ends up in a flapping or billowy condition instead, which is an unexpected complication that can lead to injury of the iris and other structures. If the ophthalmologist suspects this may happen, the physician can take the precaution of keeping the pupil open with a stronger type of dilating medication, or by using miniature hooks. Even if the patient discontinued the use of alpha-blockers as far back as five years ago, the syndrome can still occur.

H21.82 Plateau iris syndrome (post-iridectomy) (postprocedural)

Plateau iris syndrome is an uncommon anatomical condition causing angle closure glaucoma and is particularly important in those under 50. It is called 'plateau' because on gonioscopy, the central iris is flat, like a plateau, and the peripheral iris curves steeply. A large or anteriorly positioned ciliary body alters the configuration of the iris and pushes the peripheral iris up into the angle. Pupillary block pushes against the lens and stops aqueous humor from flowing into the anterior chamber from the posterior chamber. The resulting pressure in the posterior chamber pushes the peripheral iris against the trabecular meshwork, causing angle closure glaucoma. Definitive diagnosis can be made when angle closure still persists after an iridectomy/iridotomy has been done to make a hole in the iris, equalizing the pressure between the chambers and preventing pupillary block. The angle is so narrow that angle closure persists spontaneously or whenever the pupil dilates.

H25 Age-related cataract

A cataract is a partial or complete clouding over of the crystalline lens that focuses incoming light onto the retina. Cataracts obscure vision and are the leading form of preventable blindness. Cataracts often form slowly and painlessly, and can affect vision without the patient even realizing a cataract is developing. A senile, or age-related cataract is one that forms as a person gets older, due to either a build-up of dead cells within the capsule of the lens or clumping of protein deposits (which are normally spaced in such a way as to enable light to pass through and be focused).

H25.0 Age-related incipient cataract

An incipient senile cataract is one that appears in an older patient and takes up less than 15% of the lens, only slightly interfering with the patient's vision.

H25.01 Cortical age-related cataract

In a cortical senile cataract, the clouding starts at the edge of the lens and grows inward. This type of cataract typically appears as thin, ring-shaped layers that lighten towards the center of the eye.

H25.03 Anterior subcapsular polar age-related cataract

An anterior subcapsular polar senile cataract is a clouding over of the lens in an older patient that results from a defect within the front of the lens, beneath the capsule and in the central area.

H25.04 Posterior subcapsular polar age-related cataract

A posterior subcapsular polar senile cataract is a clouding over of the lens in an older patient that results from a defect within the rear of the lens, beneath the capsule, and in the central area.

H25.1 Age-related nuclear cataract

In a nuclear sclerosis cataract, the cataract forms in or near the exact center of the lens.

H25.2 Age-related cataract, morgagnian type

In an age-related morgagnian type cataract, also called a hypermature cataract, the lens itself begins to disintegrate and liquefy, giving it a wrinkled, snowflake-filled appearance.

H26 Other cataract

A cataract is a partial or complete clouding over of the crystalline lens that focuses incoming light onto the retina, causing obscured vision. They are the leading form of preventable blindness and often form slowly and painlessly over time as a person ages. Other cataracts reported in this category include those that form in an infant or very young person and not as a result of aging, trauma, adverse drug reaction, or other ocular conditions.

H26.0 Infantile and juvenile cataract

Infantile, juvenile, and presenile cataract indicate that the clouding of the lens is not due to anything occurring with the aging process, but due to a defect in the growth of the lens.

H26.01 Infantile and juvenile cortical, lamellar, or zonular cataract

In a nonsenile cortical, lamellar, or zonular cataract, the clouding starts at the edge of the lens in a young patient and grows inward. This type of cataract typically appears as thin, ring-shaped layers that lighten towards the center of the eye.

H26.03 Infantile and juvenile nuclear cataract

An infantile or juvenile nuclear cataract is a clouding over of the lens in a young patient that forms in or near the center of the lens.

H26.04 Anterior subcapsular polar infantile and juvenile cataract

An anterior subcapsular polar infantile and juvenile cataract is a clouding over of the lens in a young patient as a result of a defect within the front of the lens, beneath the capsule and in the central area.

H26.05 Posterior subcapsular polar infantile and juvenile cataract

A posterior subcapsular polar infantile and juvenile cataract is a clouding over of the lens in a young patient that occurs due to a defect in the back of the lens, beneath the capsule and in the central area.

H26.1 Traumatic cataract

A traumatic cataract results when the crystalline lens that focuses incoming light onto the retina clouds over and obscures vision due to an injury to the eye. Traumatic cataracts may be caused by blunt trauma such as a blow to the eye, and from a laceration or cut, as well as from electrocution, chemical burns, and radiation.

H26.11 Localized traumatic opacities

Localized traumatic opacities, also called Vossius' ring, occurs when blunt trauma to the eye presses the iris against the lens, resulting in a ring-shaped cataract on the exterior of the lens. This usually only slightly affects vision.

H26.12 Partially resolved traumatic cataract

In some cases, a cataract caused by an injury may partially or even completely resolve on its own. This code reports a traumatic cataract which is partially resolved, regardless of whether it is expected to continue resolving any further.

H26.13 Total traumatic cataract

A total traumatic cataract is the complete obscurement of the lens due to an injury to the eye, resulting in near-total vision loss (beyond the ability to differentiate between light and dark).

H26.2 Complicated cataract

A cataract is a partial or complete clouding over of the crystalline lens that focuses incoming light onto the retina, causing obscured vision. They are the leading form of preventable blindness and often form slowly and painlessly over time as a person ages. Complicated cataracts reported in this category include those that form in the presence of another ocular disease or associated ocular disorder, which should also be coded.

H26.211 Cataract with neovascularization, right eye

Neovascularization is the growth of new and abnormal blood vessels in the eye. When these abnormal blood vessels grow into the lens, cataracts can result.

H26.22 Cataract secondary to ocular disorders (degenerative) (inflammatory)

A partial or complete clouding of the lens or lens capsule of the eye due to the presence of another ocular disorder, such as an underlying inflammatory disorder or infection, or other degenerative condition of the eye.

H26.3 Drug-induced cataract

A drug-induced cataract, also called a toxic cataract, is a partial or complete clouding over of the lens or lens capsule of the eye due to exposure to a drug or other toxic substance, such as a miotic, antimiotic, corticosteroid, metal nitro compound, or substituted hydrocarbon.

H26.4 Secondary cataract

In some cases, a cataract may be caused following trauma affecting the eye or surgical procedures. In such cases, the clouding over of the lens is considered a secondary type cataract.Cataracts that occur due to the presence of another associated ocular disorder, however, such as glaucoma, chronic iridocyclitis, degenerative eye conditions, or specific infections of the eye are considered complicated cataracts, not secondary ones, and are coded to subcategory H26.2-.

H26.41 Soemmering's ring

Soemmering's ring is a doughnut-shaped remnant of the lens behind the pupil, which may occur after cataract surgery or secondary to trauma

H27.0 Aphakia

Aphakia is the absence of the crystalline lens of the eye, which usually occurs following the surgical removal of cataracts.

H27.11 Subluxation of lens

Subluxation of the lens is a partial displacement of the lens from its normal position that can lead to total dislocation. It is caused by a partial zonular rupture from trauma, hypermature cataract, a perforated corneal ulcer causing a sudden drop in intraocular pressure, or buphthalmos with an abnormally large globe. The displaced lens causes tremors of the iris, irregular depth in the anterior chamber, and a visible midline of the lens through a dilated pupil. The patient experiences defective vision and diplopia of that eye if the lens is clear. If it is not corrected, secondary glaucoma may result.

H27.12 Anterior dislocation of lens

In an anterior dislocation of the lens, the lens moves from its normal position into the anterior chamber from a complete rupture of the zonule. This may cause iridocyclitis, corneal edema, and pupillary block glaucoma. It is treated with mydriatics and medical control of the intraocular pressure, followed by lens extraction.

H27.13 Posterior dislocation of lens

In a posterior dislocation of the lens, the lens moves from its normal position completely away from the pupillary area and sinks in the vitreous due to a complete rupture of the zonule. The lens must be removed by vitrectomy and the liquid gel replaced.

H28 Cataract in diseases classified elsewhere

This code reports a clouding over of the crystalline lens of the eye that obscures vision or causes blindness due to an underlying disease or disorder that is not ocular, or not one that directly affects the eyes. The underlying disease must be reported first, such as hypoparathyroidism, myotonia, myxedema, and malnutrition.

Note: Diabetic cataracts are not reported with this code, but with the appropriate code in the diabetes categories E08, E09, E10, E11, and E13.

H30 Chorioretinal inflammation

Choroiditis is an inflammation of the choroid, the layer of the eye behind the retina that is firmly adhered to it and provides the retina with its blood supply. Chorioretinitis is an inflammation of both the choroid and the retina. Retinitis is an inflammation of the retina, the inward layer of the orb of the eye which receives light and transmits the information received to the brain through the optic nerve to permit vision. Retinochoroiditis is an inflammation of the retina that spreads back to the choroid. All of these conditions present with pain, floating black spots in the vision, and vision loss. These inflammations are usually due to a bacterial infection, but it is

rare that the type of bacteria involved can be identified. They are treated with anti-inflammatory medications and antibiotics.

H30.0 Focal chorioretinal inflammation

A focal chorioretinal inflammation is localized in a specific area of the eye, and is classified by location.

H30.01 Focal chorioretinal inflammation, juxtapapillary

Juxtapapillary chorioretinal inflammations occur in the area of the choroid over and immediately adjacent to the optic papillae, which is the "blind spot" where the optic nerve connects to the eye.

H30.02 Focal chorioretinal inflammation of posterior pole

Chorioretinal inflammations of the posterior pole occur at the point where the nerves of the retina cluster to form the optic nerve.

Note: This code should not be used for a juxtapapillary inflammation, which is a specified part of the posterior pole.

H30.03 Focal chorioretinal inflammation, peripheral

Peripheral chorioretinal inflammations occur around the outer edges or periphery of the retina, which provides both night vision and peripheral vision.

H30.04 Focal chorioretinal inflammation, macular or paramacular

Macular chorioretinal inflammation occur in the central part of the retina responsible for fine detailed vision such as that needed for reading. This is the area where the cones of the eye are contained that capture and transmit colored light to the optic nerve. The paramacular area is the area of the retina immediately adjacent to the macula.

H30.1 Disseminated chorioretinal inflammation

Disseminated inflammations of the choroid, retina, or both have more than a single focus, or one point of inflammation, and are spread throughout the affected eye structure.

H30.11 Disseminated chorioretinal inflammation of posterior pole

Disseminated chorioretinal inflammation of the posterior pole occurs throughout the area where the nerves of the retina cluster to form the optic nerve.

H30.12 Disseminated chorioretinal inflammation, peripheral

Disseminated peripheral chorioretinal inflammations occur around the outside area, or periphery of the retina that provides both night vision and peripheral vision.

H30.2 Posterior cyclitis

Posterior cyclitis, also called pars planitis, is an inflammation of the peripheral retina and the ciliary body, the hair-like structures that hold the lens of the eye in place. In some cases, this inflammation can cause permanent vision loss if not treated.

H30.81 Harada's disease

Harada's disease is an uncommon immune-mediated disease that causes acute inflammation that typically affects the eyes as well as other systems, such as the skin, ear, and meninges (protective lining of the brain and spinal cord) in middle-aged adults. The body attacks the uvea of the eye as well as the melanocytes in the skin, and the inner ear. It is characterized by diffuse granulomatous inflammation in the uvea in both eyes. Vision becomes blurred in the acute stage with inflammation of the vitreous, thickening of the posterior choroid that becomes elevated in the peripapillary area around the optic papillae, which is the "blind spot" where the optic nerve connects to the eye.

Diseases of the Eye and Adnexa

H31.0 – H33.05

H31.0 Chorioretinal scars

Chorioretinal scars can occur as a result of inflammation, surgery, or other trauma. These can cause blind spots ranging from inconsequential to disabling, depending on their size and location.

Note: Postsurgical chorioretinal scars are reported with H59.81-.

H31.02 Solar retinopathy

A solar retinopathy is a scar on the retina as a result of solar radiation. This is usually caused by staring directly into the sun, but is also known in those who have been in the snow or water for extended periods of time without protection, due to the reflected glare.

H31.1 Choroidal degeneration

The choroid is the layer of the eye directly beneath and adhered to the retina, providing its vascular supply. Degeneration of the choroid is a group of eye disorders characterized by a loss of cellular or tissue function and subsequent structural changes in the choroid layer that will cause corresponding damage to the retina and loss of vision.

H31.11 Age-related choroidal atrophy

Age-related atrophy of the choroid is simply a deteriorating, thinning, or wasting of the choroidal layer with advancing age, causing a slow loss of vision over time.

H31.12 Diffuse secondary atrophy of choroid

Diffuse secondary atrophy of the choroid indicates that the choroidal tissue is wasting away in a disseminated fashion due to a systemic, or other underlying disease.

H31.2 Hereditary choroidal dystrophy

This category reports inherited causes of choroidal dystrophy, a degenerative disorder of the choroid of the eye, which is a layer of blood vessels between the fibrous outer covering of the eye and the retina. The choroid is directly beneath and fused to the retina. The choroid supplies blood and nutrients to the retina, and prevents excess light from reaching the retina.

H31.21 Choroideremia

Choroidemia is a congenital condition in which the choroid begins to degenerate rapidly, usually within the first ten years of life. The patient will progressively lose peripheral vision and night vision and experience tunnel vision, with complete blindness often following. This condition is usually more severe in females.

H31.22 Choroidal dystrophy (central areolar) (generalized) (peripapillary)

Central areolar choroidal dystrophy causes severe, irreversible vision loss in the 5th to 7th decades of life due to the loss of capillary function in the choroid.

H31.3 Choroidal hemorrhage and rupture

A choroidal hemorrhage is bleeding from the choroid layer, usually into the interior of the eye.

H31.31 Expulsive choroidal hemorrhage

An expulsive choroidal hemorrhage occurs when the choroid bleeds into the interior of the eye. This often presents with floating black spots (floaters) in the vision.

H31.32 Choroidal rupture

Choroidal rupture is a break in the choroid which usually involves the retinal pigment epithelium (RPE) as well, due to a blow to the eyeball. This can lead to retinal or choroidal detachment, sometimes long after the initial injury.

H31.4 Choroidal detachment

Choroidal detachment is a condition in which the choroid detaches from the sclera, the external, white part of the eyeball. Such detachment usually extends from the initial site all the way to the iris, and like retinal detachment, can affect the patient's visual acuity to various degrees depending on the site and extent of the detachment.

H31.41 Hemorrhagic choroidal detachment

Use this code if the detachment is due to bleeding in between the sclera and choroid layers of the eye.

H31.42 Serous choroidal detachment

Detachment of the choroid from the underlying layer due to a blister filled with serous fluid that forms beneath the choroid.

H33 Retinal detachments and breaks

The retina is the inward layer of the orb of the eye which receives light and transmits the information received to the brain via the optic nerve to allow for vision. Retinal detachment occurs when a break or defect occurs in the thin layer of the retina. This may occur due to the vitreous gel, the clear fluid that fills the center of the eye, shrinking and pulling away from the retina, where it is attached firmly in several places around the back wall of the eye. This shrinkage may cause it to pull a piece of the retina away with it, leaving a break known as a tear. Retinal detachment with breaks may also occur as the retina thins and deteriorates with advancing age. The atrophy process produces a break known as a hole. Some breaks or defects may also occur due to a head injury, trauma to the orbit, or diabetes. Once the hole, break, or tear is there, vitreous fluid slowly seeps into the defect, causing the retina to separate from the choroid, the middle vascular layer of the eye, and detach, causing a blindspot in vision. The patient usually experiences loss of the peripheral vision first, since most retinal detachments occur to one side rather than in the center of the eye. If the detachment reaches and includes the macula, the central portion of the retina responsible for fine detailed vision such as that needed for reading, recognizing faces, etc., the patient will lose all central vision and become effectively completely blind.

H33.0 Retinal detachment with retinal break

Retinal detachments with retinal breaks as one or more holes or tears in the retina lining the inside of the eye are called rhegmatogenous retinal detachments and are the most common form, which can occur in healthy eyes. After the hole or tear occurs, ocular fluid from the center of the eye then migrates through the break to enter the space underneath the retina, between the retina and the choroid, causing them to peel apart. Symptoms include the sudden appearance of 'floaters' visible in the eye, a ring of hair-like floaters just to the outside of central vision, flashes, a slight feeling of heaviness in the eye, and loss of peripheral vision.

H33.01 Retinal detachment with single break

Use this code if the detachment is partial, not total (i.e., has not reached the macula) and is due to a single break or defect.

H33.02 Retinal detachment with multiple breaks

Use this code if the detachment is partial, not total (i.e., has not reached the macula) and is due to more than one small tear or hole in the retina.

H33.03 Retinal detachment with giant retinal tear

Partial detachment due to a giant tear rather than a small defect or break will cause continued retinal detachment to occur much more quickly and is a greater potential for blindness.

H33.04 Retinal detachment with retinal dialysis

Partial detachment due to retinal dialysis is a process in which the retina develops a split at the point where it attaches to the mid-eye, usually due to trauma, diabetes, or a congenital defect. Dialyses which occur at the very periphery caused by atrophy are the most common form of idiopathic retinal detachment in children.

H33.05 Total retinal detachment

Total retinal detachment occurs when a tear or break includes the macula, the central portion of the retina responsible for fine detailed vision such as that needed for reading, recognizing faces, etc. The patient will lose all central vision and become effectively completely blind.

H33.1 Retinoschisis and retinal cysts

Retinoschisis is a progressive disease characterized by splitting of the retina's neurosensory layers, usually in the outer peripheral layer, when bullous type lesions appear on the peripheral retina causing poor vascularization and fibrous traction that pulls on the retina. This can lead to loss of vision in that corresponding field in the rarer cases, although the more common form is asymptomatic. This can be very hard to differentiate from retinal detachment, but normal degenerative type of retinsoschisis by itself does not lead to separation of the retina clear through the fovea.

Note: The hereditary type of retinoschisis is reported with Q14.1 and is much less common. This type causes the retina to split into two layers and can affect the nerve tissue in the macula, resulting in loss of visual resolution needed for detailed viewing. This is not the same as retinal detachment, in which the retina pulls away from the choroid.

H33.2 Serous retinal detachment

Serous retinal detachment, the less common form of retinal detachment, occurs when fluid accumulates underneath the retina, between it and the choroid, due to an inflammatory process, injury, or vascular anomaly, rather than through a hole, tear, or break in the retina. This is also known as retinal detachment without retinal breaks, or exudative retinal detachment. Exudative detachment more commonly occurs in elderly patients and this type is made worse by surgery as opposed to detachment caused by breaks or defects, which can be repaired by surgery.

H33.3 Retinal breaks without detachment

Retinal defects which do not result in a current detachment. Because retinal detachment may develop at a later date, the surgeon may elect to seal these breaks using laser or cryo (cold) surgery before any problems develop.

H33.31 Horseshoe tear of retina without detachment

A horseshoe tear of the retina is also known as a classic flap tear. This is a tractional type tear caused when the vitreous gel of the eye pulls away from the retina in an area where it is firmly attached, pulling the retina incompletely free of the layer underneath in a triangular-shaped tear, or flap, like a horseshoe. The point of the tear is still attached to the mobile vitreous, which can act to tear the retina further from the retinal pigment epithelium.

A horseshoe tear can occur at first without detachment of the retina. If an area of retinal tissue is pulled completely free by the vitrous, it is known as an operculated tear, or operculum of the retina, and the tissue will then float in the vitreous above the retinal tear. The patient will perceive flashes of light or increase in floaters in the vision. If further separation of the retina occurs at the tear, and the liquid vitreous gel gains access to the subretinal space, then rhegmatogenous retinal detachment can form. Horseshoe tears appearing without detachment are therefore treated prophylactically with laser photocoagulation to seal the retinal break against the underlying retinal pigment epithelium before fluid leaks underneath and causes detachment.

Note: The majority of rhegmatogenous retinal detachments occur from this pathological type of vitreous detachment, or tractional pulling away, that results in horseshoe or giant retinal tears.

H33.32 Round hole of retina without detachment

Round retinal holes are another type of retinal break that occurs at first without retinal detachment. Round holes are not caused by the tractional pulling away of the vitreous gel from the retina, as in horseshoe tears, but are more like a slowly evolving detachment occuring with the vitrous gel still attached, caused by chorioretinopathy or chronic atrophy of the retina. This is thought to be associated with blood vessel sclerosis that disturbs the overlying vitreous. As the retinal tissue slowly dies dues to the shut down in blood supply, the surrounding vitreous also degenerates. The resulting round holes seem to occur mostly in younger patients with myopia. The round hole in the retina can still lead to retinal detachment and is treated with cryotherapy and scleral buckling in most cases, or laser retinopexy to keep the retina sealed against the underlying epithelium.

H33.4 Traction detachment of retina

Traction detachment of the retina occurs due to pulling on the retina from fibrous or fibro-vascular scar tissue within the inner eye caused by a chronic inflammatory process or former injury, or neovasularization. The pulling action of the scar tissue causes the sensory retina to pull away from the retinal pigment epithelium. This type of retinal detachment is most commonly seen in diabetic patients.

H34.0 Transient retinal artery occlusion

Transient arterial occlusion indicates that the blockage of blood flow to the retina is not permanent, but passes after a period of time. Nevertheless, the time during which bloodflow was decreased or stopped can cause permanent damage to the retina.

H34.1 Central retinal artery occlusion

A central retinal artery occlusion, sometimes abbreviated as CRAO, compromises the blood supply to the entire retina, and causes a sudden loss of vision.

H34.21 Partial retinal artery occlusion

A partial arterial occlusion will cause vision loss over a longer period of time that affects either the entire eye or just part of it depending on which artery is blocked. In some cases, the body may try to compensate for the partial blockage by creating new, abnormal vessels around the blockage to supply the eye.

H34.23 Retinal artery branch occlusion

A branch retinal arterial occlusion, or BRAO, compromises the blood supply to a branched area of the retina and will cause the same rapid decline as a central artery occlusion, but only to part of the field of vision.

H34.81 Central retinal vein occlusion

A central retinal vein occlusion closes off the final vein which collects all of the blood from the vessels that flow through the eye. This blockage in blood flowing freely from the eye causes pressure to build up and results in blood leaking into the interior of the eye, and permanent damage to the retina.

H34.82 Venous engorgement

Venous engorgement indicates that partial or complete blockage of the retinal veins has resulted in high pressure building up throughout the blood vessels supplying the retina, which can cause serious damage.

H34.83 Tributary (branch) retinal vein occlusion

Venous tributary, or branch, occlusion will also cause blockage in blood flowing from the eye as in central vein occlusion. The resulting pressure build up causes blood leakage into the eye and damage to the retina, but the extent depends on the location of the blockage.

H35.01 Changes in retinal vascular appearance

Changes in vascular appearance are not a disorder per se, but may be indicative of another disorder of the retina that has not yet caused significant vision loss.

H35.02 Exudative retinopathy

Exudative retinopathy, also called Coats' syndrome or disease, develops as a result of a malformation of the blood vessels of the eye, which in turn causes a buildup of fluid that is harmful to the retina. Vision loss usually begins in the first decade of life, sometimes as early as four to six months of age. This disorder is named for the fluid that exudes into the interior of the eye.

H35.03 Hypertensive retinopathy

Hypertensive retinopathy is damage to the retina due to high blood pressure.

H35.04 Retinal micro-aneurysms, unspecified

A retinal microaneurysm, the dilation of a point on one or more arteries in the eye, is another indicator of retinal disease. The point of dilation, which has the appearance of an inflated balloon, is a point of weakness in the artery wall which, if it bursts, could cause floaters due to blood entering the inner eye as well as cutting off a portion of the retina from its blood supply. If caught early enough, laser surgery can often correct the problem before the vessel bursts.

H35.05 Retinal neovascularization, unspecified

Retinal neovascularization indicates that new and abnormal blood vessels are growing in the retina or choroid, another possible precursor to retinal disease.

H35.06 Retinal vasculitis

Retinal vasculitis is a condition in which the blood vessels of the retina have become inflamed, perhaps due to an infection. The inflammation, and subsequent damage to the retina, can range from mild to a severe inflammation that can cause permanent blindness.

H35.07 Retinal telangiectasis

Retinal telangiectasia indicates that instead of dilating at a single point, one or more vessels in the eye have become dilated (enlarged) across their length. This again can be a precursor to a more serious retinal disease, such as exudative retinopathy.

H35.1 Retinopathy of prematurity

Retinopathy of prematurity (ROP) is a leading cause of childhood blindness that involves the abnormal development of blood vessels in the retina in premature babies. Eye development is disrupted when infants are born prematurely. The vessels may stop growing, or may grow into the clear gel at the back of the eye. The fragile vessels rupture and bleed and the retina may pull loose from the eye surface. The smallest and sickest preemies have the greatest risk of developing severe ROP, which results in blindness. Symptoms of severe ROP are crossed eyes, abnormal eye movement, white pupils, and severe nearsightedness.

H35.12 Retinopathy of prematurity, stage 1

Stage 1 shows mildly abnormal blood vessel growth.

H35.13 Retinopathy of prematurity, stage 2

Stage 2 shows moderately abnormal blood vessel growth.

H35.14 Retinopathy of prematurity, stage 3

Stage 3 shows severely abnormal blood vessel growth.

H35.15 Retinopathy of prematurity, stage 4

Stage 4 shows severely abnormal blood vessel growth with partial retinal detachment.

H35.16 Retinopathy of prematurity, stage 5

Stage 5 results in total retinal detachment.

H35.17 Retrolental fibroplasia

Also known as cicatricial retinopathy of prematurity, the older term 'retrolental fibroplasia' refers to the cicatricial disease that occurs when the retina is actually scarred.

H35.3 Degeneration of macula and posterior pole

The macula is the central part of the retina responsible for fine detailed vision such as that needed for reading, recognizing faces, etc. The posterior pole is the point where the nerves of the retina cluster to form the optic nerve; the pole has no sensory nerves itself, resulting in a tiny blind spot. A degeneration of either of these bodies will result in severe vision loss.

H35.31 Nonexudative age-related macular degeneration

Nonexudative senile macular degeneration, also known as dry macular degeneration, affects older adults and results in loss of vision in the central field, because of damage to the macula of the retina--the central area of vision providing the most detailed visual acuity. It begins with the accumulation of yellow deposits of cellular debris, called drusen, in the the macula between the retina and the choroid underneath. Drusens that go on developing to advanced stages cause macular degeneration and retinal detachment. Blindness occurs when the drusen become large and/

or numerous enough that they disrupt the pigmented epithelial layer of the retina beneath the macula.

H35.32 Exudative age-related macular degeneration

Exudative age-related macular degeneration, also known as wet macular degeneration, affects older adults and results in loss of vision in the central field, because of damage to the macula of the retina--the central area of vision providing the most detailed visual acuity. The wet, exudative form is more severe than the nonexudative, dry form. Vision loss in this case is due to the abnormal growth of blood vessels up from the choroid (choroidal neovasculization) behind the retina, through the Bruch's membrane that can cause retinal detachment. The abnormal vessels cause blood and protein to leak into the macula. The fluid leakage and resulting scarring eventually result in permanent damage to the photoreceptors when left untreated. Exudative macular degeneration is usually treated with laser coagulation to stop or reverse the growth of blood vessels.

H35.33 Angioid streaks of macula

Angioid streaks of the choroid are broad, irregular, red to brown to gray lines that radiate from the area around the optic nerve and which serve as an indicator of degeneration or disease of the choroid such as pseudoxanthoma, elasticum, or Paget's disease.

H35.34 Macular cyst, hole, or pseudohole

Macular cysts, holes, or pseudoholes are other possible causes of vision loss in the macula. A cyst is a fluid-filled pocket, similar to a blister on the skin. A hole indicates a small opening in the macula. A pseudohole is a pit that has not yet penetrated all layers of the retina at the macula.

H35.35 Cystoid macular degeneration

Cystoid macular degeneration causes loss of vision due to fluid-filled pockets (cysts) that form in the macular region of the retina. These can form due to other diseases, aging, inflammation, or extreme nearsightedness.

H35.36 Drusen (degenerative) of macula

Drusen are tiny, yellowish spots of cellular debris, related to cholesterol deposits that can accumulate in the optic disc or macula of the retina -- the central area of vision providing the most detailed visual acuity. Drusens go on to cause degeneration of the macula and loss of vision as they become large and numerous and disrupt the pigment epithelial layer of the retina beneath the macula.

H35.37 Puckering of macula

Macular puckering indicates that the shape of the macula has become distorted, usually due to scar tissue built up in the surrounding retina.

H35.38 Toxic maculopathy

Toxic maculopathy indicates damage affecting the macula of the retina--the central area of vision providing the most detailed visual acuity--due to a poisonous substance introduced into the body or as an adverse effect complicating the use of prescription drugs. Damage to the macula results in loss of central vision.

H35.4 Peripheral retinal degeneration

The peripheral retina, the greater portion of the retina outside of the central macular portion, is responsible for peripheral and night vision. A degeneration of this part of the eye is usually first noticed as a shadow in the peripheral vision.

H35.41 Lattice degeneration of retina

Lattice degeneration is a common form of atrophic retinal degeneration in which oval or linear patches of thinning appear in the peripheral retina in a lattice pattern. The thinning of the peripheral retina may produce breaks that progress to retinal detachment and is a common reason for detachment in young patients with myopia. The cause is thought to be vascular insufficiency that leads to ischemia or sclerosis. Laser treatment is ususally done to seal the break in lattice degeneration cases.

H35.42 Microcystoid degeneration of retina

Microcystoid degeneration, also referred to as Blessig's cysts and Iwanoff cysts, is a frequent degenerative type of intraretinal lesions on the periphery of the retina, more often seen on the temporal side than the nasal side. They appear as small bubbles or vacuoles between the outer and inner nuclear layers of the retina than can be confused with a hole, but are actually pseudoholes that rarely cause serious vision loss and do not generally predisposed to retinal detachment.

H35.43 Paving stone degeneration of retina

Paving stone degeneration affects both the retina and its vascular, choroidal layer underneath. The disease presents with multiple rounded, yellow-white lesions that appear as punched out areas through an atrophied retina and choroid, through which the sclera may be partly visible. The lesions have discete margins and appear more in outer and inner quadrants. The lesions may grow into each other and occur more commonly with age, although benign cases are not associated with complications.

H35.44 Age-related reticular degeneration of retina

Age-related reticular degeneration gives a net-like appearance to the interior of the retina, that in itself does not cause a serious impact on the patient's vision, but may be a sign of more serious degeneration of the eye.

H35.45 Secondary pigmentary degeneration

Secondary pigmentary degeneration affects the retina pigment epithelium, or RPE, the pigmented layer just beneath the outer surface of the retina which supplies blood and maintains the surface layer of neurovisual cells. The RPE is firmly attached to both the underlying choroid and the overlying layer of retinal visual cells. The RPE also shields the retina from an excess amount of incoming light; maintains the pH balance; phagocytoses the old, outer discs from the photoreceptors; and also maintains internal ocular immunity. Degeneration and dysfunction of the RPE is often found concomitant with age-related macular degeneration and retinitis pigmentosa.

H35.46 Secondary vitreoretinal degeneration

A secondary vitreoretinal degeneration is a deterioration of the vitreous gel that fills the eye along with the retina, caused by another disease or disorder.

H35.5 Hereditary retinal dystrophy

Hereditary retinal dystrophies are changes which occur in the structure of the retina due to a genetic abnormality or disorder. The effects of these dystrophies can range from inconsequential to those which cause permanent blindness.

H35.52 Pigmentary retinal dystrophy

Pigmentary retinal dystrophy is a genetic abnormality or change in the retina pigment epithelium, or RPE, the pigmented layer just beneath the outer surface of the retina which supplies blood and maintains the surface layer of neurovisual cells. The RPE is firmly attached to both the underlying choroid and the overlying layer of retinal visual cells. Dystrophy of the RPE can cause any type of visual problems from dimming of visual acuity, to bilateral cloudy or blurred vision, to progressive loss of vision. Reticular pigmentary retinal dystrophy causes the appearance of drusen and a network of black pigmented lines and knots like a fish-net appearance on the posterior pole of the retina. This also includes retinitis pigmentosa, a group of inherited degenerative retinal diseases affecting the cones and rods in the RPE. Progression of the disease leads to loss of sight and may begin in infancy or later in life. Symptoms can range from defective light and dark adaptation to night blindness, tunnel vision, loss of central vision or peripheral vision, and blindness.

H35.6 Retinal hemorrhage

A retinal hemorrhage is bleeding onto the surface of the retina due to a rupture of the blood vessels that supply it. Such a rupture requires an extremely violent blow to the head, and is often a sign of shaken baby syndrome or other child abuse when seen in children.

H35.7 Separation of retinal layers

Separation of the retinal layers due to disease is distinct from retinal detachment, in which the retina pulls away from the choroid, and from age-related retinoschisis, in which lesions on the peripheral retina appear that can cause fibrous-like traction of the retina and lead to detachment.

H35.71 Central serous chorioretinopathy

Central serous chorioretinopathy is a disorder in which fluid seeps from the choroid, the underlying layer supplying the retina with blood, into the retina above, causing the layers of the retina to become filled with fluid and separate from each other. The cause of this disorder is not presently known.

H35.72 Serous detachment of retinal pigment epithelium

The retina pigment epithelium, or RPE, is the pigmented layer beneath the outer surface of the retina which supplies blood and maintains the surface layer. In serous detachment of retinal pigment epithelium, fluid seeps from the choroid in between the layers of the retina and usually occurs without any noticeable vision loss unless it affects the macula, the central part of the retina.

H35.73 Hemorrhagic detachment of retinal pigment epithelium

Hemorrhagic detachment of the retinal pigment epithelium indicates that the retinal separation is due to bleeding into the layers of the retina, rather than fluid accumulation. This type of separation usually results in far more serious vision loss than serous detachment.

H35.81 Retinal edema

Edema is swelling due to a build-up of fluid. This includes retinal cotton wool spots, abnormal fluffy, white patches that appear on the retina caused by nerve fiber damage from the accumulations of fluid containing intracellular debris within the nerve fiber layers. Swelling in this case is caused by blockage of normal flow through ischemic areas.

H36 Retinal disorders in diseases classified elsewhere

Retinal dystrophy in systemic or cerebroretinal lipidoses or lipid storage disorders is coded here. Lipidoses are genetic, degenerative disorders in which an abnormal amount of fats accumulate in the brain, spinal cord, and/or other parts of the body. When reporting retinal changes due to this disorder, the underlying disorder must be coded first.

H40 Glaucoma

Glaucoma is a disorder in which an increase in fluid pressure in the eye causes damage to the optic nerve, leading to vision loss and, if the disorder is not treated, permanent blindness. Glaucoma is caused when the outflow of ocular fluid, called the aqueous humor or aqueous fluid, is blocked. In a normal eye, the fluid from the interior chamber of the eye flows freely between the ciliary body (the muscles and fibers that support and focus the lens) and the lens into what is called the anterior chamber, the space between the lens and the cornea. It then passes through the trabecular meshwork, a spongy tissue at the chamber angle, the border between the iris and the cornea, and out of the eye through a drainage canal called the canal of Schlemm. A blockage at any of these points can cause glaucoma, which is usually painless and initially presents with no symptoms at all. However, as it progresses, the patient initially experiences loss of peripheral vision, while the center vision remains normal. As the disease continues, vision continues to narrow until blindness results. Medication, surgery, and/or laser surgery may all be used to correct glaucoma.

H40.0 Glaucoma suspect

Glaucoma suspect, also known as borderline glaucoma is a phrase that indicates that there is strong suspicion of glaucoma developing, or a preglaucomatous state of the eye, but no absolute glaucoma present or definite evidence of vision loss.

H40.00 Preglaucoma, unspecified

Preglaucoma, open angle glaucoma suspect, or borderline glaucoma patients are characterized by one or more of these findings when gonioscopy shows normal, open angles: narrowing or notching of the optic disc rim at the poles, abnormalities of the retinal nerve fiber layer, nerve fiber layer disc hemorrhage, asymmetrical appearance of the optic disc or rim between the eyes, and intraocular pressure consistently above 21 mm Hg.

H40.01 Open angle with borderline findings, low risk

Open angle with borderline findings indicates that there is no evidence of blockage in the trabecular meshwork with normal appearing, open anterior chamber angles, but there appears to be some minor blockage at the canal of Schlemm, borderline intraocular pressure readings, or suspicious optic disc appearance. Patients at low risk for developing glaucomatous optic nerve damage have other possible risk factors such as systemic hypertension, cardiovascular disease, myopia, migraine headaches, and peripheral vasospasm.

H40.02 Open angle with borderline findings, high risk

Open angle with borderline findings indicates that there is no evidence of blockage in the trabecular meshwork with normal appearing, open anterior chamber angles, but there appears to be some minor blockage at the canal of Schlemm, borderline intraocular pressure readings, or suspicious optic disc appearance. Patients at high risk are those in whom glaucomatous damage can be reasonably expected and who have one or more of these characteristics: intraocular pressure repeatedly measured in the upper 20s or higher, racial background of African descent, a thinner corneal thickness, advanced age, any history of glaucoma, suspicious optic nerve or retinal nerve abnormalities that suggest early damage, and additional ocular conditions or systemic diseases that contribute to risk such as diabetes. Progressive loss of visual function can be prevented by early detection. Treatment is aimed at lowering the IOP below the level where damage typically occurs, and stabilizing the visual field.

H40.03 Anatomical narrow angle

An anatomical narrow angle occurs in some people of advancing age, particularly of Asian ethnicity, as the lens of the eye continues to grow and pushes the iris forward, which narrows the angle. The distance between the lens and iris is also narrow. Patients with narrow angles are suspect for primary angle closure glaucoma, as the condition can develop quickly if the iris makes contact with the lens, blocking aqueous flow.

H40.04 Steroid responder

Steroid responder indicates that the use of steriods, either medically or illicitly, is causing some increase in the interocular pressure.

Note: Glaucoma due to the therapeutic use of corticosteroids is reported with codes H40.6-.

H40.05 Ocular hypertension

Ocular hypertension indicates that there is increased ocular fluid pressure, but the reason is not known.

H40.06 Primary angle closure without glaucoma damage

Primary angle closure is caused by the iris in contact with the trabecular meshwork, blocking the outflow of aqueous humor from the eye. Primary angle closure glaucoma can occur as a narrowing angle develops over time in some people of advancing age, particularly of Asian ethnicity, as the lens of the eye continues to grow and pushes the iris forward, narrowing the angle. When this develops slowly, intraocular pressure elevation is slow and primary angle closure is diagnosed without glaucoma damage. Some patients will develop ocular redness and discomfort, and the IOP may be normal but is usually higher.

H40.1 Open-angle glaucoma

Most forms of glaucoma are classified as being either open angle or closed angle. Open angle glaucoma indicates that there is no direct blockage of the trabecular meshwork at the chamber angle, and that the problem may rather be a blockage within the canal of Schlemm.

H40.11 Primary open-angle glaucoma

Primary open angle glaucoma indicates that the patient is experiencing high ocular pressure despite an apparent free flow of fluid through the chamber angle of the cornea. This may be due to an excessive creation of ocular fluid rather than insufficient outflow.

H40.12 Low-tension glaucoma

Low tension glaucoma indicates that the damage to the optic nerve is not due to excessively high ocular pressure, but rather due to insufficient blood flow to the nerve itself. This is usually treated by using medication to further lower the ocular pressure so that there is less resistance to the blood flow.

H40.13 Pigmentary glaucoma

Pigmentary glaucoma occurs when granules of the pigment which colors the eye break off and cause blockage of the drainage canals.

H40.14 Capsular glaucoma with pseudoexfoliation of lens

Pseudoexfoliation glaucoma occurs when the support system which holds the lens of the eye in place breaks down, creating flakes of material which can block the ducts that drain the eye. It presents with a white, flaky material which floats in the anterior chamber.

H40.15 Residual stage of open-angle glaucoma

The residual stage of open angle glaucoma indicates damage done to the optical nerve due to a previous bout of open angle glaucoma.

H40.2 Primary angle-closure glaucoma

Primary angle-closure glaucoma occurs when the surface of the trabecular meshwork becomes blocked, often due to overgrowth of the chamber angle by the iris. This results in a severe, sudden increase in intraocular pressure because of the chamber angle being blocked at the iris and cornea. Rapid vision loss occurs as normal drainage of the aqueous fluid is prevented.

H40.21 Acute angle-closure glaucoma

Acute angle-closure glaucoma is a severe, sudden increase in interocular pressure due to a blockage of the chamber angle, which can cause a correspondingly rapid loss of vision.

Note: Acute angle-closure glaucoma is a medical emergency.

H40.22 Chronic angle-closure glaucoma

Chronic angle-closure glaucoma is not as severe as acute cases, but occurs over a long period of time, causing a gradual loss of vision until it is corrected.

H40.23 Intermittent angle-closure glaucoma

Intermittent angle-closure glaucoma indicates that high ocular pressure due to blockage of the flow of aqueous humor from the eye is not present continuously, but comes and goes.

H40.24 Residual stage of angle-closure glaucoma

Residual stage of angle-closure glaucoma refers to the lasting damage done to the optic nerve after or in between episodes of high intraocular pressure. The high pressure was caused by blockage of the trabecular meshwork at the chamber angle of the iris and the cornea that prevented aqueous fluid from leaving the eye.

H40.4 Glaucoma secondary to eye inflammation

Any inflammation of the eye can compress the canals which drain the aqueous fluid, causing a build-up of intraocular pressure and leadng to secondary glaucoma. One specific type of secondary glaucoma due to inflammation is glaucomatocyclitic crisis, also called Posner-Schlossman syndrome. In this uncommon form of secondary glaucoma, fluid pressure builds up in the anterior chamber due to a flow of fluid coming from the interior of the eye, causing pain and potentially (but rarely) displacing and damaging the iris, lens, and/or ciliary body.

H40.6 Glaucoma secondary to drugs

Glaucoma secondary to drugs is often caused by the use of corticosteroids, a type of hormone produced naturally in the body, that can have the effect of stimulating increased intraocular eye pressure when taken as a prescription medication.

H40.81 Glaucoma with increased episcleral venous pressure

Glaucoma with increased episcleral venous pressure is a condition in which the blood pressure of the veins of the sclera, the white of the eye, is increasing as the pressure of the fluid of the eye increases.

H40.82 Hypersecretion glaucoma

Hypersecretion glaucoma is caused by the overproduction of ocular fluid rather than insufficient drainage, and can usually be controlled with medication.

H40.83 Aqueous misdirection

Aqueous misdirection is a form of glaucoma in which fluid from the eye's inner chamber does not flow normally out into the anterior chamber, but instead is misdirected back into the posterior chamber, the part of the eye between the iris and the ciliary body, which holds the lens in place.

H43.00 Vitreous prolapse, unspecified eye

Vitreous prolapse indicates that vitreous gel is found in an abnormal position in the eye.

H43.31 Vitreous membranes and strands

A condition in which fibrous strands and/or membranes of solid material are found in the vitreous solution of the eye.

H43.39 Other vitreous opacities

Conditions in which the normally clear vitreous fluid becomes opaque, which often causes a loss of visual acuity.

H43.8 Other disorders of vitreous body

The vitreous body is the clear gel-like liquid that fills the interior of the eyeball.

H43.81 Vitreous degeneration

Vitreous degeneration is a condition in which the eye loses the proper functioning of the vitreous gel. This decreases its ability to maintain the right pressure and protect the retina, and could lead to blindness.

H43.82 Vitreomacular adhesion

Vitreomacular adhesion is a condition affecting the center of the retina, called the macula, which is important for vision. In the normal eye, vitreous gel fills the entire vitreous cavity. This gel is made up of 99% water with collagen fibers, large molecules of hyaluronic acid, hyalocytes, inorganic salts, lipids, and polysaccharides. The aging process results in typically nonpathologic posterior vitreous detachment, followed by liquefaction of the vitreous. These age-related changes cause the gel to collapse when the collagen fibers condense and cause the gel to pull forward. When only part of the membrane separating the vitreous from the retina remains attached to the macular area, adhesion occurs at the site. This incomplete detachment can progress and lead to traction syndrome, macular holes, macular edema, proliferative retinopathy, and exudative macular degeneration.

H44.0 Purulent endophthalmitis

Purulent endophthalmitis is a condition in which an inflammation of the tissues of the eye, usually due to an infection, or tumor necrosis or foreign body within the globe of the eye, results in the formation of pus. This inflammation presents with loss of visual acuity, pain, white blood cells within the orb of the eye, swelling of the eye and the eyelid, and the accumulation of fluid in surrounding tissues. In acute cases, permanent vision loss can easily take place unless the inflammation is quickly brought under control. Chronic cases still pose a threat, but are less of a risk of permanent vision loss in the short term. Chronic cases can persist for months or even years.

Note: Use another code to identify the causative organism.

H44.01 Panophthalmitis (acute)

Panophthalmitis is an inflammation that affects all the structures or tissue layers of the eye at once.

H44.02 Vitreous abscess (chronic)

A vitreous abscess is an infected pocket or cavity that appears in the vitreous humor of the eye, which is a clear, gel-like layer that covers and protects the retina in the back of the eye.

H44.1 Other endophthalmitis

Other types of endophthalmitis include those types that do not produce pus.

H44.11 Panuveitis

Panuveitis is an inflammation of all parts of the uveal tract, the front part of the eye that includes the iris, the ciliary body (the hair-like filaments that hold the lens in place), and the choroid (the layers of blood vessels between the iris and the retina that nourish the eye).

H44.12 Parasitic endophthalmitis, unspecified

Parasitic endophthalmitis is an inflammation caused by the intrusion of a parasite into the eye.

Note: This unspecified code should only be used if a more specific code for the parasite is not available.

H44.13 Sympathetic uveitis

Sympathetic uveitis is an inflammation that can sometimes occur in the uninjured eye after an injury to the other eye. This inflammation can appear anywhere from several weeks to several years after the initial injury, and is thought to be an an overreaction by the body's immune system to the original injury that causes it to attack healthy tissue.

H44.2 Degenerative myopia

Degenerative myopia, sometimes called progressive high or malignant myopia, is a condition marked by steadily increasing near-sightedness due to disease in the choroid, the middle layer of the orb of the eye which contains the layers of blood vessels that nourish the rest of the eye. If not corrected, this condition leads to detachment of the retina, the inmost layer of the eye which translates light into nerve impulses to be interpreted by the brain, resulting in permanent blindness.

H44.31 Chalcosis

Use this code for metallosis of the globe when a metal other than iron is accumulating in the eye; e.g., zinc, copper.

H44.32 Siderosis of eye

Siderosis is a condition in which iron from the bloodstream accumulates in the eye, causing degeneration. This is usually caused by a high mineral content in the blood due to a metabolic disorder, and may be treated with medication and a special diet if caught early enough.

H44.4 Hypotony of eye

Hypotony of the eye is a condition in which there is insufficient fluid within the eye to maintain its proper shape (similar to the effect of low air pressure in a tire).

H44.42 Hypotony of eye due to ocular fistula

Hypotony due to an ocular fistula indicates that an abnormal opening into the interior of the eye causes a loss of fluid and pressure. An ocular fistula is often a result of a prior acute infection. A fistula causes decreased eye pressure due to allowing ocular fluid to leak from the normal chambers of the eye, like a slow leak in the tire of a car.

H44.5 Degenerated conditions of globe

A degenerated (as opposed to a degenerative) condition of the globe of the eye is one in which vision loss is not continuing to progress or worsen; that is, that the damage to the patient's vision is done.

H44.51 Absolute glaucoma

Absolute glaucoma is the final stage of blindness in glaucoma. The abnormally high fluid pressure of the aqueous humor within the eye is so high that permanent damage to the retina, blood vessels, and the structures around the iris and lens results in a blind eye. This high pressure is usually very painful.

H44.52 Atrophy of globe

Atrophy of the globe is attributed to extremely low intraocular fluid pressure that causes the eye to lose its shape in a manner similar to the effect of low air pressure in a tire and the extremely hypotensive eye then becomes blind.

H44.53 Leucocoria

Leucocoria is a condition in which part or all of the vitreous, the fluid center of the eye, becomes white and opaque, obscuring vision. This condition is often visible on the outside as a whitish pupil. It is often indicative of retinoblastoma, a highly malignant tumor.

H44.6 Retained (old) intraocular foreign body, magnetic

A foreign body in the eye can often remain long after the initial penetration, causing irritation and infection. The following codes are used when the object is within the interior of the eye rather than on the surface. A magnetic foreign body contains some amount of iron, which is sometimes a factor in deciding how best to extract it, if necessary. Foreign bodies are classified by their location.

Note: the following codes are for "old" foreign objects in the eye only, not those from current, new injuries.

H44.61 Retained (old) magnetic foreign body in anterior chamber

An old magnetic foreign body that contains some amount of iron located within the area between the lens and the cornea.

H44.62 Retained (old) magnetic foreign body in iris or ciliary body

An old magnetic foreign body that contains some amount of iron located in the iris--the colored portion of the eye, or in the ciliary body--the hair-like filaments that hold the lens in place.

H44.65 Retained (old) magnetic foreign body in vitreous body

An old magnetic foreign body that contains some amount of iron located within the vitreous body--the fluid-filled inner chamber of the eye.

H44.7 Retained (old) intraocular foreign body, nonmagnetic

A foreign body in the eye can often remain long after the initial penetration, causing irritation and infection. The following codes are used when the object is within the interior of the eye rather than on the surface. Non-magnetic foreign bodies (e.g., a sliver of wood or plastic) are reported according to their location.

Note: the following codes are for "old" foreign objects in the eye only, not for those from current, new injuries.

H44.71 Retained (nonmagnetic) (old) foreign body in anterior chamber

An old non-magnetic foreign body such as a sliver of wood or plastic located within the area between the lens and the cornea.

H44.72 Retained (nonmagnetic) (old) foreign body in iris or ciliary body

An old, non-magnetic foreign body such as a sliver of wood or plastic located in the iris--the colored portion of the eye, or in the ciliary body--the hair-like filaments that hold the lens in place.

H44.721 Retained (nonmagnetic) (old) foreign body in iris or ciliary body, right eye

Use this code if the foreign body is caught in the colored portion or in the ciliary body, the hair-like filaments that hold the lens.

H44.75 Retained (nonmagnetic) (old) foreign body in vitreous body

An old non-magnetic foreign body such as a sliver of wood or plastic located in the fluid-filled inner chamber of the eye.

H44.81 Hemophthalmos

Hemophthalmos is a condition in which blood pools within the eyeball due to a rupture of the vessels of the choroid, the middle layer of the orb. This pool of blood blocks light from the retina, causing blindness.

Note: This code is not to be used for hemophthalmos due to a recent injury.

H44.82 Luxation of globe

Luxation of the globe means that the eye has slipped out of its proper place in its socket. This may occur as a result of weakness in the muscles that control the movement of the eye.

H46 Optic neuritis

The optic nerve is part of the central nervous system, and transmits visual impulses from the back of the eye to the brain. The visual pathways are the channels through the brain by which visual impulses travel from the eye to the visual cortex of the brain. Inflammatory disorders of these structures are often progressive, and damage to the optic nerve is typically permanent. Damage to the optic nerve and visual pathways will result in varying degrees of visual impairment.

H46.0 Optic papillitis

Optic papillitis is a swelling of the optic disc where the optic nerve connects to the retina.

H46.1 Retrobulbar neuritis

Retrobulbar neuritis is a condition in which the portion of the optic nerve directly behind the eye becomes inflamed.

H46.2 Nutritional optic neuropathy

The optic nerve is damaged due to malnutrition. This is uncommon in the U.S.

H47.01 Ischemic optic neuropathy

In ischemic optic neuropathy, the optic nerve is adversely affected and malfunctions due to a lack of blood flow.

H47.03 Optic nerve hypoplasia

Optic nerve hypoplasia is a congenital underdevelopment of the optic nerves occurring during pregnancy. The optic nerve bundles that send signals from the eye to the occipital lobe of the brain somehow do not fully develop. The condition is not hereditary and the causes are uncertain. Optic nerve hypoplasia can occur in one or both eyes and may result in only mild visual impairment or more serious impairment in decreased acuity and field of vision. Patients may also have involuntary eye movements and an aversion to light.

H47.1 Papilledema

Papilledema is a condition in which the optic disc, the part of the retina that connects to the optic nerve (the "blind spot" because it lacks any photoreceptors), swells with fluid.

H47.11 Papilledema associated with increased intracranial pressure

Swelling of the optic disc, the part of the retina that connects to the optic nerve, caused by increased intracranial pressure.

H47.14 Foster-Kennedy syndrome

Foster-Kennedy syndrome is a disease in which the patient suffers from papilledema in one eye and atrophy of the optic nerve in the other. This condition is caused by raised pressure inside the skull due to the formation of a tumor.

H47.2 Optic atrophy

Optic atrophy is a wasting of the optic nerve in which it degenerates or malfunctions.

H47.21 Primary optic atrophy

Primary optic atrophy is a condition in which the head of the optic nerve appears pale, with sharp edges. This is typically due to a loss of blood flow to the nerve.

H47.23 Glaucomatous optic atrophy

Glaucomatous atrophy of the optic disc is a condition in which abnormally high pressure inside the eye causes damage to the optic nerve at the point where it attaches to the back of the eye.

H47.29 Other optic atrophy

Other types and causes of optic atrophy include postinflammatory optic atrophy in which the optic nerve degenerates due to the effects of a previous infection or inflammation of the eye or its surrounding structures. Optic atrophy associated with a retinal dystrophy in which a disease affecting the retina results in degeneration of the optic nerve as well. Partial optic atrophy indicates a type in which only a portion of the nerve is affected.

H47.3 Other disorders of optic disc

Other disorders affecting the area in the back of the retina where the optic nerve attaches to the eye.

H47.31 Coloboma of optic disc

Coloboma of the optic disc is a congenital defect of the iris in which there is a gap, hole, or cleft in the rear of the eye that failed to close. While this is often asymptomatic, it may cause ghost images, blurred or decreased visual acuity, or a partial loss of vision in the afflicted eye.

H47.32 Drusen of optic disc

This disorder causes tiny concentrations of crystallized calcium and protein to accumulate on the optic disc. While usually asymptomatic, the patient may experience some loss of peripheral vision.

H47.33 Pseudopapilledema of optic disc

Pseudopapilledema is a condition in which the optic disc becomes swollen due to diseases affecting the optic nerve.

H47.39 Other disorders of optic disc

Other disorders of the optic disc include crater-like holes, or tiny pits that can be seen in the back of the retina.

H47.4 Disorders of optic chiasm

The optic chiasm is the point in the brain at which visual impulses cross in the middle of the brain. Impulses from the left eye are received in the right side of the visual cortex, and vice versa. These disorders are classified according to what type of disease is associated with them.

H47.41 Disorders of optic chiasm in (due to) inflammatory disorders

Inflammatory disorders which disrupt the transmission of visual impulses from the eyes to the visual cortex of the brain.

H47.42 Disorders of optic chiasm in (due to) neoplasm

Disorders in which neural impulses from the eye are interrupted by tumors or other neoplasms in the brain.

H47.43 Disorders of optic chiasm in (due to) vascular disorders

Conditions in which neural impulses from the eye are interrupted on their path to the brain due to blood-flow problems in the brain and head.

H47.6 Disorders of visual cortex

The visual cortex is the part of the cerebral cortex that processes visual stimuli collected by the eye. These type of disorders are usually classified according to their associated diseases.

H47.61 Cortical blindness

Blindness cause by a disorder or defective function of the brain, not the eyes.

H49 Paralytic strabismus

Codes in this section are used to report strabismus and other disorders in which the eyes fail to move in a coordinated fashion due to some kind of palsy or paralysis affecting eye muscles. Strabismus is a condition in which the eyes cannot focus on the same object due to an imbalance of the strength of the muscles that control eye movements.

H49.0 Third [oculomotor] nerve palsy

Third oculomotor nerve palsy is a condition in which palsy of the third pair of cranial nerves that control movements of the eye causes the eye muscles to become abnormally weak, twitch., or even completely paralyzed.

H49.1 Fourth [trochlear] nerve palsy

In palsy of the trochlear nerve, the fourth pair of cranial nerves controlling the superior oblique muscles of the eyes become abnormally weak, twitch, or become paralyzed.

H49.2 Sixth [abducent] nerve palsy

Palsy of the abducent nerve, also known as the sixth cranial nerve, affects the muscle on the lateral portion of the eye near the temple and causes twitching, weakness, and paralysis.

H49.3 Total (external) ophthalmoplegia

Paralysis of all the muscles that move the eye as well as the muscles controlling the diameter of the pupil and shape of the lens.

H49.4 Progressive external ophthalmoplegia

Progressive external ophthalmoplegia is a condition in which the muscles that move the eye slowly become paralyzed.

H50.0 Esotropia

Esotropia is a type of strabismus in which there is deviation of the visual axis of one or both eyes turning inward toward the other eye.

H50.01 Monocular esotropia

Visual axis deviation in which one eye turns inward toward the other.

H50.02 Monocular esotropia with A pattern

Visual axis deviation in which one eye turns upwards and inwards.

H50.03 Monocular esotropia with V pattern

Visual axis deviation in which one eye turns downwards and inwards.

H50.05 Alternating esotropia

In alternating esotropia, the inward visual deviation shifts from one eye to the other.

H50.06 Alternating esotropia with A pattern

A visual deviation in which the eye turning upward and inward shifts from one eye to the other.

H50.07 Alternating esotropia with V pattern

A visual deviation in which the eye turning downward and inward shifts from one eye to the other.

H50.1 Exotropia

Exotropia is a type of strabismus in which there is deviation of the visual axis of one or both eyes turning outward away from each other.

H50.11 Monocular exotropia

Visual axis deviation in which one eye turns outward away from the other.

H50.12 Monocular exotropia with A pattern

Deviation of the visual axis in which one eye turns upwards and outward away from the other.

H50.13 Monocular exotropia with V pattern

Deviation of the visual axis in which one eye turns downwards and outward away from the other.

H50.15 Alternating exotropia

In alternating exotropia, the outward visual deviation shifts from one eye to the other.

H50.16 Alternating exotropia with A pattern

A visual deviation in which the eye turning upward and outward shifts from one eye to the other.

H50.17 Alternating exotropia with V pattern

A visual deviation in which the eye turning downward and outward shifts from one eye to the other.

H50.2 Vertical strabismus

Vertical strabismus, also called hypertropia, is the condition in which an eye deviates upwards.

H50.3 Intermittent heterotropia

Intermittent heterotropia is a form of strabismus in which one or both eyes deviate outward or inward for a period of time before returning to the normal visual axis.

H50.31 Intermittent monocular esotropia

Visual axis deviation in which one eye turns inward toward the other for a period of time and then returns to the normal axis.

H50.32 Intermittent alternating esotropia

Visual axis deviation in which the left eye alternates with the right eye turning inward for a period of time before returning to its normal axis.

H50.33 Intermittent monocular exotropia

Visual axis deviation in which one eye turns outward away from the other for a period of time and then returns to the normal axis.

H50.34 Intermittent alternating exotropia

Visual axis deviation in which the left eye alternates with the right eye turning outward for a period of time before returning to its normal axis.

H50.41 Cyclotropia

Cyclotropia is a condition in which one of the eyes deviates by rotating around the anteroposterior axis (the imaginary line drawn from the center of the iris to the back of the eye). While this is not as observable as other forms of strabismus, it can still result in impaired binocular vision.

H50.42 Monofixation syndrome

Monofixation syndrome, also known as microtopia, is a condition of subnormal binocular vision in which small angle strabismus with central retina scotoma in the deviating eye that prevents bifixation, is present with central fixation in the preferred eye, and binocular peripheral fusion. Because the central retina has tiny areas of reception that are more sensitive to blurring or image disparity than the peripheral retina, when a scotoma appears in the central retina but allows for binocular fusion of the peripheral vision, monofixation syndrome results. This condition is desirable when bifixation is not possible and often results from surgical treatment for congenital esotropia.

H50.43 Accommodative component in esotropia

In an accommodative component in esotropia, the patient spontaneously attempts to accommodate for the deviating eye, but still has problems focusing.

H50.5 Heterophoria

Heterophoria is a failure of the visual axes to stay parallel when one eye is covered and the stimulus of visual fusion is taken away. The direction that the eye deviates differs.

H50.51 Esophoria

An inward deviation of the eye whenever the other is covered or fusional vision of both eyes is interrupted.

H50.52 Exophoria

An outward deviation of the eye whenever the other is covered or fusional vision of both eyes is interrupted.

H50.53 Vertical heterophoria

An upward deviation of the eye whenever the other is covered or fusional vision of both eyes is interrupted.

H50.54 Cyclophoria

Deviation of one eye around the anteroposterior axis (the imaginary line drawn from the center of the iris to the back of the eye) whenever the other eye is covered, or fusional vision of both eyes is interrupted.

H50.6 Mechanical strabismus

Deviation from the normal visual axis caused by defects of the ocular muscles that do not allow the eyes to move coherently.

H50.61 Brown's sheath syndrome

Brown's sheath syndrome is a condition in which the muscle that moves the eye upward and inward is too short, impairing eye movement.

H50.81 Duane's syndrome

Duane's syndrome is a congenital defect in which abnormal fibrous tissue is found attached to the muscles that move one of the patient's eyes, inhibiting proper movement.

H51.0 Palsy (spasm) of conjugate gaze

Palsy (spasm) of conjugate gaze is a neurological disorder affecting the ability to move both of the eyes together in a single horizontal or vertical direction. Gaze palsies most often affect horizontal gaze direction controlled by neural input from the cerebrum, cerebellum, neck, and vestibular centers. Neural input converges at the horizontal gaze center, integrates into one impulse to the adjacent sixth cranial nerve controlling lateral movement on the same side and to the contralateral third cranial nerve controlling medial rectus movement on the other side. Gaze palsy is most often caused by lesions in the cerebral hemispheres and cranial nerves, and stroke.

H51.11 Convergence insufficiency

Convergence insufficiency is a condition in which the eyes appear to move normally but have difficulty shifting inwards due to weak muscles. This often results in a headache and blurred vision, especially while reading.

H51.12 Convergence excess

A convergence excess or spasm is a condition in which the patient's eyes fail to move in a coordinated fashion when viewing objects up close.

H51.20 Internuclear ophthalmoplegia, unspecified eye

In internuclear ophthalmoplegia, the nerve fibers that control eye movements are damaged, usually due to a stroke or multiple sclerosis.

H52 Disorders of refraction and accommodation

Disorders of refraction and accommodation are those which are typically corrected by glasses or contact lenses, such as near- and far-sightedness.

H52.0 Hypermetropia

Hypermetropia, better known as hypertopia and far-sightedness, occurs when the point of focus for light entering the eye occurs behind the retinal wall of the eye. This may be because the eyeball is too short from front to back, or because the cornea and/or lens do not focus the light on the correct point. In either case, the effect is that the patient can focus on distant objects, but close objects (e.g., the text on a book held in the hand) are blurry.

H52.1 Myopia

Myopia, or near-sightedness, occurs when the point of focus is in front of the retinal wall (i.e., within the interior chamber of the eye), either because of an unusually long eyeball from front to back, or because the cornea and/or lens do not focus the light properly on the correct point. In either case, the effect is that the patient can focus on objects up close, but distant objects are blurry.

H52.2 Astigmatism

Astigmatism is a condition in which the cornea has an oval shape (i.e., almost like a football) instead of a perfectly round shape. This causes light to focus on more than one point of the retina, resulting in blurred vision. Astigmatism is often seen alongside near- or far-sightedness.

H52.21 Irregular astigmatism

In an irregular astigmatism, the meridians (lines drawn at the peak of curvature) are not 180 degrees apart.

H52.22 Regular astigmatism

In a regular astigmatism, the meridians (lines drawn at the peak of curvature) are 180 degrees apart.

H52.31 Anisometropia

Anisometropia is a condition in which the two eyes have unequal vision. For example, one may be near-sighted while the other is far-sighted, or one of two near-sighted eyes may have far less visual acuity than the other. This can cause the brain to favor the eye with better visual acuity over the other, and can cause loss of vision, or "lazy eye," in the other eye if not corrected.

H52.32 Aniseikonia

Aniseikonia causes the images received by the retinas of the two eyes to appear to be of different sizes, locations, and/or shapes. This may be due to differences in the sizes of the two eyes, surgery, and/or damage to one of the eyes causing the retina to have become stretched.

H52.4 Presbyopia

Presbyopia is a condition which typically occurs in the patient's 40s, in which the lens of the eye loses its elasticity, making it more difficult to focus the eyes on near points. For example, the patient may need to hold books further away to read them, similar to far-sightedness.

H52.5 Disorders of accommodation

Disorders of accommodation are vision disorders caused by a disorder of the ciliary muscle, a ring-shaped muscle which controls and focuses the lens.

H52.51 Internal ophthalmoplegia (complete) (total)

A total or complete internal ophthalmoplegia is a complete paralysis of the ciliary muscle, which prevents the patient from focusing his or her vision at all. This disorder may initially present as far-sightedness.

H52.52 Paresis of accommodation

A paresis of accommodation is a partial paralysis of the ciliary muscle, the ring-like muscle that controls and focuses the lens. It is often initially mistaken for far-sightedness.

H52.53 Spasm of accommodation

A spasm of accommodation is an abnormal, uncontrolled contraction of the ciliary muscle. This usually initially presents as near-sightedness.

H53.0 Amblyopia ex anopsia

Amblyopia ex anopsia is a loss of visual acuity in the absence of an organic disease. It presents in only one eye, and is uncorrectable with lenses. It occurs when one eye is heavily favored over the other during a child's visual developmental period (up to 8 years old), causing the brain to ignore the lesser eye, leading to complete vision loss in that eye.

H53.01 Deprivation amblyopia

Deprivation amblyopia occurs when cataracts or other visual problems deprive a child of normal vision in one eye during the eyes' developmental period. As the brain favors the better eye, permanent blindness can occur in the affected eye.

H53.02 Refractive amblyopia

Refractive amblyopia occurs when a refractive disorder (e.g., near- or far-sightedness) develops more severely in one eye than the other during the eyes' developmental period. As the brain favors the better eye, permanent blindness can occur in the affected eye.

H53.03 Strabismic amblyopia

Strabismic amblyopia, sometimes called lazy eye, is amblyopia which develops due to a misalignment or weakness of the muscles that control the eye, causing a crossed-eye appearance. As the brain favors one eye over the other, vision loss in the unused eye can develop.

H53.1 Subjective visual disturbances

Subjective visual disturbances are visible only to the patient, and cannot be seen by the physician unlike, for example, a cataract or an astigmatism. Visual loss, one such subjective disturbance, refers to a period during which the patient experiences blurring, fogging, or dimming of the vision. The patient may experience this visual loss only once, in repeated episodes over several years, or permanently. It is most often caused by a loss of blood flow to the eye, called ischemia.

H53.12 Transient visual loss

Transient visual loss indicates that the visual loss is temporary, and may last for anywhere from a few minutes to a few hours.

H53.13 Sudden visual loss

Sudden visual loss indicates that the visual loss had no preceding signs, appeared almost spontaneously, and is ongoing.

H53.14 Visual discomfort

Visual discomfort describes a variety of conditions, such as asthenopia (eye-strain) or photophobia (experiencing pain in bright light). These conditions are most often the result of working in poor lighting conditions.

H53.15 Visual distortions of shape and size

Visual distortions of shape and size indicate that the patient is unable to properly discern the shape and/or size of an object, which appear distorted. For example, a patient with macropsia makes objects seem unusually large, while micropsia makes them appear unusually small.

H53.16 Psychophysical visual disturbances

Psychophysical visual disturbances are caused by an error in how the brain interprets the nerve impulses from the eyes.

H53.2 Diplopia

Diplopia means that the patient is experiencing double-vision.

H53.3 Other and unspecified disorders of binocular vision

Binocular vision refers to how the eyes work together to form a single, perceived image.

Diseases of the Eye and Adnexa

H53.31 – H55.02

H53.31 Abnormal retinal correspondence

Abnormal retinal correspondence occurs when the eyes are not aligned properly, causing the brain to compensate by attempting to align the mismatched images. If the eyes are later re-aligned by surgery or other therapy, this can result in double-vision and other visual disturbances.

H53.32 Fusion with defective stereopsis

Fusion with defective stereopsis indicates that the vision of the two eyes is fused into one image by the brain, but that this fusion is imperfect, resulting in a faulty depth perception since the brain interprets depth by the differences between the images of the two eyes.

H53.33 Simultaneous visual perception without fusion

Simultaneous visual perception without fusion is a condition in which the imaging from both eyes reaches the brain and are both processed, but in which the brain does not merge them into a single image. As a result, the patient sees two side-by-side images instead of the usual one.

H53.34 Suppression of binocular vision

Suppression of binocular vision occurs when the brain ignores the image of one eye in favor of the other, usually due to the suppressed eye being the significantly weaker of the two. This condition most often occurs during childhood development of the eyes, up to eight years of age.

H53.4 Visual field defects

A visual field defect is a blind spot. This is as an area, often small, in which the patient has no vision where they normally should. A small blind-spot, which is invisible to the patient since the brain overlooks it, naturally occurs at the juncture where the optic nerve attaches to the eye. Such a defect may be referred to as a scotoma (pl. scotomata) when it is visible to the patient, such as a grayed-out or unfocused area, or as a dark spot. In some cases, such as a blind spot that appears during the course of a migraine headache, these defects are temporary, but they are more often permanent as a result of physical damage to the retina and/or optic nerves. Bilateral field defects are those which are visible in both of the eyes, and are nearly always due to a disorder or disease in the part of the brain which processes vision rather than in the retinas.

H53.41 Scotoma involving central area

A blind spot that occurs in the central five degrees of the patient's vision.

H53.42 Scotoma of blind spot area

A scotoma that occurs in the eye's natural blind-spot at the juncture where the optic nerve attaches to the eye, so that it becomes a noticeable blind spot to the patient.

H53.43 Sector or arcuate defects

A sector or arcuate defect is a blind-spot that occurs in an arc-shape, usually to one side of the central vision. This defect is caused by damage to the optic nerve rather than by the retina.

H53.46 Homonymous bilateral field defects

A homonymous bilateral field defect affects either the top or bottom half of the visual field in both eyes.

H53.47 Heteronymous bilateral field defects

A heteronymous bilateral field defect affects the opposite halves of the visual field in both eyes (e.g., the top half in one eye and the bottom in the other).

H53.48 Generalized contraction of visual field

A generalized contraction or constriction is a condition where one or both eyes experience a narrowing of the field of vision, which may or may not be visible to the patient as tunnel vision.

H53.5 Color vision deficiencies

Color vision is produced by cone-like structures on the retina of the eye. These cones are divided into three types, which receive the wavelengths of light that make up the colors red, green, and blue respectively. Color vision deficiencies, otherwise known as color-blindness, are caused by a disorder affecting one or more types of the cones.

H53.51 Achromatopsia

Achromatopsia is complete color blindness, so that the patient sees the world only as shades of gray. Because the cones provide detailed vision as well as color, a person with this disorder who has to depend entirely on the rod-like structures which provide night vision, usually also have poor visual acuity. This disorder is rare, and may be caused by disease, an injury to the retina or optic nerve, or by a genetic disorder.

H53.53 Deuteranomaly

A deutan defect is a loss or abnormality of the green-sensitive cones. This disorder affects only males, and makes it difficult to distinguish between certain shades of red and green, though an inability to distinguish at all between pure red and pure green is extremely rare.

H53.54 Protanomaly

A protan defect is a loss or abnormality of the red-sensitive cones. This disorder affects only males, and makes it difficult to distinguish between certain shades of red and green, though an inability to distinguish at all between pure red and pure green is extremely rare.

H53.55 Tritanomaly

A tritan defect, which results from a loss or abnormality in the blue cones, results in difficulty in differentiating between blue and yellow. This disorder may result from a side-effect of taking certain drugs, from retinal detachment, or due to other diseases of the nervous system.

H53.6 Night blindness

Night-blindness, in contrast with color-blindness, is the result of deficient or damaged rods instead of cones that creates severely diminished visual ability in low light that makes it difficult or impossible to see at night. When the rods in the retina lose their ability to respond to light, they may work very little or not at all and since more rods than cones are located around the outer area of the retina, the patient usually suffers loss of peripheral vision with night blindness. These patients will also need a longer time to adjust to contrasting levels of light when going from brightly lit areas to dimly lit areas.

Note: Night blindness due to a vitamin A deficiency is not coded here, but reported with E50.5.

H53.61 Abnormal dark adaptation curve

An abnormal dark-adaptation curve indicates that while the patient does have some night vision, it drops off at unusually light conditions; e.g., a patient might only see in full moonlight what a normal person could perceive in near darkness.

H53.72 Impaired contrast sensitivity

Impaired contrast sensitivity is difficulty being able to discern the differences in luminances, or different brightness levels, between adjacent areas in an image. An object is distinguishable by the difference in brightness and color of it in comparison to other objects within the same field of view.

H55.0 Nystagmus

Nystagmus is fast, uncontrollable and involuntary jerky movements of the eyes, often exaggerated by looking in a particular direction. This results in an inability to look steadily at an object.

H55.01 Congenital nystagmus

Congenital nystagmus is an inherited condition of fast, uncontrollable and involuntary jerky movements of the eyes, which is often associated with conditions such as albinism and achromatopsia.

H55.02 Latent nystagmus

In latent nystagmus, the patient exhibits nystagmus in one eye only when the other eye is covered.

H55.04   Dissociated nystagmus

In dissociated nystagmus, the eyes move in different patterns.

H55.09   Other forms of nystagmus

Nystagmus is sometimes associated with disorders of the vestibular system, which is located in the inner ear and keeps track of the motion and position of the body, and also allows for smooth vision while moving.

H55.81   Saccadic eye movements

In deficiencies of saccadic eye movements, the eyes move rapidly and involuntarily while changing which (stationary) object they are focusing on.

H55.89   Other irregular eye movements

In deficiencies of smooth pursuit movements, the patient's eyes jerk while tracking a moving object.

H57.0   Anomalies of pupillary function

Aberrant action in the opening and closing of the iris that controls pupil size and the amount of light passing to the retina.

H57.01   Argyll Robertson pupil, atypical

An atypical Argyll Robertson pupil is a condition in which the pupil does not change shape in response to light.

H57.02   Anisocoria

Anisocoria is a condition in which the pupils are of unequal size.

H57.03   Miosis

In persistent miosis, the pupils abnormally contract to less than 2 millimeters in size.

H57.04   Mydriasis

In mydriasis, a disease or medication causes the pupils to become abnormally dilated.

H57.05   Tonic pupil

In tonic pupil, sometimes called Adie's pupil or tonic pupillary reaction, parasympathetic denervation causes the pupil to react slowly in response to light, but still allows it to change somewhat better in response to accomodation (near vision). This is the most common cause of anisocoria, or unequal pupil size. The tonic pupil contracts in slow motion in response to light stimulus and becomes smaller than the normal pupil. It remains constricted while redilating only very slowly in darker surroundings. Some patients also have transient cycloplegia. Initial evaluation may show a pupil frozen to both light or accomodation and later a light-near dissociation occurs.

H59.4   Inflammation (infection) of postprocedural bleb

Postprocedural bleb, called a filtering bleb, is an auxiliary drain placed on the outside of the eyeball following certain ophthalmologic procedures, particularly trabeculetomy for glaucoma. Infection commonly occurs because the filtering bleb is extremely thin walled, which allows bacteria to invade easily. Postprocedural bleb inflammation or infection is categorized by the stage of severity.

H59.41   Inflammation (infection) of postprocedural bleb, stage 1

Stage 1 infection of posprocedural bleb is characterized by purulence, or discharge containing pus that appears with or without a mild inflammation in the anterior segment of the eye. Stage 1 infection may be resolved with topical antibiotics.

H59.42   Inflammation (infection) of postprocedural bleb, stage 2

Stage 2 infection of posprocedural bleb is characterized by purulence, or discharge containing pus that appears with moderate inflammation in the anterior segment of the eye. Stage 2 infection requires topical and oral antibiotics with frequent evaluation and a subconjunctival injection of antibiotics when improvement is not seen within 24-48 hours.

H59.43   Inflammation (infection) of postprocedural bleb, stage 3

Stage 3 infection of postprocedural bleb is characterized by a full anterior chamber reaction, vitritis, and severe pain. Stage 3 infections can develop into bleb-related endophthalmitis and acute loss of vision. Stage 3 infection may require multiple subconjunctival injections of antibiotics. After the infection is cleared, many patients require surgical revision to the bleb and may be at risk for repeat infection.

H60 **Otitis externa**

Otitis externa is an inflammation of the outer ear and ear canal. Acute otitis externa is usually associated with some type of bacterial or fungal infection, abscess, or cellulitis although acute otitis externa may also be noninfective in origin, caused by allergic or chemical contact. Symptoms include rapid onset of pain, a feeling of pressure/fullness in the ear, and difficulty hearing.

H60.2 **Malignant otitis externa**

In malignant otitis externa, a bacterial infection of the outer ear leads to tissue death.

H60.33 **Swimmer's ear**

Swimmer's ear is otitis externa caused by prolonged immersion in water which moistens the skin of the outer ear, providing a breeding ground for bacteria and fungi.

H60.39 **Other infective otitis externa**

Infective otitis externa is an infection of the outer ear canal. Symptoms of otitis externa include a painful, swollen outer ear, as well as a discharge from the ear.

H60.4 **Cholesteatoma of external ear**

A cholesteatoma of the external ear is a cyst-like growth containing cholesterol, among other substances. This condition is a rare birth defect.

H60.6 **Unspecified chronic otitis externa**

Otitis externa is an inflammation of the outer ear and ear canal. Chronic inflammation generally lasts more than 3-4 months or has more than 4 episodes in 1 year. Chronic otitis externa may be caused by some type of dermatitis (eczema) and presents with itching, a feeling of pressure/fullness in the ear, and difficulty hearing.

H61.0 **Chondritis and perichondritis of external ear**

Chondritis and perichondritis of the external ear is an inflammation of the cartilage of the outer, visible part of the ear, called the pinna, and the dense fibrous membrane that connects the cartilage to the surrounding soft tissue.

H61.01 **Acute perichondritis of external ear**

Acute perichondritis of the outer ear is a severe inflammation of the cartilage of the pinna, usually short-lived.

H61.02 **Chronic perichondritis of external ear**

In chronic perichondritis of the outer ear, the degree of inflammation of the pinna is usually less than that of an acute attack, but may linger for months or even years.

H61.03 **Chondritis of external ear**

Chondritis of the outer ear is an inflammation of the dense fibrous membrane that connects the external ear cartilage to the surrounding soft tissue.

H61.11 **Acquired deformity of pinna**

An acquired deformity of the outer portion of the ear is one caused by trauma, injury, or illness rather than a hereditary condition.

H61.12 **Hematoma of pinna**

A hematoma of the auricle or pinna is a swelling filled with blood on the outer ear.

H61.2 **Impacted cerumen**

Impacted cerumen is wax which has built up so as to block the external ear canal.

H61.3 **Acquired stenosis of external ear canal**

Narrowing of the external ear canal caused by trauma, injury, or illness rather than a hereditary condition.

H61.81 **Exostosis of external canal**

A bony growth covered with cartilage forming in the outer ear canal.

H65 **Nonsuppurative otitis media**

Nonsuppurative otitis media is an infection of the middle ear that does not produce pus.

H65.0 **Acute serous otitis media**

In acute serous otitis media, the infection of the middle ear is accompanied by a build-up of fluid, usually due to inflammation of the Eustachian tube that prevents drainage.

H65.11 **Acute and subacute allergic otitis media (mucoid) (sanguinous) (serous)**

Acute allergic serous otitis media is an inflammation of the middle ear accompanied by fluid build-up that is caused by an allergic reaction. Acute allergic mucoid otitis media is a condition in which the allergic middle ear inflammation is accompanied by the formation of mucous. Acute allergic sanguinous otitis media is an allergic infection accompanied by bleeding in the middle ear.

H65.19 **Other acute nonsuppurative otitis media**

Other acute nonsuppurative otitis media includes acute and subacute cases of middle ear infections that are not producting pus, other than allergic or serous. This includes mucoid otitis media in which the infection is accompanied by mucous, sanguinous otitis media is which there is bleeding of the middle ear's structures with the infection, and seromucinous otitis media, producing both a build-up of serum-like fluid with mucous in the middler ear.

H65.2 **Chronic serous otitis media**

In chronic serous otitis media, the middle ear infection has an extended duration, usually of several months, and is accompanied by a fluid build-up in the middle ear.

H65.3 **Chronic mucoid otitis media**

In chronic mucoid otitis media, a long-term middle ear infection causes mucous to become trapped in the middle ear, usually due to an inflammation of the Eustachian tube (which normally drains mucous into the throat).

H65.41 **Chronic allergic otitis media**

A long-term inflammation of the middle ear caused by an allergic reaction.

H65.49 **Other chronic nonsuppurative otitis media**

Use this code to report specified forms of chronic nonsuppurative otitis media, other than mucoid or serous, that are not producing pus and are not caused by an allergic reacion; for example, chronic exudative, chronic seromucinous, or chronic nonpurulent effusive otitis media.

H66 **Suppurative and unspecified otitis media**

Otitis media is an inflammation of the middle ear, between the tympanic membrane and inner ear (including the eustachian tube) and can be chronic (symptoms present for >2 weeks with eardrum perforation) or acute. Inflammation may be caused by a viral, bacterial, or fungal infection and is often precipitated by an upper respiratory infection (cold) or allergies. Symptoms can include intense pain and feeling of pressure/fullness in the ear and drainage from the ear. Suppurative otitis media is a middle ear infection that produces a discharge of pus.

H66.0   Acute suppurative otitis media

A sudden or severe middle ear infection that is producing a discharge of pus.

H66.1   Chronic tubotympanic suppurative otitis media

Chronic tubotympanic suppurative otitis media is a condition in which the middle ear infection produces pus and affects both the tympanic membrane and the Eustachian tube.

H66.2   Chronic atticoantral suppurative otitis media

In chronic atticoantral suppurative otitis media, the middle ear infection produces pus and spreads into the upper eardrum and mastoid process of the skull.

H66.9   Otitis media, unspecified

Unspecified otitis media is coded whenever otitis media is identified as either acute or chronic, but not further specified.

H68.0   Eustachian salpingitis

The Eustachian tube connects the middle ear to the pharynx and maintains proper inner-ear pressure. Eustachian salpingitis is an infection or inflammation of this tube.

H68.12   Intrinsic cartilagenous obstruction of Eustachian tube

A condition in which an overgrowth of the cartilage of the outer ear blocks the ear canal.

H68.13   Extrinsic cartilagenous obstruction of Eustachian tube

A condition in which an overgrowth of outer ear cartilage compresses the ear canal.

H69.00   Patulous Eustachian tube, unspecified ear

A patulous Eustachian tube is one which is overly expanded.

H70   Mastoiditis and related conditions

Mastoiditis is an inflammation of the mastoid process, a porous, bony structure of the skull located behind the ear. This part of the skull most often becomes infected when a bacterial infection of the middle ear is not properly treated and migrates.

H70.01   Subperiosteal abscess of mastoid

A subperiosteal abscess of the mastoid process is a pocket of pus and infected material located in the air cells of the mastoid process of the skull behind the ear.

H70.1   Chronic mastoiditis

Chronic mastoiditis is a long-term, ongoing inflammation of the mastoid process, a porous, bony structure of the skull located behind the ear. The inflammation may continue over months or years. This type of infection is normally less severe than an acute infection but usually requires surgery to drain the mastoid process before it will resolve.

H70.2   Petrositis

Petrositis is an inflammation of the dense, hard bone behind the temple that protects the inner ear.

H70.81   Postauricular fistula

A postauricular fistula is an abnormal passage that forms behind the ear and leads to another part of the skull or face, usually resulting from a severe infection.

H71   Cholesteatoma of middle ear

A cholesteatoma of the middle ear is a cyst-like mass filled with cell debris and cholesterol of the middle ear and/or mastoid process, the porous bone of the skull behind the ear.

H71.3   Diffuse cholesteatosis

Diffuse cholesteatosis is a condition in which there are multiple cholesteatomas throughout the middle ear.

H72   Perforation of tympanic membrane

The tympanic membrane is more commonly known as the eardrum. This membrane separates the middle ear from the outer ear, and vibrates to transmit sound waves through the middle ear to the inner ear. Minor perforations usually heal themselves and are not medical emergencies, while severe perforations may require surgical repair.

H72.0   Central perforation of tympanic membrane

A hole in the center of the eardrum.

H72.1   Attic perforation of tympanic membrane

A hole in the uppermost portion of the eardrum.

H72.2   Other marginal perforations of tympanic membrane

Other perforations around the margins, or edges, of the eardrum.

H72.82   Total perforations of tympanic membrane

A total, or complete, perforation of the eardrum always results in severe hearing loss and requires surgical correction.

H73   Other disorders of tympanic membrane

The tympanic membrane is more commonly known as the eardrum. This membrane separates the middle ear from the outer ear, and vibrates to transmit sound waves through the middle ear to the inner ear.

H73.01   Bullous myringitis

In bullous myringitis, the inflammation of the eardrum is caused by a virus and is characterized by blood-filled blisters.

H73.81   Atrophic flaccid tympanic membrane

An atrophic flaccid eardrum is one which has wasted away and lost its tension, resulting in severe hearing loss.

H73.82   Atrophic nonflaccid tympanic membrane

In an atrophic nonflaccid tympanic membrane, the eardrum is wasting away and weakening, but has not lost its tension. While some hearing loss results, it is usually not as dramatic as in an atrophic flaccid eardrum.

H74.0   Tympanosclerosis

Tympanosclerosis is a condition in which the eardrum thickens and hardens, reducing its ability to vibrate and transmit sound. This condition can also affect the middle ear cavity and the small bones (ossicles) that transmit sound from the eardrum to the inner ear. This condition is reported according to which part of the ear it affects.

H74.1   Adhesive middle ear disease

In adhesions of the middle ear, structures in the middle ear grow together or are connected by fibrous scar tissue, impairing their ability to function. The incus, or middle ossicle adheres to the eardrum in drum to incus adhesion; the stapes connecting to the inner ear may also adhere to the eardrum; or the promontorium, the projecting part of the cochlea of the inner ear may adhere to the eardrum.

H80   Otosclerosis

In otosclerosis, abnormal spongy bone begins to form where the stapes bone of the middle ear meets the oval window leading to the inner ear, causing progressive hearing loss.

H80.0   Otosclerosis involving oval window, nonobliterative

The oval window is the oval opening in the middle ear through which the ossicles transmit sound to the cochlea. Nonobliterative otosclerosis involves sponge-like bone formation in which the oval window is partially impeded.

H80.1   Otosclerosis involving oval window, obliterative

The oval window is the oval opening in the middle ear through which the ossicles transmit sound to the cochlea. Obliterative otosclerosis involves abnormal sponge-like bone formation to the extent that the oval window is completely blocked.

H81   Disorders of vestibular function

The vestibular system is located in the bony labyrinth of the inner ear and coordinates balance, posture, and eye moments while the body is in motion. If this system is damaged, vertiginous syndromes such as vertigo, or dizziness, can result.

H81.0   Ménière's disease

Meniere's disease is a disorder of unknown origins which presents with symptoms of vertigo, ringing in the ear (tinnitus), and progressive hearing loss for all tones. Usually only one ear is affected, although the disease can occur bilaterally. Meniere's disease may affect both the cochlea and the vestibular system. Patients with Meniere's disease that affects only the cochlea of the inner ear experience the symptoms of hearing loss and tinnitus more severely than they do vertigo. Patients with Meniere's disease that affects only the vestibular system experience vertigo more severely than they do hearing loss and tinnitus.

H81.1   Benign paroxysmal vertigo

Benign paroxysmal positional vertigo is a form of vertigo caused by calcified debris in the vestibular system. This debris can be the result of a head injury, infection, or other inner ear disorder. Vertigo is the sensation that one's body (subjective vertigo) or surroundings (objective vertigo) are in motion. Vertigo is often accompanied by nausea, vomiting, and/or problems maintaining balance. Central vertigo arises from a problem in the central nervous system, usually the brainstem or cerebellum. The cause of central vertigo can include tumors and vascular accidents.

H81.2   Vestibular neuronitis

Vestibular neuronitis is a disorder which causes transient inner ear disturbances that result in periods of vertigo, vomiting, and nausea.

H81.39   Other peripheral vertigo

Vertigo is the sensation that one's body (subjective vertigo) or surroundings (objective vertigo) are in motion. Vertigo is often accompanied by nausea, vomiting and/or problems maintaining balance. Peripheral vertigo arises from disturbances in the inner ear.

H81.4   Vertigo of central origin

Vertigo of central origin is caused by a disorder of the central nervous system, usually the brainstem or cerebellum. The cause of central vertigo can include tumors and vascular accidents rather than a disorder of the inner ear.

H83.0   Labyrinthitis

Labyrinthitis is an inflammation of the inner ear that may be accompanied by a build-up of serous fluid or a discharge of pus.

H83.1   Labyrinthine fistula

A labyrinthine fistula is an abnormal tube or passageway which forms between the inner ear and another structure in the skull, usually due to a severe infection. These fistulae can become infected themselves as well as impair inner ear function. A fistula attached to the round window of the inner ear leading into the cochlea is usually covered by a secondary tympanic membrane. A fistula may also connect to the oval window of the inner ear, which interfaces with the ossicles of the middle ear, or to the semicircular canals of the cochlea.

H83.2   Labyrinthine dysfunction

Labyrinthine dysfunction may be hyperactive or hypoactive. Hyperactive dysfunction occurs when the ear(s) are too sensitive too sound, gravitation, and pressure changes, causing pain, tinnitus, and vertigo. A hypoactive labyrinthine occurs when the inner ear structure is not sensitive enough to sound, or has lost some of its functional capabilities. A total loss of

reactivity to sound, pressure, or gravitational orientation is also included in dysfunction.

H83.3   Noise effects on inner ear

Noise effects on inner ear includes acoustic trauma that occurs whenever the inner ear is damaged due to an explosion, as well as other noise-induced hearing loss.

H90.2   Conductive hearing loss, unspecified

Conductive hearing loss is the loss of audio acuity caused by interference with the transmission of sound waves before they can reach the inner ear and the hearing nerve. The main cause in children is from otitis media with inflammation and fluid filling the Eustachian tube, preventing the ear drum from properly vibrating. In adults, the cause is mainly from otosclerosis, a build-up of calcium around the stapes in the middle ear, preventing it from vibrating. Other causes include temporary blockages from earwax, allergies, or fluid build-up in colds, outer ear swimmer's ear infection, ruptured tympanic membrane, or a fractured middle ear bone. Conductive hearing loss is often temporary and can be resolved with medical or surgical intervention, but if left untreated, it can result in permanent damage. Those with conductive hearing loss experience an overall reduction in the volume of sounds and hear most things as muffled. A conductive hearing loss that continues through a critical learning period can result in developmental problems.

H90.5   Unspecified sensorineural hearing loss

Sensorineural hearing loss is caused by damage to the auditory nerve and the microscopic, hair-like cells in the cochlea of the inner ear. The source of the problem can occur in the inner ear, in the nerve leaving the ear, or in the brain. This is often called 'nerve deafness' and the damage causing it is generally irreversible or noncurable. It is improved with hearing aids, surgery, or cochlear implants. Sensorineural hearing loss can result from tumors on the acoustic nerve; physical trauma resulting in head and ear injuries affecting the cochlea or cranial nerve VIII; exposure to rubella in the mother during pregnancy; inherited and congenital causes; aging; autoimmune reactions such as multiple sclerosis; Meniere's disease; infections such as measles, mumps, and meningitis; prolonged exposure to highly intense noise levels; ototoxic medications like tobramycin, streptomycin, gentamicin, aspirin, furosemide, cisplatin, and quinine; and cochlear otosclerosis. The hearing loss may be partial or total in both ears, or occur in only one ear, and may develop gradually or suddenly.

Unspecified sensorineural hearing loss includes congenital deafness, sensory hearing loss, central hearing loss, and neural hearing loss. Central hearing loss is caused by a disorder of the brain that affects the auditory pathway or processing of information from the acoustic nerve within the central nervous system. Neural hearing loss stems from damage to the eighth cranial (auditory) nerve, caused by conditions such as neurological disease or damage and neuromas. Tumors on the nerve may be life-threatening, but are also often curable. Sensory hearing loss results from defects or dysfunction affecting the function of the hair-like cells of the cochlea in the inner ear. This can be caused by damage from situations such as noise trauma, viral infections, drug toxicity, cochlear otosclerosis, and Meniere's disease.

H90.6   Mixed conductive and sensorineural hearing loss, bilateral

Mixed hearing loss is conductive hearing loss (CHL) in combination with sensorineural hearing loss (SNHL). Damage or a disorder is present in the outer and/or middle ear along with damage to or a disorder of the inner ear (cochlea) and/or Cranial Nerve VIII (vestibulocochlear nerve).

H91.1   Presbycusis

Presbycusis is the gradual hearing loss that often occurs with aging.

H92.0   Otalgia

Pain in the ear which may be caused by inflammation within the ear itself, or referred otogenic pain, originating from an area outside the ear, such as another part of the head.

H92.1   **Otorrhea**

A condition in which fluid leaks from the ear.

Note: When cerebrospinal fluid leaks through the ear, it is coded to G96.0.

H92.2   **Otorrhagia**

A condition in which blood that is not from any identifiable trauma or injury leaks from the ear.

H93.0   **Degenerative and vascular disorders of ear**

Degenerative and vascular disorders typically cause progressive hearing loss as the structures of the ear gradually lost their integrity and ability to function, or the blood supply to the auditory structures is reduced.

H93.01   **Transient ischemic deafness**

Transient ischemic deafness is a passing loss of hearing that occurs when the blood flow to the auditory organs is decreased due to injury or disease.

H93.1   **Tinnitus**

Tinnitus is a ringing, hissing, roaring, or other sound in the ear absent any apparent stimulus. In subjective tinnitus, the noise can only be heard by the patient. In objective tinnitus, the noise can be heard by other people as well as by the patient. This condition is usually the result of a circulatory problem (such as an aneurysm), repeating contractions of the muscles of the inner ear, or one or more structural defects of the inner ear.

H93.21   **Auditory recruitment**

Auditory recruitment is a condition in which a slight increase in sound intensity is perceived as being abnormally loud.

H93.22   **Diplacusis**

Diplacusis is a condition in which one sound is heard as two separate sounds at different tones or pitches.

H93.23   **Hyperacusis**

In hyperacusis, the sense of hearing is abnormally heightened. This can result in ear pain as normal sounds seem amplified in volume.

H93.25   **Central auditory processing disorder**

An acquired central auditory processing disorder is any type of difficulty relating to the processing of sound frequency, intensity, and information in the temporal region of the central nervous system. These types of processing disorders can be caused by neurological problems from tumors or brain injury, stroke, degenerative neurological conditions, even bacterial or viral infections of the brain or spinal cord.

H93.29   **Other abnormal auditory perceptions**

Other abnormal auditory perceptions includes an impairment of the auditory discrimination that results in the patient being unable to distinguish different sound tones. This condition may be colloquially described as tone-deafness, but that term is frequently mis- and over-used.

H93.3   **Disorders of acoustic nerve**

The acoustic nerve is cranial nerve VIII. It may also be called the auditory nerve, vestibular nerve, cochlear nerve, or vestibulocochlear nerve. Disorders of cranial nerve VIII may result from infection, inflammation, ototoxic drug use, injury, tumors, and exposure to environmental toxins.

H95.0   **Recurrent cholesteatoma of postmastoidectomy cavity**

A recurrent cholesteatoma is a cyst-like mass full of debris and cholesterol that forms in the cavity resulting from a mastoidectomy procedure.

H95.1   **Other disorders of ear and mastoid process following mastoidectomy**

A mastoidectomy is a surgical procedure in which the porous bone of the mastoid process of the skull behind the ear is drilled to drain infected material.

H95.12   **Granulation of postmastoidectomy cavity**

Granulations are small, grain-like masses which may form in the wound resulting from a mastoidectomy procedure to remove the porous bone of the mastoid process of the skull behind the ear

H95.13   **Mucosal cyst of postmastoidectomy cavity**

A mucosal cyst, a pocket of infected material lined with a mucous membrane, may sometimes form in the cavity that remains after a mastoidectomy procedure to remove the porous bone of the mastoid process of the skull behind the ear.

I00   **Rheumatic fever without heart involvement**

Rheumatic fever is an inflammatory disease that appears as a complication of untreated or undertreated infection with Group A Streptococci, the type of bacteria commonly responsible for throat infections. The onset of rheumatic fever usually develops 2-4 weeks after strep throat or even following scarlet fever. Those stricken by rheumatic fever are typically between 5-20 years of age. The inflammation of rheumatic fever may last several weeks or months and can permanently damage tissue, especially of the heart, joints, integument, and central nervous system. Symptoms of rheumatic fever without heart involvement vary and may change with the course of the disease. Signs and symptoms include fever; red, hot, swollen joints with migration of the pain from one joint to another, particularly the knees, ankles, elbows, and wrists as well as the shoulders and hips, flat or slightly raised and painless skin rash with a jagged edge appearing on the trunk and proximal extremities; nosebleeds, and bumps under the skin. Treatment is aimed at lessening the pain and other symptoms, preventing further inflammatory damage and another occurrence of rheumatic fever.

I01   **Rheumatic fever with heart involvement**

Rheumatic fever is an inflammatory disease that appears as a complication of untreated or undertreated infection with Group A Streptococci, the type of bacteria commonly responsible for throat infections. The onset of rheumatic fever usually develops 2-4 weeks after strep throat or even following scarlet fever. Those stricken by rheumatic fever are typically between 5-20 years of age. The inflammation of rheumatic fever may last several weeks or months and can permanently damage tissue, especially of the heart, joints, integument, and central nervous system. Symptoms of rheumatic fever with heart involvement vary and may change with the course of the disease. Signs and symptoms include fever; red, hot, swollen joints with migration of the pain from one joint to another, particularly the knees, ankles, elbows, and wrists as well as the shoulders and hips; flat or slightly raised and painless skin rash with a jagged edge appearing on the trunk and proximal extremities; nosebleeds, and bumps under the skin. Cardiac symptoms include chest pain and cardiac murmur, acute inflammation of the heart muscle, heart valves, or tissue surrounding the heart, and weakened heart muscle and pumping action causing fatigue and tiredness. Treatment is aimed at lessening the pain and other symptoms, preventing further inflammatory damage to the heart and joints, and another occurrence of rheumatic fever.

I01.0   **Acute rheumatic pericarditis**

Acute rheumatic pericarditis is a condition in which rheumatic fever causes a severe inflammation of the protective lining around the heart.

I01.1   **Acute rheumatic endocarditis**

Acute rheumatic endocarditis is a condition in which rheumatic fever causes a severe inflammation of the inner cavities and chambers of the heart.

I01.2   **Acute rheumatic myocarditis**

Acute rheumatic myocarditis is a condition in which rheumatic fever causes a severe inflammation of the heart muscles.

I02   **Rheumatic chorea**

Rheumatic fever is an inflammatory disease that appears as a complication of untreated or undertreated infection with Group A Streptococci, the type of bacteria commonly responsible for throat infections. The onset of rheumatic fever usually develops 2-4 weeks after strep throat or even following scarlet fever. Those stricken by rheumatic fever are typically between 5-20 years of age. The inflammation of rheumatic fever may last several weeks or months and can permanently damage tissue, especially of the heart, joints, integument, and central nervous system. Chorea is a nervous complication of rheumatic fever which causes involuntary muscle twitches in the limbs and face. Signs of rheumatic chorea include a display of Sydenham's chorea, or St. Vitus' Dance, with jerky, uncontrollable movements of the hands, feet, and face accompanied by outbursts of inappropriate or unusual behavior, such as crying or laughing suddenly out of context.

I02.0   **Rheumatic chorea with heart involvement**

Chorea is a nervous complication of rheumatic fever which causes involuntary muscle twitches in the limbs and face. Signs of rheumatic chorea include a display of Sydenham's chorea, or St. Vitus' Dance, with jerky, uncontrollable movements of the hands, feet, and face accompanied by outbursts of inappropriate or unusual behavior, such as crying or laughing suddenly out of context. Rheumatic chorea may appear with the other signs and symptoms of acute rheumatic fever with heart involvement, including red, hot, swollen joints with migration of the pain from one joint to another; flat or slightly raised and painless skin rash with a jagged edge appearing on the trunk and proximal extremities; nosebleeds; chest pain and cardiac murmur; acute inflammation of the heart muscle, heart valves, or tissue surrounding the heart; and weakened heart muscle and pumping action causing fatigue and tiredness. Treatment is aimed at lessening the pain and other symptoms, preventing further inflammatory damage to the heart and joints, and another occurrence of rheumatic fever.

I02.9   **Rheumatic chorea without heart involvement**

Chorea is a nervous complication of rheumatic fever which causes involuntary muscle twitches in the limbs and face. Signs of rheumatic chorea include a display of Sydenham's chorea, or St. Vitus' Dance, with jerky, uncontrollable movements of the hands, feet, and face accompanied by outbursts of inappropriate or unusual behavior, such as crying or laughing suddenly out of context. Rheumatic chorea may appear with the other signs and symptoms of rheumatic fever, including fever; red, hot, swollen joints with migration of the pain from one joint to another, particularly the knees, ankles, elbows, and wrists as well as the shoulders and hips; flat or slightly raised and painless skin rash with a jagged edge appearing on the trunk and proximal extremities; nosebleeds, and bumps under the skin. Treatment is aimed at lessening the pain and other symptoms, preventing further inflammatory damage to the heart and joints, and another occurrence of rheumatic fever.

I05   **Rheumatic mitral valve diseases**

Rheumatic fever is an inflammatory disease that appears as a complication of untreated or undertreated infection with Group A Streptococci, the type of bacteria commonly responsible for throat infections. The onset of rheumatic fever usually develops 2-4 weeks after strep throat or even following scarlet fever. Those stricken by rheumatic fever are typically between 5-20 years of age. The inflammation of rheumatic fever may then last several weeks or months and can permanently damage tissue, especially of the heart, joints, integument, and central nervous system. Chronic rheumatic heart disease is permanent damage to the heart from this long-term inflammation, which most commonly affects the mitral valve--the valve between the two left chambers of the heart. Rheumatic fever damage to heart valves and muscle can lead to problems later in life with arrhythmias, such as atrial fibrillation, and heart failure.

I05.0   **Rheumatic mitral stenosis**

Rheumatic mitral stenosis is permanent damage to the valve between the left chambers of the heart from long-term inflammation of rheumatic fever. The valve becomes narrowed, which restricts the forward flow of blood through the left atrium to the left ventricle. As a result of the valve not being able to open wide enough, pressure builds up and causes the upper chamber to swell. The pooling blood backed up in the left atrium may then begin to collect within the lung tissue, resulting in pulmonary edema and difficulty breathing. When caused by rheumatic fever, the valve damage usually develops between 5-10 years after the acute onset or episode of rheumatic fever. Symptoms of the valve damage may not appear until later. In adults, they usually develop between ages 20-50 and may remain mild or unnoticed often beginning with an episode of atrial fibrillation or a detected heart murmur. Other symptoms such as a noticeable cough, fatigue, swelling in the feet and ankles, difficulty breathing, heart palpitations, and chest discomfort may appear later and worsen with exercise. Treatment depends on the severity of symptoms and the condition of the heart and lungs. Medications such as diuretics, nitrates, beta blockers, digoxin, ACE inhibitors, and beta and calcium-channel blockers are used to treat symptoms of heart failure, atrial fibrillation, and high blood pressure. Anticoagulants are used to prevent blood clot formation. Percutaneous balloon mitral valvotomy or valvuloplasty may be done to open or repair a less damaged valve. In more severe cases, surgical repair or replacement of the valve is necessary.

I05.1   Rheumatic mitral insufficiency

Rheumatic mitral insufficiency is permanent damage to the valve between the left chambers of the heart from long-term inflammation of rheumatic fever. The valve becomes incompetent and leaks, allowing regurgitation, or backflow of blood in the wrong direction from the left ventricle back into the left atrium. When blood flows backwards as the heart contracts, less blood is pumped out to the rest of the body, triggering the heart to work harder, pumping with more force. This leads to congestive heart failure. Symptoms from the damaged mitral valve may be mild or go unnoticed, and generally develop gradually. They include fatigue, exhaustion, and light-headedness, cough, rapid breathing, tachycardia and/or palpitations, shortness of breath that increases both with exercise or activity and while lying down, swollen ankles, and excessive nocturia. Signs upon physical exam include a vibration over the heart, the sound of a gallop or distinctive heart murmur, crackles in the lungs, and other signs of right-sided heart failure such as an enlarged liver and bulging neck veins. Treatment depends on the type and severity of symptoms and the condition of the heart. Medications such as diuretics, anti-arrhythmia drugs, blood thinners, beta blockers, ACE inhibitors, and a low sodium diet are used to reduce high blood pressure and the strain on the heart. Catheterization is done if heart function worsens and surgical repair or replacement of the valve may eventually be needed.

I05.2   Rheumatic mitral stenosis with insufficiency

Rheumatic mitral stenosis with insufficiency is permanent damage to the valve between the left chambers of the heart from long-term inflammation of rheumatic fever. The valve becomes narrowed, restricting the forward flow of blood through the left atrium to the left ventricle, causing pressure to build up and the upper chamber to swell. The pooling blood backed up in the left atrium begins to collect within the lung tissue, resulting in pulmonary edema and difficulty breathing. The valve also becomes incompetent and leaks at the same time, allowing regurgitation, or backflow of blood in the wrong direction from the left ventricle back into the left atrium. When blood flows backwards as the heart contracts, less blood is pumped out to the rest of the body, triggering the heart to work harder, pumping with more force. This leads to congestive heart failure. Valve damage from rheumatic fever usually develops between 5-10 years after the acute onset of rheumatic fever. Symptoms may not appear until later and include fatigue, exhaustion, and light-headedness, cough, rapid breathing, tachycardia and/or palpitations, shortness of breath that increases with exercise or activity and while lying down, and swollen feet and ankles. Treatment depends on the type and severity of symptoms and the condition of the heart. Medications and a low sodium diet are used to reduce high blood pressure and the strain on the heart. Catheterization is done if heart function worsens and surgical repair or replacement of the valve may become necessary.

I06   Rheumatic aortic valve diseases

Rheumatic fever is an inflammatory disease that appears as a complication of untreated or undertreated infection with Group A Streptococci, the type of bacteria commonly responsible for throat infections. The onset of rheumatic fever usually develops 2-4 weeks after strep throat or even following scarlet fever. Those stricken by rheumatic fever are typically between 5-20 years of age. The inflammation of rheumatic fever may then last several weeks or months and can permanently damage tissue, especially of the heart, joints, integument, and central nervous system. Chronic rheumatic heart disease is permanent damage to the heart and/ or its valves from this long-term inflammation. Rheumatic aortic valve diseases affect the valve between the left ventricle of the heart and the aorta. Damage from rheumatic fever often occurs 5-10 years or more after the acute onset of rheumatic fever and can lead to serious heart problems later in life, such as arrhythmias and heart failure.

I06.0   Rheumatic aortic stenosis

Rheumatic aortic stenosis is permanent damage to the valve between the left ventricle of the heart and the aorta from long-term inflammation, subsequent scar tissue formation, and/or calcium plaque build-up due to rheumatic fever, causing the valve to become narrow, stiffen or fuse. The aortic valve is composed of three tightly-fitted, triangular shaped leaflets between the left lower chamber of the heart and the body's largest artery, the aorta. The leaflets are forced open with contraction, like a one-way gate. When the ventricle relaxes, the leaflets shut, preventing the backflow of blood. In rheumatic aortic stenosis, the valve isn't able to open wide enough, restricting the forward flow of oxygenated blood through the left ventricle into the aorta and out to the rest of the body. As a result, the ventricle has to increase pressure to pump enough blood out through the valve. This extra work thickens the walls of the ventricle and weakens the heart muscle, which in turn limits the amount of blood it can pump, leading to heart failure. Aortic valve stenosis may be mild or severe and doesn't usually produce warning signs or symptoms until it has become severe. Detecting an abnormal heart sound, or murmur, on physical exam is often the first sign. Other symptoms include fatigue, shortness of breath, or feeling faint--especially during exertion or activity, palpitations, chest pain, and swollen ankles and feet. Severe aortic stenosis often requires surgery to replace the valve before life-threatening heart problems occur.

I06.1   Rheumatic aortic insufficiency

Rheumatic aortic insufficiency is permanent damage to the valve between the left ventricle of the heart and the aorta from long-term inflammation, subsequent scar tissue formation, and/or calcium plaque build-up due to rheumatic fever, causing the valve to become incompetent and leak. The aortic valve is composed of three tightly-fitted, triangular shaped leaflets between the left lower chamber of the heart and the body's largest artery, the aorta. The leaflets are forced open with contraction, like a one-way gate. When the ventricle relaxes, the leaflets shut, preventing the backflow of blood. In rheumatic aortic insufficiency, the valve isn't able to close completely. This allows regurgitation, or the flow of blood in the wrong direction back into the left ventricle. As a result, the left ventricle dilates or widens, and a larger amount of blood is pumped through the aortic valve with each contraction, leading to a very forceful, bounding heartbeat. Other signs upon examination include hard pulses in the extremities, bobbing of the head in rhythm with the heartbeat, a murmur or other abnormal heart sound, low diastolic blood pressure, and signs of fluid build-up in the lungs. Aortic valve insufficiency often has no symptoms for years, which may appear suddenly or slowly. Symptoms include fatigue, fainting, and weakness, particularly with activity, shortness of breath that increases both with exertion and while lying down, swollen feet, legs, or abdomen, and chest pain. Severe aortic insufficiency often requires surgery to repair or replace the valve. Mild or moderate cases require monitoring with echocardiogram, limiting activity, blood pressure medication, and diuretics.

I06.2   Rheumatic aortic stenosis with insufficiency

Rheumatic aortic stenosis with insufficiency is permanent damage to the valve between the left ventricle of the heart and the aorta from long-term inflammation, subsequent scar tissue formation, and/or calcium deposits due to rheumatic fever. This causes the valve to become narrow, stiff, and incompetent. The aortic valve is composed of three tightly-fitted, triangular shaped leaflets between the left lower chamber of the heart and the body's largest artery, the aorta. The leaflets are forced open with contraction, like a one-way gate. When the ventricle relaxes, the leaflets shut, preventing the backflow of blood. In rheumatic aortic stenosis with insufficiency, the narrowed valve isn't able to open wide enough, which restricts the amount of oxygenated blood the left ventricle can pump out of the heart.

In the resting phase, the valve is not able to close completely, allowing regurgitation, or the flow of blood in the wrong direction back into the left ventricle. As a result, the ventricle has to increase pressure to pump enough blood out through the valve with each contraction as it becomes dilated with a larger amount of blood. This extra work thickens the walls of the ventricle, weakens the heart muscle, and limits the amount of blood it can pump, leading to heart failure. Aortic valve stenosis usually occurs with insufficiency and warning signs or symptoms typically appear when it has become severe. A murmur and a bounding pulse are often the first signs. Other signs include hard pulses in the extremities, bobbing of the head in rhythm with the heartbeat, low diastolic blood pressure, and fluid in the lungs. Symptoms include fatigue, fainting, and weakness, particularly with activity; shortness of breath that increases both with exertion and while lying down; swollen feet, legs, or abdomen; palpitations, and chest pain. Surgery is required in severe cases to repair or replace the valve. Mild or moderate cases require monitoring, limiting activity, blood pressure medication, and diuretics.

I10   Essential (primary) hypertension

Essential hypertension refers to high blood pressure with no identifiable cause or underlying condition causing blood pressure to increase. This is also known as primary hypertension and accounts for 95 percent of all hypertension. Blood exerts pressure on artery walls as it is pumped through the body. Systolic blood pressure is the pressure against the artery walls measured when the heart contracts, and the diastolic pressure is measured when the heart relaxes. Normal blood pressure is below 120/80. If the systolic pressure is consistently above 140 or the diastolic reading is consistently over 90, then hypertension is occurring.

Several factors contribute to high blood pressure, such as the size and condition of arteries, whether narrowed or arteriosclerotic; the volume of water and salt content in the body; the amount of blood being pumped; the action of the heart; hormone levels; and the condition of the kidneys. Other factors include being overweight, smoking, stress, heredity, and alcohol use. Blood pressure is controlled through lifestyle management, such as weight loss, exercise, and a low-fat, low-sodium diet that is rich in whole grains, chicken, fruits and vegetables, with little red meat. Medications include diuretics, beta blockers, calcium channel blockers, and angiotensin receptor blockers or enzyme converter inhibitors. Symptoms can include headaches, dizziness, confusion, visual changes, chest pain, shortness of breath, perspiration, nose bleeds, and excessive tiredness, although many people with hypertension are not aware of it and it has been called a silent disease. Untreated hypertension can lead to heart attacks, stroke, kidney damage, vision loss, and congestive heart failure.

Malignant essential hypertension is also included. Malignant hypertension is severely elevated arterial blood pressure without apparent physiologic cause accompanied by papilledema, swelling of the optic nerve behind the eye. This is also known as accelerated hypertension or arteriolar necrosclerosing hypertension and is a medical emergency affecting about one percent of those with high blood pressure. Permanent organ damage of the kidneys, heart, brain, and eyes can result. Hospitalization is necessary until the severe high blood pressure is under control. Symptoms include blurred vision, change in mental status, stupor, lethargy, anxiety, confusion, chest pain, decreased urinary output, weakness, nausea, vomiting, and seizure.

I11   Hypertensive heart disease

This category reports heart disease, with or without heart failure that has resulted from the effects of systemic hypertension over time. Hypertensive heart disease is often manifested as cardiomegaly affecting the left ventricle in particular, as it must pump harder to move blood through arteries at high pressure, and can eventually lead to heart failure.

Note: In order to assign codes from category I11, there must be a cause and effect relationship between the heart disease and the hypertension.

Note: The heart disease in this category includes myocarditis, myocardial degeneration, cardiomegaly, cardiopathy, and other carditis or ill-defined heart disease when they are specified as due to hypertension.

I12   Hypertensive chronic kidney disease

This category reports chronic kidney disease related to or due to systemic hypertension. Elevated blood pressure is a major contributor to kidney function decline in hypertensive patients and to the development of chronic kidney disease as well as a strong risk factor and underlying cause for progression to end stage renal disease, requiring dialysis and/or transplant. Since advanced kidney failure also causes hypertension, these conditions are related whether the hypertension is identified as the cause or the consequence of the impaired kidney function. Any kidney condition classifiable to N18 stated as with hypertension is automatically presumed to be related to or due to the hypertension. No cause and effect relationship need be implied or stated.

Note: Renal disease that is not stated as related to, due to, or with hypertension is not coded within this category.

Note: If the patient also has acute kidney failure, a sudden failure of kidney function that may or may not be reversible, stemming from more immediate causes such as shock, dehydration, septicemia, blood clots, toxins, or obstructed urine outflow, then an additional code for the acute renal failure is also required.

Note: Secondary renovascular hypertension caused by a narrowing of the arteries carrying blood to the kidneys themselves is not included in this category. Only essential forms of systemic hypertension without apparent underlying organic cause are included.

I13   Hypertensive heart and chronic kidney disease

This category reports heart disease, with or without heart failure, with chronic kidney disease that has resulted from the effects of essential hypertension, whether benign or accelerated, malignant, or arteriolar necrosclerosing hypertension. Kidney damage is brought on by hypertensive changes in the small arteries and arterioles of the kidney, resulting in ischemic atrophy and degeneration of the renal tubules with fibrosis of the interstitial tissue. Arteriolar nephrosclerosis, or hardening of the arterioles of the kidney, is often associated with both benign and malignant hypertension. It can have an insidious onset associated with edema, urinary casts, tubule degeneration, glomerulonephritis, and cardiac hypertrophy, and can lead to renal insufficiency and congestive heart failure. Untreated malignant hypertension almost always leads to kidney damage and can permanently damage other organs as well. Hypertensive heart damage includes conditions such as myocarditis, myocardial degeneration, cardiomegaly, cardiopathy, and other carditis or ill-defined heart disease that can lead to heart failure.

I15   Secondary hypertension

Secondary hypertension is abnormally high blood pressure caused by another underlying physiological condition or disease. These can include: renal (kidney) disease, adrenal gland tumors, congenital malformation of blood vessels, sleep apnea, medications (hormone contraceptives, decongestants, steriods), recreation drug use (cocaine), thyroid and parathyroid gland disorders. Renovascular hypertension is the most common cause of secondary hypertension.

I15.0   Renovascular hypertension

Renovascular hypertension is caused by narrowing or stenosis of the arteries supplying blood to the kidneys. Atherosclerosis may cause plaque deposits to build up on the artery walls. Fibromuscular dysplasia may cause cells of the artery wall to overgrow and narrow the lumen. The artery may also be compressed from injury, tumor, or blood clots. When blood flow to the kidney is reduced, the kidney responds by producing the protein, renin, which converts into an enzyme in the bloodstream that causes the body to retain salt and water. The arterioles then become restricted and cause the symptoms of renovascular hypertension, which leads to many serious complications, including heart disease, congestive heart failure, stroke, blindness, and kidney failure. Renovascular hypertension occurs in a very small percentage of those with hypertension, usually in men over 45 with atherosclerosis, and in those with fibromuscular dysplasia.

I20   Angina pectoris

Angina pectoris is severe chest pain associated with a lack of blood flow to the heart, usually from a spasm or occlusion in the coronary arteries and is aggravated by physical exertion, stress, or excitement.

I20.0   Unstable angina

Unstable angina is also known as crescendo angina, accelerated angina, worsening effort angina, preinfarction syndrome, and intermediate coronary syndrome. Chest pain occurs at rest or with minimal exertion and follows a pattern of increasing severity and duration, threatening to escalate into a myocardial infarction.

I20.1   Angina pectoris with documented spasm

Angina pectoris with documented spasm is also known as angiospastic angina, variant angina, and Prinzmetal angina. This is a severe from of the condition that occurs while the patient is at rest, and not only when they are active or under stress. Patients suffering from this condition usually suffer from long bouts of chest pain.

I20.8   Other forms of angina pectoris

This includes angina decubitus, which is severe chest pain that occurs when the patient is lying down.

Note: Use this code for angina equivalent and report any additional codes for associated symptoms.

I25   Chronic ischemic heart disease

Chronic ischemic heart disease is a long-term or possibly permanent condition that occurs when the heart is deprived of oxygen, usually due to coronary disease which obstructs the flow of blood to the heart.

I25.1   Atherosclerotic heart disease of native coronary artery

Also known as coronary atherosclerosis, coronary artery disease, CAD, and atherosclerotic cardiovascular disease, this is a syndrome affecting arterial blood vessels in the heart. The syndrome is characterized by inflammation and accumulation of macrophage white blood cells and low-density lipoproteins along the arterial walls. This leads to narrowing of the vessels and decreased blood flow to the heart muscle and may cause angina (chest pain).

I25.82   Chronic total occlusion of coronary artery

An artery supplying blood to the heart that is completely blocked for an extended period of time. Although collateral blood flow around the blocked area may avoid infarction, the blocked artery still increases the risk of myocardial infarction or death. This condition also severely limits activity, particularly because the compensating blood flow cannot increase in proportion to exercise or increased work load. The chronically blocked artery can be treated with angioplasty or drug-eluting stent placement.

Note: Coronary atherosclerosis for the affected vessel(s) needs to be coded first. Acute coronary occlusions are excluded from chronic total occlusion of a coronary artery.

I25.83   Coronary atherosclerosis due to lipid rich plaque

Coronary artery disease is a leading cause of death in the U.S. Most myocardial infarctions are caused by the rupture of plaque in the coronary arteries, with subsequent blood clot formation that blocks the flow of blood to the heart muscle. Lipid-rich plaques are those suspected of being vulnerable to rupture and causing thrombosis and myocardial infarction.

Note: Identifying the type of plaque in coronary arteries is important for choosing a treatment stent, whether bare metal or drug-eluting.

I25.84   Coronary atherosclerosis due to calcified coronary lesion

Calcified coronary lesions are caused by calcium deposited in the coronary arteries. These are different from other ischemic coronary lesions formed by the build-up of lipid rich plaque. Calcium plaque deposits in coronary arteries are very hard and often cannot be crossed, blocking stents from reaching the targeted treatment area, and preventing full expansion of stents. This makes treatment with interventional or intraluminal procedures such as angioplasty and stent placement difficult or impossible. Calcified coronary lesions are often treated by CABG or cleared with atherectomy. An increased amount of calcium deposited in arteries can also lead to a higher incidence of major cardiac events than lipid type plaques.

I26   Pulmonary embolism

Pulmonary embolism (PE) occurs when a clump of material migrates and forms a blockage in the main artery to the lungs or arterial branches in the lungs. The most common cause of blockage is a blood clot from the legs (deep vein thrombosis) but air, fat, amniotic fluid, and talc (intravenous drug use) can also cause a PE. Symptoms include difficulty breathing, low oxygen saturation levels, chest pain (especially with inspiration), cough, and elevated heart and respiratory rates.

I26.90   Septic pulmonary embolism without acute cor pulmonale

A septic pulmonary embolus arises from a localized infection elsewhere in the body, like cellulitis or oral/dental infections. Pieces of the infectious material break loose from the original site and travel through the venous system to the heart and then into the pulmonary arteries where the embolus gets lodged in the small vessels there. Septic pulmonary emboli then cause lung abscesses or necrotizing pneumonia. A lung abscess entails a localized infection with necrosis in a cavity at least 2 cm. Necrotizing pneumonia has multiple, localized, infected cavities smaller than 2 cm, with necrosis.

Note: The underlying infection causing the embolism needs to be coded first.

I26.92   Saddle embolus of pulmonary artery without acute cor pulmonale

A saddle embolus is a large thromboembolus that straddles a dividing artery at the bifurcation point and blocks both branches of the vessel. A saddle embolus of the pulmonary artery bridges across the artery from the heart as it divides into the left and right main pulmonary arteries, blocking both. A large pulmonary saddle embolus causes sudden death. These emboli originate in the lower extremity veins and travel through the venous system to the vena cava, through the right atrium and ventricle into the pulmonary artery. The thrombus becomes lodged where the larger vessel divides into smaller ones and there it occludes the pulmonary artery and its branches, preventing blood from entering the lungs.

I27.0   Primary pulmonary hypertension

Primary pulmonary hypertension is a rare disease in which the pulmonary artery becomes constricted, restricting the flow of blood to the lungs. Symptoms of this condition include chronic shortness of breath, chest pain, dizziness, and fainting.

I27.1   Kyphoscoliotic heart disease

Kyphoscoliotic heart disease is a rare condition in which the blood pressure of the lungs is elevated due to an abnormal curvature of the spine.

I27.82   Chronic pulmonary embolism

A pulmonary embolism is a blood clot that has broken away from the wall of a vein in one location and traveled to the lungs where it gets lodged in the arteries, blocking blood flow to the heart and lungs. Nearly 90 percent of pulmonary emboli have formed from deep vein thrombosis in the legs, but can also be caused by pieces of atherosclerotic plaque, cellular debris in conditions such as sickle cell anemia, fat escaping from the bone marrow when a fracture occurs, or from amniotic fluid during childbirth. Emboli occur as complications of surgery, bed confinement, severe varicose veins or phlebitis, recent heart attack or stroke, and chronic illness, like congestive heart failure. Oral contraceptives, obesity, broken leg, clotting disorders, sitting for long periods of time, and congenital heart defects all cause increased risk. Chronic pulmonary embolism occurs when small blood clots travel repeatedly to the lungs over a period of several years. Symptoms of shortness of breath, leg swelling, and general weakness build up gradually. Emboli cause rapid breathing, chest pain, anxiousness, increased pulse rate, dizziness, and fainting. Sudden death can occur. Patients are hospitalized, given anticoagulants to dissolve clots and prevent new ones, and oxygen therapy to increase blood levels. Some patients will require surgical removal of the clot and some require placement of a device that filters blood returning to the heart and lungs until the clot dissolves.

I28.1   Aneurysm of pulmonary artery

An aneurysm of the pulmonary artery that supplies blood to the lungs indicates that a portion of the artery becomes enlarged and engorged with blood, forming a pouch or sac. If not surgically corrected, this aneurysm can rupture, causing severe internal bleeding and possibly death.

I30.0   Acute nonspecific idiopathic pericarditis

Acute idiopathic pericarditis is a severe inflammation of the membranous sac encasing the heart which has no apparent cause.

I31.2   Hemopericardium, not elsewhere classified

Hemopericardium is a condition in which internal bleeding causes the pericardial sac to fill with blood.

I31.4   Cardiac tamponade

Cardiac tamponade is increased pressure on the heart due to fluid accumulating in the pericardial sac. The increased pressure impairs the ventricles' filling action and results in decreased cardiac output with symptoms similar to heart failure or cardiogenic shock: tachycardia, dyspnea, and orthopnea. The fluid accumulation can be caused by different conditions, including effusion resulting from infection or malignancy, a cardiac surgery post-operative complication, aortic dissection, penetrating trauma, or rupture of the heart. Treatment requires removing the fluid from the sac around the heart, either by pericardiocentesis, placing a drainage catheter, creating a pericardial window, or even surgery in emergencies.

I34.0   Nonrheumatic mitral (valve) insufficiency

Nonrheumatic mitral valve insufficiency is the most common type of heart valve disorder in which the valve becomes incompetent and leaks, allowing regurgitation, or backflow of blood in the wrong direction from the left ventricle back into the left atrium. When blood flows backwards as the heart contracts, less blood is pumped out to the rest of the body, triggering the heart to work harder, pumping with more force. This leads to congestive heart failure. Mitral valve insufficiency may be due to many different conditions that weaken or damage the valvular tissue such as degenerative diseases, mitral valve prolapse, infection of the valves or heart muscle, swelling, heart disease with high blood pressure, and the use of certain FDA banned appetite suppressants for more than 4 months. If mitral valve insufficiency is caused by a heart attack, an infection that has destroyed valvular tissue, or a disease condition that causes the cords attaching the heart muscle to the valve to break, symptoms will come on suddenly. They include fatigue, exhaustion, light-headedness, cough, rapid breathing, tachycardia and/or palpitations, shortness of breath that increases both with exercise or activity and while lying down, and swollen ankles. Signs include a vibration over the heart, the sound of a gallop or distinctive heart murmur, crackles in the lungs, and other signs of right-sided heart failure such as an enlarged liver and bulging neck veins. Treatment depends on the condition and function of the heart. Medications such as diuretics, anti-arrhythmia drugs, blood thinners, beta blockers, ACE inhibitors, and a low sodium diet are used to reduce high blood pressure and the strain on the heart. Catheterization is done if heart function worsens surgical repair or replacement of the valve may become necessary.

I34.2   Nonrheumatic mitral (valve) stenosis

Nonrheumatic mitral valve stenosis is a narrowed opening in the valve between the left chambers of the heart that is not a result of damage from rheumatic fever. Although causative factors other than rheumatic fever are rare, mitral valve stenosis may result from radiation treatment to the chest, iatrogenic causes, and the formation of calcium deposits around the valve. The narrowed valve restricts the forward flow of blood through the left atrium to the left ventricle. As a result of the valve not being able to open wide enough, pressure builds up and causes the upper chamber to swell. The pooling blood backed up in the left atrium may then begin to collect within the lung tissue, resulting in pulmonary edema and difficulty breathing, and leading to congestive heart failure. In adults, symptoms

of a stenosed valve may remain mild or unnoticed and often begin with an episode of atrial fibrillation or a detected heart murmur. Other symptoms such as a noticeable cough, fatigue, swelling in the feet and ankles, difficulty breathing, heart palpitations, and chest discomfort may appear later and worsen with exercise. Treatment depends on the severity of symptoms and the condition of the heart and lungs. Medications such as diuretics, nitrates, beta blockers, digoxin, ACE inhibitors, and beta and calcium-channel blockers are used to treat symptoms of heart failure, atrial fibrillation, and high blood pressure. Percutaneous balloon mitral valvotomy or valvuloplasty may be done to open or repair a valve. In more severe cases, surgical repair or replacement of the valve is necessary.

I35.0   Nonrheumatic aortic (valve) stenosis

Nonrheumatic aortic valve stenosis is damage to the valve between the left ventricle of the heart and the aorta, most often due to aging and the accumulation of calcium deposits, which causes the valve to become narrowed, stiffened, or fused. The aortic valve is composed of three tightly-fitted, triangular shaped leaflets between the left lower chamber of the heart and the body's largest artery, the aorta. The leaflets are forced open with contraction, like a one-way gate. When the ventricle relaxes, the leaflets shut, preventing the backflow of blood. The narrowed valve isn't able to open wide enough and restricts the forward flow of oxygenated blood through the left ventricle into the aorta and out to the rest of the body. As a result, the ventricle has to increase pressure to pump enough blood out through the valve. This extra work thickens the walls of the ventricle and weakens the heart muscle, which in turn limits the amount of blood it can pump and leads to heart failure. Aortic valve stenosis may be mild or severe and doesn't usually produce warning signs or symptoms until it has become severe. Stenosis from aging usually appears around age 70. Detecting an abnormal heart sound, or murmur, on physical exam is often the first sign. Other symptoms include fatigue, shortness of breath, or feeling faint--especially during exertion or activity, palpitations, chest pain, and swollen ankles and feet. Severe aortic stenosis often requires surgery to replace the valve before life-threatening heart problems occur.

I35.1   Nonrheumatic aortic (valve) insufficiency

Nonrheumatic aortic insufficiency is damage to the valve between the left ventricle of the heart and the aorta, causing it to become incompetent and leak. Any condition damaging the valve can cause insufficiency, which is often due to deterioration with age and high blood pressure, calcium deposits on the valve, and endocarditis. The aortic valve is composed of three tightly-fitted, triangular shaped leaflets between the left lower chamber of the heart and the body's largest artery, the aorta. The leaflets are forced open with contraction, like a one-way gate. When the ventricle relaxes, the leaflets shut, preventing the backflow of blood. In rheumatic aortic insufficiency, the valve isn't able to close completely. This allows regurgitation, or the flow of blood in the wrong direction back into the left ventricle. As a result, the left ventricle dilates or widens, and a larger amount of blood is pumped through the aortic valve with each contraction, leading to a very forceful, bounding heartbeat. Other signs include hard pulses in the extremities, bobbing of the head in rhythm with the heartbeat, a murmur or other abnormal heart sound, low diastolic blood pressure, and signs of fluid build-up in the lungs. Aortic valve insufficiency often has no symptoms for years, which may appear suddenly or slowly. Symptoms include fatigue, fainting, and weakness, particularly with activity, shortness of breath that increases both with exertion and while lying down, swollen feet, legs, or abdomen, and chest pain. Severe aortic insufficiency often requires surgery to repair or replace the valve in severe cases, as well as repair the aorta, if it has become dilated. Mild or moderate cases require monitoring with echocardiogram, limiting activity, blood pressure medication and diuretics.

I35.2   Nonrheumatic aortic (valve) stenosis with insufficiency

Nonrheumatic aortic stenosis with insufficiency is damage to the valve between the left ventricle of the heart and the aorta, most often due to deterioration with age and high blood pressure, the accumulation of calcium deposits, or endocarditis. The valve becomes narrowed and stiff, as well as incompetent, and leaks. The aortic valve is composed of three tightly-fitted, triangular shaped leaflets between the left lower chamber of the heart and the body's largest artery, the aorta. The leaflets are forced open with contraction, like a one-way gate. When the ventricle relaxes, the leaflets shut, preventing the backflow of blood. In rheumatic aortic insufficiency, the valve isn't able to close completely. This allows regurgitation, or the flow of blood in the wrong direction back into the left ventricle. As a result, the left ventricle dilates or widens, and a larger amount of blood needs to be pumped through the aortic valve with each contraction, leading to a very forceful, bounding heartbeat. The narrowed valve also isn't able to open wide enough and restricts the forward flow of blood out to the rest of the body. The ventricle has to increase pressure to pump the blood out through the valve. This extra work thickens the walls of the dilated ventricle and weakens the heart muscle more, which leads to heart failure. Other signs include hard pulses in the extremities, bobbing of the head in rhythm with the heartbeat, a murmur or other abnormal heart sound, low diastolic blood pressure, and signs of fluid build-up in the lungs. Aortic valve stenosis with insufficiency often has no symptoms for years, and doesn't usually produce warning signs until it has become severe. Detecting an abnormal heart sound, or murmur, on physical exam is often the first sign. Symptoms include fatigue, fainting, and weakness, particularly with activity, shortness of breath, swollen feet, legs, or abdomen, and chest pain. Severe aortic insufficiency often requires surgery to repair or replace the valve. Mild or moderate cases require monitoring, limiting activity, blood pressure medication, and diuretics.

I36 Nonrheumatic tricuspid valve disorders

The tricuspid valve is located between the right atrium and right ventricle of the heart and is formed by 3 leaflets.

I36.0 Nonrheumatic tricuspid (valve) stenosis

Tricuspid valve disorders include stenosis, or narrowing, which restricts the forward flow of blood through the atrium to the ventricle.

I36.1 Nonrheumatic tricuspid (valve) insufficiency

Tricuspid valve disorders include insufficiency, or regurgitation, which is characterized by leakage of blood backward into the ventricle during diastole (resting phase).

I37 Nonrheumatic pulmonary valve disorders

The pulmonary valve is located between the right ventricle of the heart and the pulmonary artery and is formed by 3 leaflets.

Note: Pulmonary valve disorders are rare and most are present at birth and are coded in the congenital anomalies chapter.

I37.0 Nonrheumatic pulmonary valve stenosis

Pulmonary valve disorders include stenosis, or narrowing, which restricts the forward flow of blood from the ventricle to the lungs.

I37.1 Nonrheumatic pulmonary valve insufficiency

Another pulmonary valve disorder is insufficiency or regurgitation which is characterized by leakage of blood backward into the ventricle during diastole (resting phase).

I42.1 Obstructive hypertrophic cardiomyopathy

Hypertrophic cardiomyopathy is an abnormal thickening of the heart that is usually inherited and occurs in both men and women equally. Genetic mutations make heart muscle grow abnormally thick with an abnormal arrangement of heart muscle fibers and muscle cells in disarray. The severity varies widely. Some people have few, if any, symptoms and lead normal lives. Blood flow may be reduced or even obstructed through the left ventricle. The hypertrophied heart muscle can also affect the heart's electrical conduction system and cause irregular heart beats or even dangerous ventricular fibrillation or tachycardia. Many people with hypertrophic cardiomyopathy will have the obstructive form of the disease in which the septum between the left and right ventricles, the two bottom chambers of the heart, becomes enlarged enough to obstruct blood flow being pumped out to the body. This causes shortness of breath with exertion, chest pain, dizziness, and syncope. Heart failure can result when the thickened heart muscle becomes too stiff to fill effectively and

can't meet the body's needs. The abnormal structure of heart muscle cells can also cause fast or irregular heartbeats and arrhythmias with the risk of sudden cardiac death.

I42.2 Other hypertrophic cardiomyopathy

Hypertrophic cardiomyopathy is an abnormal thickening of the heart that is usually inherited and occurs in both men and women equally. Genetic mutations make heart muscle grow abnormally thick with an abnormal arrangement of heart muscle fibers and muscle cells in disarray. The severity varies widely. Some people have few, if any, symptoms and lead normal lives. Nonobstructive hypertrophic cardiomyopathy makes the left ventricle pumping chamber stiff, reducing the amount of blood the chamber can hold, and how much blood gets pumped out to the body upon contraction. In a few cases, the thickened heart muscle causes shortness of breath, chest pain and/or fainting with exertion, dizziness, fatigue, and palpitations or other life-threatening types of abnormal heart rhythms. The smaller space available through which blood can flow also causes blood to move more forcefully through the valves, which can prevent the mitral valve from closing properly, leading to regurgitation, causing dilated and weakened cardiac muscle, and even heart failure.

I42.4 Endocardial fibroelastosis

Endocardial fibroelastosis is a condition in which the inner lining of the heart becomes abnormally thick, especially in the left ventricle. Patients diagnosed with this condition rarely survive more than a couple of years.

I44.0 Atrioventricular block, first degree

An atrioventricular block is a disorder which impairs the conduction or impulses from the atria of the heart to the ventricles. A first degree atrioventricular block is the least severe form of the condition. Patients with this disorder will often show no symptoms except a decreased tolerance for exercise and exertion. A first degree atrioventricular block is a very rare condition which is usually benign.

I44.1 Atrioventricular block, second degree

In a second degree atrioventricular block, some electrical impulses from the atrium fail to reach the heart ventricles, causing most patients to experience fainting, chest pain, and/or dizziness. Second degree atrioventricular block can result in heart failure.

I44.2 Atrioventricular block, complete

An atrioventricular block is a disorder which impairs the conduction or impulses from the atria of the heart to the ventricles. In a complete atrioventricular block, the electrical impulses are completely cut off.

I44.4 Left anterior fascicular block

Left anterior fascicular block (LAFB), also known as left anterior hemiblock (LAHB), is the most common partial block of the left bundle branch and involves the electrical conduction of impulses from the atrioventricular node. In a LAFB (LAHB) the anterior half of the left bundle branch is defective causing the impulse to pass first to the posterior area of the ventricle and delaying activation of the anterior and upper ventricle. It can be observed on an EKG tracing as left axis deviation.

I44.5 Left posterior fascicular block

Left posterior fascicular block (LPFB), also known as left posterior hemiblock (LPHB) is a less common partial block of the left bundle branch and involves the electrical conduction of impulses from the atrioventricular node. In LPFB (LPHB) the posterior half of the left bundle branch is defective causing the impulse to pass first to the anterior and upper ventricle and delaying activation of the posterior ventricle. It can be observed on an EKG tracing as right axis deviation.

I44.60 Unspecified fascicular block

An unspecified left bundle branch hemiblock occurs when the conduction of electrical signals from the left bundle branch, which further divides into two fascicles for the left ventricle--the left anterior fascicle and the left posterior fascicle, is partially blocked somewhere on this path. This condition is often indicative of coronary heart disease. When the heart's electrical conduction system at these specialized conduction fibers for the left ventricle is partially blocked, it disrupts the near simultaneous contraction of the left and right ventricles and results in an un-coordinated and inefficient heartbeat. The partially blocked left ventricle then contracts slightly after the right.

I44.7 Left bundle-branch block, unspecified

An unspecified left bundle branch block is a condition in which the heart's electrical conduction system at the specialized fibers for the left ventricle is defective and either slows down or blocks the electrical impulse going to the left ventricle. This disrupts the normal, nearly simultaneous contraction of both ventricles together and causes an un-coordinated and inefficient heartbeat. After traveling through the left and right atria, the electrical impulse travels from the atrioventricular node down the Bundle of His, which divides into the left and right bundle branches, which send the impulse into the left and right ventricles, respectively. The left bundle branch further divides into two fascicles and on into millions of Purkinje fibers, which coordinate the electrical impulse with millions of heart muscle cells to produce a co-ordinated and synchronous heartbeat. In a left bundle branch block, the partially blocked left ventricle contracts after the normally stimulated right ventricle.

I45.0 Right fascicular block

Right fascicular block is a defect in the heart's electrical conduction system. The right ventricle is not activated by an impulse from the right bundle branch but does depolarise when impulses from the left bundle branch travel through the myocardium and finally reach the right ventricle. It can be observed on an EKG tracing as a wide QRS complex.

I45.10 Unspecified right bundle-branch block

An unspecified right bundle branch block is a condition in which a portion of the heart's electrical conduction system at the specialized conduction fibers for the right ventricle is defective and either slows down or blocks the electrical impulse to the right ventricle. This causes an un-coordinated and inefficient heartbeat. After traveling through the left and right atria, the electrical impulse travels from the atrioventricular node down the Bundle of His, which divides into the left and right bundle branches, that send the impulse into the left and right ventricles, respectively. When the right bundle branch is blocked, the normal, nearly simultaneous contraction of both ventricles is disrupted. The right ventricle is not activated at the same time as the left by an impulse coming from the right bundle branch, but it does depolarise when the impulse from the left bundle branch travels through the myocardium, and finally makes its way to the right ventricle. The right ventricle then contracts after the left ventricle. It can be observed on an EKG tracing as a wide QRS complex.

I45.4 Nonspecific intraventricular block

Nonspecific intraventricular block includes an unspecified bundle branch block, a condition in which a portion of the heart's electrical conduction system at the specialized conduction fibers for the ventricles is defective and either slows down or blocks the electrical impulses to the ventricles, causing an un-coordinated and inefficient heartbeat. After traveling through the left and right atria, the electrical impulse travels from the atrioventricular node down the Bundle of His, which divides into the left and right bundle branches, which send the impulse into the left and right ventricles, respectively. When both bundle branches are functioning normally, the two ventricles contract nearly simultaneously.

I45.6 Pre-excitation syndrome

Pre-excitation syndrome includes anomalous atrioventricular excitation, or Lown-Ganong-Levine syndrome, a condition in which the patient has an extra electrical conduit between the atria of the heart and the ventricles. This condition can remain asymptomatic, or result in an irregular heartbeat, as well as heart failure.

I45.81 Long QT syndrome

This hereditary disorder is a defect of the heart's electrical conduction system. Patients with this condition will have an abnormally long gap between the time it takes for the heart ventricles to contract. Common symptoms include abnormally fast heart rate and fainting. Attacks may be brought on by intense emotional or physical activity.

I46 Cardiac arrest

Cardiac arrest is the failure of the heart muscle to contract effectively which impedes the normal circulation of blood and prevents oxygen delivery to the body.

I47 Paroxysmal tachycardia

Paroxysmal tachycardia is a heart rhythm disorder characterized by recurrent episodes of rapid heartbeats, usually with an abrupt onset and a spontaneous return to a normal. The condition is caused by an abnormal electrical focus that can originate in the atrium, atrioventricular node or ventricle.

I47.0 Re-entry ventricular arrhythmia

Re-entry ventricular arrhythmias occur when the conduction system in the heart does not complete a circuit but instead loops back on itself, it may be anatomically or functionally defined. Anatomically defined re-entry has a fixed anatomic pathway with conduction via accessory pathways through bypass tracts in the atria and ventricles. Wolff-Parkinson-White syndrome (WPW) is an anatomically defined re-entry ventricular arrhythmia. Functionally defined re-entry has a circuit of assorted pathways arising from multiple locations. Ventricular fibrillation that follows ventricular tachycardia is a functionally defined re-entry ventricular arrhythmia. Causes can include ischemia of the heart muscle, electrolyte/pH imbalance, or bradycardia.

I47.1 Supraventricular tachycardia

Supraventricular tachycardia (SVT) is a heart rhythm disorder characterized by rapid heart rate that arises from an area above the ventricles. In normal conduction, the electrical impulse arises from the sinoatrial node (SA node) to depolarizes and contract the atria followed by the ventricles. SVT with a sinoatrial origin is called sinoatrial nodal reentrant tachycardia (SNRT). SVT with an atrial origin includes: Ectopic (unifocal) atrial tachycardia (EAT), Multifocal atrial tachycardia (MAT), atrial fibrillation (or flutter) with rapid ventricular response. SVT with an atrioventricular origin (junctional tachycardia) includes: AV nodal reentrant tachycardia (AVNRT) or junctional reciprocating tachycardia (JRT), AV reciprocating tachycardia (AVRT) visible or concealed (including Wolff-Parkinson-White syndrome) and junctional ectopic tachycardia (JET). SVT is not usually life threatening and may be caused by medications/drugs, thyroid disorders, emotional stress, and structural anomalies of the heart (Wolff-Parkinson-White syndrome).

I47.2 Ventricular tachycardia

Ventricular tachycardia (V-tach, VT) is a heart rhythm disorder characterized by rapid heart rate, usually >100 beats per minute (bpm), with 3 or more successive beats originating from the ventricles. VT can be monomorphic, where all of the beats look the same in all leads of a surface electrocardiogram (ECG, EKG), or polymorphic, with beat to beat variability. VT that lasts <30 seconds is considered to be non-sustained and VT with a duration of >30 seconds is sustained. VT may be a complication of a myocardial infarction (MI, heart attack), cardiomyopathy (enlarged heart), myocarditis (heart inflammation), low blood levels of potassium (hypokalemia), lack of oxygen (hypoxia, hypoxemia), or certain medications. Symptoms can include dizziness, fainting (syncope), chest pain (angina), and shortness of breath.

I48.0 Paroxysmal atrial fibrillation

Atrial fibrillation is a rapid, irregular heartbeat of the atrium.

I49.01 Ventricular fibrillation

Ventricular fibrillation (V-fib) is a serious, life threatening heart rhythm disorder characterized by rapid, irregular heartbeat of the ventricles and failure of the heart to pump blood effectively which can lead to cardiac arrest and death if a regular heartbeat is not restored quickly. Myocardial infarction is the most common cause of V-fib. Other causes include electrocution accidents, cardiomyopathies, other arrythhmias, and heart surgery.

I49.02 Ventricular flutter

Ventricular flutter (V-flutter) is a critically unstable heart rhythm disorder often observed between ventricular tachycardia and ventricular fibrillation as a rapid, regular heartbeat of the ventricles. The ventricular rate is >250 beats per minute (bpm) with surface tracing on electrocardiogram (ECG, EKG) characterized by a sinusoidal waveform without clearly defined QRS complex and T waves.

I49.40 Unspecified premature depolarization

Premature depolarization, or ectopic beats, may arise from the atria or the ventricle and is characterized by extra or skipped heartbeats. There is usually no cause atributed to the irregularity and the condition is benign. Premature depolarizations have been observed in patients with low blood potassium levels (hypokalemia), cardiomyopathy, and ingestion of caffeine, alcohol, nicotine, and other stimulant substances.

I50.9 Heart failure, unspecified

Unspecified congestive heart failure occurs when the heart is unable to pump enough blood to the extremities and the lungs, resulting in edema in these areas of the body, but the part of the heart which has failed is not specified.

I51.1 Rupture of chordae tendineae, not elsewhere classified

A rupture of chordae tendineae is a tear in the fibrous tissue which connects the heart valves to the papillary muscles that anchor the valves.

I51.2 Rupture of papillary muscle, not elsewhere classified

A rupture of papillary muscle is a tear in the muscle which connects the chordae tendineae to the wall of the heart.

I51.81 Takotsubo syndrome

Takotsubo syndrome is a reversible type of left ventricular dysfunction brought on by emotional or physiological stress in the absence of obstructive coronary artery disease. This syndrome has been reported with more frequency in the United States and Europe in the last few years, although it was recognized and reported first within the Japanese poplulation. The name comes from a Japanese fishing pot that is round-bottomed and narrow in the neck, designed for catching octopus. Takotsubo syndrome is also referred to as transient left ventricular apical ballooning syndrome, making reference to the morphological shape features of this syndrome affecting the left ventricular apex and midventricle. Studies will show an elevated ST segment in the precordial leads, cardica enzyme and biomarker level elevation, and transient apical systolic left ventricular function with chest pain. Resolution is usually rapid after the onset and the exact cause is unknown, but thought to be brought on by simultaneous spasms in multiple coronary vessels. Complications can develop that need to be treated, such as arrythmias and left heart failure.

I60 Nontraumatic subarachnoid hemorrhage

Nontraumatic, spontaneous subarachnoid hemorrhage is an extravasation of blood that occurs between the middle (arachnoid) and inner (pial) layers of the protective membrane covering the brain. Spontaneous hemorrahage into this area, referred to as the subarachnoid space, is most often caused by a ruptured cerebral aneurysm or an arteriovenous malformation.

I61 Nontraumatic intracerebral hemorrhage

Nontraumatic, spontaneous intracerebral (intraparenchymal) hemorrhage is an extravastion of blood that occurs within the brain tissue. The most common cause of nontraumatic intracerebral bleeding is hemorrhagic stroke, but aneurysm and ateriovenous malformation may also cause the condition.

I62.0 Nontraumatic subdural hemorrhage

Nontraumatic, spontaneous subdural hemorrhage is an extravastion of blood that occurs between the dura mater--the very outer layer of the protective membrane covering the brain, and the arachnoid mater--the middle layer of the covering around the brain. The arachnoid mater is attached very closely to the inside of the dura mater and is much more delicate. The bleeding in spontaneous subdural hemorrhage most often arises from bridging veins that cross the subdural space. It can increase intracranial pressure, leading to compression of brain tissue, and may cause the brain to shift inside the skull.

I62.1 Nontraumatic extradural hemorrhage

Nontraumatic, spontaneous extradural (epidural) hemorrhage is an extravastion of blood that occurs between the dura mater--the outer layer of the protective covering around the brain, and the skull. Extradural bleeding is usually arterial and can increase intracranial pressure leading to compression of brain tissue and may cause the brain to shift inside the skull.

I67.2 Cerebral atherosclerosis

Cerebral atherosclerosis is a condition in which some blood vessels of the brain become coated with plaque.

I67.4 Hypertensive encephalopathy

Hypertensive encephalopathy occurs when high blood pressure interferes with the proper function of the brain. The patient may experience headaches, loss of vision, or dizziness.

I67.5 Moyamoya disease

In Moyamoya disease, blood vessels at the base of brain become blocked and rupture. This disease occurs primarily in people of Japanese descent.

I69.022 Dysarthria following nontraumatic subarachnoid hemorrhage

Dysarthria is a motor speech disorder caused by neurological injury of some type that results in the inability to control or coordinate the muscles used in speaking. It can be brought about by stroke, brain tumor, or traumatic brain injury. The muscles of the mouth, face, or throat may not move, move only slowly, or become weak. Symptoms appear as slow, slurred speech; soft or whispering speech; rapid, mumbling speech; abnormal rhythm and intonation; limited tongue, jaw, and/or lip movement; drooling; and hoarseness, depending on the location and extent of neurological damage. Dysarthria also occurs in Parkinson s disease, amyotrophic lateral sclerosis, multiple sclerosis, neurological conditions leading to facial weakness and paralysis, or excessive use of alcohol, sedatives, or narcotics. This code is used to report dysarthria that occurs specifically as a late effect of cerebrovascular disease that results in hemorrhaging, occlusion, and/or stenosis, and not from trauma.

I69.023 Fluency disorder following nontraumatic subarachnoid hemorrhage

Also known as stuttering, fluency disorders are recognized by characteristic disruptions in speech production such as sound and syllable repetitions, articular blocks or fixations preventing one from moving forward with speech, and inappropriately prolonged speech sounds.

Note: This type is subsequent to a brain lesion or disease, causing bleeding into the subarachnoid space, typically a late effect of a cerebrovascular accident, and is sometimes called neurogenic stuttering.

I70.92 Chronic total occlusion of artery of the extremities

A chronic total occlusion of an extremity artery usually develops slowly over a period of time as an initial partial blockage. When this happens in the leg, the first symptom may be pain upon exercise, graduating to pain at rest, as the blockage worsens. Chronic symptoms vary depending on the collateral blood flow. Collateral blood flow can compensate somewhat for the blockage, but actually allows it to grow worse with relatively mild symptoms, whereas acute total occlusion cases usually present with sudden onset of severe pain. The thrombus in the chronic blockage often has hard, fibrotic, or calcified caps at the proximal and distal ends. Treatment with surgical stenting or angioplasty is more difficult in these cases because it is hard to cross the blockage. Thrombectomy or bypass surgery may also be done.

I71.4 Abdominal aortic aneurysm, without rupture

An aneurysm of the aorta occurs when an abdominal section of the aorta becomes abnormally enlarged due to weakening of the vessel wall, forming a sac or pouch. Symptoms include diffuse pain in the abdomen and lower back and a feeling of abdominal bloating.

I73.00 Raynaud's syndrome without gangrene

Raynaud's disease is a condition characterized by insufficient blood supply to the hands and feet, which may turn bluish. Typical symptoms include pain, tingling, and numbness in the hands and feet. In some cases, gangrene may develop.

I73.1 Thromboangiitis obliterans [Buerger's disease]

In Buerger's disease, the medium-sized arteries and veins of the hands and feet become inflamed and blocked by blood clots. This disease is typically the result of decades of tobacco use, and usually results in gangrene developing in the extremities.

I73.81 Erythromelalgia

Erythromelalgia, also known as Mitchell's disease or red neuralgia, is a condition marked by abnormal dilation of the blood vessels of the extremities, especially in the feet, causing a painful, burning sensation, as well as redness of the skin.

I74.01 Saddle embolus of abdominal aorta

A saddle embolus is a large thromboembolus that straddles a dividing artery at the bifurcation point and blocks both branches of the vessel. A saddle embolus of the abdominal aorta lodges at the aortoiliac bifurcation, causing rest pain, motor sensory deficits, and bilateral lower extremity ischemia that can become irreversible very quickly. Acute embolic occlusion of the terminal aorta at its bifurcation is a life-threatening crisis. Most of these emboli are from cardiac origin, almost always caused by dislodged intracardiac mural thrombi from the left ventricle or atrium, particularly in patients who have had a recent myocardial infarction. Emboli may also originate in the lower extremities in those with chronic lower extremity ischemia. The embolus travels through the abdominal aorta until it lodges at the terminal point dividing into smaller vessels. A saddle embolus can be caught before it becomes lethal if the patient experiences symptoms in time for treatment. High-dose heparinization is given and bilateral catheter embolectomy or direct aortic embolectomy is done.

I75 Atheroembolism

An atheroembolism is an obstruction of an artery by a fat deposit. This generally occurs when a clump of fat cells detaches from the wall of a large artery, and travels through blood vessels until it becomes lodged in a smaller artery. This condition should be coded according to the site of the blockage.

I76 Septic arterial embolism

Septic arterial emboli originate from some other centralized infection, such as one affecting the heart, like infective endocarditis, or an abscess in the lungs. Some of that infectious matter breaks away from the original site and travels as an embolus through the arterial system until it reaches a vessel too small for it to pass through, where it becomes lodged. This may happen in any of the small arterioles throughout the body, particularly in the brain, the extremities, and the retina of the eye. The infectious embolism can cause tissue death within the blocked area due to the presence of bacteria and lack of blood supply or oxygen.

I77.0 Arteriovenous fistula, acquired

An acquired arteriovenous fistula is an abnormal passage between an artery and a vein that was not present at birth.

I77.1 Stricture of artery

An abnormal narrowing of the lumen of an artery, which allows less blood to flow through the vessel.

I77.2 Rupture of artery

The spontaneous, erosive, or ulcerative disruption of an artery.

I77.4 Celiac artery compression syndrome

Celiac artery compression syndrome occurs when the celiac artery, which runs through the abdomen, is crushed inside the body. The most common symptom of this condition is abdominal pain.

I77.81 Aortic ectasia

Ectasia is a dilation or distention of a tubular structure. Aortic ectasia is a diffuse or irregular dilation of the aorta less than 3 cm in diameter that is usually identified either by screening for abdominal aortic aneurysm (AAA) or as an incidental finding. The ectasia may be idiopathic or associated with aging and other co-existing risk factors such as hypertension, ischemic heart disease, peripheral vascular disease, or chronic obstructive pulmonary disease. Patients with aortic ectasia do not currently have an aortic aneurysm, but ectatic aortas do expand very slowly over time, and approximately 20% of patients go on to develop an aneurysm within 2-3 years.

Note: Report aortic ectasia by the location of the dilation, either unspecified in site, abdominal, thoracic, or both.

I78.0 Hereditary hemorrhagic telangiectasia

Hereditary hemorrhagic telangiectasia is a genetic disorder which results in small vascular malformations on the patient's body, most notably on the tongue, hands, nose, and mucous membranes in the mouth and nose. These malformations cause bleeding into the skin and mucous membranes.

I78.1 Nevus, non-neoplastic

A non-cancerous nevus on the skin is a mole or a birthmark which is present from birth and results from an overgrowth of melanin.

I80 Phlebitis and thrombophlebitis

Phlebitis is the inflammation of a vein. Thrombophlebitis is vein inflammation with formation of a blood clot within the vessel. Inflammation can be caused by bacteria, chemicals, mechanical injury, prolonged immobilization, certain medications, genetic disorders, alcohol and drug abuse. Phlebitis of superficial veins is usually characterized by tenderness, redness, warmth and swelling in the skin overlying the inflamed vessel. Deep vein phlebitis usually manifests with widespread pain and swelling in the affected limb. Thrombophlebitis poses a risk of the blood clot breaking free of the vessel wall and becoming an embolus that circulates to other areas of the body including the lungs and brain, where it causes a blockage and infarction of tissue.

I80.00 Phlebitis and thrombophlebitis of superficial vessels of unspecified lower extremity

Inflammation and thrombus formation in veins close to the skin surface in the lower extremities, including the greater and lesser saphenous vein.

I81 Portal vein thrombosis

In portal vein thrombosis, a blood clot forms in the main vein of the liver.

I82 Other venous embolism and thrombosis

An embolism is a sudden obstruction of a blood vessel caused by a detached blood clot, air bubble, foreign substance, or other material. Thrombosis occurs when a blood clot forms attached to the wall of a blood vessel.

I82.0 Budd-Chiari syndrome

Budd-Chiari syndrome is a condition which occurs with obstruction or occlusion of the main vein of the liver when it becomes blocked by the formation of an attached blood clot. The blockage causes an enlarged liver, sudden, progressive abdominal pain and tenderness, intractable ascites, mild jaundice, portal hypertension, and eventually liver failure.

I82.1 Thrombophlebitis migrans

Thrombophlebitis migrans is an inflammation of a vein that is related to the formation of a blood clot that starts in one vein and spreads to another.

I82.22 Embolism and thrombosis of inferior vena cava

The inferior vena cava (IVC) is the large vein that drains the deoxygenated blood from the lower extremities, abdomen, and iliac veins into the right atrium of the heart. The IVC is formed by the junction of the right and left common iliac veins and lies posterior to the abdominal cavity, running along the right side of the vertebral column. Although it is a rare occurrence, if an embolism or thrombosis severely restricts or occludes blood flow through the IVC, it causes an immediate life-threatening condition.

I82.40   Acute embolism and thrombosis of unspecified deep veins of lower extremity

This subcategory reports the formation of a blood clot or subsequent traveling emboli in the deep veins of the lower extremities. Deep venous thrombosis in itself is not as dangerous as the life-threatening condition it can precipitate when the thrombus dislodges, creating an embolism, that can travel to the lungs. The embolism becomes lodged in one of the branches of the pulmonary artery, clogging the supply of blood to the lungs and heart.

Note: Codes in subcategory I82.40 are used to report acute cases of embolism or deep vein thrombosis in unspecified deep veins of the lower extremity. When this occurs in the distal or proximal lower extremity, select codes from I82.4Z or I82.4Y.

I82.61   Acute embolism and thrombosis of superficial veins of upper extremity

This code reports the formation of a blood clot or subsequent embolism within the superficial veins of the arm. The cephalic and basilic veins are the two main superficial veins beginning in the forearm that run laterally (cephalic) and medially (basilic) to join the axillary vein at different levels. These veins are preferred access sites for PICC line (peripherally inserted central venous catheter) insertion, the most common cause of thrombus formation, and for blood draws, also closely related to the likelihood of thrombosis. Unlike superficial thrombi of the lower extremities, superficial thrombi caused by blood draws or PICC lines in the upper extremities are likely to spread to the deep venous system and involve the axillary vein.

I82.62   Acute embolism and thrombosis of deep veins of upper extremity

Deep vein thrombosis (DVT) of the upper extremity is the formation of a blood clot within a vein deep in the arm. The deep venous system of the upper extremity consists of the paired radial and ulnar veins below the elbow that form the paired brachial veins, which then join with the basilic vein to form the axillary vein, and continue on to the subclavian.

Note: The radial, ulnar, and brachial veins included under this code are rarely the primary site of idiopathic or spontaneous DVT. Typically, thrombosis occurs in the more proximal deep veins, such as the axillary, subclavian, and internal jugular veins (coded elsewhere). This is particularly due to the fact that the subclavian and internal jugular veins are used for the insertion of pacemakers and indwelling lines or central venous access catheters, which are a common cause of thrombus formation.

I82.81   Embolism and thrombosis of superficial veins of lower extremities

Superficial veins in the leg lie just below the skin and are easily visible. Blood flows from the superficial veins through perforator veins into the deep venous system. The perforator veins have one-way valves that only allow blood to flow in the direction of the heart when the veins are squeezed in normal pumping action. Venous thrombosis is the formation of a blood clot within these vessels. Even when the thrombus dislodges and forms an embolism that can travel, superficial venous embolism and thrombosis of the lower extremity does not pose the life-threatening danger of becoming pulmonary emboli because of the perforator valves that act like a sieve and filter clots from entering the deep venous system.

I82.A1   Acute embolism and thrombosis of axillary vein

This subcategory reports the formation of a blood clot or subsequent traveling embolus within the axillary vein, which is considered a proximal deep vein. The paired brachial veins join the basilic vein to form the axillary vein. Both the superficial basilic and cephalic veins join the axillary vein, which continues on to the subclavian. A thrombus that forms in the

superficial cephalic or basilic vein is likely to travel to the deep venous system and involve the axillary vein.

Note: Idiopathic or spontaneous DVT formation typically occurs more often in the proximal axillary vein than in the radial, brachial, or ulnar veins (coded elsewhere).

I82.A2   Chronic embolism and thrombosis of axillary vein

This subcategory reports the chronic, recurring formation of blood clots or subsequent traveling emboli within the axillary vein over a period of time. The axillary vein is considered a proximal deep vein. The paired brachial veins join the basilic vein to form the axillary vein. Both the superficial basilic and cephalic veins join the axillary vein, which continues on to the subclavian. The thrombi that form in the superficial cephalic or basilic veins are likely to travel to the deep venous system and involve the axillary vein.

I82.B1   Acute embolism and thrombosis of subclavian vein

This subcategory reports the formation of a blood clot or subsequent traveling embolus within the subclavian vein, which is considered a proximal deep vein. The subclavian vein is fed by the axillary vein and is a typical site of DVT formation. This is due to the fact that the subclavian veins are used for the insertion of pacemakers and indwelling lines or central venous access catheters, which are a common cause of thrombus formation.

I82.B2   Chronic embolism and thrombosis of subclavian vein

This subcategory reports the chronic, recurring formation of blood clots or subsequent traveling emboli over a period of time within the subclavian vein, which is considered a proximal deep vein. The subclavian vein is fed by the axillary vein and is a typical site of DVT formation. This is due to the fact that the subclavian veins are used for the insertion of pacemakers and indwelling lines or central venous access catheters, which are a common cause of thrombus formation.

I82.C1   Acute embolism and thrombosis of internal jugular vein

This subcategoy reports the formation of a blood clot or subsequent traveling embolus within the internal jugular vein. The internal jugular is a deep vein that is a typical site of DVT formation, particularly due to the fact that it is used for the insertion of pacemakers and indwelling lines or central venous access catheters, which are a common cause of thrombus formation. Jugular deep vein thrombosis becomes complicated by the life-threatening condition of pulmonary emboli in about 36 percent of cases, which is close to the same percentage observed in those with lower extremity DVT.

I82.C2   Chronic embolism and thrombosis of internal jugular vein

This subcategory reports chronic, recurring formation of blood clots or subsequent traveling emboli within the internal jugular vein over a longer period of time. The internal jugular is a deep vein that is a typical site of DVT formation, particularly due to the fact that it is used for the insertion of pacemakers and indwelling lines or central venous access catheters, which are a common cause of thrombus formation. Jugular deep vein thrombosis becomes complicated by the life-threatening condition of pulmonary emboli in about 36 percent of cases, which is close to the same percentage observed in those with lower extremity DVT.

I83   Varicose veins of lower extremities

Varicose veins are swollen, dilated, twisted veins, which most commonly occur in the lower extremities, but can occur anywhere in the body. Varicose veins result from valve incompetence. Leaflet valves in the vein which normally open and close to move blood forward do not function properly allowing retrograde (backward) flow and pooling of blood in the vessels. This causes the vein to become enlarged, tortuous, and painful. The condition is more common in women, with pregnancy often a precipitating factor. Symptoms include itching and pain in the affected area, as well as heaviness or weakness in the affected limb.

Note: Varicose veins complicating pregnancy or the puerperium is coded to O22.0- and O87.4 respectively.

I85 Esophageal varices

Esophageal varices are dilated, submucosal veins in the lower part of the esophagus, the tube that connects the throat and stomach. Esophageal varices occur when veins in the lower esophagus near the stomach become swollen and twisted, usually due to high blood pressure in the hepatic vein (portal hypertension) and are prone to bleeding. Causes include cirrhosis, thrombosis, schistosomiasis or other parasitic infection, and Budd-Chiari syndrome, or hepatic vein obstruction.

I86.1 Scrotal varices

Scrotal varices, or varicoceles, are enlarged veins along the spermatic cord. The condition may be visible, underlying the skin of the scrotum, or invisible but palpable when the testicles are manually examined. Varicoceles form slowly over time and appear most often between the ages of 15 and 25. The sudden appearance of a varicocele in older males may indicate a kidney tumor. Varicoceles have been associated with male infertility.

I86.4 Gastric varices

Gastric varices are dilated, submucosal veins in the stomach that are prone to bleeding. Causes include portal hypertension, cirrhosis of the liver, and thrombosis in the splenic vein, which frequently occurs as a complication of pancreatitis, pancreatic cancer, or other abdominal tumor.

I87.0 Postthrombotic syndrome

In postphlebitic or postthrombotic syndrome, the patient experiences harmful symptoms due to the formation of blood clots in veins deep within the lower legs. It may remain asymptomatic but can also cause ulceration and/or inflammation from the lack of proper blood circulation.

I87.1 Compression of vein

In compression of a vein, other bodily tissue exerts pressure on a vein, reducing its capacity.

I87.2 Venous insufficiency (chronic) (peripheral)

Chronic insufficiency of the peripheral veins is a condition in which the veins of the extremities are not able to drain blood sufficiently over a longer period of time, resulting in an accumulation of fluids in the afflicted area of the body.

I88.0 Nonspecific mesenteric lymphadenitis

Nonspecific mesenteric lymphadenitis is an inflammation of the lymph nodes in the folds of the membrane that encloses the abdominal organs. This condition presents with symptoms similar to appendicitis.

I89 Other noninfective disorders of lymphatic vessels and lymph nodes

The lymphatic channels transport lymph fluid throughout the body, where it delivers nutrients to cells and removes waste products. Reservoirs in the lymph system called lymph nodes filter bacteria and other waste products out of the lymph fluid before it is dumped back into the bloodstream. Noninfectious disorders result from a cause other than bacteria, viruses, or parasites.

I89.0 Lymphedema, not elsewhere classified

Lymphedemas occur when the lymph system is blocked by a blood clot, foreign debris, or other material backing up the flow of lymph and causing swelling from the accumulation of lymphatic fluid.

I89.1 Lymphangitis

Lymphangitis is an inflammation affecting a lymph vessel.

I95 Hypotension

Hypotension is abnormally low blood pressure.

I95.0 Idiopathic hypotension

Idiopathic hypotension is low blood pressure occurring without any apparent cause.

I95.1 Orthostatic hypotension

Orthostatic hypotension is abnormally low blood pressure that occurs when a person moves to a standing or upright position.

I96 Gangrene, not elsewhere classified

Gangrene is a complication of prolonged lack of blood flow to tissue causing cell death or necrosis. The ischemic tissue dies off and decays, becoming black and malodorous.

I97.2 Postmastectomy lymphedema syndrome

Postmastectomy lymphedema syndrome is localized edema in the upper arm that occurs following breast removal along with the underlying lymph nodes. This decreases the circulation of lymph fluid through the chest area, causing fluid back-up and swelling.

J00   Acute nasopharyngitis [common cold]

Acute nasopharyngitis, or the common cold, is caused by a virus, and results in inflammation of the mucous membranes from the nasal cavities to the back of the throat.

J02   Acute pharyngitis

Acute pharyngitis is a severe inflammation of the oropharynx in the throat. This condition is the most common cause of a sore throat. Symptoms include cough, painful swallowing, headache, and fever.

J02.0   Streptococcal pharyngitis

Strep throat presents with fever, swollen glands, and a sore throat that appears red with white patches on the tonsils. Nausea, vomiting, and abdominal pain are sometimes present, most often in children. Untreated cases can cause a later onset of rheumatic fever. Streptococcus is a gram positive bacteria, sub-classified by hemolytic properties (alpha hemolytic and beta hemolytic). The most commonly identified pathological groups in medical settings are *S. pneumoniae* and *S. viridans* (alpha hemolytic) and Groups A and B streptococci (beta hemolytic).

J03   Acute tonsillitis

Acute tonsillitis is a severe inflammation of the tonsils. Many conditions can cause inflammation of the tonsils, including several common diseases of early childhood. Symptoms of this condition are sore throat, headache, high fever, and coughing. The tonsils will be visibly swollen and red.

J04   Acute laryngitis and tracheitis

Inflammation of the larynx and trachea, producing symptoms such as headache, fever, and sore throat. Many diseases and conditions can cause laryngitis and tracheitis, especially diseases of the upper respiratory system.

J04.2   Acute laryngotracheitis

An inflammation of the larynx, trachea, and the vocal cords.

J04.3   Supraglottitis, unspecified

Supraglottitis is a bacterial infection of unknown origin that causes swelling of the larynx, vocal cords, epiglottis, and other structures of the throat. The hallmark symptoms of this condition are difficulty swallowing and talking, labored breathing, and drooling. Also of note is the absence of coughing.

J05.0   Acute obstructive laryngitis [croup]

Croup is an infectious disease occurring in young children which involves the vocal cords, trachea, and bronchial tubes. The most common symptoms of this condition are sore throat, dry, hacking cough, and a fever. Many different bacteria and viruses can cause inflammation in the larynx, blocking off the throat.

J05.1   Acute epiglottitis

An inflammation of the epiglottis, the fold at the back of the tongue which prevents food from spilling into the airway. Due to its position in the throat, an inflamed epiglottis can easily block the airway, resulting in a serious condition.

J09.X   Influenza due to identified novel influenza A virus

The influenza virus has three different types: A, B, and C. Types B and C are specific to humans. Type A affects mainly birds and is called avian influenza (A/H5N1). There are, however, three subtypes of A known to circulate in humans. The highly pathogenic strain spreads quickly among birds and can be 100% deadly in 48 hours. It was reported causing disease in humans in Asia in 1997. Since influenza viruses are constantly changing, they may have adapted to infect humans and there is little immunity against the new virus. Most cases of bird flu in humans come from contact with infected domestic poultry or surfaces contaminated with infected bird secretions or excretions. Contacting the virus from another person is extremely rare. Symptoms depend upon the particular virus and include normal flu-like symptoms to pneumonia and other severe respiratory diseases.

Note: Only influenza A types normally affecting birds, swine, or other animals should be reported here, not cases of flu due to other common kinds of influenza viruses. Also, the specifically identified 2009 H1N1 influenza virus that caused the epidemic outbreak of 2009 is classified in the ICD-10-CM index under category J10. Other new influenza A viruses now being identified as causing the flu in swine as well as other animals and transmitted to humans is coded in this subcategory.

J09.X1   Influenza due to identified novel influenza A virus with pneumonia

Use this code to report human influenza cases due to novel influenza A viruses occurring in pigs or other animals that have not been previously found in humans when it is occurring with any form of pneumonia or bronchopneumonia.

Note: Use an additional code to report the specific type of pneumonia.

J09.X2   Influenza due to identified novel influenza A virus with other respiratory manifestations

Use this code to report human influenza cases due to novel influenza A viruses occurring in pigs or other animals that have not been previously found in humans when it is occurring with respiratory conditions such as laryngitis, pharyngitis, sinusitis, or other acute upper respiratory condition.

Note: Additional codes are necessary for associated sinusitis or pleural effusion.

J09.X3   Influenza due to identified novel influenza A virus with gastrointestinal manifestations

Use this code to report human influenza cases due to novel influenza A viruses occurring in pigs or other animals that have not been previously found in humans when it is occurring with gastrointestinal manifestations caused by the novel influenza A virus, such as gastritis, enteritis, and gastroenteritis.

Note: Viral gastroenteritis is sometimes identified as 'intestinal flu' and is not coded here as a gastrointestinal tract manifestation of the novel influenza A virus disease, but is reported with a code from the infectious disease chapter.

J09.X9   Influenza due to identified novel influenza A virus with other manifestations

Use this code to report human influenza cases due to novel influenza A viruses occurring in pigs or other animals that have not been previously found in humans when it is occurring with other manifestations caused by the novel influenza A virus, such as encephalopathy, middle ear infections, and myocarditis.

Note: Other manifestations, such as acute suppurative otitis media, require that another code is assigned to identify the condition.

J12   Viral pneumonia, not elsewhere classified

Pneumonia is a serious infection and inflammation of the lungs caused by invading organisms, such as bacteria, viruses, fungi, mycoplasma, and rickettsia. Air is inhaled through the trachea into the two major airways, or bronchi, which subdivide in the lungs into numerous smaller airways, called bronchioles that end in tiny clusters of air sacs, called alveoli. When microorganisms get past the body's defense mechanisms and invade the lung tissue, the immune system defenses cause inflammation in the air sacs, which fill with fluid and pus, making breathing difficult. Lobar pneumonia affects only one section, or lobe, of a lung. Bronchial pneumonia can affect many patches of tissue throughout both lungs. Death can result because oxygen is not reaching the blood, and infection spreads throughout the body.

Viral pneumonia is believed to account for half of all pneumonia cases. There are about a dozen different viruses causing pneumonia and more and more are being identified as causing respiratory infections. Viral pneumonia tends to strike primarily in winter and is usually less severe than bacterial pneumonia. The symptoms are very similar to influenza and include a dry cough, fever, headache, muscle pain, and increasing breathlessness that may become extreme. Viral pneumonia has the added risk of complication by bacterial invasion and the development of secondary bacterial pneumonia.

Note: Pneumonia may also be caused by the inhalation or aspiration of irritant substances, such as food, vomitus, liquids, gastric juices, gases, dust, and harmful chemicals or toxic fumes. Aspiration type pneumonias, as well as allergic or eosinophilic, newborn or congenital pneumonia, are not included here, which reports pneumonia caused by invading living viruses other than influenza viruses.

J12.0 Adenoviral pneumonia

The human adenoviruses are grouped into six subgenera A–F within the mammalian genus of the family *Adenoviridae*. Most adenovirus infections are mild and require no therapy. Adenoviruses commonly cause respiratory infections, but also gastroenteritis, conjunctivitis, cystitis, and rashes. These viruses are unusually stable to chemical or physical agents and adverse pH conditions, so they have a longer survival time outside of a host. Adenoviruses are transmitted by direct contact, fecal-oral route, and sometimes waterborne transmission, such as inadequately chlorinated swimming pools. In the United States, adult respiratory distress is most often caused by serotypes 4 and 7. When type 7 is inhaled, it is associated with severe cases of pneumonia that must be managed by treating symptoms and complications.

J12.1 Respiratory syncytial virus pneumonia

Respiratory syncytial virus, or RSV, is the most common cause of pneumonia in infants and children under 1 year. Most children have been infected with it by age 2. It also infects adults and older children, but tends to mimic the common cold in those age groups. In infants, particularly premature infants and those with underlying conditions, the RSV infection can be severe and requires hospitalization. Pneumonia symptoms include high fever, severe cough, wheezing, bluish color to the skin, and difficulty breathing, making the child prefer to sit up. Infants may have markedly drawn in chest muscles and skin between the ribs when breathing and breaths are short, shallow, and rapid. The virus is contracted through the eyes, nose, and mouth by direct contact through shaking hands or touching a contaminated object, or by inhaling infected respiratory secretions in the form of coughs or sneezes.

J12.2 Parainfluenza virus pneumonia

The four types of human parainfluenza viruses (HPIV) are second to respiratory syncytial virus (RSV) as the most common cause of serious lower respiratory tract disease in young children. HPIV can cause repeated infection and usually manifests as a common cold and/or sore throat in older children and adults but can also cause serious lower respiratory infections and pneumonia in the elderly and immune-compromised as well as the very young. HPIV-3 is the type commonly associated with pneumonia and other severe pulmonary disease. Pneumonia symptoms overlap with bronchiolitis, including tachypnea, wheezing, cyanosis, crackles on auscultation, and radiological findings of peribronchial and interstitial consolidation. The peak occurrence of HPIV-3 is usually in the spring and early summer months. The virus is spread whenever it reaches mucous membranes through close contact with infected respiratory secretions from people or on contaminated objects. It is unstable in the environment, but can survive a few hours on inanimate surfaces and is easily inactivated with soap and water.

J12.81 Pneumonia due to SARS-associated coronavirus

SARS-associated coronavirus, SARS-CoV has been confirmed as a previously unrecognized virus responsible for severe adult respiratory syndrome. Although human coronaviruses are responsible for up to 30 percent of colds, they rarely cause lower respiratory disease. The SARS-CoV is new to the human population and its gene sequence differs substantially from all known coronaviruses. It is spread primarily by respiratory droplets propelled through the air by sneezing or coughing that contact the mucous membranes of another person and by touching contaminated surfaces and then the eyes, nose, or mouth. Illness usually begins with a high fever, chills, body aches, headache, and sometimes diarrhea. Mild respiratory symptoms at onset and a dry, nonproductive cough may progress to a state of hypoxemia requiring mechanical ventilation in a few cases and later, the development of pneumonia.

J13 Pneumonia due to Streptococcus pneumoniae

This type of pneumonia is caused by the *Streptococcus pneumoniae* bacteria, called pneumococcus. This is the most common cause of community acquired bacterial pneumonia, estimated to be responsible for 500,000 cases every year in the United States, mostly in children under 2 and adults over 65. Up to 70 percent of healthy people carry pneumococcus in the nose and throat. Pneumonia occurs when the bacteria is breathed in and invades the lungs, bypassing the normal immune system. Pneumococcal pneumonia may come on suddenly with a severe, shaking chill followed by high fever, cough, rapid breathing, chest pains and shortness of breath, sometimes with muscle aches, nausea and vomiting, and headache. *S. pneumoniae* is becoming more and more resistant to antibiotics due to their widespread overuse and misuse.

J14 Pneumonia due to Hemophilus influenzae

H. influenzae is the second most common type of community acquired pneumonia, after *Streptococcus pneumoniae*, particularly affecting those over 65, people with coexisting medical diseases, and children under 5 years of age. *H. influenzae* is a gram-negative anaerobic coccobacillus that causes pneumonia and other invasive infections. The most virulent type is encapsulated type b (Hib). The other nonencapsulated strains are known as nontypeable. The success of the Hib conjugate vaccine has significantly lowered the number of cases in children under 5 years old in the U.S. since 2000, and most infections are now caused by the nonencapsulated strains. Pneumonia is characterized by acute, severe inflammation in the bronchial tree and parenchyma with infiltration and destruction of respiratory epithelium. Purulent substance can discharge into the tracheobronchial tree or pleural space, infect the blood, and spread to extrapulmonary sites. Infection is usually acquired by direct inhalation of the inoculate or by pulmonary aspiration from the upper respiratory tract, where nontypeable strains colonize the nasopharynx in 80% of people.

Note: It is important to distinguish that the patient has pneumonia due to *H. influenzae* infection and not a case of influenza accompanied by pneumonia, which may often be acquired with the flu.

J15 Bacterial pneumonia, not elsewhere classified

Bacterial pneumonia is a serious infection and inflammation of the lungs. Some bacteria causing pneumonia are already present in healthy throats. When the body's defenses are weakened by other viral or respiratory illness, old age, malnutrition, or an impaired or immature immune system, bacteria can get past the body's defense mechanisms and invade the lung tissue. The immune system causes inflammation in the air sacs, which fill with fluid and pus (consolidation), making breathing difficult. This may affect one part of or an entire lobe, called lobar pneumonia, or many patches of tissue throughout all five lobes of both lungs, called bronchial pneumonia. Infection may spread throughout the body, sometimes causing septicemia or meningitis. Death can result because oxygen is not reaching the blood. Pneumonia acquired in an institution is normally far more severe, aggressive, and harder to treat than community acquired pneumonia and because the patients are sicker even without the pneumonia, they are not as capable of fighting off the infection. Symptoms of bacterial pneumonia can come on gradually or very suddenly. In serious cases, the person experiences a fever as high as 105 degrees F, shaking chills, chattering teeth, chest pain, productive cough, profuse sweating, and rapid breathing. Patients may have a blue tinge to the skin. High risk groups, such as the elderly and people with chronic illness, may actually have milder symptoms. Older people may even have a lower temperature than normal instead of the high fever that typically characterizes bacterial pneumonia.

Note: This category includes specific types of bacterial pneumonia other than that due to *Streptococcus pneumoniae* and *H.influenzae.*

J15.0 Pneumonia due to Klebsiella pneumoniae

Klebsiella is a part of normal intestinal flora found in most human colons. This is a nasty opportunistic pathogen that produces an enterotoxin and causes serious infection when it enters another part of the body. *Klebsiella pneumoniae* infections are more common in hospitals. Pneumonia is the most common Klebsiella infection also acquired outside the hospital and tends to infect those with underlying conditions, such as alcoholism, diabetes, and chronic lung disease. Symptoms present as flu-like with high fever, chills, and a cough that produces a lot of thick sputum tainted with blood resembling current jelly in appearance. Mortality can be around 50% due to the underlying disease that tends to be present in patients. This type of pneumonia is aggressive with rapid onset, frequently causing destruction and necrosis in the lung more than other types of pneumonia due to the formation of pus pockets and empyema which may also surround the lung and cause scar tissue to form. Surgery may be needed to save a lung. Klebsiella is also developing antibiotic resistance as are many other bacteria.

J15.1 Pneumonia due to Pseudomonas

Pneumonia due to *Pseudomonas aeruginosa* is a leading cause of gram-negative nosocomial pneumonia. *P. aeruginosa* can survive in almost any moist environment and does not usually infect healthy persons, but can be a lethal pulmonary pathogen. Endotracheal intubation, long term steroid use, compromised immune systems, and age are risk factors. Symptoms include cough, fever and chills, shortness of breath, hypoxia, and sputum containing pus. Bacteria confirmation is isolated from sputum cultures. *P. aeruginosa* is spread mainly from contact with moisture-containing environmental reservoirs, particularly in a hospital setting. The bacterium produces the enzyme collagenase that breaks down collagen fibers. It attaches itself to mucous tissue through tiny, hair-like fimbriae. Treatment is crucial for survival, but the bacteria can exist with a biofilm coating that makes it more resistant to antibiotics.

J15.2 Pneumonia due to staphylococcus

Staphylococcal pneumonia tends to develop mainly in people with chronic lung conditions such as bronchitis and emphysema or those with influenza. This type of pneumonia is both community and hospital acquired. Staphylococcus causes typical pneumonia symptoms, however, the fever and chills tend to be more persistent in staphylococcal pneumonia than with pneumococcal pneumonia. Symptoms can worsen rapidly with severely deteriorating lung function that could be fatal. Abscesses occasionally form in the lung tissue and air-filled lung cysts may develop in children. The bacteria may be spread in the bloodstream. Pus in the pleural cavity (empyema) may need to be drained with a chest tube or by needle aspiration.

J15.21 Pneumonia due to staphylococcus aureus

Staph aureus is most likely to occur in those who are hospitalized and accounts for approximately 15% of hospital acquired pneumonias and about 2% of community acquired pneumonias. It tends to strike the very young, very old, those with other illnesses, and alcoholics. *S. aureus* is not very common, but serious enough to have a mortality rate anywhere from 15% to 40%.

J15.212 Pneumonia due to Methicillin resistant Staphylococcus aureus

Pneumonia caused by a strain of *Staphyloccocus aureus,* known as MRSA, that is resistant to, or unaffected by, the broad-spectrum antibiotics used to treat it. Most MRSA infections are acquired in hospitals, dialysis centers, and nursing homes with the elderly and immune compromised at greatest risk, but another type also occurs among otherwise healthy people in the community. Both community-associated and hospital-associated MRSA infections can be fatal.

J15.3 Pneumonia due to streptococcus, group B

Group B species, *S. agalactiae,* is most commonly seen in postpartum women and in neonates. Pneumonia from this species can be seen in newborns.

J15.4 Pneumonia due to other streptococci

Group A Streptococcus is the one responsible for strep throat, skin infections, life-threatening toxic shock syndrome, and necrotizing fasciitis, as well as rheumatic and scarlet fever. Infection can spread along lymphatic channels and through the blood. Although pneumonia caused by this strain is rare, localized tissue like the lungs can also become infected. The most significant streptococcal species belonging to Group A is the beta hemolytic type, *S. pyogenes.*

Other streptococcal strains include Group C and G, known as *S. equi* and *S. canis* species, which can also cause pneumonia as well as sore throats, skin infections, and neonatal and puerperal sepsis. Other streptococcal strains include the Viridians group and Group D Streptococci. Group D includes the enterococcal species, which are more prevalent in hospitalized patients and can be very difficult to eradicate, requiring a combination of cell-wall acting drug, like ampicillin, and an aminoglycoside, such as gentamicin. Vancomycin resistant strains may also be resistant to cell-wall acting drugs, aminoglycosides, and other glycopeptides. These pneumonia cases require strict isolation and the use of streptogramins and oxazolidinones.

J15.5 Pneumonia due to Escherichia coli

E. coli is a bacterium commonly found in the intestines as a normal part of the flora that helps digest food. Most *E. coli* is harmless and does not cause disease in humans, but when the bacteria invade other areas of the body, or a person becomes infected with one of the dangerous strains, serious illness can result. Respiratory tract infections from *E. coli* are very uncommon and are almost always connected with an *E. coli* infection of the urinary tract. Bacteremia due to *E. coli* precedes pneumonia and is connected to another focus of infection in the urinary or gastrointestinal tract. Nosocomial *E. coli* pneumonia may be due to microaspiration of already colonized upper airway secretions in patients who are very ill. *E. coli* pneumonia tends to manifest as a bronchopneumonia affecting the lower lobes with the presence of empyema.

J15.6 Pneumonia due to other aerobic Gram-negative bacteria

Gram negative bacteria such as Proteus, Serratia, and Acinetobacter cause serious pneumonia that almost always occurs in hospitalized people or nursing home residents, especially those on respirators. Others at risk are older people, infants, those with chronic diseases, and alcoholics. Gram negative pneumonia is frequently so severe that patients can rapidly develop acute respiratory failure. Lung tissue can be rapidly destroyed by the bacteria. Symptoms progress more quickly than with gram-positive pneumonia and patients tend to be sicker. Sputum coughed up is thick and blood-tinged, resembling current jelly. Gram negative pneumonia requires treatment in the hospital and often requires the person to be on a ventilator. Even with expert care, between 25%-50% of patients with gram-negative pneumonia do not survive.

Note: Gram negative pneumonias caused by Klebsiella, Pseudomonas, Legionella, or gram negative anaerobes are not included here.

J15.7 Pneumonia due to Mycoplasma pneumoniae

Mycoplasma pneumoniae are the smallest, free-living, disease-causing agents in humans, unclassified as bacteria or viruses and having characteristics of both. This organism lacks a peptidoglycan cell wall, instead it has a cell membrane incorporating a sterol compound. The lack of a cell wall makes this organism resistant to many antibiotics. Symptoms of infection may be mild and come on gradually. *Mycoplasma pneumoniae* causes mild but widespread pneumonia with a cough that can come in violent attacks and produce sparse mucus. Chills and fever occur as early symptoms and sometimes people experience nausea and vomiting. Some people may not feel sick enough to seek medical care or stay in bed. A "walking pneumonia" diagnosis is probably due to mycoplasma. Profound weakness may last for a long time along with a dry, nagging cough.

Diseases of the Respiratory System

J15.8 – J21.0

J15.8 Pneumonia due to other specified bacteria

Anaerobes are microorganisms that live and grow best within an environment that is completely or almost completely devoid of oxygen. Moderate anaerobes can survive with some oxygen in their environment while microaerophillic anaerobes can grow in air, but poorly. Obligate anaerobes are unable to grow in or are killed by the presence of oxygen. Facultative anaerobes live and grow both in the presence or absence of oxygen. Anaerobes can be gram positive or gram negative and are a part of normal human flora. Most infections, including pneumonia are caused by endogenous flora of the host when conditions change to profoundly favor the growth of anaerobes or to allow the development of opportunistic infection in other areas. Anaerobes produce exotoxins and will form lung abscesses or empyema in pneumonia.

Note: Anaerobes causing pneumonia reported with this code include Bacteroides, Butyrivibrio, Clostridium, Eubacterium, Fusobacterium, Peptococcus, Peptostreptococcus, Proprionibacterium, and Veillonella.

J16.0 Chlamydial pneumonia

Chlamydia bacteria cause pneumonia symptoms similar to mycoplasma pneumonia. The Chlamydia that causes pneumonia is not the same as the type that causes sexually transmitted diseases. This kind of pneumonia is the most common in school age children and can be more serious when it does afflict older adults, but will usually respond to antibiotics.

J17 Pneumonia in diseases classified elsewhere

This category includes several types of infectious diseases known to be associated with acquiring pneumonia or having pneumonia appear as an aspect of the primary disease. Pneumonia occurring with disseminated types of invasive fungal infections that are not specifically identified with a code from the infectious disease chapter is reported here. Only a few fungi cause opportunistic fungal infections. Systemic mycoses usually present as endogenous infections, but some may be caused by circumstances such as the presence of an infected catheter with dissemination into multiple organs, like the lungs. This code also reports rheumatic pneumonia that occurs when nodules and occlusions form in the tissue that separates the lungs, usually resulting in death. This condition is a complication of severe rheumatic fever, which occurs due to an untreated streptococcal throat infection.

Note: The underlying condition must be coded first, such as Q fever, rheumatic fever, or schistosomiasis.

J18.0 Bronchopneumonia, unspecified organism

In the lungs, air is inhaled through the trachea into the two major airways, or bronchi, which subdivide in the lungs into many smaller airways, called bronchioles, that end in tiny clusters of air sacs, called alveoli. When microorganisms get past the body's defense mechanisms and invade the lung tissue, the immune system defenses cause inflammation in the air sacs, which fill with fluid and pus, making breathing difficult. Bronchopneumonia is the type that originates from those many smaller branching ducts of the bronchial tubes, the bronchioles. Bronchopneumonia spreads from the bronchioles to the nearby alveoli and affects many patches of tissue throughout both lungs, most often bilaterally.

Note: Use this code to report bronchopneumonia with no further description of types of bronchopneumonia when the infecting organism is not specified, such as hemorrhagic bronchopneumonia, terminal bronchopneumonia, or pleurobronchopneumonia.

Note: Bronchiolitis is not coded as bronchopneumonia.

J20 Acute bronchitis

Acute bronchitis is an inflammation of the mucous membranes lining the bronchi, the two main airways that branch from the trachea carrying air to distal portions of the lungs. Acute bronchitis usually occurs with a viral or bacterial infection with symptoms that include cough with production of bloody mucous, wheezing, fever, malaise, and fatigue.

J20.0 Acute bronchitis due to Mycoplasma pneumoniae

Acute bronchitis is a condition in which the bronchi, the two main passages that lead from the trachea to the lungs, become inflamed. Primary symptoms include bloody mucous, wheezing, fever, malaise, and fatigue. Mycoplasma, also called Eaton's agent, is an infection by the *Mycoplasma pneumoniae* bacterium, which may be called Pleuropneumonia-like organisms (PPLO). It most commonly affects the lungs, usually causing a mild pneumonia over a course of one to three weeks.

J20.1 Acute bronchitis due to Hemophilus influenzae

Acute bronchitis is a condition in which the bronchi, the two main passages that lead from the trachea to the lungs, become inflamed. *Hemophilus influenzae* is a bacterium with six encapsulated strains (a-f) and some untypable, unencapsulated strains. H. influenzae is an opportunistic pathogen known to cause pneumonia, as well as meningitis, epiglottitis, and other infection/illness, most often in children.

J20.2 Acute bronchitis due to streptococcus

Acute bronchitis is a condition in which the bronchi, the two main passages that lead from the trachea to the lungs, become inflamed. Streptococcus is a gram positive bacteria, sub-classified by hemolytic properties (alpha hemolytic and beta hemolytic). The most commonly identified pathological groups in medical settings are *S. pneumoniae* and *S. viridans* (alpha hemolytic) and Groups A and B streptococci (beta hemolytic).

J20.5 Acute bronchitis due to respiratory syncytial virus

Acute bronchitis is a condition in which the bronchi, the two main passages that lead from the trachea to the lungs, become inflamed. Respiratory syncytial virus (RSV) infections occur most often in infants and young children. RSV usually causes mild cold-like symptoms in the respiratory tract, however, premature infants and immunocompromised individuals can develop bronchitis requiring hospitalization with RSV infection.

J20.6 Acute bronchitis due to rhinovirus

Acute bronchitis is a condition in which the bronchi, the two main passages that lead from the trachea to the lungs, become inflamed. Rhinovirus is the most frequent cause of upper respiratory infections. There are at least 100 identified types of human rhinovirus that differ by their surface proteins. Rhinovirus is spread by respiratory droplets in the air, on contaminated surfaces and via direct (person to person) contact with an infected individual.

J20.7 Acute bronchitis due to echovirus

Acute bronchitis is a condition in which the bronchi, the two main passages that lead from the trachea to the lungs, become inflamed. Echovirus (enteric cytopathic human orphan virus) is found primarily in the gastrointestinal (GI) tract. It is a highly infectious but largely opportunistic virus that usually affects children as an acute febrile illness.

J21 Acute bronchiolitis

Acute bronchiolitis is an inflammation and swelling of the mucous membranes lining the bronchioles, the smallest passages which carry air in the lungs. This disease occurs most commonly in infants and children under the age of 2 years, and is most often caused by viral illness. Typical symptoms are productive coughing, wheezing, tachypnea, nasal flaring, and shortness of breath.

J21.0 Acute bronchiolitis due to respiratory syncytial virus

Acute bronchiolitis is an inflammation and swelling of the mucous membranes lining the bronchioles, the smallest passages which carry air in the lungs. Respiratory syncytial virus (RSV) infections occur most often in infants and young children. RSV usually causes mild cold-like symptoms in the respiratory tract, however, premature infants and immunocompromised individuals can develop bronchiolitis that requires hospitalization with an RSV infection.

J30.0   Vasomotor rhinitis

Vasomotor rhinitis is a kind of nonallergic rhinitis, characterized by an ongoing runny nose with constant watery nasal discharge, stuffiness, and sneezing that is not caused by hay fever, other allergies, or an infection. Even though the exact cause isn't identified, certain irritant act as triggers for the symptoms: dry or polluted air, ingesting alcohol, certain medications, or spicy foods, and even experiencing strong emotions. The trigger causes the blood vessels in the mucous membrane tissues lining the nasal passageways to become inflamed and results in rhinitis symptoms.

J30.1   Allergic rhinitis due to pollen

Allergic rhinitis is a chronic runny nose with constant watery nasal discharge, itchy, watery eyes, stuffiness, sneezing, and sinus pressure caused by inflammation of the nasal mucous membranes. This is triggered by pollen, which is released into the air by plants as part of their reproductive process. Hay fever caused by pollen begins immediately after exposure to tree pollen, grasses, or weeds and the symptoms remain as long as the person is exposed to the pollen inducing the allergic response. Hay fever occurs at certain times of the year when particular plants are in bloom, and their pollen is carried by the wind. It is more likely to affect children and young adults. The severity of allergic symptoms tends to lessen with age over decades. Treatments include nasal wash with saline solution, antihistamines, nasal corticosteroid sprays, decongestants, prescription medicine leukotriene inhibitors, and immunotherapy with a series of allergic shots in severe cases.

J30.2   Other seasonal allergic rhinitis

Other seasonal allergic rhinitis is a chronic runny nose with constant watery nasal discharge, itchy, watery eyes, stuffiness, sneezing, and sinus pressure caused by inflammation of the nasal mucous membranes triggered by other seasonal allergens besides pollen. Seasonal allergic rhinitis begins immediately after exposure to the particular allergen and the symptoms remain as long as the allergen is present during certain times of the year. It is more likely to affect children and young adults. The severity of symptoms from seasonal allergies tends to lessen with age over decades. Treatments include nasal wash with saline solution, antihistamines, nasal corticosteroid sprays, decongestants, prescription medicine leukotriene inhibitors, and immunotherapy with a series of allergic shots in severe cases.

J30.5   Allergic rhinitis due to food

Allergic rhinitis due to food is an allergic reaction from food that causes inflammation of the nasal mucous membranes and resulting allergic symptoms such as an itchy, runny nose with watery nasal discharge; itchy, watery, puffy eyes; nasal congestion and clogged ears; sneezing; sinus pressure; cough, and itchy or sore throat and roof of the mouth. The allergic response begins immediately after exposure to the allergen in the food. Symptoms last until the allergen is removed from the system.

J30.81   Allergic rhinitis due to animal (cat) (dog) hair and dander

Allergic rhinitis is a chronic runny nose with constant watery nasal discharge, itchy, watery eyes, stuffiness, sneezing, and sinus pressure caused by inflammation of the nasal mucous membranes triggered by contact with hair or dander of animals. The allergic response begins immediately after exposure to the allergen from the animal. Symptoms last until the person is no longer exposed to the particular allergen and the allergic response has cleared from the system. Treatments include measures to prevent or reduce exposure to the particular animal, such as removal of the animal from the area, and washing clothes, linens, and carpets. Nasal washes with saline solution, eye drops, antihistamines, nasal corticosteroid sprays, decongestants, and prescription medicine leukotriene inhibitors may also be used as well as immunotherapy in severe cases.

J30.89   Other allergic rhinitis

Other specified allergic rhinitis is a chronic runny nose with constant watery nasal discharge, itchy, watery eyes, stuffiness, sneezing, and sinus pressure caused by inflammation of the nasal mucous membranes triggered by allergens that are nonseasonal, also known as perennial. Other specified nonseasonal allergic rhinitis may be due to indoor allergens that are continually present, such as common house dust, dust mites, and even cockroaches. Symptoms begin immediately after exposure to the particular allergen. Because perennial allergic rhinitis is caused by nonseasonal allergic triggers, some may suffer symptoms year round. Treatments include measures to prevent or reduce exposure to the causative allergen(s), such as pest control and frequent washing of walls, linens, and carpets; nasal washes with saline solution, antihistamines, nasal corticosteroid sprays, decongestants, prescription medicine leukotriene inhibitors, and immunotherapy in severe cases.

J30.9   Allergic rhinitis, unspecified

Allergic rhinitis is an inflammation of the mucous membranes of the nose due to an allergic reaction. An allergic reaction occurs when the immune system exhibits an abnormal sensitivity to a substance that would normally not cause it to react. The chief symptom is a constant runny nose and itchy, watery eyes.

J31.0   Chronic rhinitis

Chronic rhinitis is a long-term, persistent inflammation of the nasal mucous membranes from many potential causes, that may eventually lead to wasting of the mucosal tissues and glands. Rhinitis is marked by symptoms of constant runny nose, nasal congestion and discharge, itchy, watery, puffy eyes, sneezing, and sinus pressure. Chronic may be defined somewhat broadly, but usually entails symptoms that are present for some part of the day, often lasting an hour or longer, for most days of the year. The inflammation may be chronic if symptoms are not controlled using medication for over 4 weeks. Obstructive causes of chronic rhinitis result in nasal air flow disorders, headache, olfactory disorders, and sleep disturbances, greatly affecting health and quality of life. In obstructive or hypertrophic cases, treatment is often laser turbinate or mucotomy surgery. Granulomatous (chronic) rhinitis is caused by an inflamed granulomatous formation within the nasal lining that may resemble a tumor or be associated with ulcerative rhinitis. Granulomatous rhinitis can appear in those who are constantly exposed to a polluted environment or suffer a long-term infection with conditions such as tuberculosis or syphilis.

J31.1   Chronic nasopharyngitis

Chronic nasopharyngitis is long-term inflammation of the entire upper respiratory system, including the nose, sinuses, larynx, and bronchial tubes.

J31.2   Chronic pharyngitis

Chronic pharyngitis is a long-term inflammation of the pharynx, resulting in a sore throat.

J32   Chronic sinusitis

Chronic sinusitis is a long-term inflammation of the lining of a sinus cavity. Sinusitis is reported by the location of the infected sinus.

J32.0   Chronic maxillary sinusitis

The maxillary sinuses are located beneath the eyes in the cheekbones.

J32.1   Chronic frontal sinusitis

The frontal sinuses are located behind the eyebrows in the forehead.

J32.2   Chronic ethmoidal sinusitis

The ethmoidal sinuses are located between the bridge of the nose and the eyes.

J32.3   Chronic sphenoidal sinusitis

The sphenoidal sinuses are behind the temples in the sides of the skull.

J33   Nasal polyp

Nasal polyps are benign tumors that grow on mucous membrane tissue of the nose.

J33.1   Polypoid sinus degeneration

In polypoid sinus degeneration, a polyp in a sinus cavity leads to the deterioration of the lining of the sinus.

J34.2   Deviated nasal septum

A deviated nasal septum is a condition in which the cartilage flap that separates the right and left nostril is shifted out of place, usually due to trauma. Complications of this condition include difficulty breathing through the nose and recurrent sinus infections.

J34.3   Hypertrophy of nasal turbinates

The nasal turbinates are coiled bony structures inside the nasal cavities. Hyptertrophic, or enlarged, turbinates can lead to headache, snoring, stuffy nose, and difficulty breathing through the nose.

J34.81   Nasal mucositis (ulcerative)

Mucositis is a common complication of cancer treatment, causing inflammation and severely painful ulcerative sores in the soft tissues of mucous membranes throughout the body. The cells in mucosal surfaces divide rapidly which is why they suffer damage from chemotherapy and radiation. Treatment for nasopharyngeal carcinoma particularly may result in ulcerative nasal mucositis.

J35   Chronic diseases of tonsils and adenoids

The tonsils and adenoids are composed of lymph tissue and form a ring around the top of the throat. The tonsils are easily visible through the mouth as two masses of tissue on either side of the back of the throat. The adenoids are harder to see, and are located behind the nose and roof of the mouth high in the throat. They can threaten to close the airway if they become infected, inflamed, and severely swollen.

J35.0   Chronic tonsillitis and adenoiditis

Chronic infection and inflammation of the tonsils and adenoids that continues to occur over a longer period of time. This may be caused by bacteria or viruses. Common symptoms of infection include drooling, trouble breathing, bad breath, and problems with the ears. Inflammation of the tonsils is easily seen through the mouth.

J35.1   Hypertrophy of tonsils

A non-tumorous enlargement of the tonsils without an increase in the number of constituent cells; an increase in the volume of tonsillar tissue due to enlargement or overgrowth of the existing, component cells.

J35.3   Hypertrophy of tonsils with hypertrophy of adenoids

An increase in the size of the tonsils and adenoid tissue due to enlargement or overgrowth of the existing, component cells. The most common symptom of this condition is difficulty breathing as the abnormally large structures obstruct the airway.

J35.8   Other chronic diseases of tonsils and adenoids

Other chronic diseases of tonsils and adenoids includes adenoid vegetations in which fungus grows around the adenoids at the top of the throat; calculus or scar formation of the tonsils or adenoids; and tonsillar tag or ulcer.

J36   Peritonsillar abscess

In a peritonsillar abscess, a pus-filled sore extends into the roof of the mouth. The primary symptom of this condition is pain and inflammation at the top of the throat.

J37.0   Chronic laryngitis

Chronic laryngitis is a long-term inflammation of the vocal cords. Usually, the only symptom of laryngitis is the partial or total loss of the ability to speak. Chronic laryngitis is usually caused by a bacterial or viral infection.

J37.1   Chronic laryngotracheitis

Chronic laryngotracheitis is similar to chronic laryngitis, but the inflammation extends past the vocal cords and into the trachea.

J38.0   Paralysis of vocal cords and larynx

Paralysis of the larynx or vocal cords usually occurs due to damage of the muscles and/or nerves that control these structures.

J38.4   Edema of larynx

Edema of the larynx is a condition in which the larynx becomes swollen due to a buildup of fluids in the afflicted tissue.

J38.5   Laryngeal spasm

In spasms of the larynx, the muscles of the larynx contract involuntarily.

J38.6   Stenosis of larynx

An abnormal narrowing, or constriction, of the larynx.

J38.7   Other diseases of larynx

Other diseases of the larynx include an abscess, ulcer, perichondritis, necrosis, and cellulitis of the larynx. Cellulitis and perichondritis of the larynx are conditions in which the soft tissue and connective tissue beneath the mucous membranes of the larynx become inflamed.

J39.0   Retropharyngeal and parapharyngeal abscess

A pus-filled sore at the back of the throat behind the pharynx or around the pharyngeal tissue.

J39.2   Other diseases of pharynx

Other diseases of the pharynx include a pharyngeal cyst and edema of the pharynx in which the space at the top of the throat swells due to an accumulation of bodily fluids in the afflicted tissue.

J41.1   Mucopurulent chronic bronchitis

Mucopurulent chronic bronchitis is a condition in which the bronchial tubes secrete pus as well as mucous. This type of bronchitis tends to alternate between dormant and active periods.

J42   Unspecified chronic bronchitis

Chronic bronchitis is a long-term, ongoing inflammation of the main bronchial tubes that branch off from the throat and carry air to the lungs. The bronchial tubes are lined with mucous and tiny hairs that help to filter dirt particles and other impurities out of the air before it enters the lungs. Bronchitis results in an inflammation of the mucous membranes that line the inside of the bronchial tubes, which impairs their ability to function effectively. If left untreated, chronic bronchitis can damage the lungs and lead to life-threatening complications. The chronic form of bronchitis is diagnosed when the patient has a mucous-producing cough most days of the month for three months of the year, for two consecutive years. Other potential causes must be eliminated before chronic bronchitis can be diagnosed. Smoking is the most common cause of chronic bronchitis by a wide margin. Other causes include the inhalation of harmful fumes or particles in the workplace and air pollution.

J43   Emphysema

Emphysema is a type of chronic obstructive pulmonay disease (COPD) characterized by the slow destruction of elastic tissue of the alveoli (air sacs) in the lungs. The air sacs become abnormally enlarged. The lungs begin to lose their elasticity, causing subsequent wall collapse with expiration, trapping air (carbon dioxide) and limiting oxygen availability, making breathing difficult. This condition is almost always associated with smoking, and typically occurs after age 45. Other causes include pollution and exposure to coal or silica dust. A genetic form of the disease also exists. Common symptoms are shortness of breath during exertion, coughing which brings up sticky phlegm, and hyperventilation.

J43.9   Emphysema, unspecified

This includes emphysematous bleb, which is a thin, air filled sac that forms in the lung of an emphysema patient.

J44   Other chronic obstructive pulmonary disease

Chronic obstructive (asthmatic) (emphysematous) bronchitis occurs when chronic bronchitis causes a permanent airway obstruction, resulting in labored breathing and an exacerbation of the symptoms of chronic bronchitis. Patients suffering from this disease will feel short of breath, and may experience hypoxia. This is a progressive disease, and if steps are not taken to treat it, respiratory failure can result.

Note: Additional codes need to be reported for the type of asthma, when applicable, and to identify exposure to or use of tobacco.

J45   Asthma

Asthma is a condition of diffuse airway inflammation making it very difficult to breathe that may be triggered by a variety of stimuli that include household and environmental allergens, infections, exercising, emotional upset or excitement, inhaled irritants like perfumes, cigarette smoke, and air pollution, and even aspirin. An attack causes the bronchial tubes to spasm and constrict. If the hyperreactive bronchial tubes are severely constricted, carbon dioxide can accumulate in the lungs and cause unconsciousness or death. Airway remodeling involving fibrosis, hypertrophy of pulmonary smooth muscle, and desquamation caused by extensive inflammatory infiltrate also occurs with asthma.

J45.991   Cough variant asthma

In cough variant asthma, the only manifestation of an asthma attack is persistent coughing.

J47   Bronchiectasis

Bronchiectasis is a localized, irreversible dilation, or overstretching, of the bronchial tubes or large airways due to destruction of muscle and elastic tissue in the airway lining. Causes include inhaled foreign objects, respiratory infections, inhalation of chemicals, allergies, inflammatory bowel disease, hiatal hernia, immunodificiency, and genetic disorders such as cystic fibrosis and ciliary dyskinesia. Symptoms include cough (dry or productive of sputum), shortness of breath, and fatigue.

J60   Coalworker's pneumoconiosis

Pneumoconiosis is a condition in which the inhalation of dust or other small particles causes the formation of nodules and scar tissue in the lungs. Also known as black lung or miners' asthma, coal workers' pneumoconiosis (CWP) is caused by the long-term inhalation of smoke or coal dust which results in discoloration and eventual degradation of the lungs. CWP is strictly a result of environment; therefore progression is determined by factors such as length of exposure, concentration and type of dust inhaled, and smoking history. Due to the time required for the dust to accumulate in the lungs, CWP is rarely diagnosed in people under the age of fifty. There is no remedy for this condition other than treating the symptoms and avoiding further exposure to dust. Simple coal workers' pneumoconiosis (SCWP) is frequently asymptomatic. Reports of cough or shortness of breath generally indicate a secondary condition such as bronchitis or smoking. SCWP is rarely debilitating. In contrast, complicated coal workers' pneumoconiosis (CCWP) with wheezing and shortness of breath can indicate that lung function has become impaired. CCWP is often disabling; it has also been linked to heart failure and pulmonary tuberculosis. Many times CCWP will be referred to as pulmonary massive fibrosis (PMF).

J61   Pneumoconiosis due to asbestos and other mineral fibers

Asbestosis is a chronic lung disease caused by inhaling asbestos particles over a prolonged period. The asbestos particles lodge in the alveoli of the lungs, causing the lungs to become inflamed and less able to transfer oxygen to the blood. Over time, scar tissue develops on the lungs. The primary symptom of this condition is progressive shortness of breath, while many other symptoms common with pulmonary disease, such as coughing, will not appear. Patients with this disease are at increased risk of lung cancer, mesothelioma, and death due to respiratory failure.

J62   Pneumoconiosis due to dust containing silica

As the silica-containing dust accumulates in the lungs, the lungs become inflamed and begin to lose their elasticity as reactive fibrous tissue builds up. Common signs of this condition are heavy or labored breathing, shortness of breath, coughing, and difficulty bringing up mucous. Patients suffering from this disease are also at a higher risk of lung infections.

J62.0   Pneumoconiosis due to talc dust

When talc dust accumulates in the lungs, the lungs become inflamed and begin to lose their elasticity as reactive fibrous tissue builds up. Common signs of this condition are heavy or labored breathing, shortness of breath, coughing, and difficulty bringing up mucous. Patients suffering from this disease are also at a higher risk of lung infections.

J63   Pneumoconiosis due to other inorganic dusts

When dust accumulates in the lungs, the lungs become inflamed and begin to lose their elasticity as reactive fibrous tissue builds up. Common signs of this condition are heavy or labored breathing, shortness of breath, coughing, and difficulty bringing up mucous. Patients suffering from this disease are also at a higher risk of lung infections.

J64   Unspecified pneumoconiosis

Pneumoconiosis is a condition in which the inhalation of dust or other small particles causes the formation of nodules and scar tissue in the lungs. As the dust accumulates in the lungs, they become inflamed and begin to lose their elasticity as reactive fibrous tissue builds up. Common signs of this condition are heavy or labored breathing, shortness of breath, coughing, and difficulty bringing up mucous. Patients suffering from this disease are also at a higher risk of lung infections.

J67   Hypersensitivity pneumonitis due to organic dust

Hypersensitivity pneumonitis is allergic alveolitis/pneumonitis caused by inhaling organic dust, or fungal, actinomycotic, or other particles from the external environment. The inner air sacs of the lungs become inflamed because of an allergic reaction to the organic substance being inhaled, particularly when the lungs' exposure is intense and/or prolonged. Common symptoms of this condition are dry cough, tightness in the chest, muscle aches, malaise, sore throat, headache, and shortness of breath. If the condition is chronic, permanent lung damage or even death due to respiratory failure can result. The specific conditions in this category are classified by the particular organic allergen which triggers the condition.

J67.0   Farmer's lung

In farmers' lung, the allergic pneumonitis is triggered by inhaling moldy dust present in hay.

J67.1   Bagassosis

Bagassosis is an allergic pneumonitis triggered by inhaling dust from sugar cane.

J67.2   Bird fancier's lung

In bird-fanciers' lung, the allergic pneumonitis is caused by inhaling particles from bird droppings and dander.

J67.3   Suberosis

Suberosis is an allergic pneumonitis triggered by moldy cork dust.

J67.4   Maltworker's lung

Malt workers' lung is an allergic pneumonitis triggered by spores of the mold *Aspergillus clavatus*, which is found in malt.

J67.5   Mushroom-worker's lung

Mushroom workers' lung is an allergic pneumonitis caused by the chemical urethanes in fungi.

J67.6   Maple-bark-stripper's lung

Maple bark strippers' lung is an allergic pneumonitis due to inhaling moldy wood bark.

J67.7   Air conditioner and humidifier lung

Ventilation pneumonitis is a condition in which the patient has an allergic pneumonitis response to the mold, fungus, or other particles found in the ventilation system of a building or humidifer.

J67.8 Hypersensitivity pneumonitis due to other organic dusts

This code include cheese-washer's lung, furrier's lung, coffee worker's lung, and fish meal worker's lung.

J70.5 Respiratory conditions due to smoke inhalation

Respiratory conditions due to smoke inhalation are caused by breathing in smoke from a fire. The smoke is a mixture of heated particles and gases, some of which may be toxic, or contain certain chemicals that injure the mucous membrane lining the respiratory tract. This causes airway collapse and respiratory distress. The smoke also fills the space needed for oxygen and causes asphyxiation. The throat and airways can be burned if the smoke is hot. Symptoms include coughing, bronchospasm, increased mucus production, soot in the air passages that causes the mucus to be streaked with grey or black, hoarseness, shortness of breath with rapid breathing, and swollen nostrils and nasal passages.

J80 Acute respiratory distress syndrome

Acute respiratory distress syndrome (ARDS) is a life threatening condition that can occur with trauma (injury), infection or aspiration (inhalation) of foreign matter to the lungs. This leads to acute inflammation of lung tissue and impairs the exchange of oxygen and carbon dioxide and causing hypoxia (low oxygen levels) and/or hypercapnia (high carbon dioxide levels). Symptoms include shortness of breath (SOB), tachypnea (fast rate of breathing) and mental confusion (from lack of oxygen or build up of carbon dioxide).

J81.0 Acute pulmonary edema

A sudden, severe accumulation of fluid in the lungs.

J82 Pulmonary eosinophilia, not elsewhere classified

Pulmonary eosinophilia is thought to be an allergic reaction to the parasitic worm *Ascaris lumbricoides* as it travels through the respiratory system. Common symptoms include malaise, wheezing, shortness of breath, dry cough, and fever.

J84.01 Alveolar proteinosis

Pulmonary alveolar proteinosis is a condition in which abnormally high amounts of surfactant, a substance secreted by the lungs to help the alveoli stay open, are produced. This reduces the ability of the lungs to oxygenate the blood. Symptoms of this condition include shortness of breath, persistent dry cough, weight loss, and low grade fever. This condition is often mistaken for chronic pneumonia.

J84.02 Pulmonary alveolar microlithiasis

Pulmonary alveolar microlithiasis is a rare disease in which small calcium deposits form in the alveoli in the lungs. Patients with this condition are usually asymptomatic.

J84.03 Idiopathic pulmonary hemosiderosis

A condition in which repeated episodes of bleeding from the alveoli causes a buildup of hemosiderin in the lungs. Hemosiderin is a protein that stores iron until it is needed in the blood, but its buildup in the lungs causes difficulty breathing. This condition primarily effects children and young adults. Common symptoms include bleeding from the lungs, bloody mucous, and fluid accumulations in the lungs.

Note: This does not include acute idiopathic pulmonary hemorrhage in infants (R04.81).

J84.11 Idiopathic interstitial pneumonia

Idiopathic interstitial pneumonias encompass a clinical group of scarring lung diseases that have distinctive presentation, pathophysiology, and differing outcomes or clinical courses. Even after comprehensive evaluation, patients do not have any known specific exposure to environmental agents, drugs, or toxins; there is no systemic illness identified; and no underlying genetic condition.

J84.112 Idiopathic pulmonary fibrosis

Idiopathic pulmonary fibrosis is a type of chronic fibrosing interstitial pneumonia occurring without an identified cause, usually presenting after age 50. When drug toxicity, environmental exposure, radiation, certain medications, and other medical conditions are ruled out, the condition is called idiopathic. Pulmonary fibrosis scars and thickens the lung tissue surrounding the delicate air sacs. The damage is irreversible. The stiff, thickened tissue makes it difficult for the lungs to function and get oxygen into the bloodstream. Chest x-rays and CT scans will show the scar tissue and its extent. The histological pattern from biopsy demonstrates what pathologists call a usual interstitial pattern. Pulmonary function studies may demonstrate restriction and reduced total lung capacity or vital capacity and impaired gas exchange. Symptoms come on gradually and include prominent, even debilitating dyspnea and a nonproductive cough that does not respond to antitussives. Treatment cannot stop the ultimate progression of the disease. Pulmonary rehab and oxygen therapy aim at improving daily functioning, making breathing easier, reducing blood pressure in the heart as it has to work harder, and lessening complications from reduced oxygen levels. Lung transplantation is a last resort.

J84.113 Idiopathic non-specific interstitial pneumonitis

Non-specific interstitial pneumonitis (NSIP) is a type of idiopathic interstitial pneumonia with a more favorable prognosis than other interstitial pneumonias. The amount of fibrosis varies between patients. Lung biopsy shows diffuse inflammation. CT scans show mainly ground glass abnormalities in more cellular inflamed NSIP and both ground glass abnormalities and scarring fibrosis in more fibrotic NSIP. A combination of fibrosis and inflammation is most common. NSIP usually occurs between 40 and 50 years of age, often 10 years earlier than idiopathic pulmonary fibrosis, and can also happen in children. The onset is gradual and symptoms include breathlessness, chronic or subacute cough, fatigue, dyspnea, and sometimes weight loss. Symptoms may be present up to 3 years before a diagnosis. Pulmonary function tests show restrictive ventilation in most patients and mildly decreased airflow with hypoxemia occurring when exercising. Treatment involves immunosuppression with oral corticosteroids. Patients usually survive 7-10 years. There is a clinical overlap with idiopathic pulmonary fibrosis and surgical biopsy is often needed to distinguish the two. The histologic pattern is not unique and also appears in connective tissue disease and hypersensitivity pneumonitis, which also need to be ruled out.

J84.114 Acute interstitial pneumonitis

Acute interstitial pneumonitis, or Hamman-Rich syndrome, is an accelerated form of interstitial lung disease with diffuse, damaging infiltrates that progress rapidly in a distinct, organizing histologic pattern like that found in cases of acute respiratory distress from sepsis and shock. The cause of acute interstitial pneumonitis is not known. This is a rare, but severe interstitial lung disease that affects otherwise healthy people. Symptoms of cough, fever, and dyspnea often occur for only a week before seeking medical attention and hospitalization with mechanical ventilation is often necessary after only a few days or weeks after the onset.

J84.115 Respiratory bronchiolitis interstitial lung disease

This is a manifestation of interstitial lung disease that occurs in rare cases when significant pulmonary symptoms and abnormal lung function develop in association with a lesion of respiratory bronchiolitis that normally remains asymptomatic. The lesion is found in smokers and is composed of pigmented macrophages within the bronchioles. Nonspecific symptoms of dyspnea and cough are gradual in onset in current smokers in their 40s or 50s with a history of heavy smoking. Men are more affected than women. Lungs show patchy changes with infiltrates of brownish macrophages, lymphocytes, and histiocytes clustered in the bronchioles, alveolar ducts, and peribronchiolar alveolar spaces. Fibrosis around the bronchioles is seen expanding into the alveolar walls.

J84.116 Cryptogenic organizing pneumonia

Cryptogenic organizing pneumonia usually presents with varying degrees of cough and dyspnea in patients that have had an illness for around

3 months without response to antibiotics. About one third of patients describe having had a previous viral illness, but there are no known risk factors. CT scans show alveolar filling in an organizing pneumonia pattern and there may be polyps in the bronchioles. Diagnosis may require biopsy to see very small patches of organizing pneumonia. Pulmonary function tests show restrictive ventilatory pattern and reduced diffusing capacity with airflow obstruction in some. Resting hypoxemia may occur mildly. The average age of onset is 55 yrs, in both men and women. Most patients recover with oral corticosteroids, but many relapse within 3 months when the corticosteroids are stopped, so treatment may be prolonged for 6 months. Some may require long-term immunosuppression with cytotoxic agents, and a very few will continue to develop fibrosis even with aggressive therapy and require a transplant.

Note: Cryptogenic organizing pneumonia (COP) is the revised, modern nomenclature for bronchiolitis obliterans with organizing pneumonia. This change in terminology is preferred because it rests on the essential features of the condition while avoiding confusion with the airway disease constrictive bronchiolitis obliterans. Because it is of unknown cause, it excludes organizing pneumonia, NOS or due to known, underlying cause, which is coded to J84.89.

J84.117 Desquamative interstitial pneumonia

Desquamative interstitial pneumonia is often considered an extended form of respiratory bronchiolitis interstitial lung disease when pigmented macrophages accumulate in the distal airspaces. The inflammatory infiltrate often includes plasma cells, eosinophils, and lymphocytes, and fills the alveolar spaces diffusely throughout large areas of the lungs in a uniform manner. The infiltrate is no longer centered around the bronchioles. It is also called alveolar macrophage pneumonia and primarily affects males smokers in their 40s and 50s. Dry cough and dyspnea are insidious, lasting over months and may progress to respiratory failure. Most patients improve with smoking cessation and corticosteroids.

J84.2 Lymphoid interstitial pneumonia

Lymphoid interstitial pneumonia is a rare disorder marked by the infiltration of lymphocytes and plasma cells into the interstitium that accumulate diffusely. Diagnosis almost always requires surgical biopsy. Symptoms present as subacute dyspnea and cough of slow onset that gradually increases breathlessness over 3 or more years accompanied by fever, weight loss, chest pain, and pain in the joints. It is more common in women in their 50s, but it can present at any age. Lung nodules and widespread consolidation occur with dense interstitial lymphoid infiltrate extensive throughout alveolar walls. Infiltrate also includes histiocytes with type II cell hyperplasia and increased macrophages. The cause may be unknown, but associated conditions such as collagen vascular disease, immunodeficiency, infective pneumonia, drug or toxin exposure are often investigated first as the cause.

J84.81 Lymphangioleiomyomatosis

Lymphangioleiomyomatosis (LAM) is a rare, often fatal lung disease affecting women almost exclusively. This disease behaves like a kind of interstitial lung disease. The lungs become infiltrated with neoplastic smooth muscle cells of unknown origin. The abnormal smooth muscle proliferates in disorderly growth throughout the lungs, destroying the normal lung tissue, and preventing air from moving in and out. This disease may be sporadic and also occurs in women with tuberous sclerosis complex. LAM can cause pneumothorax and air leaks out of the lung into the pleural space when the lung is collapsed, causing pain and shortness of breath. One lung may collapse over and over again. The disease worsens over time and progresses at different rates. Lung transplant may be an option for severe damage.

J84.82 Adult pulmonary Langerhans cell histiocytosis

Adult pulmonary Langerhans cell histiocytosis is a rare interstitial lung disorder that occurs almost exclusively in smokers, but the underlying etiology is unknown. The morbidity peak is between 20 and 40 years and the chief characteristic is Langerhans' cell granulomas infiltrating and destroying distal bronchioles. CT is necessary for diagnosis and shows a mix of nodules, cavitating nodules, and cysts mainly in the upper lungs with the lung bases spared. Fluid from bronchoalveolar lavage shows nonspecific high macrophage count and some Langerhans' cells. Definitive diagnosis requires surgical biopsy in an area identified by CT. There is no effective treatment and the mechanisms of this orphan disease are not very well known, although it acts like a single-system disease as opposed to multisystem involvement in other histiocytic diseases affecting young people.

J84.83 Surfactant mutations of the lung

Surfactant mutations of the lung are a group of disorders caused by inborn genetic errors of surfactant metabolism that result in significant morbidity and mortality in children. Surfactant is the lipid-rich coating of the lungs' airways that is critical for proper inflation and function of the lungs. Surfactant dysfunction leads to childhood interstitial lung disease, but each mutation type presents with a characteristic clinical picture, course, and prognosis. Symptoms usually present as a newborn, but may appear later in childhood as unknown chronic lung disease. Surfactant protein B deficiency is invariably fatal within the first few months. It is refractory to surfactant replacement and ventilation therapy. Lung transplantation is the only effective treatment. Surfactant protein C deficiency causes acute and chronic interstitial lung disease in infants and children, even into adulthood. Surfactant protein ABCA3 mutations cause varying presentations and is now known to cause interstitial lung disease even in older patients. Children have survived up to 18 years without transplant, but ABCA3 mutations can still cause severe respiratory cases leading to death.

Note: The different types of surfactant lung mutation include surfactant protein B mutation (SPB), surfactant protein C mutation (SPC), surfactant associated ATP binding cassette A3 mutation (ABCA3), and surfactant associated thyroid transcription factor 1 mutation (TTF-1).

J84.841 Neuroendocrine cell hyperplasia of infancy

Neuroendocrine cell hyperplasia of infancy (NEHI) is a rare disorder causing tachypnea, retractive sinking in areas of the ribs and neck, low oxygen in the blood, lung crackles, growth problems, gastric reflux of food and drink. These symptoms appear in otherwise healthy babies in the first year. Respiratory symptoms are present continually, even into adolescence, but slowly get better over years. Prolonged use of oxygen may be required for years, starting in the first year. Additional nutrition helps with weight gain and growth, and flu shots help lower chance of infection. High resolution CT scans and surgical biopsy are done for diagnosis. The cause is unknown and long-term results are not known, but babies with NEHI have specialized neuroendocrine cells in the bronchioles. NEHI may occur in more than one member of a family and may have a genetic link. There have been no deaths or need for transplant reported.

J84.842 Pulmonary interstitial glycogenosis

Pulmonary interstitial glycogenosis (PIG) is a very rare disorder causing newborns to have trouble breathing. Symptoms usually appear at birth or after birth and include tachypnea, low oxygen saturation and hypoxemia, retractive sinking in areas of the ribs and neck, pulmonary hypertension. The cause is unknown but many babies with PIG were born prematurely and have congenital heart disease. A lung biopsy is required for diagnosis and shows a proliferation of poorly defined clear cells containing glycogen infiltrating the alveolar interstitium that causes significant thickening and has major implications for newborns in neonatal or cardiac ICU.

J84.843 Alveolar capillary dysplasia with vein misalignment

Alveolar capillary dysplasia with vein misalignment is a disorder that affects the development of the lungs and their blood vessels. The tiny alveolar capillaries in the small air sacs where oxygen and carbon dioxide are exchanged fail to develop. The number of capillaries are severely reduced and also malpositioned. The pulmonary veins from the lungs into the heart are also malpositioned or bundled together with the pulmonary arteries flowing the other direction. Respiratory distress develops shortly after birth with cyanosis and severe pulmonary hypertension that progresses rapidly even with advanced ventilation and extracorporeal membrane oxygenation.

Death usually occurs within the first 2 months. Some cases have a family history and it is believed to be an autosomal recessive genetic disorder.

J86 Pyothorax

Pyothorax includes empyema, pyopneumothorax, thoracic or pleural abscess, septic pleurisy, and any type of purulent pleurisy. Empyema is a condition in which pus discharges into the space between the lungs and the chest wall, usually due to an infection of the lungs.

J86.0 Pyothorax with fistula

Use this code to report empyema, purulent pleurisy, or a pleural or thoracic abscess occurring together with the formation of a fistula, which is an abnormal passage between the infected area and another structure inside the body.

J90 Pleural effusion, not elsewhere classified

Pleurisy is a condition in which the fluid-filled sacs that separate the lungs from the chest wall become inflamed. The hallmark symptom of this condition is a sharp chest pain while inhaling deeply. Patients with pleurisy tend to take rapid shallow breaths. Other symptoms include chills, coughing, and fever. This code reports pleurisy with effusion when there is seepage of fluid into the chest cavity.

J91.0 Malignant pleural effusion

Malignant pleural effusions are a devastating complication of cancer patients. This is a dangerous fluid accumulation between the layers of the membrane lining the chest cavity and lungs, most often caused by cancers of the breast and lung, lymphomas, or any tumor that metastasizes to the mediastinal lymph nodes. The fluid build-up results from disturbance in the normal reabsorption of fluid from obstructed mediastinal lymphatics. A sample of fluid is removed first via thoracentesis to determine the type of effusion. Once diagnosed, aggressive treatment is done to drain the fluid by chest tube thoracostomy or thoracentesis and treating the underlying tumor. Medication to prevent re-accumulation of fluid after drainage may be used.

J93.0 Spontaneous tension pneumothorax

Spontaneous tension pneumothorax is a disorder in which the lung collapses due to air leaking from the lung into the chest cavity.

J93.11 Primary spontaneous pneumothorax

Pneumothorax is a collapsed lung caused by air within the pleural space between the two layers that line the outside of the lung and the inside of the chest wall. The air expands the pleural space and pushes against the lung, causing it to collapse, producing sudden chest pain on the affected side with shortness of breath. A primary spontaneous pneumothorax occurs for no obvious reason, without underlying pulmonary disease or any preceding traumatic event, although it typically results from the rupture of tiny, subclinical blebs or bullae, causing symptoms without warning. The typical age is from 18-40. Treatment ranges from observation to more aggressive intervention to restore complete lung expansion. Smaller, uncomplicated cases may heal quickly on their own as the air reabsorbs. A tube and one-way valve or a suction tube thoracostomy may be inserted between the ribs to remove the excess air. Surgical removal of a part of the lung may also be necessary.

J93.12 Secondary spontaneous pneumothorax

Pneumothorax is a collapsed lung caused by air within the pleural space between the two layers that line the outside of the lung and the inside of the chest wall. The air expands the pleural space and pushes against the lung, causing it to collapse, producing sudden chest pain on the affected side with shortness of breath. A secondary spontaneous pneumothorax occurs in the presence of another underlying lung disease with structural pathology. The air leaks into the pleural space through damaged or compromised alveoli. This kind of pneumothorax presents a much more serious clinical case because of the comorbidity. The least invasive procedure is used to re-expand the lung, such as insertion of a thoracoscope, resecting

a bleb, removing a portion of the pleura, and using sclerotherapy or laser cautery to seal the pleural cavity.

Note: The underlying, causative disease must be coded first. One of the most common causes of secondary spontaneous pneumothorax is chronic obstructive pulmonary disease.

J93.81 Chronic pneumothorax

Chronic pneumothorax is a long-standing collapsed portion of the lung which may be clinically stable and affect only a small portion of the lungs, causing month-long history of dyspnea with exertion. This is a rare complication of a spontaneous pneumothorax resolved after chest-tube insertion. The affected lung margins show chronic status by appearing thick and lobulated while underlying lung is normal.

J93.82 Other air leak

Other air leak includes persistent air leak which can lead to a life-threatening tension pneumothorax, or collapse of the lung through pressure exerted by continuous air leaking into the pleural space that cannot escape. Persistent air leaks are a significant risk following lung resections or after a primary or secondary spontaneous pneumothorax. When the conventional treatments fail to resolve a persistent pulmonary air leak, an alternative to prolonged use of chest tube drainage involves blocking the bronchus endoscopically to reduce the flow of air through the leak and facilitate closure. Another treatment involves collecting the patient's own blood from a peripheral vein and introducing it through a pleural drain with an inverted siphon that impedes the return of the blood but not the escape of air.

J93.83 Other pneumothorax

Other pneumothorax is used to report any acute or spontaneous pneumothorax that is not further specified.

J93.9 Pneumothorax, unspecified

Pneumothorax is a collapsed lung caused by air within the pleural space between the two layers that line the outside of the lung and the inside of the chest wall. The air expands the pleural space and pushes against the lung, causing it to collapse, producing sudden chest pain on the affected side with shortness of breath.

J95.1 Acute pulmonary insufficiency following thoracic surgery

Acute cases of post-thoracic surgery pulmonary insufficiency may progress rapidly and become fatal. Treatment consists of aggressive supportive measures to reverse the hypoxia, mechanical ventilation, broad-spectrum antibiotics, diuresis, and use of low-dose steroids. There may be impaired perfusion with the development of edema, and the collapse of alveoli. Operative injury that damages the tiny capillaries where they meet the alveoli and oxygen passes into the blood, allows blood and tissue fluid to leak into the lungs, blocking air from entering, causing excess fluid and respiratory distress.

J95.4 Chemical pneumonitis due to anesthesia

Chemical pneumonitis is a lung irritation and inflammation due to breathing in toxins, gases, fumes, or vapors. This code reports chemical pneumonitis specifically due to anesthesia administered during a procedure. When anesthesia causes pneumonitis, the severity of symptoms may depend upon the individual's response to the exposure as well as the time of exposure and how much of the gas was breathed in. Symptoms include a wet-sounding gurgling noise in the lungs while breathing; coughing and an irritated throat; pain, tightness, or burning sensation in the lungs and/or the throat; nausea and vomiting; headaches; dizziness; difficulty thinking clearly; and blue lips and fingernails. The airways and lungs may swell with fluid accumulating in the lungs in acute cases.

This code also includes postprocedural aspiration pneumonia. Most postoperative cases acquired in a hospital environment after a procedure are ventilator-associated and occur when the airway becomes colonized with pathogenic bacteria in the presence of endotracheal or nasogastric tubing that desiccates the patient's airway. The normal ciliary process of removing pathogens and mucous secretions is ineffective, allowing pathogens to flourish in the respiratory tract, particularly with the use of broad spectrum antibiotics that allow the pathogens to replace normal flora. Infected secretions are then aspirated into the tracheobronchial tree. Aspiration of secretions occurs anytime the glottis is bypassed or there is inadequate subglottic suctioning. Medical devices also become contaminated with the pathogenic secretions, and added risk factors such as lying in the supine position and enteral feedings, also contribute to aspiration into the tracheobronchial tree. Aspiration pneumonia can also occur when postoperative vomiting is breathed into the lungs.

J95.812 Postprocedural air leak

Postoperative air leak is a condition that frequently occurs after a thoracic procedure, particularly following pulmonary resections, in which chest tubes have been placed to reduce the risk of an iatrogenic pneumothorax, or collapsed lung, but an air leak is still present without a significant amount of air in the pleural space. The majority will stop spontaneously but some can become a cause of other postoperative morbidity. The size of the air leak is quantified in ml/min or ml/breath to eliminate the subjectivity of its size and help determine chest tube setting changes and healing. A complicated postoperative air leak requires more than chest tube drainage, such as the use of a chest seal or sterile occlusive dressing with a one-way valve.

J95.821 Acute postprocedural respiratory failure

This is a condition of rapid, significant failure in the lungs' ability to exchange carbon dioxide and oxygen that occurs soon after a procedure. Impaired gas exchange and ventilation causes a lack of oxygen in the arterial blood (hypoxemia), too much carbon dioxide (hypercapnia), or both together. Symptoms include wheezing, tight chest, rapid breathing and heartbeat, coughing, sweating, confusion, and accessory muscle use. Postoperative respiratory failure is a relatively common and potentially fatal complication, usually defined as the need for intubation and prolonged mechanical ventilation to correct hypercapnia and assure adequate oxygenation. Risk factors for the surgical patient include age, smoking, obesity, prolonged anesthesia time, chronic pulmonary conditions such as COPD, and upper abdominal, thoracic, or emergency surgeries.

Note: Postprocedural respiratory failure that is not further specified is coded to acute as the default.

J95.822 Acute and chronic postprocedural respiratory failure

This is a failure in the lungs' ability to exchange carbon dioxide and oxygen that occurs after a surgical procedure with an acute form in the presence of chronic development. Impaired gas exchange and ventilation causes a lack of oxygen in the arterial blood (hypoxemia), too much carbon dioxide (hypercapnia), or both together. Symptoms include wheezing, tight chest, rapid breathing and heartbeat, coughing, sweating, confusion, and accessory muscle use. Postoperative respiratory failure is a relatively common and potentially fatal complication, usually defined as the need for intubation and prolonged mechanical ventilation to correct hypercapnia and assure adequate oxygenation. Risk factors for the surgical patient include age, smoking, obesity, prolonged anesthesia time, chronic pulmonary conditions such as COPD, and upper abdominal, thoracic, or emergency surgeries.

J95.84 Transfusion-related acute lung injury (TRALI)

Transfusion related acute lung injury (TRALI) is a devastating, but rare complication of transfusion therapy that can be fatal. TRALI typically develops within six hours of transfusion, but most cases present inside of two hours. Damage to the alveolar capillary membrane is caused by antibodies and other biologically active mediators in the inflammatory process in a susceptible person. The clinical presentation of mild or moderate reactions mimic adult respiratory distress syndrome with tachycardia, fever, chills, dyspnea, hypotension and hypoxemia. Severe reactions reveal acute pulmonary edema and diffuse pulmonary infiltrates in both lungs and requires mechanical ventilation.

J95.851 Ventilator associated pneumonia

Acquiring ventilator assisted pneumonia (VAP) is a risk that comes with the use of long-term ventilation and the required endotracheal intubation necessary for respiratory support for patients unable to breathe on their own. Patients with a new or persistent lung infiltrate and purulent tracheal aspirate are suspected of having VAP. This is confirmed by positive blood culture and bacterial culture of protected catheter brushings. The most common isolated micro-organisms include *Pseudomonas aeruginosa*, MRSA, or *Acinetobacter baumannii*.

Note: The causative organism must be identified with an additional code.

J96 Respiratory failure, not elsewhere classified

Respiratory failure involves the inadequate exchange of gases by the respiratory system leading to hypoxia (PaO2 < 60 mmHg) and/or hypercapnia (PaCo2 >50 mmHg).

J96.01 Acute respiratory failure with hypoxia

Hypoxia without hypercapnia and is most often due to ventilation/perfusion (V/Q) mismatch (air volume in the lungs does not match blood flow through the lungs). This type of acute respiratory failure can be caused by parenchymal disease, vascular disease (shunting, pulmonary embolism), and interstitial lung disease (ARDS, emphysema).

J98.01 Acute bronchospasm

Acute bronchospasm is a constriction or contraction of the smooth muscle in the large air passages, severely limiting airflow. Report bronchospasm when it is not otherwise specified as due to asthma or other identifiable obstructive pulmonary disease.

J98.11 Atelectasis

Atelectasis happens when a lung becomes either totally or partially deflated. This can occur for a variety of reasons, such as lung cancer, trauma, or changes in pressure due to altitude or submersion. Symptoms of a collapsed lung include sharp chest pain, trouble breathing or labored breathing, and coughing.

J98.2 Interstitial emphysema

Interstitial emphysema is a condition in which air builds up inside lung tissue due to the rupture of alveoli in the lungs. A labored cough is the typical symptom.

J98.3 Compensatory emphysema

Compensatory emphysema occurs when an otherwise healthy lung suffers reduced capacity as the result of a disease or surgical procedure reducing lung capacity in the other lung.

J98.6 Disorders of diaphragm

The diaphragm is the muscular structure that separates the abdominal organs from the organs of the chest. The diaphragm expands and contracts to move air into and out of the lungs.

K00.0 Anodontia

Anodontia is a congenital defect in which many (partial anodontia) or all (complete anodontia) of the teeth do not develop and are absent from the mouth. This may affect both the baby (or deciduous) and permanent teeth, or may affect the permanent teeth only.

K00.1 Supernumerary teeth

Supernumerary teeth are teeth which appear in addition to the normal numbers of teeth. These usually appear at the time the permanent teeth grow in and are often removed to prevent crowding of the other teeth.

K00.2 Abnormalities of size and form of teeth

Three common forms of abnormalities include concrescence, in which the roots of two or more teeth become joined; fusion of two or more teeth, so that the patient appears to have one less tooth than normal; and gemination, in which two or more teeth grow from the same tooth bud. Other types of abnormalities may change the shape of a tooth, such as a normally square-topped molar forming into a conical shape instead, or one or more teeth may grow unusually large (macrodontia) or small (microdontia).

K00.3 Mottled teeth

Mottled teeth is a disorder linked to drinking water with high flourine content during tooth formation. This can cause the teeth to suffer from defective calcification, the process which uses calcium to form hard tissues such as tooth and bone, giving the tooth an initial chalky white appearance which gradually turns brown.

K00.4 Disturbances in tooth formation

Disturbances of tooth formation includes any deformity of the tooth that is present from the time the tooth is formed in the jaw, as opposed to due to disease, injury, or tooth decay.

K00.6 Disturbances in tooth eruption

Tooth eruption is the process by which teeth appear from beneath the gum. Disturbances of this process can include structural disturbances, such as impacted teeth, as well as premature or late occurrence of tooth growth and eruption.

K00.7 Teething syndrome

Teething syndrome refers to the pain and discomfort an infant experiences as their baby teeth erupt from the gum.

K02 Dental caries

Dental caries are more commonly known simply as cavities, holes which damage the structure of the teeth. These are caused by bacteria which live in the mouth that convert food, particularly sugars and starches, into acid. This acid combines with food particles and saliva to form a sticky substance called plaque, which adheres to the teeth and allows the acid to erode holes into them over time. Cavities are most common on the back molars, just above the gum line, and at the edges of existing fillings. Caries are reported to the depth of tooth tissue affected: The hard tissues of the teeth include the enamel, or surface layer; the dentin, the hard but porous tissue that connects the enamel to the pulp (the fleshy interior that contains the blood vessels and nerves that supply the tooth); the root of the tooth; and the cementum, a layer of tough, yellowish, bone-like tissue that covers the root of the tooth.

K02.3 Arrested dental caries

Arrested dental caries are those which were caught at an early stage, before they damaged enough of the enamel to require filling.

K02.5 Dental caries on pit and fissure surface

Pit and fissure cavities appear in tiny cracks or in natural pits such as the tops of the molars.

K02.7 Dental root caries

Cavities in the root surface, inside the gumline.

K03 Other diseases of hard tissues of teeth

The hard tissues of the teeth include the enamel, or surface layer; the dentin, the hard but porous tissue that connects the enamel to the pulp (the fleshy interior that contains the blood vessels and nerves that supply the tooth); the root of the tooth; and the cementum, a layer of tough, yellowish, bone-like tissue that covers the root of the tooth.

K03.0 Excessive attrition of teeth

Excessive attrition is a term that simply means that the patient's teeth exhibit excessive wear and tear as a result of tooth-to-tooth contact, often due to a habit of grinding the teeth. This may give the patient's smile a "gummy" appearance due to the shortened tooth length. Excessive attrition may be described as approximal, meaning that it affects two or more teeth that are side-by-side, and/or occlusal, meaning that it is affecting the biting surface of one or more molars.

K03.1 Abrasion of teeth

Abrasion of teeth is differentiated from attrition in that the source of the wear-and-tear is not contact with the other teeth, but contact with other objects. The most common culprits are metal objects held in the teeth (e.g., bobby pins and nails) or excessively hard brushing.

K03.2 Erosion of teeth

Erosion of teeth is differentiated from attrition and abrasion in that it is caused by chemical or bacterial action from sources such as food, drugs or medicines, or persistent vomiting. Whereas a dental cavity is a single site of damage, erosion is more widespread, affecting a large surface area instead of a single pit.

K03.3 Pathological resorption of teeth

Pathological resorption of the hard tissues of the teeth is the loss of the material of the dentin and/or cementum due to a disease.

K03.4 Hypercementosis

Hypercementosis is an excessive deposit of cementum on the surface of the root of the tooth. It usually presents with no signs or symptoms, and is only discovered by x-ray imaging. This condition often requires the extraction of the affected tooth, which may be difficult due to the altered root shape.

K03.5 Ankylosis of teeth

Ankylosis of the teeth is a condition in which the roots of the teeth grow into and merge with the bone of the jaw. This most often occurs during development of the tooth and is more common in the baby teeth than in permanent teeth. This most often presents with the tooth appearing sunk into the gum, as the ankylosis prevents it from erupting correctly. Extraction of the tooth is problematic, but is usually required.

K03.6 Deposits [accretions] on teeth

Accretions on the teeth, also called dental calculus or tartar, are deposits that resist removal by normal brushing and require removal by a professional dental cleaning. These deposits, which often form in between teeth and can extend into pockets created between the tooth and gum, can cause swelling, bleeding, and weakening of the gums.

K03.7 Posteruptive color changes of dental hard tissues

Intrinsic posteruptive color changes, also called staining or discoloration of the teeth, can result from a number of factors. This may be caused by heredity, drugs, metabolic disorders, or other factors. Staining rarely affects the function of the tooth (except in some cases where bleeding from the pulp is at fault), but it is often treated for cosmetic purposes.

K03.81 Cracked tooth

Cracking of a tooth occurs because human teeth actually flex during the process of chewing or biting down. Cracks occur most often in multicusped teeth like molars and premolars because this flexing forces the cusps apart like a wedging action on the surfaces that make contact. This kind of cracking results from the normal wear and tear on a tooth, not from traumatic injury. Cracking can result in incomplete fractures if the crack continues through the enamel into the dentin, the living part of the tooth. A cracked tooth becomes symptomatic, causing pain, when the flexing causes the cracked portions of tooth to move. Extensive cracking can lead to devitalization of the tooth.

K04 Diseases of pulp and periapical tissues

The pulp is the soft center of the tooth which contains the nerves as well as the blood vessels which nourish the dentin. The periapical tissues are those at the apex, or points, of the roots of the teeth.

K04.0 Pulpitis

Pulpitis is an inflammation of the pulp that may present with varying degrees of pain in the affected tooth. Note that pulpitis may be anywhere from acute and short-lived to chronic or even irreversible. In the latter cases, a root canal or extracting the tooth may be necessary.

K04.1 Necrosis of pulp

Necrosis of the pulp indicates that the pulp of the tooth has died, which can lead to infection in the jaw and/or adjoining teeth. Removal of the affected tooth is usually necessary.

K04.2 Pulp degeneration

Pulp degeneration indicates wasting away of the pulp, which will cause death of the surrounding dentine. In some cases, this wasting away may be accompanied by hardening of the tissue of the pulp, forming stones of calcified material within it.

K04.3 Abnormal hard tissue formation in pulp

In abnormal hard tissue formation in the pulp, the dentine grows into the pulp, constricting and ultimately killing it.

K04.4 Acute apical periodontitis of pulpal origin

Acute apical periodontitis of pulpal origin is a severe inflammation of the periodontal ligament, which connects the tooth to the jawbone. This may be due to infection or necrosis (death) of the pulpal tissue.

K04.5 Chronic apical periodontitis

Chronic apical periodontitis is a slowly expanding, spherical, infected wound that can form at the apex, or point, of the root of a tooth. It usually forms as a complication of pulpitis.

K04.6 Periapical abscess with sinus

A periapical abscess with a sinus originates in the pulp and carves a cavity to the surface of the tooth.

K04.8 Radicular cyst

A radicular cyst is a fluid-filled pocket that forms in the jaw beneath one or more teeth which can displace the teeth if it is not drained.

K05 Gingivitis and periodontal diseases

Gingival and periodontal diseases affect the gums and the tendon that holds the teeth to the jaw, respectively. For example, gingivitis is an inflammation of the gums caused by a bacterial infection which presents with sores in the mouth, swollen and bright red or purple gums that have a shiny appearance, bleeding gums, and gums that are tender to the touch.

K05.00 Acute gingivitis, plaque induced

Acute gingivitis is a sudden or severe inflammation of the gums that presents with red or purplish swollen gum tissue with a shiny appearance or sores in the mouth, bleeding, and tenderness. This code reports plaque-induced acute gingivitis, which is of bacterial origin and the most common form. Plaque is a thin film deposit on teeth composed of food debris, dead epithelial cells, and mucin that becomes a growth medium for bacteria.

K05.01 Acute gingivitis, non-plaque induced

Non-plaque induced acute gingivitis is not of a bacterial origin. Since there are many nonbacterial origins of acute gingivitis, distinguishing between plaque and non-plaque induced etiologies helps provide a more precise approach to therapy to interrupt the gingival lesions and stop progression of the disease. Nonbacterial origins of gingivitis may be of multiple pathologies, particularly of many systemic diseases or disorders involving other major body systems, metabolic control in diabetic patients, and even adverse affects of pregnancy. These pathologies present complex diagnostic and management challenges that require establishing collaboration between other care providers as diverse as dermatologists and gastroenterologists.

K05.10 Chronic gingivitis, plaque induced

Chronic inflammation of the gums may appear less severe than acute cases, but remains persistent over a course of months or years despite treatment and can result in gingival recession, exposed teeth, and progression to periodontal disease affecting the ligaments and alveolar bony structures that support the teeth. Plaque induced chronic gingivitis stems from a bacterial etiology.

K05.11 Chronic gingivitis, non-plaque induced

Chronic inflammation of the gums may appear less severe than acute cases, but remains persistent over a course of months or years despite treatment and can result in gingival recession, exposed teeth, and progression to periodontal disease affecting the ligaments and alveolar bony structures that support the teeth. Non-plaque induced chronic gingivitis is not of bacterial origin. Since there are many nonbacterial origins of gingivitis, distinguishing between plaque and non-plaque induced etiologies helps provide a more precise approach to therapy in order to interrupt the gingival lesions and stop progression of the disease.

K05.2 Aggressive periodontitis

Aggressive periodontitis is a serious disease affecting the gums, ligaments, and alveolar bony structures that hold and support the teeth. Receding gums leave teeth exposed where infection reaches deeper into the pockets created around the teeth and requires immediate oral hygiene enforcement for the control of plaque levels; professional root scaling and planing to remove the bacterial plaque and calculus; and periodontal surgery as necessary to help save the teeth. Aggressive periodontitis has a rapid rate of disease progression in persons who may otherwise appear healthy. It may appear within a family group and can be seen in localized (K05.21) and generalized (K05.22) patterns.

K05.21 Aggressive periodontitis, localized

Localized aggressive periodontitis usually has a childhood onset, appearing around puberty. Damage occurs mostly in the permanent first molars and incisors, although many different patterns of affected teeth are seen. There is a strong microbial etiology connected to the pathogen *Actinobacillus actinomycetemcomitans* and abnormal functioning of neutrophils. The blood produces a strong antibody response to infecting agents. Therapy is aimed at altering and hopefully eliminating the microbial cause and any other identifiable systemic or immune contributing factors.

K05.22 Aggressive periodontitis, generalized

Generalized aggressive periodontitis is most often seen in people under age 30. A loss of gum attachment between teeth affects at least 3 other permanent teeth besides the first molars and incisors. Loss of tooth attachment happens in pronounced episodes or periods of destruction. Generalized aggressive periodontitis is also associated with the pathogen *Actinobacillus actinomycetemcomitans,* abnormal functioning of neutrophils, and the presence of *Porphyromonas gingivalis.* The blood produces a poor serum antibody response to the infecting agents. Therapy is aimed at arresting the progression of the disease by eliminating the pathogenic microbes, controlling other systemic or immune contributing factors, and preserving the teeth.

K05.3 Chronic periodontitis

Chronic periodontitis is an ongoing inflammatory disease of the gums, ligaments, and alveolar bony structures that hold and support the teeth. Gum tissue recedes, creating pockets where infection can invade deeper around the tooth, causing a progressive loss of bone and tooth attachment. Chronic periodontitis is the most commonly appearing form of periodontitis and is most prevalent in adults. The resulting loss in tooth attachment progresses slowly, although there can be periods of faster progression. The many contributing factors that increase the risk of periodontitis in addition to microbial infection include smoking, genetic susceptibility, hormonal changes such as during pregnancy, stress, medications, systemic disease like diabetes and rheumatoid arthritis, and poor nutrition. Chronic periodontitis may appear as generalized (K05.32) or in localized (K05.31) areas of the mouth.

K05.31 Chronic periodontitis, localized

Localized chronic periodontitis appears with inflamed gums and gingival recession that slowly progresses to a loss of bone and tooth attachment occurring in one particular, isolated segment of the mouth.

K05.32 Chronic periodontitis, generalized

Chronic periodontitis is an ongoing inflammatory disease of the gums, ligaments, and alveolar bony structures that hold and support the teeth. Gum tissue recedes and slowly progresses to a loss of bone and tooth attachment affecting the entire mouth, putting all teeth at risk.

K05.4 Periodontosis

Periodontosis is an older dentistry term for the chronic degenerative disease of the periodontal soft tissue and supporting tooth sockets without accompanying inflammation. This also reports juvenile periodontosis, which is a rare and destructive infectious periodontal disease that can progress rapidly and affects the front teeth and first permanent molars in children.

K06.0 Gingival recession

In minimal gingival recession, the gumline has receded 1-2 mm. In moderate recession, the gumline has receded 3-4 mm. In severe recession, the gumline has receded 5 or more mm. This severity of recession requires surgical correction in order to protect the roots of the teeth. A localized gingival recession effects only one or a few neighboring teeth. A generalized recession affects the whole mouth.

K08.0 Exfoliation of teeth due to systemic causes

Exfoliation of the teeth due to systemic causes simply indicates that the teeth and surrounding structures are deteriorating due to an underlying, system-wide disease.

K08.1 Complete loss of teeth

Complete edentulism is a condition in which the patient has lost all of his or her teeth. Teeth may be lost due to trauma, periodontal disease, tooth decay, or other cause. Edentulism is reported with a class level used to determine how easily the patient can be treated with prosthodontic techniques, e.g., dentures. There are four criteria used to judge how well a candidate presents for prosthetic replacement: bone height of the jaw, the alignment of the upper and lower jaw, the morphology of the residual gum line, and the muscle attachments in the jaw.

Class I patients have a fully or almost fully intact dental structure and are the most apt to respond well to prosthetic treatment.

Class II patients suffer from some degradation of the supporting dental structures or present with early onset of a disease process which is expected to damage those structures. Dentures may require special modifications to fit properly.

Class III patients require surgical revision of the dental supporting structures of the jaw in order to be fitted with dentures due to severe deterioration and/or an ongoing disease process.

Class IV patients have the most seriously degraded dental support structures. Surgical intervention is required before dentures can be fitted, but is not always possible or successful due to the condition of the jaw.

K08.2 Atrophy of edentulous alveolar ridge

Alveolar ridge atrophy is a wasting away of the bony ridge that supports the root structure of teeth. An edentulous alveolar ridge has already suffered loss of the teeth. Continued atrophy of the bony ridge is coded by degree of its wasting and which jaw is affected.

K08.3 Retained dental root

A retained dental root indicates that part or all of the root structure of a tooth remains in the jaw after the tooth is extracted or otherwise lost. The root may remain where it is and fuse to the bone of the jaw, or it may eventually work its way out to the surface, where it can be easily removed. In many cases, the retained root can be the cause of infection and inflammation, requiring surgical removal. In this case, the problem usually presents with pain at the site, which can range from dull and infrequent to a nagging, deep pain, and may also present with a bitter taste or smell emerging from an unknown area of the mouth.

K08.4 Partial loss of teeth

In partial edentulism, the patient is missing some of his or her teeth, but not all. Teeth may be lost due to trauma, periodontal disease, tooth decay, or other cause. A class level is used to determine the severity of the patient's tooth loss and how easily the patient can be treated with prothodontic techniques, e.g., dentures. There are four criteria used in this determination: the location and extent of the tooth loss; the condition of the teeth next to the area of tooth loss; the condition of the contacting surfaces of the teeth; and the condition of the gum line.

Class I patients have a fully or almost fully intact dental structure and are the most apt to respond well to prosthetic treatment.

Class II patients suffer from some degradation of the supporting dental structures or present with early onset of a disease process which is expected to damage those structures. Dentures may require special modifications to fit properly.

Class III patients require surgical revision of the dental supporting structures of the jaw in order to be fitted with dentures due to severe deterioration and/or an ongoing disease process.

Class IV patients have the most seriously degraded dental support structures. Surgical intervention is required before dentures can be fitted, but is not always possible or successful due to the condition of the jaw.

K08.5 Unsatisfactory restoration of tooth

Because materials used to restore teeth are not permanent, they can suffer failure, which then becomes failure in the dentition itself after these prosthetic materials have been used to replace the surface of the tooth. Failed restorations have a clinical significance when it comes to function and tissue pathology. Defective bridges, crowns, fillings, or other dental restorations occasion more dental care, including not only repeat procedures, but procedures that must address additional dental, oral, or systemic problems occasioned by the failed restoration.

K08.50 Unsatisfactory restoration of tooth, unspecified

Unsatisfactory or defective outcome of a tooth restoration procedure may include bridges, crowns, and fillings. Because materials used to restore teeth are not permanent, they can suffer failure, which then becomes failure in the dentition itself after these prosthetic materials have been used to replace the surface of the tooth. Unsatisfactory or failed restorations have a clinical significance when it comes to loss of proper function and tissue pathology.

K08.51 Open restoration margins of tooth

The margin of the restorative material is not continuous with the natural contours of the tooth, possibly with pits at the margin line. An open margin discrepancy creates an open door for bacteria and their toxins to invade the tooth and penetrate the dentin where they cause inflammation of the pulp and secondary decay.

K08.52 Unrepairable overhanging of dental restorative materials

Overhanging tooth restoration occurs when the restorative material is not confined to the prepared site and overhangs the margins. This can cause problems with the occlusal contours, and irritation of neighboring soft tissues.

K08.530 Fractured dental restorative material without loss of material

This reports a fracture or crack within dental restorative material (not the tooth itself) without any loss of material. The durability of a dental restoration depends not only on the physical properties of the material itself but also on other factors such as the technique used when placing the restorative material, other ancillary materials used, patient cooperation during the procedure, patient hygiene, chewing or biting habits, and diet. A fracture in the dental restorative can occur when the material is stressed beyond its capacity to maintain integrity.

K08.531 Fractured dental restorative material with loss of material

A fracture in dental restorative material accompanied by a loss of some portion of the material used occurs when the material is stressed beyond its capacity to maintain integrity. It then becomes compromised enough to allow some portion or piece of the material itself to break loose.

K08.54 Contour of existing restoration of tooth biologically incompatible with oral health

The contours of an existing restoration are biologically incompatible with oral health when the restoration is responsible for producing any type of complication that affects the periodontal or soft tissue structures of the mouth, or the overall health and viability of the teeth. Over or undercontouring causes different degrees of lack of contact, which affects the form and function of the tooth, causing mild to serious or critically traumatic occlusal problems.

K08.55 Allergy to existing dental restorative material

Use this code when the dental restorative material placed in the mouth is causing the patient to have an allergic reaction. All restorative materials have the potential to elicit allergic responses in patients who are hypersensitive. The nickel-chromium-beryllium alloys used in making crowns and bridges are of particular concern, since many people are allegedly allergic to nickel. Manifestations may present differently for each patient, but can include skin rashes, inflammation, and toxicity-type responses. Hypersensitivity reactions require removal and replacement with alternative materials.

K08.56 Poor aesthetic of existing restoration of tooth

Poor aesthetics of an existing restoration are reported when the appearance of the dental restoration is inadequate and the patient finds it too displeasing or unsatisfactory to accept.

K08.8 Other specified disorders of teeth and supporting structures

Vertical displacement of the alveolus and teeth indicates that one or more teeth as well as their sockets have been separated from the bone of the jaw, usually by trauma to the face. An occlusal plane deviation indicates that one or more of the patient's alveoli is not in its proper place in the jaw. This usually presents with the tooth being out of place and crowding the teeth on one side with an excessively large gap on the other, or being loose due to not fitting into the socket properly.

K09 Cysts of oral region, not elsewhere classified

A cyst is a fluid-filled pocket in the tissue, which can cause infection and may result in other tissues being pushed out of the way as the cyst expands. In many cases, a cyst presents similarly to a benign tumor.

K09.0 Developmental odontogenic cysts

A developmental odontogenic cyst appears in the cells that produce the teeth and their associated structures.

K09.1 Developmental (nonodontogenic) cysts of oral region

This includes a fissural cyst of the jaw that appears at the junction of two or more structures which may or may not be developing, such as globulomaxillary cyst, nasoalveolar cyst, nasolabial cyst, or nasopalatine cyst.

K11 Diseases of salivary glands

The salivary glands secrete saliva, a fluid which contains water, electrolytes, mucus, and enzymes, which in turn begin the digestive process as food is being chewed.

K11.0 Atrophy of salivary gland

Atrophy, or wasting away, of the saliva glands results in insufficient saliva being produced. This presents with extreme dryness of the mouth and lips, causing difficulty in chewing and swallowing and promoting tooth decay due to undigested sugars and other foods remaining on the teeth. In some cases, the senses of taste and scent may be diminished.

K11.1 Hypertrophy of salivary gland

Hypertrophy of the saliva glands indicates overgrowth of the glands with a corresponding increase in saliva production. Though rarely harmful, the excess saliva can be inconvenient.

K11.2 Sialoadenitis

Sialoadenitis is an inflammation and/or infection of one or more of the salivary glands. The condition is fairly common, often recurrent with both viruses and bacteria as causative agents. Parotitis is an infection of the parotid glands, the largest pair of salivary glands. The other two pairs of glands that may become infected are the submandibular and sublingual glands. Symptoms include submandibular pain and swelling, inflammation of buccal mucosa, and drainage (often purulent) from Stensen and Wharton ducts.

K11.3 Abscess of salivary gland

An abscess of the salivary glands is a pocket of infected material surrounded by inflamed tissue that has formed in the glandular tissue. An abscess must usually be treated by draining it and/or using antibiotics to fight the infection.

K11.4 Fistula of salivary gland

A fistula is an abnormal tract that has developed between the salivary gland and another structure or organ to which it does not normally connect.

K11.5 Sialolithiasis

Sialolithiasis is a calculus, or stone, that has developed in the salivary gland. This often presents with pain and can block the salivary duct, leading to dry-mouth and inflammation. In some cases, the stone may need to be removed surgically.

K11.6 Mucocele of salivary gland

A mucocele is a type of cyst (a pocket filled with fluid, usually infected and swollen) which fills with mucus. A mucocele can occur when a salivary gland duct ruptures, causing inflammation and blue-white or translucent nodules that usually appear on the inside of the lip. This condition is most common in young adults.

K11.7 Disturbances of salivary secretion

Disturbances of salivary secretion includes hypoptyalism or hyposalivation (also called hyposialosis), sialorrhea or hypersalivation (also called ptyalism), and xerostomia. Sialorrhea is an increased production of saliva from the salivary glands, resulting in an abnormal amount of saliva in the mouth. Hypersalivation may also occur due to a decreased ability to clear out the saliva that is produced from the mouth. Both causes can result in drooling or difficulty swallowing. Hypersalivation is often a precursor to vomiting or oncoming nausea. Hypoptyalism is an abnormally diminished secretion of saliva, which can result in xerostoma, or dry mouth. Dry mouth occurs whenever the salivary glands are not working properly, such as not enough saliva being produced, or a diminished flow of saliva prevents it from entering the mouth. This makes chewing and swallowing difficult and also leads to an increased risk of tooth decay.

K11.8 Other diseases of salivary glands

Other diseases of salivary glands include sialectasia, stenosis or stricture of a salivary duct, necrotizing sialometaplasia, benign lymphoepithelial lesions, and Mikulicz' disease. Sialectasia is a dilation of the salivary duct that usually begins with a purulent inflammation that remains chronic and destroys the gland's acini, which are the basic secretory units in the gland formed by clusters of cells, leaving a localized dilatation. Necrotizing sialometaplasia is an uncommon type of benign inflammatory lesion that simulates a malignancy and is most often caused by ischemia of salivary gland tissue. Many cases remain painless and seem to appear spontaneously, typically manifesting as an ulcerated, crater-like lesion of the palate that mimicks malignancy, but also as a submucosal swelling with intact mucosal surface. Either types may lead to bony erosion of the palate. Mikulicz' disease is a rare, chronic condition marked by abnormal enlargement of the glands in the head and neck. It is usually benign but occurs in conjunction with underlying diseases such as Hodgkin's disease, leukemia, SLE, and Sjögren's syndrome, and puts the patient at greater risk for lymphoma.

K12 Stomatitis and related lesions

Stomatitis is an inflammation of the mucosal soft tissues of the mouth and includes the inside of the cheeks, the palate, tongue, gums, and floor of the mouth. It is usually caused by a viral infection and most commonly seen in childhood. It presents with fever, excessive saliva (drooling), and sometimes with visible sores within the mouth.

K12.0 Recurrent oral aphthae

Recurrent oral aphthae, also called recurrent aphthous stomatitis, aphthous ulceration, and stomatitis herpetiformis is a common condition in which noncontagious canker sores form repeatedly on the epithelial surfaces in the mouth. These ulcers may have a red perimeter and exude a gray/white material. They may appear either singly or in groups, normally lasting for a week or longer and healing completely in between occurrences. The condition is thought to be a T-cell mediated immune response to different triggers, some of which include local trauma, malnutrition, stress, and even allergies. The aphthae are frequently painful and may interfere with eating or drinking. Treatment is aimed at reducing pain and promoting healing as no cure is known.

K12.1 Other forms of stomatitis

Stomatitis is an inflammation of the mucosal soft tissues of the mouth and includes the inside of the cheeks, the palate, tongue, gums, and floor of the mouth. Other specified forms of this inflammation and irritation can cause ulcers or vesicular lesions in the affected tissue.

K12.2 Cellulitis and abscess of mouth

Cellulitis is a potentially serious infection which appears as a swollen area of soft tissue that feels hot and is tender to the touch. An abscess is a pocket of infected material surrounded by inflamed tissues which usually requires drainage in order to heal. Left untreated, either can cause a spreading infection or even sepsis.

K12.31 Oral mucositis (ulcerative) due to antineoplastic therapy

Mucositis is a common complication of cancer treatment, causing inflammation and ulcerative sores in the soft tissues of mucous membranes, such as those in the mouth and lining the entire alimentary tract. The cells in mucosal surfaces divide rapidly which is why they suffer damage from

chemotherapy and radiotherapy. Mucositis causes severe pain and the inability to swallow or take oral medications.

Note: An additional code must be assigned to identify the antineoplastic or immunosuppressive drug (T45.1x5) or other cancer therapy, such as a radiological procedure and radiotherapy (Y84.2).

K12.32 Oral mucositis (ulcerative) due to other drugs

Oral ulcerative mucositis is inflamed mucosal soft tissues of the mouth with severely painful erosive lesions.

Note: This reports cases caused by drugs other than those used in antineoplastic or chemotherapy. Assign an additional code to identify the adverse effect of the drug.

K12.33 Oral mucositis (ulcerative) due to radiation

Oral ulcerative mucositis is inflamed mucosal soft tissues of the mouth with severely painful erosive lesions. The cells in mucosal surfaces divide rapidly which is why they suffer damage from radiation. Mucositis causes severe pain and the inability to swallow or take oral medications.

Note: This code is reported for cases caused by exposure to ionizing, nonionizing, or natural radiation (radon), and man-made visibile and ultraviolet light, not for reporting mucositis in response to radiological procedures or radiotherapy treatment for cancer (K12.31). An additional code must be assigned to identify the type of radiation exposure.

K12.39 Other oral mucositis (ulcerative)

Oral ulcerative mucositis is inflamed mucosal soft tissues of the mouth with severely painful erosive lesions.

Note: This reports cases caused by a viral infection rather than cancer treatment, drugs, or radiation.

K13.0 Diseases of lips

Diseases of the lips includes such conditions as fistula, cellulitis, abscess, hypertrophy, and cheilosis, or cheilitis. Cheilosis is a painful inflammatory condition of the lips caused by a candida yeast infection that results in scaling, cracking, and weeping at the corners. This can occur with ill-fitting dentures, licking, or otherwise irritating the corners of the mouth where the yeast then collects and grows, particularly in those with diabetes, anemia, or immune deficiencies. Angular cheilitis or cheilosis, also called perleche and commissural cheilitis, is a fissure running in the corner of the mouth with reddened, irritated, or inflamed skin adjacent to the fissure.

K13.1 Cheek and lip biting

Biting the insides of the cheeks and the lips is a body-focused repetitive behavior that is extremely common. Many people are unaware of when or how often they are biting. Although it is not considered an obsessive compulsive behavior, it generally occurs with nervous tension, stress, or feeling that something isn't right as well as with anxiety. Severity may range from biting chapped skin from the lips to biting healthy skin, causing rawness and bleeding. Lip and cheek biting can become a long-term, chronic habit that leads to sore, peeling, inflamed, dry, or raw lips and cheeks. Healing will occur on its own when the habit is stopped. Some may require therapy aimed at controlling the causative trigger.

K13.21 Leukoplakia of oral mucosa, including tongue

Oral leukoplakia is a condition of the mouth in which lesions of thickened, white or grayish plaques form on the mucous membranes of the tongue, gums, insides of the cheeks, and bottom of the mouth that cannot be scraped off. It is most common in the elderly, particularly those with a history of tobacco use. The plaques are benign, but can become serious in some cases, as a precursor to cancer, particularly on the floor of the mouth where cancer is known to occur next to areas of leukoplakia.

K13.22 Minimal keratinized residual ridge mucosa

Keratin is a tough protein substance which is the main component in hair and nails in humans, and horns and hooves in other animals. The residual ridge is the portion of the tooth's support structure that remains even after the tooth itself has been lost. A minimally keratinized residual ridge will be soft and prone to develop sores under the pressure of dentures.

K13.23 Excessive keratinized residual ridge mucosa

Keratin is a tough protein substance which is the main component in hair and nails in humans and horns and hooves in other animals. The residual ridge is the portion of the tooth's support structure that remains even after the tooth itself has been lost. An excessively keratinized residual ridge may be unusually large, making denture fitting problematic.

K13.24 Leukokeratosis nicotina palati

Leukokeratosis nicotina palati is known as smoker's palate. This is a type of leukoplakia that appears as a diffuse white or grayish patch on the hard palate containing many slightly raised papules or nodules with red spots in the center. The red spots are the tiny ducts of inflamed minor salivary glands. The condition is painless and caused by the palatal mucosa response to chronic heat exposure coming from pipe or cigar smoking. Any mucosa underneath dentures, if worn, remains unaffected. Severe cases cause a dry lake bed appearance and fissuring or the palatal mucosa. When the mucosal response is triggered by reverse smoking, and not heat alone, it tends to be premalignant.

K13.3 Hairy leukoplakia

Oral hairy leukoplakia is an uncommon form of leukoplakia caused by the Epstein-Barr virus (EBV), which remains in the body for life once a person is infected, although normally in a dormant state. Whitish, fuzzy plaques that resemble folds or ridges appear mainly on the side of the tongue, but also other sites in the oral cavity. Hairy leukoplakia is seen mostly in those with HIV/AIDS infection or other severe immune deficiency and is often mistaken for thrush. The appearance of hairy leukoplakia can actually signify that antiretroviral drugs are not working.

K13.5 Oral submucous fibrosis

Oral submucosal fibrosis (OSF) is a chronic and debilitating disease which presents with the buildup of fibrous (scar-like) tissue in the soft tissue of the mouth, which causes rigidity and a progressive inability to open the mouth. This disease is most common in those who chew tobacco and similar substances.

K14.0 Glossitis

Glossitis indicates changes in the appearance of the tongue due to an inflammation. The inflammation might be due to a bacterial or viral infection; an injury, such as a burn or cut; exposure to irritants such as tobacco, alcohol, or heavily-spiced food; an allergic reaction; or another disorder that isn't localized to the tongue. It presents with swelling, soreness, tenderness, and an unusually smooth appearance to the tongue, which is usually a dark, "beefy" red color. The patient may also experience difficulty with chewing, swallowing, or speaking. Glossitis is treated by treating the underlying cause.

K14.1 Geographic tongue

A geographic tongue is covered with smooth, red, beefy patches, giving it a map-like appearance. It may also be sore or present with a burning pain. Geographic tongue may be the result of the same irritants that can cause glossitis.

K14.2 Median rhomboid glossitis

Median rhomboid glossitis presents as a large, smooth, reddish patch in the center of the back of the tongue. This patch may be rhomboid (roughly rectangular) or circular. This disorder is usually congenital (present from birth), and while it has no cure, it is not usually debilitating either. The most common side-effect is that the patient may complain of a burning sensation when he or she eats spicy food.

K14.3 Hypertrophy of tongue papillae

Papillae are the tiny bumps or buds on the tongue that contain the taste buds. There is a V-shaped row of 8-12 papillae towards the back known as the circumvallate papillae. Hypertrophy of the tongue papillae indicates that these papillae have grown to an unusually large size, though not due to a tumor.

K14.4 Atrophy of tongue papillae

Papillae are the tiny bumps or buds on the tongue that contain the taste buds. There is a V-shaped row of 8-12 papillae towards the back known as the circumvallate papillae. Atrophy of the tongue papillae indicates that they have diminished in size or are in the process of shrinking. This condition may be a symptom for other disorders.

K14.5 Plicated tongue

A plicated tongue, more commonly called a fissured tongue, is one in which the tongue presents with numerous deep grooves or fissures on the top surface. These furrows may differ in size and depth, and give the tongue a wrinkled appearance. This condition is often present from birth, although it is not uncommon to see it develop in childhood or even later. In some cases, these fissures are indicative of malnutrition or another disease.

K14.6 Glossodynia

Glossodynia simply indicates pain and/or a burning sensation on the tongue which is not accompanied by any visible symptoms. This is most often caused by a vitamin B12 deficiency and is often seen in otherwise healthy women, in particular.

K20 Esophagitis

Esophagitis is an inflammation of the mucosal lining or submucosal coat of the esophagus. These layers are closest to the interior passage of the esophagus and protect the esophageal muscles underneath. Esophagitis usually occurs as a result of bacterial or viral infection, but may also occur as a result of an allergic reaction, or exposure to stomach acid.

K20.0 Eosinophilic esophagitis

Also known as allergic esophagitis, eosinophilic esophagitis affects both children and adults and was previously connected to acid reflux esophagitis, but is now identified as a different clinical pathology that does not respond to proton pump inhibitors. Associated symptoms include severe dysphagia, food impaction, proximal esophageal strictures, and food allergies. Clinical findings following an endoscopy and mucosal biopsy include dense eosinophilic infiltration of the squamous epithelium, whitish exudates, ringed esophagus, fragile mucosa, vertical lines in the mucosa, and narrow lumen. The disease is thought to be connected to an exaggerated response to food antigens.

K20.8 Other esophagitis

Note: This includes an abscess of the esophagus.

K21 Gastro-esophageal reflux disease

Gastroesophageal reflux disease (GERD) is a chronic digestive disorder that occurs when the muscular valve between the esophagus and the stomach fails to function properly. Gastric acid is able to flow backward (reflux) from the stomach into the esophagus. The mucosal tissue lining the esophagus becomes irritated causing symptoms such as frequent heartburn, difficulty swallowing, chronic cough, and laryngitis.

K21.0 Gastro-esophageal reflux disease with esophagitis

Reflux esophagitis is an inflammation of the esophagus due to reflux of the gastric acid in the stomach back up into the esophageal tube. This inflammation is usually isolated to the lower parts of the esophagus.

K21.9 Gastro-esophageal reflux disease without esophagitis

Esophageal reflux is a disorder in which gastric acid from the stomach has washed backwards into the esophagus, either due to the sphincter (ring-shaped) muscle that separates the esophagus and the stomach not closing all the way, allowing seepage, or due to a muscle spasm of the sphincter which allows a greater volume of the acid to wash into the esophagus over a shorter period of time. This causes a burning sensation, usually centered in the middle of the chest near the breast bone.

K22.0 Achalasia of cardia

Achalasia of the cardia is a rare disorder that presents with an abnormal enlargement of the esophagus, which impairs its ability to push food down towards the stomach, and with failure of the sphincter (ring-shaped) muscle to relax so as to allow food to pass through into the stomach.

K22.1 Ulcer of esophagus

An ulcer of the esophagus is an erosive lesion that develops on the interior wall of the esophagus, usually as a result of gastric acid from the stomach causing damage when it seeps past the ring-shaped sphincter muscle that separates the stomach from the esophagus.

K22.2 Esophageal obstruction

Stricture and stenosis of the esophagus causees the muscles of the esophagus which normally guide food to the stomach to become thickened and/or tight and narrow so as to reduce the space within the lumen of the espophagus.

K22.3 Perforation of esophagus

A perforation of the esophagus is a hole in the esophagus which penetrates the surrounding muscle so that food can enter the mediastinum, the surrounding area of the chest cavity. This usually results in infection and inflammation of the chest (mediastinitis). A perforation is most often the result of an injury during a medical procedure involving the esophagus, such as the placement of a nasogastric feeding tube.

K22.4 Dyskinesia of esophagus

Dyskinesia of the esophagus is a disorder in which the muscles of the esophagus that normally guide food to the stomach are weakened or paralyzed and are not able to contract in the normal coordinated fashion, causing difficulty in swallowing.

K22.5 Diverticulum of esophagus, acquired

A diverticulum is a pouch or sac that forms in a tubular organ. An acquired diverticulum of the esophagus is a cul-de-sac that forms in the side of the esophagus, which can trap food diverted to it and ultimately become infected. This must be corrected surgically.

K22.6 Gastro-esophageal laceration-hemorrhage syndrome

Gastroesophageal laceration-hemorrhage syndrome, also called Mallory-Weiss syndrome, is a condition in which the esophagus becomes torn and bleeds near the area where it connects to the stomach due to prolonged vomiting, hiccuping, or other spasming activity.

K22.7 Barrett's esophagus

There is a clear distinction in the type of cells that line the stomach and intestines and the type of cells that line the esophagus. Barrett's esophagus occurs when the gastro-intestinal cells grow up into the esophagus. Since the cells lining the stomach have protection against gastric acid, this is often a defense mechanism the body uses to protect the esophagus from acid reflux; however the displacement of cells may also cause dysplasia or abnormal cell growth. These changes increase the risk of developing a rare esophageal adenocarcinoma. There are no discrete symptoms for Barrett's esophogus, but GERD symptoms can include frequent heartburn, difficulty swallowing, chronic cough, and laryngitis.

K25 Gastric ulcer

A gastric ulcer, or stomach ulcer, is a break in the normal tissue that lines the stomach to protect the outer layers from the stomach's acid. An ulcer most commonly presents with abdominal pain, nausea, indigestion, vomiting (which may or may not include blood), blood in the stool, weight loss, and fatigue. The chances of getting an ulcer are increased by long-term stress, certain infections, smoking, taking certain medications (including aspirin), age, and being put on a ventilator. Gastric ulcers are classified according to severity or duration and the complications present. An acute ulcer appears suddenly with severe symptoms, while a chronic ulcer may be less severe, but continue over a long period of time for months or even years. Hemorrhage is an instance of bleeding, in this case due to

the damage done to the stomach wall by the ulcer. Perforation means that the ulcer has created a hole that allows gastric acid and food to leak into the surrounding abdominal cavity, which almost always results in serious infection and inflammation.

K26 Duodenal ulcer

A duodenal ulcer is an erosive lesion which occurs in the duodenum, the short length of small intestine that connects with the stomach. It is in this length that the gastric acids of the stomach are neutralized before the partially-digested food is carried to the rest of the intestine. The same conditions that can cause a gastric ulcer can contribute to an ulcer in the duodenum, and like a gastric ulcer, a duodenal ulcer is classified according as to severity or duration, and the complications that are present. An acute ulcer appears suddenly with severe symptoms, while a chronic ulcer may be less severe, but continue over a long period of time, for months or even years. Hemorrhage is an instance of bleeding, in this case due to the damage done to the intestinal wall by the ulcer. Perforation means that the ulcer has created a hole that allows gastric acid and food to leak into the surrounding abdominal cavity, which almost always results in serious infection and inflammation.

K27 Peptic ulcer, site unspecified

A peptic ulcer is one which appears in either the stomach and/or the duodenum (the section of small intestine immediately adjacent to the stomach). Peptic ulcers are classified according to severity or duration, and the complications that are present. An acute ulcer appears suddenly with severe symptoms, while a chronic ulcer may be less severe, but continue over a long period of time, for months or even years. Hemorrhage is an instance of bleeding, in this case due to the damage done to the stomach and/or intestinal wall by the ulcer. Perforation means that the ulcer has created a hole that allows gastric acid and food to leak into the surrounding abdominal cavity, which almost always results in serious infection and inflammation.

Note: Use the codes in this category only if the exact location of the ulcer is not otherwise specified. If the ulcer is known to be in the duodenum, a code from category K26 should be used, while one known to be in the stomach should be reported with category K25.

K28 Gastrojejunal ulcer

A gastrojejunal ulcer takes place in the small intestine below the level of the duodenum. These are far more rare than ulcers of the stomach or duodenum, but are classified similarly, according to severity or duration, and the complications that are present. An acute ulcer appears suddenly with severe symptoms, while a chronic ulcer may be less severe, but continue over a long period of time, for months or even years. Hemorrhage is an instance of bleeding, in this case due to the damage done to the intestinal wall by the ulcer. Perforation means that the ulcer has created a hole that allows gastric acid and food to leak into the surrounding abdominal cavity, which almost always results in serious infection and inflammation.

K29 Gastritis and duodenitis

Gastritis and duodenitis are inflammation of the stomach and duodenum of the small intestine, respectively, due to any of several causes. This inflammation most commonly presents with abdominal pain, nausea, indigestion, vomiting, which may or may not include blood, melena, loss of appetite and weight, and fatigue. The chances of getting an ulcer are increased by long-term stress, certain infections, smoking, taking certain medications (including aspirin), age, and severe injury.

K29.0 Acute gastritis

Acute gastritis is a severe, usually sudden, appearance of stomach inflammation and its attendant symptoms.

K29.2 Alcoholic gastritis

Inflammation of the stomach associated with the overuse of alcohol.

K29.4 Chronic atrophic gastritis

Chronic atrophic gastritis is a common condition in the elderly in which both the peptic gland, which produces gastric acid, and the protective membrane of the stomach waste away. As a result, there is insufficient acid to kill many types of bacteria, which in turn leads to an inflammation of the stomach and possibly the small intestine.

K29.8 Duodenitis

Duodenitis is an inflammation of the duodenum, the part of the small intestine immediately adjacent to the stomach.

K30 Functional dyspepsia

Dyspepsia is a chronic pain and/or uncomfortable feeling in the upper middle part of the stomach. It can come and go, but is usually there most of the time and may be accompanied by bloating, heartburn, nausea, vomiting, and excessive burping. It may be caused by an ulcer or acid reflux disease, in which case the underlying cause should be coded first, and in some cases may be a prelude to cancer of the stomach.

K31.0 Acute dilatation of stomach

Acute dilation of the stomach, sometimes called acute distension of the stomach, is a condition in which the stomach becomes bloated due to an excessive build-up of gas or a bowel obstruction preventing food from passing out of it. In the latter case, the patient may present with spells of vomiting every few days in which the food is seen to be fermented rather than digested.

K31.1 Adult hypertrophic pyloric stenosis

Acquired hypertrophic pyloric stenosis is a blockage of the sphincter muscle that separates the stomach from the small intestine due to an overgrowth in the size of the pyloric cells. This blockage can typically be felt through the skin over the stomach as an olive-shaped mass. Surgical intervention is usually required to remove it.

K31.2 Hourglass stricture and stenosis of stomach

An hourglass stricture or stenosis of the stomach indicates that an abnormal narrowing of the stomach has given it an hourglass-shape. This is sometimes referred to as "cascade stomach," and interferes with the stomach's ability to process food.

K31.3 Pylorospasm, not elsewhere classified

A pylorospasm is an uncontrolled muscle spasm of the pyloric sphincter, which separates the stomach from the duodenum. This causes pain and vomiting due to the resulting inability of the stomach to move food through to the intestine.

K31.4 Gastric diverticulum

A gastric diverticulum is an abnormal cul-de-sac, or outpouching, that forms in the side of the stomach, which can trap food diverted to it and ultimately become infected. This must be corrected surgically.

K31.81 Angiodysplasia of stomach and duodenum

Angiodysplasia of the stomach and duodenum is a condition in which the blood vessels around these parts of the digestive tract become dilated and fragile due to thinning of the vessel walls. This results in intermittent bleeding into the GI tract, and is usually due to wear-and-tear from age.

K31.82 Dieulafoy lesion (hemorrhagic) of stomach and duodenum

A Dieulafoy lesion is an abnormality in a small artery that supplies blood to the gastrointestinal tract, usually in the stomach or duodenum, which causes the artery to appear abnormally large and extruded (similar to a hemorrhoid). It rarely causes symptoms or requires treatment, but rarely may cause severe bleeding and require emergency surgical repair.

K31.83 Achlorhydria

Achlorhydria is a condition in which the stomach does not produce enough acid; specifically, the condition is defined as the pH of the stomach falling to less than 4.0, which in turn can lead to an inflammation of the stomach and possibly the small intestine.

K31.84 Gastroparesis

Gastroparesis results from a malfunction of the stomach's natural pacemaker, which serves pretty much the same function as the heart's pacemaker in that it controls the involuntary contractions of the stomach muscles, which in turn grind food down before it enters the small intestine. This condition occurs when the rate of the electrical waves from the pacemaker slows down, causing the stomach to contract less frequently. It usually presents with a feeling of fullness after only a few bites of food, bloating, excessive belching, and nausea, though abdominal ache, vomiting, and heartburn may also occur.

Note: The underlying disorder should be coded first, such as diabetes mellitus with neurological manifestations or anorexia nervosa.

K35 Acute appendicitis

The vermiform appendix, usually referred to as simply the appendix, is a small sac or blind-ended tube averaging 10 cm in length that connects to the cecum of the large intestine (which in turn is immediately below the junction with the small intestine). Its function is debated, but it is widely believed to be a vestigial organ that served a function in an earlier time in history. Removal of the appendix does not seem to present any problem to the patient. Acute appendicitis is a severe inflammation of the appendix, which may occur due to obstruction by fecal matter or a tumorous growth. Obstruction leads to infection, which causes the characteristic inflammation, and if not treated by removing the appendix, tissue death with dissemination of the infection to the rest of the body can threaten the life of the patient. Appendicitis presents with severe abdominal pain and tenderness, one or two episodes of vomiting, slight to moderate fever, an elevated white blood cell count, and constipation (or diarrhea in some cases). Acute appendicitis is classified by whether the inflammation includes the peritoneum, the thin membrane that lines the abdominal and pelvic cavities and which supports and protects the internal organs.

K35.3 Acute appendicitis with localized peritonitis

Appendicitis presents with severe abdominal pain and tenderness, one or two episodes of vomiting, slight to moderate fever, an elevated white blood cell count, and constipation (or diarrhea in some cases). Localized peritonitis includes an abscess, or area of inflamed tissue within one area of the peritoneum.

K36 Other appendicitis

Note: Other appendicitis includes chronic or recurrent cases.

K37 Unspecified appendicitis

Unspecified appendicitis is less severe than acute appendicitis, though it presents with much the same symptoms, and can often be treated with antibiotics rather than surgery.

K38.0 Hyperplasia of appendix

Hyperplasia is another common disorder of the appendix in which the constituent cells of the appendix divide too rapidly and continue to divide long after the appendix has reached its normal size. This causes an enlarged appendix, due to an increase in the number of component cells. In some cases, this may be indicative of cancer. Surgically removing the appendix is usually the preferred method of treatment.

K40 Inguinal hernia

A hernia is a condition in which a weakness in the muscle wall of the abdomen allows an organ, usually the intestine, to protrude through it. A hernia is usually harmless in and of itself, but presents the risk of cutting off the blood supply to the organ that is protruding, at which point it becomes a medical emergency. In many cases, the physician may choose surgery to treat a hernia in order to prevent this from happening. An inguinal hernia is one which pushes through a weak spot in the inguinal canal, a triangle-shaped opening in the muscles of the groin. It presents as a lump in the groin near the thigh, possibly with pain and, in severe cases, blockage in the intestine.

K40.0 **Bilateral inguinal hernia, with obstruction, without gangrene**

An inguinal hernia on both sides that presents with a bowel obstruction. Part of the bowel is completely pinched off where it extrudes through the herniated muscle wall, preventing material from passing through, but without mention of gangrene.

Note: This includes incarcerated, irreducible, and strangulated hernia.

K40.1 **Bilateral inguinal hernia, with gangrene**

An inguinal hernia on both sides that present with gangrene, a condition where part of the bowel develops dead and decaying tissue due to a loss of blood supply reaching that portion of intestine protruding through the herniated muscle wall. This condition is usually lethal unless the gangrenous tissue is surgically removed.

K40.3 **Unilateral inguinal hernia, with obstruction, without gangrene**

An inguinal hernia on one side only that presents with a bowel obstruction. Part of the bowel is completely pinched off where it extrudes through the herniated muscle wall, preventing material from passing through, but without mention of gangrene.

Note: This includes incarcerated, irreducible, and strangulated hernia.

K40.4 **Unilateral inguinal hernia, with gangrene**

An inguinal hernia on one side only that present with gangrene, a condition where part of the bowel develops dead and decaying tissue due to a loss of blood supply reaching that portion of intestine protruding through the herniated muscle wall. This condition is usually lethal unless the gangrenous tissue is surgically removed.

K44 **Diaphragmatic hernia**

A diaphragmatic hernia is a muscle weakness which does not appear in the outer abdominal wall, but appears in the diaphragm, the powerful muscle that enables breathing. These are most commonly congenital conditions (coded elsewhere), and are not usually immediately apparent on a standard exam. The acquired type reported here iclude hiatal hernia, esophageal sliding hernia, or paraesophageal hernia.

K50 **Crohn's disease [regional enteritis]**

Regional enteritis, also called granulomatous enteritis or, more commonly, Crohn's disease, is a chronic inflammation of the intestinal tract that occurs due to a malfunction of the body's immune system, which causes it to attack its own healthy cells. This inflammation is most common at the junction of the small and large intestines, but is not limited to that area. As a result of the inflammation, the intestinal wall becomes thick, interfering with normal digestion, and may form deep ulcers. Crohn's disease may also present with one or more of the following: a skin rash; abnormal connections between the intestines and other organs or the skin (fistulas); inflammation of the liver, joints, gums, and/or eyes; kidney stones; and blood-clotting disorders. It commonly presents with abdominal pain, fever, diarrhea or constipation, a loss of appetite and corresponding weight loss, a tumor-like abdominal mass, fatigue, bleeding into the intestinal tract as ulcers form, bloating and flatulence, unusually foul-smelling and/or bloody stool, and pain when passing the stool. The patient may also suffer from nutritional deficiencies due to inadequate digestion of food.

K51 **Ulcerative colitis**

Ulcerative colitis is a chronic inflammation of the large intestine, including the rectum, which causes erosive lesions to form in the lining. This inflammation causes the colon to empty frequently from diarrhea. The condition is usually intermittent with exacerbation of symptoms (diarrhea with/without blood and/or mucus) and then extended periods without symptoms. Other symptoms include fatigue, loss of appetite, weight loss, rectal bleeding, dehydration and malnutrition due to the loss of body fluids and nutrients, fever, nausea, and severe abdominal cramps. In some cases, the patient may also experience inflammation in other areas of the body, such as the eyes or joints, as well as skin rashes and anemia.

K51.0 **Ulcerative (chronic) pancolitis**

Universal ulcerative colitis, also called pancolitis, is an ongoing inflammation affecting the entire large intestine and causing sores anywhere in the lining.

K51.2 **Ulcerative (chronic) proctitis**

Ulcerative chronic proctitis is an ongoing inflammation of the mucous membrane of the rectum, causing open, erosive sores to form in the lining.

K51.3 **Ulcerative (chronic) rectosigmoiditis**

Chronic ulcerative proctosigmoiditis, or rectosigmoiditis, is an ongoing inflammation of the mucous membrane of the rectum and sigmoid colon, the S-shaped intestinal portion between the descending colon and the rectum, that causes erosive sores to form in the lining.

K51.5 **Left sided colitis**

Left sided colitis is an inflammation that affects the entire left-hand side of the colon, including the rectum, the sigmoid colon, and the descending colon.

K52.0 **Gastroenteritis and colitis due to radiation**

An inflammation of the stomach and intestines in general or the large bowel in particular due to radiation--either accidental exposure, or radiation therapy in the treatment of cancer.

K52.1 **Toxic gastroenteritis and colitis**

An inflammation of the stomach and intestines in general or the large bowel in particular due to exposure to a toxic substance or poison.

K52.81 **Eosinophilic gastritis or gastroenteritis**

Eosinophilic gastritis or gastroenteritis is an extremely rare disorder associated with selective eosinophilic infiltration of layers of the stomach and/or small intestine with increased immunoglobulin E, and the exclusion of eosinophils involved in any other organ outside the GI tract. Eosinophilic involvement in the GI tract may be mucosal, muscularis, or serosal. The clinical symptoms are determined by the location of the infiltrates. Mucosal type presents with abdominal pain, diarrhea, vomiting, blood loss, and malabsorption. The muscularis type presents with symptoms of obstruction and pyloric stenosis. The serosal type presents with eosinophilic ascites. The cause of the eosinophilia remains unknown, although about half of patients have a history of asthma, hay fever, or food allergies.

K52.82 **Eosinophilic colitis**

An extremely rare disorder associated with selective eosinophilic infiltration of layers of the colon with increased immunoglobulin E and the exclusion of eosinophils involved in any other organ outside the GI tract. Eosinophilic involvement in the GI tract may be mucosal, muscularis, or serosal. The clinical symptoms are determined by the location of the infiltrates. Mucosal type presents with abdominal pain, diarrhea, vomiting, blood loss, and malabsorption. The muscularis type presents with symptoms of obstruction and pyloric stenosis. The serosal type presents with eosinophilic ascites. The cause of the eosinophilia remains unknown, although about half of patients have a history of asthma, hay fever, or food allergies.

K55.0 **Acute vascular disorders of intestine**

Acute vascular insufficiency of the intestine is caused when damage occurs to one or more major vessels, partially or completely cutting off the blood flow from part or all of the intestine. This can very rapidly cause tissue death and gangrene, requiring surgical removal of the dead tissue.

K55.1 **Chronic vascular disorders of intestine**

Chronic vascular insufficiency of the intestine is usually the result of aging and/or degeneration of the blood vessels feeding the intestines. It presents with a decline in the nutrients absorbed by the intestines, abdominal pain, and diarrhea or constipation.

K55.20 **Angiodysplasia of colon without hemorrhage**

Angiodysplasia of the colon is a condition in which the blood vessels that supply the colon and carry away nutrients become dilated, with a corresponding thinning and weakening of the vessel walls, which can cause occasional bleeding into the intestinal tract. Use this code if there is no mention of bleeding.

K55.21 Angiodysplasia of colon with hemorrhage

Angiodysplasia of the colon is a condition in which the blood vessels that supply the colon and carry away nutrients become dilated, with a corresponding thinning and weakening of the vessel walls, which can cause occasional bleeding into the intestinal tract. Use this code if there is bleeding.

K56.0 Paralytic ileus

Paralytic ileus is a blockage of the connection between the small and large intestine due to the intestine's muscle wall not working properly to move food through. This may occur due to a fluid imbalance, damage to the nerves, a loss of blood supply, or to a toxin.

K56.1 Intussusception

Intussusception is a condition in which a section of the small intestine prolapses into an adjoining section and folds into it as one section of a telescope folds into a larger section. It is most often seen in children from three months to six years of age, and causes a blockage which in turn presents with swelling, inflammation, intermittent pain, vomiting, shallow breathing as the gastrointestinal tract pushes up on the diaphragm, a rapid heartbeat, and lethargy. It may be treated with an air enema or surgically.

K56.2 Volvulus

Volvulus is a condition in which the intestine becomes twisted, constricting the passageway and preventing food from moving through it normally. This presents with sudden, severe abdominal pain, vomiting, and abdominal distention. Blockage also causes dehydration and a loss of blood supply to the affected area, eventually causing tissue death if not corrected.

K56.3 Gallstone ileus

Impaction caused by a gallstone which has passed into the intestinal tract.

K56.41 Fecal impaction

Fecal impaction is a development of chronic constipation and decreased colon motility causing dry, hard stools to become a large, solid mass in the rectum that cannot be expelled. There may be paradoxical fecal incontinence as watery stool from higher in the bowel passes around the obstruction as diarrhea. Bedridden patients and those with severe nervous system disorders, or those taking medications such as anticholinergics, narcotics, and antidiarrheals are at risk. Treatment involves removing the impacted stool and taking preventive measures against constipations and future impactions.

K56.5 Intestinal adhesions [bands] with obstruction (postprocedural) (postinfection)

Intestinal adhesions are abnormal, fibrous, scar-like bands of tissue that form around the intestine, binding sections together or joining the intestine to the abdominal wall. The adhesive bands result from abnormal healing after surgery or infection and can constrict the intestines enough to cause a blockage or obstruction.

K57 Diverticular disease of intestine

Diverticular disease is a condition occurring when an outpouching or sac, called a diverticulum (plural: diverticula), forms in the wall of the intestines. Most people with a diverticulum in the intestinal tract do not experience any symptoms, though mild cramps, bloating, and constipation can occur. The condition of having one or more diverticula is called diverticulosis. Bleeding from a diverticulum is a rare but known complication which results from a small blood vessel within the diverticulum weakening and breaking open. It presents with blood in the stool and usually resolves itself without treatment. Diverticulitis is an inflammation of a diverticulum, which can present with abdominal pain and tenderness In the region of the diverticulum. In cases where the inflammation is due to infection, fever, nausea and vomiting, cramping, and constipation may also occur. Diverticular disease is coded by location and whether it is occurring with or without perforation or abscess, and with or without bleeding.

K58 Irritable bowel syndrome

Irritable bowel syndrome, a functional disorder rather than a disease, results from hypersensitive nerves and muscles in the large intestine, which in turn cause cramping, pain, gas and bloating, diarrhea, and/or constipation, which often alternate. This syndrome, while uncomfortable, does not cause any damage to the intestinal tract. There is no cure, but medication, dietary changes, and relief from stress may reduce the symptoms. Onset is usually before age 35, with women affected more often than men and often a positive family history of the condition.

K59.0 Constipation

Constipation is a condition in which the stool moves more slowly through the bowel (i.e., the large intestine, or colon) than it should, resulting in infrequent bowel movements and hard, dry stool (due to more moisture being absorbed from the stool the longer it is in the bowel).

K59.01 Slow transit constipation

Slow transit constipation is a dysfunction of the smooth muscles that surround the intestine and push matter through, causing the movement of stool to slow down significantly or stall.

K59.02 Outlet dysfunction constipation

Outlet dysfunction constipation occurs when the pelvic muscles contract at the time that the rectal sphincter muscle opens to enable stool to leave the bowel, causing the bowel movement to be slow and difficult.

K59.1 Functional diarrhea

Functional diarrhea indicates that the cause of the patient's diarrhea is not due to an infection or other organic cause, but rather to dysfunction of the digestive tract.

K59.2 Neurogenic bowel, not elsewhere classified

Neurogenic bowel is a dysfunction of the large intestine due to damage to the spinal cord. It presents with many of the same symptoms as irritable bowel syndrome and is often misdiagnosed as the latter.

K59.3 Megacolon, not elsewhere classified

Megacolon is a condition in which the large intestine becomes extremely distended and stretched so that it is much larger than usual. This may be an acute, sudden and severe condition due to infection, or a chronic condition due to abnormal growth.

Note: Congenital megacolon and that due to exposure to toxins is classified by separate codes.

K59.4 Anal spasm

An anal spasm indicates that the rectal sphincter muscle, which controls defecation, will not open properly. This is often due to a wound in the skin over the muscle (an anal fissure), which can cause pain which causes the muscles in the area around it to reflexively contract.

K60.0 Acute anal fissure

An acute anal fissure is a small tear or break in the skin lining the anus. It presents with pain during defecation along with red blood streaking the stool, and is usually caused by passing unusually hard, dry stool. In some cases, it may interfere with normal bowel movements and in 10% of cases, requires surgical closure to heal properly.

Note: Nontraumatic, healed, or old anal sphincter tear is coded to K62.81.

K60.3 Anal fistula

Anal fistula is an abnormal, inflammatory connection between the anal canal and the skin surrounding the anal opening. Fistulas usually originate in the anal glands located between the layers of the anal sphincter muscles and are frequently a complication of an anal abscess. Symptoms include pain, itching and (purulent) drainage.

K60.4 Rectal fistula

A rectal fistula is an abnormal, inflammatory connection between the rectum and the surrounding skin surface and are frequently a complication of a rectal abscess. Symptoms include pain, itching and (purulent) drainage.

K61   Abscess of anal and rectal regions

An abscess is a pocket of infected material surrounded by inflamed tissue. When an abscess forms in the anal or rectal regions, it presents with tenderness, swelling, and pain which clear up when the abscess is drained. The patient may also experience fever, chills, and fatigue.

K61.0   Anal abscess

An anal abscess is a pocket of infection collected near the anal opening or inside the anus. The condition usually occurs in the presence of an anal fissure or as a result of a blocked anal gland. Symptoms can include pain, swelling, and (purulent) drainage from the anal area. Fistula development is common following anorectal abscess.

K62.0   Anal polyp

An anal polyp is a common type of stalk-like tissue growth arising from the wall of the anus and can be benign or become cancerous. There may be a hereditary predisposition to the development of polyps and polyps also occur more frequently in the presence of inflammatory bowel disease. The condition is largely asymptomatic but bleeding, crampy abdominal pain, diarrhea, and even intestinal obstruction may occur with large polyps.

K62.1   Rectal polyp

A rectal polyp is a common type of stalk-like tissue growth arising from the wall of the rectum and can be benign or become cancerous. There may be a hereditary predisposition to development of polyps and polyps also occur more frequently in the presence of inflammatory bowel disease. The condition is largely asymptomatic but bleeding, crampy abdominal pain, diarrhea, and even intestinal obstruction may occur with large polyps.

K62.2   Anal prolapse

Anal prolapse is a condition in which the anus turns itself inside out by sagging and dropping from its normal anatomical position, protruding through the anal opening in later stages. It is usually associated with weakness in the anal sphincter muscle in the latter stage, which may result in leakage of stool and/or mucus. The condition is found most often in older adults with a history of chronic constipation and/or diarrhea. It occurs more commonly in women where weakness of the pelvic floor muscles or nerve damage from pregnancy or vaginal delivery may be causative factors. Symptoms include pain, rectal bleeding, and fecal incontinence. This condition often requires surgery to correct.

K62.3   Rectal prolapse

Rectal prolapse is a condition in which the rectum turns itself inside out by sagging and dropping from its normal anatomincal position into the anal canal and may even protrude through the anal opening in later stages. It is usually associated with weakness in the anal sphincter muscle in the latter stage, which may result in leakage of stool and/or mucus. The condition is found most often in older adults with a history of chronic constipation and/or diarrhea. It occurs more commonly in women where weakness of the pelvic floor muscles or nerve damage from pregnancy or vaginal delivery may be causative factors. Symptoms include pain, rectal bleeding, and fecal incontinence. This condition often requires surgery to correct.

K62.4   Stenosis of anus and rectum

Stenosis of the rectum and anus indicates that either an abnormal narrowing of the rectum has given it an hourglass-shape, or that the anus has become constricted. In either case, difficulty in passing stool is the primary symptom, which leads to pain and bloating in the abdomen. The condition may be acquired following trauma, surgical procedures (such as hemorrhoidectomy), cancerous tumors, radiation therapy, or inflammatory bowel disease (Crohn's disease). Symptoms can include thin (narrow) appearing feces, feeling of resistance or pain with defecation (bowel movement). This is usually treated by gently dilating the affected organ twice per day until the condition is corrected, though surgical intervention is sometimes required.

K62.6   Ulcer of anus and rectum

An ulcer of the anus and rectum is an open, erosive lesion within the lining of the rectum and/or anus. This may present with general pain which becomes worse during defecation as well as blood and/or mucus in the stool.

K62.7   Radiation proctitis

Radiation proctitis is inflammation and tissue damage of the lower colon following exposure to x-ray or ionizing radition to treat certain cancers, such as cervical, prostate, and colon cancer. The condition may be acute, occurring during or closely following radiation therapy, and involve direct damage to the epithelial lining of the intestine. Symptoms include diarrhea, defecation urgency, and the inability to defecate (tenesmus). The condition may also be chronic, occuring months or years following radiation therapy with damage to the blood vessels of the colon. In chronic cases, the symptoms include diarrhea, rectal bleeding, pain with defecation, and intestinal obstruction.

K62.81   Anal sphincter tear (healed) (nontraumatic) (old)

Anal sphincter tears usually occur in pregnancy during delivery and can occur independently of perineal lacerations. The anal tear may not be diagnosed until later when an old tear in a nongravid patient causes fecal incontinence or other complications, especially when not quite healed.

K62.82   Dysplasia of anus

Dysplasia is the growth of abnormal cell structure that is not dangerous in itself, but is considered a potential precursor to cancer. Also known as anal intraepithelial neoplasia, both levels I and II (mild and moderate dysplasia) are coded here when histologically confirmed, as diagnosed by cytological smear. Once the dysplasia has become severe, it is considered a carcinoma in situ.

Note: Severe dysplasia of the anus, also known as intraepithelial neoplasia III, is considered carcinoma in situ and is reported within the neoplasm chapter.

K63.0   Abscess of intestine

An abscess is a pocket of infected material (pus) surrounded by inflamed tissue. An abscess of the intestine presents with pain and tenderness in the affected area, and may also present with fever, fatigue, nausea and vomiting. An abscess must usually be treated by a combination of antibiotics and surgical draining to heal.

K63.1   Perforation of intestine (nontraumatic)

Perforation of the intestine indicates that a hole in the intestinal wall is allowing food and/or fecal matter to leak into the abdominal cavity. This can cause life-threatening infection. A perforation is usually due to trauma, though in some cases, can be caused by an untreated abscess, ulcer, or fistula, and requires emergency surgical closure.

K63.2   Fistula of intestine

An intestinal fistula is an abnormal passage between the intestine and another organ in the body such as the bladder, urethra, or vagina; between two separate loops of intestine; or between the intestine and the abdominal wall, often in response to infection and inflammation. There may be drainage from the fistua due to ongoing inflammation, which can irritate the openings. Surgical drainage and closure is usually required.

K63.3   Ulcer of intestine

An ulcer of the intestine is an open, erosive lesion within the lining of the intestines that may present with a general, burning pain in the abdomen that may increase shortly after a meal, as well as blood and/or mucus in the stool.

K63.81   Dieulafoy lesion of intestine

A Dieulafoy lesion of the intestine is an abnormality in one of the small arteries that supplies blood to the intestine. It normally doesn't present any symptoms or difficulties and doesn't need treatment, but in some cases, it can cause severe bleeding into the intestine if the artery should burst. In these cases, emergency endoscopic surgery may be needed to stop the bleeding.

Diseases of the Digestive System

K61 – K63.81

K64 Hemorrhoids and perianal venous thrombosis

Hemorrhoids are clumps of dilated, swollen veins in the anus which are painful and itchy. They may appear inside or outside of the body, and may bleed slightly.

K65 Peritonitis

Peritonitis is an inflammation of the peritoneum, a membrane which lines the walls of the abdomen and protects and supports the abdominal organs. It presents with abdominal pain and swelling, fever, decreased urination and constipation, nausea and vomiting, tenderness and swelling in the joints, and excessive thirst.

K66.0 Peritoneal adhesions (postprocedural) (postinfection)

Peritoneal adhesions are fibrous, scar-like bands of tissue that join organs whjch are normally separated together, or bind organs to the abdominal wall. This may present with no symptoms at all, or may cause pain and abnormal functioning of the affected tissues. This condition is usually the result of abnormal healing after abdominal surgery or serious infection.

K66.1 Hemoperitoneum

Hemoperitoneum is a condition in which there is bleeding into the peritoneal cavity, whether due to trauma (injury) or another disorder.

K70.0 Alcoholic fatty liver

Alcoholic fatty liver is the accumulation of fats and fatty acids in the liver caused by excessive alcohol consumption. This sometimes presents with no symptoms, but more often presents as an enlarged liver, sometimes accompanied by nausea and vomiting and pain at the site of the liver. The liver usually recovers provided that the patient abstains from alcohol, but left untreated, this disorder can result in permanent damage.

K70.1 Alcoholic hepatitis

Alcoholic hepatitis is a severe inflammation of the liver caused by excessive alcohol consumption. It presents with fever, swelling of the liver, an increased white blood cell count, impairment of the normal liver function (e.g., insufficient bile being produced), and high blood pressure in the portal vein, which supplies the liver with blood. The inflammation may be controlled and/or eliminated by abstention from alcohol combined with nutritional therapy.

K70.2 Alcoholic fibrosis and sclerosis of liver

An intermediate stage liver disease in which normal, healthy tissue in the liver is replaced by scar tissue due to long-term, excessive alcohol consumption.

K70.3 Alcoholic cirrhosis of liver

Alcoholic cirrhosis of the liver is a late-stage disease condition in which the normal, healthy tissue of the liver is replaced by scar tissue due to long-term excessive alcohol consumption (as little as two to three drinks a day for women, or three to four drinks a day for men). The scar tissue prevents the proper flow of blood as well as decreases the liver's ability to perform its function. Cirrhosis presents with fatigue and weakness, loss of appetite and a corresponding weight loss, nausea, abdominal pain, and the appearance of spider-like blood vessels on the surface of the skin. This liver damage cannot be reversed, but treatment can slow or halt further growth of scar tissue. Treatment varies depending on the extent of the damage and other factors, but abstaining from alcohol is required.

K71 Toxic liver disease

The liver plays a key role in concentrating and metabolizing ingested nutrients and chemicals. Many substances can cause damage to the liver in both theraputic doses and with overdose. Damage may be widespread but is more commonly confined to a zone or lobe of the liver. Biochemical markers for liver damage include elevated aspartate aminotransferase (AST), alanlne transferase (ALT), alkaline phosphatase (ALP), and bilirubin. The condition may be asymptomatic but common symptoms include jaundice (yellow discoloration of eyes and skin), anorexia (loss of appetite), fatigue, and fever.

K72.91 Hepatic failure, unspecified with coma

Hepatic encephalopathy is hepatic failure that results in a brain disorder and coma caused by chronic liver failure. Some subtle signs of hepatic encephalopathy are seen in nearly 70% of all cirrhosis patients. Signs may also manifest in patients with spontaneous or surgically created portosystemic shunts. A variety of neuropsychiatric abnormalities occurs, including personality changes, intellectual impairment, and a depressed level of consciousness, explained by the build up of neurotoxins that are no longer being cleaned out of the system. Toxins are no longer being removed from the bloodstream because liver function is impaired. Toxins may also bypass the liver altogether by other connections formed between the portal and the systemic venous systems. Toxins then reach the brain. This syndrome is also the hallmark of fulminant hepatic failure, usually accompanied by dangerous brain swelling and edema, rarely reported in cirrhosis cases. Hepatic coma is a condition caused by severe liver dysfunction that results in complete unresponsiveness on the part of the patient and marks the prelude of mortality.

K73 Chronic hepatitis, not elsewhere classified

Chronic hepatitis is an inflammation of the liver that lasts for at least six months, and which can last for years or even decades. It ia characterized by hepatocellular necrosis with infiltration of inflammatory cells. Biochemical markers for liver damage include elevated aspartate aminotranserase (AST), alanine transferase (ALT), alkaline phosphatase (ALP), and bilirubin. The condition may be asymptomatic but common symptoms include jaundice (yellow discoloration of eyes and skin), loss of appetite, and fatigue. Other signs include swelling of the liver, an increased white blood cell count, impairment of the normal liver function (e.g., insufficient bile being produced), and high blood pressure in the portal vein, which supplies the liver with blood.

K73.0 Chronic persistent hepatitis, not elsewhere classified

Chronic persistent hepatitis is generally more mild than other forms of chronic hepatitis, but more resistant to treatment.

K74 Fibrosis and cirrhosis of liver

Liver fibrosis is a histological change in liver cells caused by liver inflammation. This change is characterized by an increase in collagen fiber deposits in the extra-cellular spaces of the liver causing a decrease in blood perfusion and hardening of the liver cells. Liver cirrhosis arises from liver fibrosis and is characterized by pseudo-lobule formation with changes to the livers fundamental structure and subsequent framework collapse. Biochemical markers for fibrostic activity include hyaluronic acid (HA), laminin (LA), collagen IV (CIV) and procollagen type III (PCIII).

K74.3 Primary biliary cirrhosis

Biliary cirrhosis causes scar tissue to form around and on the biliary ducts, which carry bile from the liver to the small intestine. This results in bile building up in the liver and damaging it, often causing cirrhosis to develop in the rest of the liver as well. It most often presents with itchy skin and fatigue, but may also present with yellowing of the skin and eyes (jaundice), cholesterol deposits on the skin, fluid retention, dry eyes or mouth, osteoporosis, arthritis, and thyroid problems.

K74.60 Unspecified cirrhosis of liver

Cirrhosis of the liver that is not otherwise specified in which there is no mention of alcohol use is a condition in which the normal, healthy tissue of the liver is replaced by scar tissue. The scar tissue prevents the proper flow of blood as well as decreases the liver's ability to perform its function. Cirrhosis presents with fatigue and weakness, loss of appetite and a corresponding weight loss, nausea, abdominal pain, and the appearance of spider-like blood vessels on the surface of the skin. This liver damage cannot be reversed, but treatment can slow or halt further growth of scar tissue. Treatment varies depending on the extent of the damage and other factors.

K75.0 Abscess of liver

An abscess is a pocket of infected material surrounded by inflamed tissue. An abscess of the liver presents with fever, fatigue, nausea, abdominal pain and tenderness in the area of the liver, loss of appetite and weight loss. An abscess is usually treated by antibiotics and surgical draining.

K75.1 Phlebitis of portal vein

Portal pyemia is a severe infection and inflammation of the portal veins which supply the liver with blood. It presents with the usual signs of septicemia (blood poisoning), such as fever and chills, jaundice (yellowed skin and eyes), sweating, and abscesses that appear in other parts of the body as the infection spreads.

K75.4 Autoimmune hepatitis

Autoimmune hepatitis is marked by continuous inflammation and necrosis of liver cells that progress to cirrhosis, often in association with other autoimmune diseases. The resulting necrosis and cirrhosis is not caused by a chronic viral infection, alcohol consumption, or previous toxic exposure to chemicals. Immune markers are found in blood serum.

K76.1 Chronic passive congestion of liver

Chronic passive congestion of the liver indicates that blood is not flowing out of the liver properly, causing it to accumulate and pool within the organ. This is usually a symptom of another disorder, such as cirrhosis.

K76.3 Infarction of liver

An hepatic infarction is a condition in which the liver is not receiving an adequate blood supply due to inflammation compressing the vessels.

K76.6 Portal hypertension

Portal hypertension indicates abnormally high blood pressure in the portal vein, which supplies blood to the liver, usually as a result of blockage in the vein or degeneration (such as cirrhosis) in the liver.

K76.7 Hepatorenal syndrome

Hepatorenal syndrome is a condition in which a person with a liver disorder also experiences a decrease in kidney function or kidney failure due to a drastic reduction in blood flow to the kidneys. The exact reason for the loss of kidney function is unknown. The symptoms include decreased urine production, a dark-colored urine, yellow (jaundiced) skin, weight gain and abdominal swelling, a change of mental status such as confusion or delirium, jerking muscle movements, and nausea and vomiting.

K76.81 Hepatopulmonary syndrome

Hepatopulmonary syndrome is a complication of chronic liver disease, especially cirrhosis, but it also occurs with acute ischemic hepatitis and non-cirrhotic portal hypertension. It affects both pediatric and adult patients and occurs when the liver disease has progressed far enough to begin affecting the lungs, resulting in pulmonary vasodilation, dyspnea, and hypoxemia. One of the liver's functions is to help regulate the tone of the blood vessels within the lungs, which become abnormal in size and number and are seen on echocardiogram with contrast or a nuclear medicine lung scan. The only effective treatment is liver transplantation.

K80 Cholelithiasis

Cholelithiasis is more commonly known simply as gallstones. The gallbladder, in which the stones can form, is a small, pear-shaped organ on the underside of the liver that is used to store excess bile until it is needed. Gallstones, which may also be called a calculus (stone) of the gallbladder, present with sporatic pain in the abdomen, which may appear to move to other parts of the body, such as the right shoulder or between the shoulder blades. This pain may be accompanied by nausea and vomiting, and may be triggered by eating fatty foods.

K81 Cholecystitis

Cholecystitis is inflammation and/or infection of the gallbladder. The condition may be acute or chronic and often involves the presence of stones or calculi (cholelithiasis). Biochemical markers include elevated white blood cell count (WBCs) and C-reactive protein (CRP), elevated aspartate aminotransferase (AST), alanine transferase (ALT), alkaline phosphatase

(ALP), and bilirubin. Symptoms of acute cholecystitis include nausea and vomiting, diarrhea, right upper quadrant (RUQ) pain and/or right scapular pain (Boas' sign). The symptoms of chronic cholecystitis may include nausea, vague abdominal pain, belching, gas, and diarrhea.

K81.0 Acute cholecystitis

Acute cholecystitis is a severe inflammation of the gallbladder, which presents with pain in the abdomen similar to that of having gallstones. This code includes specific forms of inflammation such as having an abscess or a pocket of infected material surrounded by inflamed tissue.

K81.1 Chronic cholecystitis

Chronic inflammation of the gallbladder persists for a period of several months or longer and is resistant to normal treatment.

K81.2 Acute cholecystitis with chronic cholecystitis

Acute cholecystitis with chronic cholecystitis is a long term, ongoing inflammation of the gallbladder that flares up suddenly and becomes more severe than usual.

K82.1 Hydrops of gallbladder

Hydrops of the gallbladder is a condition in which the gallbladder becomes overfull and extended due to an accumulation of mucous and other watery material rather than due to the development of stones. It generally presents with minimal signs of inflammation, such as pain in the region, fever, and fatigue. The gallbladder can usually be felt through the skin to be enlarged and tender.

K82.2 Perforation of gallbladder

A perforation of the gallbladder indicates that the wall of the sac has been broken, either by trauma or due to another condition such as gallstones. As a result, infected bile can spread to the abdominal cavity, threatening the patient's life. This condition is usually treated by emergency surgery to remove the damaged gallbladder.

K82.3 Fistula of gallbladder

A fistula of the gallbladder is an abnormal connection between the gallbladder and another organ, often as a result of an abscess or other concentrated infection. The fistula can carry bile to an area where it doesn't belong, damaging other organs as well as become infected itself, and must usually be surgically closed.

K82.4 Cholesterolosis of gallbladder

Cholesterolosis of the gallbladder is a condition in which cholesterol deposits build up on the surface of the gallbladder, giving it a "strawberry" appearance.

K83 Other diseases of biliary tract

The biliary tract connects the liver to the gallbladder and both of those organs to the small intestine, transporting bile, a substance critical for the digestion of fats.

K83.0 Cholangitis

Cholangitis is an infection of the biliary tract, which presents with pain in the upper-right abdomen and may grow worse after a fatty meal. The general indications are signs of infection (fever, nausea, vomiting, etc.), flatulence and a pale-colored stool, jaundice (yellowing of the eyes and skin), and itchiness. It is usually treated with antibiotics and anti-inflammatory medications.

K83.2 Perforation of bile duct

A perforation, or hole, in the bile duct will allow bile to enter the abdominal cavity, causing damage to the organs and possible infection, and must be closed surgically.

K83.3 Fistula of bile duct

A fistula of the bile duct is an abnormal connection between the bile duct and another organ. In addition to delivering bile to the wrong location, the fistula is prone to infection and must usually be closed surgically.

Diseases of the Digestive System

K83.4 – K92.0

K83.4 Spasm of sphincter of Oddi

The sphincter of Oddi is the muscular valve that surrounds the exit of the bile duct into the duodenum of the small intestine, a junction called the papilla of Vater. A spasm of this sphincter will prevent bile from properly flowing into the digestive tract, causing it to back up in the gallbladder and liver (and possibly casing damage to one or both of those organs as well as causing jaundice), and preventing bile from entering the small intestine, which in turn causes fats to be improperly digested.

K85 Acute pancreatitis

The pancreas is an elongated organ that rests behind the stomach and attaches to the duodenum of the small intestine via the pancreatic duct, which runs the length of the pancreas and accesses the intestine via the ampulla of Vater. The pancreas produces pancreatic juice, which contains several crucial enzymes for digesting food, as well as producing several important hormones, such as insulin and glucagon that regulate blood glucose levels. Inflammation of the pancreas usually occurs when the enzymes it produces activate while still in the organ and begin to digest pancreatic tissue. The most common cause of acute pancreatitis is biliary gallstones, but the cause may be unknown (idiopathic), or related to use of drugs or medicaments, alcohol, or autoimmune disorders. Biochemical markers include elevated amylase or lipase levels. Symptoms of acute pancreatitis include pain in the abdomen often radiating to the back, nausea, and vomiting. In severe cases, acute pancreatitis can result in bleeding and tissue damage to the pancreas as well as to the heart, lungs, kidneys, and/or the other organs as enzymes enter the bloodstream.

K86.1 Other chronic pancreatitis

The pancreas is an elongated organ that rests behind the stomach and attaches to the duodenum of the small intestine via the pancreatic duct, which runs the length of the pancreas and accesses the intestine via the ampulla of Vater. The pancreas produces pancreatic juice, which contains several crucial enzymes for digesting food, as well as producing several important hormones, such as insulin and glucagon that regulate blood glucose levels. Chronic inflammation of the pancreas does not resolve itself quickly, possibly lasting months or years, and results in the slow destruction of the pancreas.

K86.3 Pseudocyst of pancreas

A pseudocyst is similar to a cyst, but lacks the membranous lining that characterizes a normal cyst.

K90 Intestinal malabsorption

Intestinal malabsorption is a disease or condition which prevents nutrients from being properly absorbed through the intestinal wall into the bloodstream.

K90.0 Celiac disease

Celiac disease is a chronic autoimmune disorder in which the body's immune system mistakenly attacks its own healthy tissues. It causes damage to the inner surface of the small intestine in response to the ingestion of gluten, a type of starch common to wheat. Celiac disease presents with weight loss, constipation or diarrhea, deficiencies in vitamins B, D, and K, abdominal pain, bloating and gas, fatigue, and anemia.

K90.1 Tropical sprue

Tropical sprue is a malabsorption disorder common in the tropics and subtropics which may be related to an infectious organism. It primarily presents with diarrhea, but may also present with indigestion, gas, abdominal and/or muscle cramps, weight loss, paleness of the skin, irritability, and numbness. It is usually treated with antibiotics.

K90.2 Blind loop syndrome, not elsewhere classified

Blind loop syndrome is a disorder in which part of the intestine becomes blocked so that food can no longer move through it freely, though it may do so slowly. This results in a buildup of bacteria, which in turn causes nutrients not to be properly absorbed by the intestinal wall. This disorder is most commonly caused by a reaction of the body after abdominal surgery.

K90.3 Pancreatic steatorrhea

Pancreatic steatorrhea is a condition in which insufficient enzymatic pancreas secretions flow into the intestine during digestion causing severe malabsorption and nutrient deficiencies with loose stools containing unabsorbed fat as a result.

K90.81 Whipple's disease

Whipple's disease, also called intestinal lipodystrophy, is an infection of the intestinal tract by the *Tropheryma whippelii* bacteria. It interferes with the body's ability to absorb certain nutrients, particularly carbohydrates and fats. It can also create a resistance to insulin and a depression of the immune system. It is easily treated with antibiotics, but is usually fatal if no treatment is given. Symptoms of Whipple's disease include diarrhea, abdominal bloating and cramps, intestinal bleeding, loss of appetite and weight loss, muscle weakness, and fatigue. Arthritis and fever often occur several years before the intestinal symptoms develop. Because these symptoms are non-specific, a biopsy of tissue from the small intestine is needed to make the final diagnosis.

K91.1 Postgastric surgery syndromes

Postgastric surgery syndrome, more commonly known as dumping syndrome or jejunal syndrome, is a condition in which the lower end of the small intestine fills too quickly with undigested food from the stomach, which is called dumping, usually shortly after stomach surgery. Dumping that begins right after a meal, or "early" dumping, presents with nausea and vomiting, bloating, diarrhea, and shortness of breath. Dumping which occurs one to three hours later, called "late" dumping, typically presents with weakness, excessive sweating, and dizziness. The patient may suffer from one or both.

K91.5 Postcholecystectomy syndrome

Postcholecystectomy syndrome describes the presence of symptoms following removal of the gallbladder. These symptoms may include nausea, vomiting, gas, bloating, diarrhea, and/or a persistent pain in the upper-right part of the abdomen. These symptoms usually fade over time on their own.

K91.850 Pouchitis

Pouchitis is an inflammation of a surgically created internal ileoanal pouch following removal of part of the colon. The colectomy may be done to treat ulcerative colitis or familial adenomatous polyposis. The creation of the pouch is a restorative proctocolectomy with anastomosis of the ileal pouch to the anus, in order to allow the patient to preserve continence. The ileoanal pouch prevents the patient from needing a permanent ileostomy. Common complications of the pouch creation include diarrhea, which is sometimes bloody, with urgency and fecal incontinence. Fever, loss of appetite, abdominal pain, and general fatigue and malaise are also present. The pouchitis can be treated successfully with antibiotics, although relapses are common. The direct cause of the pouchitis is not understood.

K91.86 Retained cholelithiasis following cholecystectomy

The spilling of gallstones during a laparoscopic cholecystectomy occurs when the stones, or fragments of stones, fall inadvertently into the peritoneum, ducts, or abdomen. This is nearly considered a common occurrence and the consequences of retained gallstones can be severe. In the pelvis, gallstones or stone fragments can cause gynecologic pathology such as adhesive pelvic disease, dysmenorrhea, and infertility. In the abdomen, complications include intraabdominal and port site abscess formation, sinus tract formation that may persist, inflammatory masses, and pain. Stones that fall into the bile duct cause blockages, infection, and pain. Symptoms of retained gallstones after surgery may not even present until about 27 weeks later, which is the average time.

K92.0 Hematemesis

Hematemesis is vomiting blood, usually due to a bleeding ulcer or perforation of the stomach.

K92.1   Melena

Blood in the stool.

K92.81   Gastrointestinal mucositis (ulcerative)

Gastrointestinal mucositis is a common complication of cancer treatment, causing inflammation and ulcerative sores in the soft tissues of the mucous membranes lining the stomach and the intestines. This is a painful condition that hampers the patient's ability to receive proper nutrition and continue with the therapeutic doses of therapy.

K94.02   Colostomy infection

An infected colostomy generally presents with pain, tenderness, swelling, and redness at the site of the stoma, and can usually be treated with antibiotics.

K94.03   Colostomy malfunction

This code should be used to report a mechanical complication at the site of the stoma; for example, the intestine might pull away from the abdominal wall, requiring emergency surgical repair.

K95.0   Complications of gastric band procedure

Gastric banding is a type of restrictive weight loss procedure in which an adjustable silicone band lined with an inflatable balloon is placed laparoscopically around the upper part of the stomach to create a smaller pouch for food. This limits the amounts that can be eaten. The balloon is connected to a small reservoir or port under the skin in the abdomen through which the doctor can adjust the band to allow food to pass more quickly or slowly into the lower part of the stomach. This is considered a less invasive procedure than a bypass as there is no cutting or stapling done inside the patient.

K95.01   Infection due to gastric band procedure

Infections due to a gastric band procedure can occur in the band area internally, at the port area in the abdomen through which the band is adjusted, and at incision sites, particularly if the laparoscopic approach was converted to an open approach.

Note: The specified type of infection must be identified with another code.

K95.09   Other complications of gastric band procedure

Other complications of gastric band procedure include gastric perforation, stenosis of the stoma where the band restricts food from the upper pouch to the lower stomach, slippage of the band device or stomach prolapse,

leakage of the balloon or tubing, and later erosion of the band into the stomach.

Note: Use additional codes as necessary to identify the nature of the complication.

K95.8   Complications of other bariatric procedure

Other bariatric procedures for weight loss include gastric bypass and biliopancreatic diversion. A traditional Roux-en-Y gastric bypass may be done either openly or laparoscopically while the diversion is done openly with one long incision. Both use bypass. In a Roux-en-Y, a small pouch is created by stapling a portion of the stomach and a Y-shaped part of the intestine is attached to the stomach pouch and the jejunum, bypassing the duodenum. In the diversion, a portion of the stomach is removed and the bypass is attached to the distal ilium. This procedure is not commonly used as the risk is much greater. These other types of bariatric surgery not only significantly reduce food intake, but decrease the absorption of food nutrients by bypassing the small intestine. The risk of complications with these types of surgery is much greater than with banding.

K95.81   Infection due to other bariatric procedure

Infections due to other bariatric procedures could be incisional or internal. Surgeries that are performed openly present a greater risk of incisional infection than those done laparoscopically.

Note: The specified type of infection must be identified with another code.

K95.89   Other complications of other bariatric procedure

Other complications of other bariatric procedures include mechanical malfunctions such as a leak at the staple lines in the stomach, or a malfunction that develops over a longer time period. These kind of malfunctions include an ulcer at the site of the bypass anastomosis, a narrowing or stricture of the opening from the stomach, or herniation at the incision site.

Note: Use additional codes as necessary to identify the nature of the complication.

L00 Staphylococcal scalded skin syndrome

Staphylococcal scalded skin syndrome (SSSS) or Ritter's disease is a potentially serious side effect of an infection with staphylococcal bacteria that usually affects young children under the age of 5. The staph bacteria produce a protein that lyses the cellular structure holding the skin layers intact. This causes large sections of the epidermis to slough off and peel away, leaving raw, exposed areas beneath that are prone to infection. If this occurs over a large percentage of body surface area, it can become deadly, like a large burn, causing dehydration and further infection. SSSS is treated with intravenous antibiotics to prevent large areas from sloughing off.

Note: Identify percentage of skin exfoliation with an additional code from category L49.

L01.0 Impetigo

Impetigo is a highly infectious bacterial skin infection commonly acquired by children. The primary symptoms are small, painless, pustules over a red sore, usually on the face, especially around the nose and mouth. The sore will burst quickly, ooze, and leave a yellow crust over the affected area that eventually disappears leaving a red mark that heals later without scarring. Two types of bacteria cause impetigo, *Staphylococcus aureus* and *Streptococcus pyogenes*. Although anyone can contract impetigo, children are commonly affected through cuts, scrapes, insect bites, and repetitive scratching. Adults contract it through injured skin.

L01.00 Impetigo, unspecified

Impetigo is a superficial, highly contagious bacterial skin infection seen most commonly in children. *Staphylococcus aureus* is the most common cause, including MRSA, or methicillin resistant strains, which is now seen in up to 20% of cases. *Streptococcus pyogenes* is also a causative bacteria. The blisters produced by the rash can appear anywhere, but usually on the face, hands, forearms, and diaper area. The pustules will burst, ooze, and crust over. Skin that is already irritated by other conditions such as insect bites, scrapes, poison ivy, or repetitive scratching is most susceptible. The rash itself may itch and spread quickly to other areas by scratching and then touching another body part. It is also spread to others by contact with the infected skin or towels, linens, or clothing that has been contaminated. Impetigo is usually diagnosed by appearance. Cultures may be taken to identify the causative bacteria, if the patient does not respond to usual therapy. The sores may be treated with an antibiotic cream or oral medication and kept covered.

L01.01 Non-bullous impetigo

Impetigo is a highly infectious, superficial, bacterial skin infection commonly acquired by children. Non-bullous impetigo, also called crusted impetigo, is the most common type. It begins by forming tiny blisters over a red sore area, usually on the face, especially around the nose and mouth. The blisters will burst quickly, and leave a small, wet spot on the red patch that weeps fluid, then gradually forms a yellowish brown or tan crust over the affected area. The crusting eventually disappears, leaving a red mark that heals later without scarring. Non-bullous impetigo can be caused by either *Staphylococcus aureus* or *Streptococcus pyogenes*, although *S. aureus* is more common. The non-bullous type is most often treated with an antibiotic cream placed on the sores, gentle washing of the crusted area, and gauze coverings.

L01.02 Bockhart's impetigo

Bockhart's impetigo is actually a form of superficial folliculitis caused by *Staphylococcus aureus* and characterized by small, painful, tense pustules at the follicular orifices, especially on the scalp and limbs. It is also seen on the face, particularly around the mouth. The fragile, thin-walled pustules are purulent, appearing as yellowish-white domed pustules that develop in crops around the follicles and then heal in a few days. Like other types of impetigo, the infection often develops secondarily in skin that is already irritated due to injuries, insect bites, and repeated scratching.

L01.03 Bullous impetigo

Impetigo is a highly infectious, superficial, bacterial skin infection commonly acquired by children. Bullous impetigo produces larger, fluid-filled blisters on red sores that usually occur on the trunk, arms, or legs. The bullous form is almost always caused by *Staphylococcus aureus*. The bacteria releases toxins that cause the larger, fluid-filled blisters, which first appear clear, and then become cloudy. The bullous type blisters usually remain longer than the smaller, non-bullous type before they break open, ooze, and leave a larger base to scab over with the characteristic yellowish crust, which may also last longer than the sores in other types of impetigo. Bullous impetigo is usually treated with oral antibiotics for 7-10 days and careful management of sores with gentle washing and coverings over the infected area.

L01.09 Other impetigo

Impetigo is a highly infectious bacterial skin infection commonly acquired by children and caused by *Staphylococcus aureus* or *Streptococcus pyogenes*. Blisters produced by the rash can appear anywhere, but usually on the face. Normally a superficial skin infection, the pustules will burst, ooze, and crust over before eventually disappearing, leaving a red mark that heals later without scarring as the erosion is at the stratum corneum level. Other types of impetigo, however, include ulcerative impetigo, also known as a type of ecthyma extending into the dermis. Ulcerative impetigo is a deeper form of impetigo, characterized by small and shallow, purulent ulcers that have a thick, brownish-black crust within a surrounding area of erythema. The ulcers form under a crusted surface infection and often appear on the lower extremities, particularly of children, elderly, diabetics, and those with an ignored minor injury or previous insect bite. The ulcers are usually found to be teeming with bacteria, and although it may begin more like superficial impetigo, either from initial inoculation or secondary infection, it progresses deep into the dermis, often through neglect. It is treated with antibiotics and because the ulcer is full thickness, it heals with scarring.

L01.1 Impetiginization of other dermatoses

Impetiginization of other dermatoses is the occurrence of impetigo via infection of an area of skin that is already experiencing a pre-existing dermatosis, such as lesions of atopic or allergic contact dermatitis. The dermatitis predisposes the area to infection with *Staphylococcus aureus*. The enhanced susceptibility to bacteria is thought to be due to a lack of antimicrobial peptides in the inflamed skin. The resulting impetigo rash produces blisters over the affected area that burst and leave a weeping wet patch, which gradually forms a yellowish brown or tan crust over the affected area, making the existing skin disease much worse. Treatment usually consists of topical corticosteroids to inhibit the aberrant inflammation and oral antibiotics, such as cephalexin.

L02.01 Cutaneous abscess of face

An abscess is a collection of pus that accumulates within tissue as an inflammatory response precipitated by an infectious agent or foreign body. The formation of an abscess is part of the body's defense mechanism to keep infection localized. The healthy tissue around the infection forms a wall or capsule that prevents bacteria from spreading to other areas of the body. A cutaneous abscess of the face is characterized by redness, swelling, and warmth in a circumscribed area of the facial skin that may drain pus, blood, or fluid.

L02.02 Furuncle of face

A furuncle, or boil, of the face is a painful, pustulent infection of a facial hair follicle that involves all layers of the skin down to the subcutaneous layer, and extends into the sebaceous gland. The condition is characterized by a red, swollen bump filled with fluid, pus, and dead tissue that may appear white or yellow at the center. The bump can be as small as a pea or as large as a golf ball. Furuncle is caused by a bacterial infection. The bacteria invade through hair follicles or ducts of the sebaceous glands. *Staphylococcus aureus* and Group A Streptococcus bacteria are common causes.

L02.03   Carbuncle of face

A carbuncle of the face is a large infection of several furuncles that come together in the same area of the face. A furuncle is a painful, pustulent infection of a hair follicle that involves all layers of the skin down to the subcutaneous layer, and extends into the sebaceous gland, caused by a bacterial infection. The bacteria invade through hair follicles or ducts of the sebaceous glands. *Staphylococcus aureus* and Group A Streptococcus bacteria are common causes. A carbuncle is a grouping of infected hair follicles with more than one opening or duct to drain pus. The resulting lump may be quite large with inflammation and infection extending into deeper tissue, which can lead to cellulitis and lymphangitis.

L02.11   Cutaneous abscess of neck

An abscess is a collection of pus that accumulates within tissue as an inflammatory response precipitated by an infectious agent or foreign body. The formation of an abscess is part of the body's defense mechanism to keep infection localized. The healthy tissue around the infection forms a wall or capsule that prevents bacteria from spreading to other areas of the body. A cutaneous abscess of the neck is characterized by redness, swelling, and warmth in a circumscribed area of skin on the neck that may drain pus, blood, or fluid.

L02.12   Furuncle of neck

A furuncle, or boil, of the neck is a painful, pustulent infection of a hair follicle on the neck that involves all layers of the skin down to the subcutaneous layer, and extends into the sebaceous gland. The condition is characterized by a red, swollen bump filled with fluid, pus, and dead tissue that may appear white or yellow at the center. The bump can be as small as a pea or as large as a golf ball. Furuncle is caused by a bacterial infection. The bacteria invade through hair follicles or ducts of the sebaceous glands. *Staphylococcus aureus* and Group A Streptococcus bacteria are common causes.

L02.13   Carbuncle of neck

A carbuncle of the neck is a large infection of several furuncles that come together in the same area of the neck. A furuncle is a painful, pustulent infection of a hair follicle that involves all layers of the skin down to the subcutaneous layer, and extends into the sebaceous gland, caused by a bacterial infection. The bacteria invade through hair follicles or ducts of the sebaceous glands. *Staphylococcus aureus* and Group A Streptococcus bacteria are common causes. A carbuncle is a grouping of infected hair follicles with more than one opening or duct to drain pus. The resulting lump may be quite large with inflammation and infection extending into deeper tissue, which can lead to cellulitis and lymphangitis.

L02.21   Cutaneous abscess of trunk

An abscess is a collection of pus that accumulates within tissue as an inflammatory response precipitated by an infectious agent or foreign body. The formation of an abscess is part of the body's defense mechanism to keep infection localized. The healthy tissue around the infection forms a wall or capsule that prevents bacteria from spreading to other areas of the body. A cutaneous abscess of the trunk is characterized by redness, swelling, and warmth in a circumscribed area of skin on the trunk that may drain pus, blood, or fluid. This includes the skin of the abdominal or chest wall, back, groin, perineum, or umbilicus.

L02.22   Furuncle of trunk

A furuncle, or boil, of the trunk is a painful, pustulent infection of a hair follicle on the abdominal or chest wall, back, groin, perineum, or umbilicus that involves all layers of the skin down to the subcutaneous layer, and extends into the sebaceous gland. The condition is characterized by a red, swollen bump filled with fluid, pus, and dead tissue that may appear white or yellow at the center. The bump can be as small as a pea or as large as

a golf ball. Furuncle is caused by a bacterial infection. The bacteria invade through hair follicles or ducts of the sebaceous glands. *Staphylococcus aureus* and Group A Streptococcus bacteria are common causes.

L02.23   Carbuncle of trunk

A carbuncle of the trunk is a large infection of several furuncles that come together in the same area of the trunk, such as on the abdominal or chest wall, back, groin, perineum, or umbilicus. A furuncle is a painful, pustulent infection of a hair follicle that involves all layers of the skin down to the subcutaneous layer, and extends into the sebaceous gland, caused by a bacterial infection. The bacteria invade through hair follicles or ducts of the sebaceous glands. *Staphylococcus aureus* and Group A Streptococcus bacteria are common causes. A carbuncle is a grouping of infected hair follicles with more than one opening or duct to drain pus. The resulting lump may be quite large with inflammation and infection extending into deeper tissue, which can lead to cellulitis and lymphangitis.

L02.31   Cutaneous abscess of buttock

An abscess is a collection of pus that accumulates within tissue as an inflammatory response precipitated by an infectious agent or foreign body. The formation of an abscess is part of the body's defense mechanism to keep infection localized. The healthy tissue around the infection forms a wall or capsule that prevents bacteria from spreading to other areas of the body. A cutaneous abscess of the buttock is characterized by redness, swelling, and warmth in a circumscribed area of skin in the gluteal region that may drain pus, blood, or fluid.

L02.32   Furuncle of buttock

A furuncle, or boil, of the buttock is a painful, pustulent infection of a hair follicle anywhere in the gluteal region that involves all layers of the skin down to the subcutaneous layer, and extends into the sebaceous gland. The condition is characterized by a red, swollen bump filled with fluid, pus, and dead tissue that may appear white or yellow at the center. The bump can be as small as a pea or as large as a golf ball. Furuncle is caused by a bacterial infection. The bacteria invade through hair follicles or ducts of the sebaceous glands. *Staphylococcus aureus* and Group A Streptococcus bacteria are common causes.

L02.33   Carbuncle of buttock

A carbuncle of the buttock is a large infection of several furuncles that come together in the same area of the gluteal region. A furuncle is a painful, pustulent infection of a hair follicle that involves all layers of the skin down to the subcutaneous layer, and extends into the sebaceous gland, caused by a bacterial infection. The bacteria invade through hair follicles or ducts of the sebaceous glands. *Staphylococcus aureus* and Group A Streptococcus bacteria are common causes. A carbuncle is a grouping of infected hair follicles with more than one opening or duct to drain pus. The resulting lump may be quite large with inflammation and infection extending into deeper tissue, which can lead to cellulitis and lymphangitis.

L02.41   Cutaneous abscess of limb

An abscess is a collection of pus that accumulates within tissue as an inflammatory response precipitated by an infectious agent or foreign body. The formation of an abscess is part of the body's defense mechanism to keep infection localized. The healthy tissue around the infection forms a wall or capsule that prevents bacteria from spreading to other areas of the body. A cutaneous abscess of the limb is characterized by redness, swelling, and warmth in a circumscribed area of skin in the axilla, the upper or lower arm, or the upper or lower leg that may drain pus, blood, or fluid.

L02.42   Furuncle of limb

A furuncle, or boil, of the limb is a painful, pustulent infection of a hair follicle located either in the axilla or the arm or leg that involves all layers of the skin down to the subcutaneous layer, and extends into the sebaceous gland. The condition is characterized by a red, swollen bump filled with fluid, pus, and dead tissue that may appear white or yellow at the center. The bump can be as small as a pea or as large as a golf ball. Furuncle is caused by a bacterial infection. The bacteria invade through hair follicles or ducts of the sebaceous glands. *Staphylococcus aureus* and Group A Streptococcus bacteria are common causes.

L02.43 **Carbuncle of limb**

A carbuncle of the limb is a large infection of several furuncles that come together in the same area either in the axilla, the upper or lower arm, or the upper or lower leg. A furuncle is a painful, pustulent infection of a hair follicle that involves all layers of the skin down to the subcutaneous layer, and extends into the sebaceous gland, caused by a bacterial infection. The bacteria invade through hair follicles or ducts of the sebaceous glands. *Staphylococcus aureus* and Group A Streptococcus bacteria are common causes. A carbuncle is a grouping of infected hair follicles with more than one opening or duct to drain pus. The resulting lump may be quite large with inflammation and infection extending into deeper tissue, which can lead to cellulitis and lymphangitis.

L02.51 **Cutaneous abscess of hand**

An abscess is a collection of pus that accumulates within tissue as an inflammatory response precipitated by an infectious agent or foreign body. The formation of an abscess is part of the body's defense mechanism to keep infection localized. The healthy tissue around the infection forms a wall or capsule that prevents bacteria from spreading to other areas of the body. A cutaneous abscess of the hand is characterized by redness, swelling, and warmth in a circumscribed area of skin on the hand that may drain pus, blood, or fluid.

L02.52 **Furuncle hand**

A furuncle, or boil, of the hand is a painful, pustulent infection of a hair follicle on the hand that involves all layers of the skin down to the subcutaneous layer, and extends into the sebaceous gland. The condition is characterized by a red, swollen bump filled with fluid, pus, and dead tissue that may appear white or yellow at the center. The bump can be as small as a pea or as large as a golf ball. Furuncle is caused by a bacterial infection. The bacteria invade through hair follicles or ducts of the sebaceous glands. *Staphylococcus aureus* and Group A Streptococcus bacteria are common causes.

L02.53 **Carbuncle of hand**

A carbuncle of the hand is a large infection of several furuncles that come together in the same area of the hand. A furuncle is a painful, pustulent infection of a hair follicle that involves all layers of the skin down to the subcutaneous layer, and extends into the sebaceous gland, caused by a bacterial infection. The bacteria invade through hair follicles or ducts of the sebaceous glands. *Staphylococcus aureus* and Group A Streptococcus bacteria are common causes. A carbuncle is a grouping of infected hair follicles with more than one opening or duct to drain pus. The resulting lump may be quite large with inflammation and infection extending into deeper tissue, which can lead to cellulitis and lymphangitis.

L02.61 **Cutaneous abscess of foot**

An abscess is a collection of pus that accumulates within tissue as an inflammatory response precipitated by an infectious agent or foreign body. The formation of an abscess is part of the body's defense mechanism to keep infection localized. The healthy tissue around the infection forms a wall or capsule that prevents bacteria from spreading to other areas of the body. A cutaneous abscess of the foot is characterized by redness, swelling, and warmth in a circumscribed area of skin on the foot that may drain pus, blood, or fluid.

L02.62 **Furuncle of foot**

A furuncle, or boil, of the foot is a painful, pustulent infection of a hair follicle on the foot that involves all layers of the skin down to the subcutaneous layer, and extends into the sebaceous gland. The condition is characterized by a red, swollen bump filled with fluid, pus, and dead tissue that may appear white or yellow at the center. The bump can be as small as a pea or as large as a golf ball. Furuncle is caused by a bacterial infection. The bacteria invade through hair follicles or ducts of the sebaceous glands. *Staphylococcus aureus* and Group A Streptococcus bacteria are common causes.

L02.63 **Carbuncle of foot**

A carbuncle of the foot is a large infection of several furuncles that come together in the same area of the foot. A furuncle is a painful, pustulent

infection of a hair follicle that involves all layers of the skin down to the subcutaneous layer, and extends into the sebaceous gland, caused by a bacterial infection. The bacteria invade through hair follicles or ducts of the sebaceous glands. *Staphylococcus aureus* and Group A Streptococcus bacteria are common causes. A carbuncle is a grouping of infected hair follicles with more than one opening or duct to drain pus. The resulting lump may be quite large with inflammation and infection extending into deeper tissue, which can lead to cellulitis and lymphangitis.

L02.811 **Cutaneous abscess of head [any part, except face]**

An abscess is a collection of pus that accumulates within tissue as an inflammatory response precipitated by an infectious agent or foreign body. The formation of an abscess is part of the body's defense mechanism to keep infection localized. The healthy tissue around the infection forms a wall or capsule that prevents bacteria from spreading to other areas of the body. A cutaneous abscess of the head is characterized by redness, swelling, and warmth in a circumscribed area of skin on the head, except the face, that may drain pus, blood, or fluid.

L02.821 **Furuncle of head [any part, except face]**

A furuncle, or boil, of the head is a painful, pustulent infection of a hair follicle on the scalp or other part of the head, except the face, that involves all layers of the skin down to the subcutaneous layer, and extends into the sebaceous gland. The condition is characterized by a red, swollen bump filled with fluid, pus, and dead tissue that may appear white or yellow at the center. The bump can be as small as a pea or as large as a golf ball. Furuncle is caused by a bacterial infection. The bacteria invade through hair follicles or ducts of the sebaceous glands. *Staphylococcus aureus* and Group A Streptococcus bacteria are common causes.

L02.831 **Carbuncle of head [any part, except face]**

A carbuncle of the head is a large infection of several furuncles that come together in the same area of the head, such as on the scalp or other area, except the face. A furuncle is a painful, pustulent infection of a hair follicle that involves all layers of the skin down to the subcutaneous layer, and extends into the sebaceous gland, caused by a bacterial infection. The bacteria invade through hair follicles or ducts of the sebaceous glands. *Staphylococcus aureus* and Group A Streptococcus bacteria are common causes. A carbuncle is a grouping of infected hair follicles with more than one opening or duct to drain pus. The resulting lump may be quite large with inflammation and infection extending into deeper tissue, which can lead to cellulitis and lymphangitis.

L03.0 **Cellulitis and acute lymphangitis of finger and toe**

Note: Cellulitis and acute lymphangitis of finger and toe also include infections of the nail, nailbed, and cuticle.

L03.01 **Cellulitis of finger**

Cellulitis is a spreading infection of the connective soft tissue often extending into the deep dermal and subcutaneous layers of the skin, resulting in fever and swollen lymph nodes near the site of infection. The condition may be localized or diffuse and is characterized by redness, swelling, and warmth in a circumscribed area, often accompanied by an abscess, or pocket of pus. Cellulitis is caused by bacteria, usually Staphylococcus or Group A Streptococcus, that is introduced through a cut, scrape, or break in the skin. Cellulitis of the finger includes felon and whitlow. Felon is a deep, enclosed abscess of the fingertip on the palmar side that is very painful as it expands. Felon is usually caused by Staphylococcus aureus and begins with a puncture wound, particularly from wood. As the pocket of bacteria grows, it can compress blood vessels and cut off circulation, resulting in permanent damage, and/or spread to the bone, causing osteomyelitis. Whitlow is a similar, painful infection of the fingertip caused by the herpes simplex virus.

L03.02 **Acute lymphangitis of finger**

Acute lymphangitis of the finger is an infection of the lymph vessels appearing as painful, red streaks visible through the skin surface on the finger, most commonly caused by a streptococcal infection. Bacteria enter through a cut or break in the skin, where they multiple rapidly and spread so fast through the lymphatic vessels that the immune system may not be able to respond fast enough to stop the infection. The bacteria can cause tissue destruction at the site of the infection, an abscess, or cellulitis in the deeper skin layers. The infection often spreads quickly into the blood stream, resulting in serious sepsis that can be fatal.

L03.03 Cellulitis of toe

Cellulitis of the toe is a spreading infection of the connective soft tissue of the toe caused by bacteria, usually Staphylococcus or Group A Streptococcus, that was introduced through a cut, scrape, or break in the skin. Cellulitis often extends into the deep dermal and subcutaneous layers of the skin, resulting in fever and swollen lymph nodes near the site of infection. The condition may be localized or diffuse and is characterized by redness, swelling, and warmth in a circumscribed area, often accompanied by an abscess, or pocket of pus.

L03.04 Acute lymphangitis of toe

Acute lymphangitis of the toe is an infection of the lymph vessels appearing as painful, red streaks visible through the skin surface on the toe, most commonly caused by a streptococcal infection. Bacteria enter through a cut or break in the skin, where they multiple rapidly and spread so fast through the lymphatic vessels that the immune system may not be able to respond fast enough to stop the infection. The bacteria can cause tissue destruction at the site of the infection, an abscess, or cellulitis in the deeper skin layers. The infection often spreads quickly into the blood stream, resulting in serious sepsis that can be fatal.

L03.11 Cellulitis of other parts of limb

Cellulitis of other parts of a limb is a spreading infection of the connective soft tissue of the axilla, upper limb, or lower limb except fingers and toes, that is caused by bacteria, usually Staphylococcus or Group A Streptococcus, which has been introduced through a cut, scrape, or break in the skin. Cellulitis often extends into the deep dermal and subcutaneous layers of the skin, resulting in fever and swollen lymph nodes near the site of infection. The condition may be localized or diffuse and is characterized by redness, swelling, and warmth in a circumscribed area, often accompanied by an abscess, or pocket of pus.

L03.12 Acute lymphangitis of other parts of limb

Acute lymphangitis of other parts of a limb is an infection of the lymph vessels of the axilla, upper limb, or lower limb except fingers and toes, appearing as painful, red streaks visible through the skin surface on the limb, most commonly caused by a streptococcal infection. Bacteria enter through a cut or break in the skin, where they multiple rapidly and spread so fast through the lymphatic vessels that the immune system may not be able to respond fast enough to stop the infection. The bacteria can cause tissue destruction at the site of the infection, an abscess, or cellulitis in the deeper skin layers. The infection often spreads quickly into the blood stream, resulting in serious sepsis that can be fatal.

L03.211 Cellulitis of face

Cellulitis of the face is a spreading infection of the connective soft tissue of the face caused by bacteria, usually Staphylococcus or Group A Streptococcus, that was introduced through a cut, scrape, or break in the skin. Cellulitis often extends into the deep dermal and subcutaneous layers of the skin, resulting in fever and swollen lymph nodes near the site of infection. The condition may be localized or diffuse and is characterized by redness, swelling, and warmth in a circumscribed area, often accompanied by an abscess, or pocket of pus.

L03.212 Acute lymphangitis of face

Acute lymphangitis of the face is an infection of the lymph vessels appearing as painful, red streaks visible through the skin surface on the face, most commonly caused by a streptococcal infection. Bacteria enter through a cut or break in the skin, where they multiple rapidly and spread so fast through the lymphatic vessels that the immune system may not be able to respond fast enough to stop the infection. The bacteria can cause tissue destruction at the site of the infection, an abscess, or cellulitis in

the deeper skin layers. The infection often spreads quickly into the blood stream, resulting in serious sepsis that can be fatal.

L03.221 Cellulitis of neck

Cellulitis of the neck is a spreading infection of the connective soft tissue of the neck caused by bacteria, usually Staphylococcus or Group A Streptococcus, that was introduced through a cut, scrape, or break in the skin. Cellulitis often extends into the deep dermal and subcutaneous layers of the skin, resulting in fever and swollen lymph nodes near the site of infection. The condition may be localized or diffuse and is characterized by redness, swelling, and warmth in a circumscribed area, often accompanied by an abscess, or pocket of pus.

L03.222 Acute lymphangitis of neck

Acute lymphangitis of the neck is an infection of the lymph vessels appearing as painful, red streaks visible through the skin surface on the neck, most commonly caused by a streptococcal infection. Bacteria enter through a cut or break in the skin, where they multiple rapidly and spread so fast through the lymphatic vessels that the immune system may not be able to respond fast enough to stop the infection. The bacteria can cause tissue destruction at the site of the infection, an abscess, or cellulitis in the deeper skin layers. The infection often spreads quickly into the blood stream, resulting in serious sepsis that can be fatal.

L03.311 Cellulitis of abdominal wall

Cellulitis of the abdominal wall is a spreading infection of the connective soft tissue of the abdominal wall caused by bacteria, usually Staphylococcus or Group A Streptococcus, that was introduced through a cut, scrape, or break in the skin. Cellulitis often extends into the deep dermal and subcutaneous layers of the skin, resulting in fever and swollen lymph nodes near the site of infection. The condition may be localized or diffuse and is characterized by redness, swelling, and warmth in a circumscribed area, often accompanied by an abscess, or pocket of pus.

L03.312 Cellulitis of back [any part except buttock]

Cellulitis of the back is a spreading infection of any of the connective soft tissue in the back except the buttock. It is caused by bacteria, usually Staphylococcus or Group A Streptococcus, that was introduced through a cut, scrape, or break in the skin. Cellulitis often extends into the deep dermal and subcutaneous layers of the skin, resulting in fever and swollen lymph nodes near the site of infection. The condition may be localized or diffuse and is characterized by redness, swelling, and warmth in a circumscribed area, often accompanied by an abscess, or pocket of pus.

L03.313 Cellulitis of chest wall

Cellulitis of the chest wall is a spreading infection of the connective soft tissue in the chest wall caused by bacteria, usually Staphylococcus or Group A Streptococcus, that was introduced through a cut, scrape, or break in the skin. Cellulitis often extends into the deep dermal and subcutaneous layers of the skin, resulting in fever and swollen lymph nodes near the site of infection. The condition may be localized or diffuse and is characterized by redness, swelling, and warmth in a circumscribed area, often accompanied by an abscess, or pocket of pus.

L03.314 Cellulitis of groin

Cellulitis of the groin is a spreading infection of the connective soft tissue of the groin area caused by bacteria, usually Staphylococcus or Group A Streptococcus, that was introduced through a cut, scrape, or break in the skin. Cellulitis often extends into the deep dermal and subcutaneous layers of the skin, resulting in fever and swollen lymph nodes near the site of infection. The condition may be localized or diffuse and is characterized by redness, swelling, and warmth in a circumscribed area, often accompanied by an abscess, or pocket of pus.

L03.315 Cellulitis of perineum

Cellulitis of the perineum is a spreading infection of the connective soft tissue of the perineal area caused by bacteria, usually Staphylococcus or Group A Streptococcus, that was introduced through a cut, scrape, or break in the skin. Cellulitis often extends into the deep dermal and subcutaneous layers of the skin, resulting in fever and swollen lymph nodes near the site of infection. The condition may be localized or diffuse and is characterized by redness, swelling, and warmth in a circumscribed area, often accompanied by an abscess, or pocket of pus.

L03.316   Cellulitis of umbilicus

Cellulitis of the umbilicus is a spreading infection of the connective soft tissue of the umbilical area of the abdomen caused by bacteria, usually Staphylococcus or Group A Streptococcus, that was introduced through a cut, scrape, or break in the skin. Cellulitis often extends into the deep dermal and subcutaneous layers of the skin, resulting in fever and swollen lymph nodes near the site of infection. The condition may be localized or diffuse and is characterized by redness, swelling, and warmth in a circumscribed area, often accompanied by an abscess, or pocket of pus.

L03.317   Cellulitis of buttock

Cellulitis of the buttock is a spreading infection of the connective soft tissue of the buttock caused by bacteria, usually Staphylococcus or Group A Streptococcus, that was introduced through a cut, scrape, or break in the skin. Cellulitis often extends into the deep dermal and subcutaneous layers of the skin, resulting in fever and swollen lymph nodes near the site of infection. The condition may be localized or diffuse and is characterized by redness, swelling, and warmth in a circumscribed area, often accompanied by an abscess, or pocket of pus.

L03.319   Cellulitis of trunk, unspecified

Cellulitis of the trunk is a spreading infection of the connective soft tissue of the trunk that is only reported when no further specification is made as to location. The infection is caused by bacteria, usually Staphylococcus or Group A Streptococcus, that was introduced through a cut, scrape, or break in the skin. Cellulitis often extends into the deep dermal and subcutaneous layers of the skin, resulting in fever and swollen lymph nodes near the site of infection. The condition may be localized or diffuse and is characterized by redness, swelling, and warmth in a circumscribed area, often accompanied by an abscess, or pocket of pus.

L03.321   Acute lymphangitis of abdominal wall

Acute lymphangitis of the abdominal wall is an infection of the lymph vessels appearing as painful, red streaks visible through the skin surface on the abdomen, most commonly caused by a streptococcal infection. Bacteria enter through a cut or break in the skin, where they multiple rapidly and spread so fast through the lymphatic vessels that the immune system may not be able to respond fast enough to stop the infection. The bacteria can cause tissue destruction at the site of the infection, an abscess, or cellulitis in the deeper skin layers. The infection often spreads quickly into the blood stream, resulting in serious sepsis that can be fatal.

L03.322   Acute lymphangitis of back [any part except buttock]

Acute lymphangitis of the back is an infection of the lymph vessels appearing as painful, red streaks visible through the skin surface anywhere on the back, except the buttock, most commonly caused by a streptococcal infection. Bacteria enter through a cut or break in the skin, where they multiple rapidly and spread so fast through the lymphatic vessels that the immune system may not be able to respond fast enough to stop the infection. The bacteria can cause tissue destruction at the site of the infection, an abscess, or cellulitis in the deeper skin layers. The infection often spreads quickly into the blood stream, resulting in serious sepsis that can be fatal.

L03.323   Acute lymphangitis of chest wall

Acute lymphangitis of the chest wall is an infection of the lymph vessels appearing as painful, red streaks visible through the skin surface on the chest, most commonly caused by a streptococcal infection. Bacteria enter through a cut or break in the skin, where they multiple rapidly and spread so fast through the lymphatic vessels that the immune system may not be able to respond fast enough to stop the infection. The bacteria can cause tissue destruction at the site of the infection, an abscess, or cellulitis in the deeper skin layers. The infection often spreads quickly into the blood stream, resulting in serious sepsis that can be fatal.

L03.324   Acute lymphangitis of groin

Acute lymphangitis of the groin is an infection of the lymph vessels appearing as painful, red streaks visible through the skin surface in the groin area, most commonly caused by a streptococcal infection. Bacteria enter through a cut or break in the skin, where they multiple rapidly and spread so fast through the lymphatic vessels that the immune system may not be able to respond fast enough to stop the infection. The bacteria can cause tissue destruction at the site of the infection, an abscess, or cellulitis in the deeper skin layers. The infection often spreads quickly into the blood stream, resulting in serious sepsis that can be fatal.

L03.325   Acute lymphangitis of perineum

Acute lymphangitis of the perineum is an infection of the lymph vessels appearing as painful, red streaks visible through the skin surface on the perineal area, most commonly caused by a streptococcal infection. Bacteria enter through a cut or break in the skin, where they multiple rapidly and spread so fast through the lymphatic vessels that the immune system may not be able to respond fast enough to stop the infection. The bacteria can cause tissue destruction at the site of the infection, an abscess, or cellulitis in the deeper skin layers. The infection often spreads quickly into the blood stream, resulting in serious sepsis that can be fatal.

L03.326   Acute lymphangitis of umbilicus

Acute lymphangitis of the umbilicus is an infection of the lymph vessels appearing as painful, red streaks visible through the skin surface in the umbilical area, most commonly caused by a streptococcal infection. Bacteria enter through a cut or break in the skin, where they multiple rapidly and spread so fast through the lymphatic vessels that the immune system may not be able to respond fast enough to stop the infection. The bacteria can cause tissue destruction at the site of the infection, an abscess, or cellulitis in the deeper skin layers. The infection often spreads quickly into the blood stream, resulting in serious sepsis that can be fatal.

L03.327   Acute lymphangitis of buttock

Acute lymphangitis of the buttock is an infection of the lymph vessels appearing as painful, red streaks visible through the skin surface on the buttock, most commonly caused by a streptococcal infection. Bacteria enter through a cut or break in the skin, where they multiple rapidly and spread so fast through the lymphatic vessels that the immune system may not be able to respond fast enough to stop the infection. The bacteria can cause tissue destruction at the site of the infection, an abscess, or cellulitis in the deeper skin layers. The infection often spreads quickly into the blood stream, resulting in serious sepsis that can be fatal.

L03.329   Acute lymphangitis of trunk, unspecified

Acute lymphangitis of the trunk is an infection of the lymph vessels appearing as painful, red streaks visible through the skin surface on the trunk, and is only reported when no further specification is made as to location. It is most commonly caused by a streptococcal infection. Bacteria enter through a cut or break in the skin, where they multiple rapidly and spread so fast through the lymphatic vessels that the immune system may not be able to respond fast enough to stop the infection. The bacteria can cause tissue destruction at the site of the infection, an abscess, or cellulitis in the deeper skin layers. The infection often spreads quickly into the blood stream, resulting in serious sepsis that can be fatal.

L03.811   Cellulitis of head [any part, except face]

Cellulitis of the head, except the face, is a spreading infection of the connective soft tissue of the scalp caused by bacteria, usually Staphylococcus or Group A Streptococcus, that was introduced through a cut, scrape, or break in the skin. Cellulitis often extends into the deep dermal and subcutaneous layers of the skin, resulting in fever and swollen lymph nodes near the site of infection. The condition may be localized or diffuse and is characterized by redness, swelling, and warmth in a circumscribed area, often accompanied by an abscess, or pocket of pus.

L03.891 Acute lymphangitis of head [any part, except face]

Acute lymphangitis of the head is an infection of the lymph vessels appearing as painful, red streaks visible through the skin surface of the scalp or other part of head except the face, most commonly caused by a streptococcal infection. Bacteria enter through a cut or break in the skin, where they multiple rapidly and spread so fast through the lymphatic vessels that the immune system may not be able to respond fast enough to stop the infection. The bacteria can cause tissue destruction at the site of the infection, an abscess, or cellulitis in the deeper skin layers. The infection often spreads quickly into the blood stream, resulting in serious sepsis that can be fatal.

L04 Acute lymphadenitis

The lymphatic system is comprised of lymph nodes, ducts, and vessels forming an organ that produces and moves fluid from body tissue into the bloodstream. Lymphadenitis is an infectio or inflammation of the lymph nodes--small structures containing white blood cells that filter lymph fluid. Lymphadenitis is a common complication of bacterial, viral, parasitic, and fungal infections. The condition is characterized by swollen, tender, hard lumps that can be palpated in a localized area and sometimes throughout the body.

L04.0 Acute lymphadenitis of face, head and neck

Lymphadenitis is an enlargement or inflammation of the lymph nodes—small, oval clusters of highly organized immune cells grouped along the course of lymphatic vessels that filter microorganisms and abnormal cells from extracellular fluid. Lymphadenitis may affect one node or a group of nodes, unilaterally or bilaterally. Most acute cases are a benign response to infection that has entered the node, and have a sudden onset with pain, tenderness, and overlying streaking or erythema of the skin. Acute nodes usually present as soft, tender, warm to the touch, and fluctuating. Lymphadenitis of the face, head, and neck may affect several different nodal groups such as the submandibular nodes, the submental nodes, cervical or jugular nodes, occipital or suboccipital nodes, pre- and postauricular nodes, and the supraclavicular nodes. Acute, enlarged lymph nodes in these areas are usually associated with particular localized or systemic infections such as sinusitis, otitis media, conjunctivitis, pharyngitis, cat scratch fever, infectious mononucleosis, cytomegalovirus, toxoplasmosis, tinea capitis, rubella, serum sickness, and severe drug allergies. Other cases may be caused by dental abscesses and different kinds of throat masses or malignancy. Severely swollen nodes in the head and neck can cause dysphagia, dyspnea, cough, headache, and torticollis. Treatment depends on the cause and usually consists of the appropriate antimicrobial with incision and drainage of any suppurative node(s).

L04.1 Acute lymphadenitis of trunk

Lymphadenitis is an enlargement or inflammation of the lymph nodes— small, oval clusters of highly organized immune cells grouped along the course of lymphatic vessels that filter microorganisms and abnormal cells from extracellular fluid. Lymphadenitis may affect one node or a group of nodes, unilaterally or bilaterally. Most acute cases are a benign response to infection that has entered the node, and have a sudden onset with pain, tenderness, warmth, and overlying streaking or erythema of the skin. Lymphadenitis of the trunk may affect nodes in the intrathoracic, retroperitoneal, or iliac area. Acute, enlarged intra-abdominal or retroperitoneal lymph nodes are uncommon and may be associated with Yersinia enterocolitica infection, tuberculosis, deep abscesses, and lymphomas. Lymphadenitis of the inguinal nodes may be associated with venereal disease, cellulitis in the lower extremities, localized abscesses or infections of the skin, genitals, or perineum, as well as lymphomas. Intrathoracic lymph node enlargement can be caused by mycobacterial or fungal infections, sarcoidosis, and malignancy. Treatment depends on the underlying cause.

L04.2 Acute lymphadenitis of upper limb

Lymphadenitis is an enlargement or inflammation of the lymph nodes— small, oval clusters of highly organized immune cells grouped along the course of lymphatic vessels that filter microorganisms and abnormal cells

from extracellular fluid. Lymphadenitis may affect one node or a group of nodes, unilaterally or bilaterally. Most acute cases are a benign response to infection that has entered the node, and have a sudden onset with pain, tenderness, and overlying streaking or erythema of the skin. Acute nodes usually present as soft, tender, warm to the touch, and fluctuating. Lymphadenitis of the upper limb affects the shoulder and axillary area. Axillary lymphadenitis is commonly associated with cat scratch disease, localized staph and strep infections of the skin, tularemia, sporotrichosis, lymphoma, breast carcinoma, and melanoma. Treatment depends on the underlying cause and may include antibiotics and incision and drainage for suppurative nodes.

L05 Pilonidal cyst and sinus

A pilonidal cyst is a fluid and/or debris-filled cavity that forms over the spine at the top of the crease of the buttocks. The cyst is typically deep within the tissue of the lumbar region, often forming an abscess. An abnormal pilonidal sinus tract or fistula may also form in the tailbone area, connecting the cyst or abscess to the skin surface where drainage can occur. The cyst, abscess, of sinus tract forms due to irritation and debris accumulating in the hair follicles of the natal cleft, and can be very painful.

L05.01 Pilonidal cyst with abscess

A pilonidal cyst is an abnormal fluid-filled cavity containing debris of hair and skin cells that forms over the tailbone at the top of the buttock crease. Rare cases occur in other parts of the body, such as the crease between fingers, seen with sheep shearers, dog groomers, and barbers. Pilonidal cysts tend to occur after loose hair has broken through the skin and become embedded. This may occur with skin rubbing skin, friction from tight clothing, bicycling, and long periods of sitting, such as truck driving. Another causative explanation is that stretching motion in the deep dermal layers causes a hair follicle to rupture, and the cyst forms around the ruptured follicle, filling with cellular debris and hair. When the cyst becomes infected, a pocket of pus forms with swelling, redness, and extreme pain around the abscess. Most cases are seen in young men and have a tendency to recur. Surgical treatment usually consists of shaving the area around the cyst and draining it with a small incision, or removing the cyst entirely, particularly upon recurrence. The wound from infected pilonidal cysts is normally left open to drain and packed with a dressing, to allow it to heal from the inside out and reduce the risk of recurrence.

L05.02 Pilonidal sinus with abscess

A pilonidal sinus, also called a sacrococcygeal fistula, is a small channel, or tunnel, through the skin at or near the cleft at the top of the buttocks, which may appear as a dimple-like depression on the surface of the skin over the tailbone. There may be more than one sinus tract formed out to the skin and connecting in the deeper dermis. These sinus tracts are thought to be formed when loose hair punctures through the skin and works its way inside, or possibly when a ruptured hair follicle within the dermis pushes its way to the surface in conjunction with changing hormones, excess hair growth, and friction. Most cases are seen in young men. A pilonidal sinus often forms in conjunction with a cyst when fluid and cellular debris build up around the trapped hair. Pilonidal sinus with abscess can develop quickly once the tract becomes infected. Symptoms of an infected fistula include redness, swelling, pus or blood draining from the tract, particularly with a foul odor, hair protruding from the lesion, and severe pain. Treatment of an abscessed sinus tract includes lancing for drainage and scraping out any hair, blood, pus, and cellular debris from the tract. The wound is packed with a sterile dressing and left open to heal, usually taking about 4 weeks.

L05.91 Pilonidal cyst without abscess

A pilonidal cyst is an abnormal fluid-filled cavity containing debris of hair and skin cells that forms over the tailbone at the top of the buttock crease. Rare cases occur in other parts of the body, such as the crease between fingers, seen with sheep shearers, dog groomers, and barbers. Pilonidal cysts tend to occur after loose hair has broken through the skin and become embedded. This may occur with skin rubbing skin, friction from tight clothing, bicycling, and long periods of sitting, such as truck driving. Another causative explanation is that stretching motion in the deep dermal layers causes a hair follicle to rupture, and the cyst forms around the ruptured follicle, filling with cellular debris and hair. Most cases are seen in young men and have a tendency to recur. Surgical treatment usually consists of shaving the area around the cyst and draining it with a small incision, using careful, hygienic wound care to prevent infection.

L05.92   Pilonidal sinus without abscess

A pilonidal sinus, also called a sacrococcygeal fistula, is a small channel, or tunnel, through the skin at or near the cleft at the top of the buttocks, which may appear as a dimple-like depression on the surface of the skin over the tailbone. There may be more than one sinus tract formed out to the skin and connecting in the deeper dermis. These sinus tracts are thought to be formed when loose hair punctures through the skin and works its way inside, or possibly when a ruptured hair follicle within the dermis pushes its way to the surface in conjunction with changing hormones, excess hair growth, and friction. A pilonidal sinus often forms in conjunction with a cyst when fluid and cellular debris build up around the trapped hair. Treatment for an early pilonidal sinus without abscess is often a broad-spectrum antibiotic, regular shaving of the area, and careful hygiene to prevent development of an abscess.

L08.0   Pyoderma

Pyoderma, or pyogenic dermatitis, is any acute, inflammatory infection of the skin and subcutaneous tissue that produces pus. This includes purulent, septic, or suppurative dermatitis connected with a superficial bacterial infection in a localized area. This cutaneous condition is fairly nonspecific and the causative pathogen may remain unidentified.

L08.1   Erythrasma

Erythrasma is a chronic, localized, superficial skin infection caused by the gram-positive bacterium, Corynebacterium minutissimum. The most common sites infected are the intertriginous areas of the armpit, groin, underneath the breast, and the webbed spaces between the toes. This condition is most often seen in people who are obese, diabetic, or live in warm climates. The initial patches appear pink and progress to reddish-brown, scaly, sharply defined patches as the skin sheds. The patches often look similar to ringworm or other fungal infections. A special Wood's lamp, is often used for diagnosis as the lesions caused by this organism will fluoresce a bright, coral red color when exposed to ultraviolet light. Erythrasma may be treated by keeping the area clean and dry, using antibacterial soap or gels and topical aluminum chloride applications, or taking oral antibiotics such as erythromycin or azithromycin.

L08.81   Pyoderma vegetans

Pyoderma vegetans is a rare, chronic, inflammatory disorder characterized by an eruption of large, exudative, verruca-like plaques with elevated borders and multiple pustular ulcerations. Some plaques may appear hyperkeratotic. Etiology is attributed to bacterial infection in immunocompromised individuals. Fungal infections have also been noted. Pyoderma vegetans is frequently associated with ulcerative colitis, Crohn's disease, HIV infection, alcoholism with nutritional deficit, T cell lymphomas, and chronic myeloid leukemia. Some patients have a history of hidradenitis suppurativa. Histology findings are necessary for diagnosis and include pseudocarcinomatous hyperplasia, numerous abscesses within the hyperplastic (epi)dermis containing neutrophils or eosinophils. No standardized treatment is available. Antibiotics, laser debridement or curettage, topical wound therapies such as copper sulfate dressings, aluminum acetate soaks, zinc oxide or disodium chromoglycate applications, intralesional corticosteroid injections, systemic steroids, and surgical excision and skin grafting have all been used as treatment to induce healing.

L08.82   Omphalitis not of newborn

Omphalitis is an infection of the umbilical stump or belly button. Omphalitis not of the newborn is an acquired condition affecting young children or infants past the first 28 days of life, who are no longer considered neonates. Omphalitis presents as redness, warmth, swelling, pain or tenderness, and discharge of the periumbilical area. Fever, fast heart rate, poor feeding, excessive sleeping or drowsiness, and low blood pressure are also symptoms. The most common infectious agents are Staphylococcus, Streptococcus, and E.coli. Omphalitis can spread quickly, become septic, and be potentially life-threatening, especially in developing countries. Preventive measures consist of medicinal washes and keeping the umbilical stump

or belly button dry and exposed to the air. Treatment for infection consists of intravenous antibiotic therapy aimed at the particular causative agent, sometimes requiring insertion of a central catheter, and supportive care for any other complications such as hypotension or respiratory failure.

L10   Pemphigus

Pemphigus is actually a group of chronic, relapsing, autoimmune blistering diseases of the skin and mucous membranes in which serum autoantibodies are present against antigens within the cells or zones of the epidermis.

Note: Pemphigus used alone usually denotes pemphigus vulgaris, that can sometimes be fatal.

L10.0   Pemphigus vulgaris

Pemphigus vulgaris is the most common, severe from of these blistering diseases that may be fatal if not treated. Circulating antibodies against keratinocyte cell surfaces are present in this disease. It appears to affect men and women equally, usually occurring between ages 40 and 60, and is more common in persons of Mediterranean and Jewish descent. Painful erosions begin in the mouth, particularly on the buccal mucosa, and are seen in nearly all patients, causing dyphagia and poor oral intake. Mucous membrane involvement of the pharynx and larynx may cause hoarseness. Skin lesions appear months later and may remain localized, then become widespread. The skin lesions are flaccid, fragile blisters that rupture easily, but are not noticed as much as the large, painful erosions that they leave behind which weep, bleed easily, and become crusted without healing. The round or oval lesions tend to appear on the scalp, face, chest, axillae, umbilicus, groin, and mucous membranes of genitourinary areas and enlarge by joining together. Corticosteroids, immunosuppressive agents, and plasmapheresis are used in treatment. Because of the serious side effects of the treating agents, there is still significant morbidity and mortality associated with pemphigus vulgaris. Hypertension, diabetes, renal and liver abnormalities, gastrointestinal bleeding, and even death may occur from side affects and infection secondary to the immunosuppression treatment.

L10.1   Pemphigus vegetans

Pemphigus vegetans is a variant of pemphigus vulgaris that may resemble it very closely or be more benign in its course. It causes hypertrophic vegetations in the form of proliferating verrucous granulations, sometimes with pustules in the periphery after bullae rupture. The vegetations tend to coalesce into patches.

L10.2   Pemphigus foliaceous

Pemphigus foliaceous is a rare but superficial, relatively mild, chronic bullous disease covering an extensive area of skin in symmetrical formation. Lesions begin as small vesicles, gradually exfoliating and becoming crusted, and are difficult to differentiate from exfoliative dermatitis. Itching is not particularly intense, but still commonly causes secondary bacterial infections. Hair and nails may also fall out.

L10.3   Brazilian pemphigus [fogo selvagem]

Fogo selvagem, also called Brazilian pemphigus foliaceous, is an endemic form of pemphigus foliaceous that occurs in the river valleys of rural Brazil. It has also been seen in some countries of Central and South America. This type of pemphigus is considered a true autoimmune disease with highly specific autoantibodies that cross-react with the epidermis to produce the disease. The patient is sensitized to produce the antibodies specific for this disease possibly through environmental agents and/or genetic markers. Fogo selvagem means wild fire and is a description of the condition's common symptom of severe cutaneous burning or stinging with exposure to ultraviolet light. UV light induces epidermal binding of specific autoantibodies and neutrophil attachment leading to loss of intercellular adhesion of the keratinocytes and cell detachment (acantholysis). Small, superficial blisters form on the face, neck, and trunk in a seborrheic type pattern. The blisters rupture easily, leaving small erosions. Pressure or rubbing on perilesional and nonlesional skin extends blistering erosions and epidermal detachment into uninvolved skin. The lesions can become generalized, turning into exfoliative erythroderma with a small mortality risk. Protection from sunlight, topical treatment with cortisone and antibiotics, systemic corticosteroids with gradual dose reduction to the minimally effective dose, and plasmapheresis are treatments employed in fogo selvagem.

L10.4 Pemphigus erythematosus

Pemphigus erythematosus begins with a butterfly-shaped rash on the face over the nose and cheeks resembling lupus erythematosus and lesions on the chest and elsewhere that resemble the scaly, crusted, erythematous lesions of seborrheic dermatitis. Histological findings of complement and granular immunoglobulin deposits at the junction of the dermis and epidermis suggest that lupus co-exists in these patients.

L10.5 Drug-induced pemphigus

Pemphigus foliaceous and pemphigus vulgaris are commonly seen types of drug-induced pemphigus. Thiol drugs such as penicillamine, bucillamine, captopril, enalapril, and lisinopril, and are the most often reported drugs causing pemphigus. They appear to induce acantholysis directly by interfering with or activating critical endogenous enzymes, or binding with pemphigus antigens, affecting their normal function. Acantholysis is the loss of intercellular adhesion of keratinocytes in the upper epidermis that causes blister formation and epidermal detachment. Nonthiol, sulfur-containing drugs such as penicillins and cephalosporins are thought to cause acantholysis through immune mechanism production of new autoantibodies that recognize pemphigus antigens. Penicillamine seems to account for about 50% of all reported cases of drug-induced pemphigus. Cutaneous lesion eruption develops weeks to months after beginning therapy. The mechanism involved will determine the clinical appearance of the lesions. Thiol drugs tend to produce foliaceous type lesions with initial fluid-filled blisters that rupture and form erythematous, scaly or crusted plaques, mainly over the trunk. Nonthiol drug tends to produce vulgaris type lesions of flaccid bullae and erosions appearing on normal skin and in the mouth. Remission usually occurs when the offending drug is stopped. Some patients experience a chronic course of pemphigus requiring systemic corticosteroids and immunosuppressants.

L10.81 Paraneoplastic pemphigus

Malignant or paraneoplastic pemphigus is extremely rare, having an onset after 60, and affecting more women than men. It is distinguished from the classic forms of pemphigus as characterized by extensive, painful, severe, persistent mucous membrane erosions commonly involving the lips, oropharyngeal mucosa, and conjuctiva in the presence of a neoplasm, such as a leukemia or lymphoma, sarcoma, or thymoma. Skin lesions vary in shape and size. Blisters and erosions form on redness of the trunk and red, maculopapular lesions with dark centers or vesicles in the middle sometimes appear on the extremities that mimick the target-like lesions seen in erythema multiforme. They may be pruritic. Histologically, paraneoplastic pemphigus appears to be a combination of pemphigus vulgaris and erythema multiforme.

L11.1 Transient acantholytic dermatosis [Grover]

Transient acantholytic dermatosis, or Grover disease, is also known as benign papular or persistent acantholytic dermatosis. This is a benign, self-limiting disorder with a pruritic rash that usually begins by affecting the upper back and chest with widespread, discrete, red or reddish-brown keratotic papules that itch. The lesions may spread to the abdominal area or become more disseminated in severe cases onto the neck, shoulders, arms, and legs. Lesions may also appear vesicular, pustular, or acneiform, or have an unusual unilateral or zosteriform distribution. Varying degrees of itching occur in all cases. Some experience severe itching, although the cutaneous lesions are limited. Increased heat and sweating tend to increase symptoms. Etiology and pathogenesis remain unknown, and it most commonly affects middle-aged caucasian men. There are different histological patterns that closely resemble several other distinct conditions making it difficult to diagnose, and because of its transient, although persistent nature, Grover disease can also be difficult to treat. Strong topical corticosteroids, oral corticosteroids, high doses of retinoids like vitamin A, UV-B exposure, psoralen with ultraviolet A light, methotrexate, and radiation have all been used. Some cases remain refractory to treatment.

L12 Pemphigoid

Pemphigoid is actually a group of dermatological syndromes that resemble, but are distinguished from the pemphigus group.

Note: Pemphigoid used alone usually denotes bullous pemphigoid.

L12.0 Bullous pemphigoid

Bullous pemphigoid is a relatively mild, self-limiting form of a benign, subepidermal blistering disease mostly affecting the elderly between 60 and 80 years of age and is the most common form of the autoimmune bullous dermatoses. Large, tense bullae with clear fluid rupture and leave denuded areas which heal spontaneously. They may begin as red, urticarial, itchy plaques localized at sites such as the scalp, trunk, or extremity or generalized on the lower legs, forearms, thighs, groin, abdomen, but not usually on mucous membranes.

L12.1 Cicatricial pemphigoid

Cicatricial pemphigoid is also known as benign mucous membrane pemphigoid. This is a rare, subepidermal blistering disease with severe, erosive lesions primarily involving mucous membranes, chiefly of the mouth and eye. Mucous membranes of the larynx, nasopharynx, esophagus, genitalia, and rectal mucosa may also be affected. Pain in the throat and mouth causes weight loss. The patient may also lose speech. Erosions, scarring, and edema in severe cases may cause esophageal strictures or complete occlusion, or suproglottic stenosis that necessitate a tracheostomy. Oral blisters and erosions can cause adhesions between different structures in the mouth and cause dental problems. Skin involvement occurs in a third of patients and is usually focused around the face and scalp with the upper trunk. The tense vesiculobullous lesions rupture in a few hours, leaving painful, ulcer-like erosions that may easily become infected, and heal with scars. It affects women twice as much as men and typically appears in late adulthood, between 40 and 60. When the conjunctiva of the eye is affected in ocular cicatricial pemphigoid, chronic conjunctivitis leads to decreased vision with photosensitivity. Symblepharon formation may be seen as adhesions of the conjunctiva between the lid and the eyeball occurs. The scarring and fibrosis can eventually cause blindness.

L13 Other bullous disorders

Bullous dermatoses are debilitating, blistering skin diseases, some of which have serious sequelae and may possibly be fatal. Many bullous diseases are autoimmune in nature and require early interventional treatment to prevent further morbidity or mortality.

L13.0 Dermatitis herpetiformis

Dermatitis herpetiformis is a chronic skin disease that can persist indefinitely, characterized by intensely pruritic excoriations or lesions that are grouped together symmetrically, giving a 'herpetiform' appearance on the extensor surfaces of elbows, knees, lower back, buttocks, and shoulders. The lesions usually begin as vesicles or erythematous papules, urticarial wheals, crusts, or more rarely, even as large bullae. The intensely itchy lesions are usually accompanied by burning and stinging and all of these sensations may occur up to 12 hours before an eruption of the lesions. The localized areas may be left with transient hypo- or hyperpigmentation after the lesions have resolved. This condition affects twice as many males as females, usually occurring between 20 and 40 years of age, but may also appear in children and it mostly affects caucasians. Dermatitis herpetiformis lasts years and follows a prolonged course, although about one third of patients will experience spontaneous remission. Patients with this disease have a higher incidence of other autoimmune disorders such as thyroid disease, diabetes mellitus, and systemic lupus erythematosus; and most patients also suffer a gluten-sensitive enteropathy. Patients receive relief from medications such as dapsone and sulfapyridine and following dietary stipulations closely, such as a gluten-free diet, and the more difficult elemental diet, which alleviate both skin and intestinal lesions over time.

L13.1 Subcorneal pustular dermatitis

This is a rare disease of unknown etiology characterized by chronic vesicopustular eruptions along the groin, axillae, submammary areas, and the flexor areas of limbs where skin stretches. The lesions usually resolve in a few days leaving superficial scaly crusts. Synonyms of this disease are Sneddon-Wilkinson syndrome and pustulosis subcornealis.

L13.8 Other specified bullous disorders

This code includes linear IgA dermatosis, which is another type of rare, subepidermal, autoimmune bullous disorder that was previously thought to be a manifestation of dermatitis herpetiformis. It is now known to be distinct because immunopathology has demonstrated the deposition of IgA in a linear pattern along the basement membrane, sometimes also IgG. This type of dermatosis usually affects those over 30, but may appear as a chronic bullous disease in childhood, particularly in those under five. The pruritic lesions are papules, vesicles, or bullae found in groups in symmetrical distribution over extensor surfaces, particularly on the elbows, knees, and buttocks. Excoriations from scratching lead to crusted papules. The chronic childhood form of IgA dermatosis appears with abrupt onset of tense bullae on an inflamed based with itching and burning, frequently on or near the genitalia, face, and perioral region. Oral ulcers may occur as well as collars of new blisters around the periphery of old lesions.

L20 Atopic dermatitis

Atopic dermatitis is a chronic, inflammatory, non-contagious skin disorder characterized by pruritis, or itching, that precedes redness or rash, with flaking and cracking of the top layer of skin that is susceptable to infection. The rash may actually arise from scratching in response to the itch. Oily discharge may also accompany a flare-up of the condition, which will then crust over. This condition is commonly called eczema, even though it is only one form of eczema. Atopic dermatitis is found commonly in the flexural (inner) area of the elbow and knees but may also occur on hands, feet, face, neck, and chest. The condition usually begins in childhood as a reaction to irritants, food, or environmental allergens and is often outgrown by adolescence or adulthood.

L21 Seborrheic dermatitis

Seborrheic dermatitis is an inflammatory skin disorder caused by over production of sebum, from oil producing sebaceous glands found in the scalp, face, and torso. The condition is characterized by oily scaling or flaky skin, itching, and redness. The areas most commonly affected are the scalp and nasolabial folds of the face. Bacterial infections may be a complication of the condition.

L21.0 Seborrhea capitis

Cradle cap is a condition in which an infant suffers from yellow, crusted lesions of the scalp.

L21.9 Seborrheic dermatitis, unspecified

Seborrhea is a condition in which the skin becomes oily due to overproduction of the sebaceous glands. The sebum may become dry and flake off, and can seem to make the skin dry.

L23 Allergic contact dermatitis

Allergic contact dermatitis is inflammation of the skin with redness, swelling, and itching that may include blisters with fluid drainage or oozing. This occurs at any point where contact is made with an allergenic agent, such as nickel, adhesive glue, latex, make-up, dyes, and plants or animals due to hypersensitization of the patient to that particular allergen.

L24 Irritant contact dermatitis

Contact dermatitis is an inflammation of the skin characterized by redness, swelling, and itching that may include lesions with drainage or oozing. Irritant contact dermatitis can occur following direct contact over a period of time. Common irritants include laundry soaps, skin soaps, lotions and cleaning fluids. The symptoms usually go away once the irritating substance is removed from contact with the skin.

L28 Lichen simplex chronicus and prurigo

Lichen simplex chronicus is skin disorder characterized by leathery, pigmented areas caused by repetitive scratching to relieve itching. The condition is most common in children and may be triggered by tactile irritation (from clothing, etc), insect bites, or stress. Affected areas include ankles, legs, wrists, arms, genitals, and anal area. The inner area of elbow and knees are also common areas for the condition to occur.

L28.0 Lichen simplex chronicus

Lichen simplex chronicus is a skin disorder marked by thickening and scaling of the skin caused by prolonged scratching, rubbing, or itching. It usually occurs in people with other chronic skin problems, such as psoriasis, atopic dermatitis (eczema), or allergies, and in those with nervous, anxious, or depressive conditions who demonstrate repetitive movements. Lichen is more common in children who cannot stop scratching at insect bites, or other itchy skin conditions.

L28.1 Prurigo nodularis

Prurigo nodularis is a skin disease marked by hard, sore, crusty lumps or nodules about half an inch in size appearing on the extremities that cause intense bouts of itching. The itching may remain constant, occur mostly at night, or whenever any touch stimulates the sore and sets off a round of severe itching. Scratching causes excoriated lesions that often bleed and appear with old, white sores. The sores are actually the result of scratching that stimulates the nerves to thicken and send off stronger and stronger itch signals the more they are 'stimulated' by being scratched. Treatment involved potent steroid or anithistamine creams or pill, and cryotherapy in resistant cases.

L28.2 Other prurigo

Prurigo is a chronic inflammatory skin disease featuring blistered papules and severe itching.

L29 Pruritus

Pruritus is severe itching of the skin with no apparent cause.

L29.0 Pruritus ani

Pruritus ani describes severe itching of the perianal region.

L29.1 Pruritus scroti

Severe itching of the scrotal area.

L29.2 Pruritus vulvae

Severe itching of the external female genitalia.

L30.1 Dyshidrosis [pompholyx]

Dyshidrosis is an eruption of small blisters of the feet and hands caused by the sweat glands.

L40 Psoriasis

Psoriasis is a chronic, non-contagious, immune mediated skin disorder characterized by thick silvery scales and dry, red, itchy patches that may be painful. This autoimmune disorder causes scaling and inflammation of the top layer of skin, usually occurring on the face, palms, lower back, scalp, elbows, knees, and soles of the feet. The affected patches of skin may itch and burn, and may also cause restricted motion when large patches of skin (over joint areas in particular) are affected, causing a loss of normal skin elasticity and resulting in pain with movement. This condition is rarely considered serious, but can be emotionally distressing.

L40.0 Psoriasis vulgaris

Psoriasis vulgaris, or plaque psoriasis, is the most common form of psoriasis. This is a non-contagious, immune-mediated disease affecting the skin in which the normal growth cycle of skin cells is sped up. Rapidly accumulating skin cells cause lesions that initially appear as small, red spots and enlarge into patchy lesions of raised, red skin called plaques. The plaques often occur over a joint and have a silvery-white scale on top composed of the rapidly dying skin cells. The scales will continually come loose and shed off the plaques.

L40.1 Generalized pustular psoriasis

This includes impetigo herpetiformis, a rare condition affecting pregnant women that typically begins in the last trimester and resembles pustular psoriasis, although the women affected usually have no personal history of psoriasis. The rash begins as little pustules on the edges of erythematous skin on the inner thighs and groin area. The pustules join together and spread to the trunk, arms, and legs and may also spread to oral mucous membranes and nail beds. The pus-filled lesions are not initially infected with bacteria, but may become infected later. Significant symptoms are usually present along with the rash, such as fever, chills, fatigue, nausea and vomiting, and low levels of calcium and phosphate. The disease is treated with oral steroids. The rash usually resolves following delivery.

L40.4 Guttate psoriasis

Guttate psoriasis is a relatively uncommon form of psoriasis characterized by the acute appearance of small, salmon pink, tear-drop shaped spots covered with silvery, flaky scales on the trunk and extremities. It often develops suddenly, after an infection, such as strep throat, possibly due to the immune system mistaking skin cells for a harmful substance.

L40.50 Arthropathic psoriasis, unspecified

Arthropathic psoriasis, also called psoriatic arthritis, is a type of inflammatory arthritis affecting the ligaments, tendons, fascia, and joints that develops in a small percentage of those affected with the chronic skin condition, psoriasis. It can involve a few or many joints and may occur in multiple, symmetric pairs of joints bilaterally or any joint that is not the same on both sides of the body. It causes warmth, tenderness, swelling, and restricted movement in the affected joints with periodic pain that responds to medical treatment. Affected hands and feet can have enlarged "sausage" digits.

L40.51 Distal interphalangeal psoriatic arthropathy

This is considered the classic type of psoriatic arthropathy, although it occurs in about 5% of people with psoriatic arthropathy. It affects the distal joints of the fingers and toes with scaling skin, and prominent nail changes such as pitted, ridged, yellow nails.

L40.52 Psoriatic arthritis mutilans

Psoriatic arthritis mutilans is a severely deforming and destructive form of psoriatic arthropathy that mainly affects the small joints of the hands and feet, often with lower back and neck pain.

L40.53 Psoriatic spondylitis

Psoriatic spondylitis is inflammation of the spinal column in those with psoriatic arthropathy. This type is diagnosed when the predominant symptom is inflammation and stiffness occurring in the neck, lower back, sacroiliac area, and spinal vertebrae causing pain and difficulty with movement.

L41 Parapsoriasis

Parapsoriasis is a more severe form of psoriasis that is resistant to treatment. Papular lesions may appear, and the affected skin patches tend to grow with time.

L42 Pityriasis rosea

Pityriasis rosea is a common, but harmless kind of skin condition seen in young adults. This skin disease forms a pink, oval-shaped, scaly, itchy rash that begins as a single, large patch and later appears with more skin rashes on the chest, back, and extremities. It is thought to be caused by a virus. The patient may also experience headache or fever.

L43 Lichen planus

Lichen planus is a skin condition that forms an itchy rash on the skin and in the mouth, most commonly in middle-aged adults. The cause is unknown, although it is thought to be related either to an allergic or immune response. Skin rashes are often on the inner wrist, legs, torso, or genital area. The sores are symmetrical and have well-defined borders. They may appear with white streaks or striae, and be shiny or scaly with a dark-reddish purple color. Mouth sores may appear as grayish-white, or bluish-white pimples on the sides of the tongue and inside of the cheek and may be tender or painful. The affected area gradually increases in size and forms lacy, 'network' type looking lines.

L44.0 Pityriasis rubra pilaris

Pityriasis rubra pilaris is a skin disorder that causes chronic inflammation and scaling of the skin. Pink, scaly patches develop, covering much of the body, including the hands and feet, with small areas of normal skin left within the pink, scaling areas. Thickened skin also appears on the hands

and feet. The cause is unknown and treatment consists of topical creams containing urea or lactic acid as well as oral tablets, such as methotrexate.

L44.1 Lichen nitidus

Lichen nitidus is a chronic inflammatory skin eruption that is relatively rare in which tiny, 1-2 mm, discrete, whitish or flesh colored papules form on the skin, usually on the penis, inner thighs, buttocks, and abdomen. The tiny papules are flat-topped and shiny or glistening in appearance. It usually affects children and young adults, and is normally painless and nonpruritic and clears on its own without treatment.

L44.2 Lichen striatus

Lichen striatus is a benign, self-limiting, unilateral skin eruption of unknown etiology that normally affects children. Discrete, 1-3 mm, red or flesh colored, flat-topped papules with a scale erupt and then form into a linear pattern that can extend down the entire length of an extremity. In darker skinned patients, the eruption appears as white or light marks. Lesions can also affect the nail, even before the linear eruption appears on the extremity. Itching can be intense, although the lesions do not normally cause irritation. The condition can last from 4 months to 3 years, after which the skin will darken temporarily. Topical or intralesional steroids are given for treatment.

L49 Exfoliation due to erythematous conditions according to extent of body surface involved

The sloughing off or loss of skin caused by another underlying disease. The percentage of body surface area involved in the progressive spectrum of erythema multiforme grouped diseases is directly related to the correct diagnosis and is also an important clinical factor in the care that is required, such as in a burn unit.

Note: L49.- codes should not be used as a first-listed diagnosis, but are only assigned in addition to the code for the specific erythematous condition causing the exfoliation, such as Ritter's disease or scalded skin syndrome, Stevens-Johnson syndrome, or toxic epidermal necrolysis.

L50.0 Allergic urticaria

Allergic urticaria is the most common form of hives in which smooth, raised pink or white, itchy welts appear on or beneath the skin. This is a hypersensitivity response to a trigger such as food or medication, animal dander, and insect bites that occurs when the immune system releases histamines and other chemicals into the bloodstream. The hives can also have a burning or stinging sensation and will normally blanch white when pressed. Hives can change shape, enlarge and join together to form larger areas of welts, even disappear and reappear later. Mild cases are not treated and will disappear on their own. Reducing itching and swelling by taking antihistamines can help and more severe cases may need to be treated with epinephrine.

L50.1 Idiopathic urticaria

Idiopathic urticaria is a condition in which the appearance of hives has no apparent physical cause. This type of hives is usually brought on by stress.

L50.2 Urticaria due to cold and heat

Hives that appear in response to external cold or heat and typically fade quickly once the patient moves to a place with a more comfortable temperature.

L50.3 Dermatographic urticaria

A condition in which hives occur in one particular area due to scratching or continued irritation of the skin.

L50.4 Vibratory urticaria

Hives brought on by intense, prolonged vibration, usually that which occurs with the use of heavy mechanical equipment.

L50.5 Cholinergic urticaria

Cholinergic urticaria is a condition in which hives appear on the skin in response to a rise in body temperature. Causative increases in body heat typically occur with exercise, stress, excitement, or agitation, and overheating.

L51 Erythema multiforme

Note: Multiple conditions may manifest as a result of the disease processes diagnosed in this category. Such manifestations should be coded in addition: mucositis, stomatitis, inflammation or edema of the eyelid or conjunctiva, corneal ulcer, scarring, or perforation, or symblepharon.

Note: Since the disease processes involved here may be a result of adverse drug reactions and also involve the sloughing of skin, use additional codes to identify the causative drug and an additional code to mark the percentage of skin lost.

L51.0 Nonbullous erythema multiforme

Nonbullous erythema multiforme is a type of acute, self-limiting skin disease with distinctive target lesions that occur as an immune-mediated response. Although the etiology is unknown, it is often connected to infection in most adult cases, especially herpes simplex virus, and to medication in most pediatric cases, particularly penicillin. Other drugs that may cause this hypersensitivity reaction include sulfonamides, NSAIDS, hydantoins, phenothiazines, and barbiturates. Other pathogens that may be a precipitating factor include fungal infections, Epstein-Barr virus, Streptococcus A, and Mycoplasma pneumoniae. The characteristic target-like blotches have a regular round shape with a peripheral red ring around a pale center and sometimes a central dark area. Classical target lesions may not be visible until several days after the onset when various other lesions are present, such as sharply demarcated macules or papules that may gradually darken, enlarge, or become purpuric. Itching and burning can occur with the eruption. The lesions are generally distributed in a symmetrical pattern with a tendency to appear on the lower legs. There is no formation of fluid-filled blisters in nonbullous erythema multiforme, a minimal amount of any epidermal detachment, and no mucous membrane involvement. Mild cases do not require treatment and usually resolve without a problem. Treatment is aimed at the infectious agent or discontinuing the causal drug. Recurrent, herpes-associated cases may be treated with acyclovir, valacyclovir, or famciclovir.

L51.1 Stevens-Johnson syndrome

Stevens-Johnson syndrome (SJS) was previously thought to be synonymous with erythema multiforme major, but is now noted as a clinically distinct disorder. SJS is often caused by adverse drug reactions and also presents with similar mucosal erosions but widespread distribution of painful, blistering, flat, atypical, target-like cutaneous lesions or purpuric macules over the trunk, arms, legs, and face. There is also epidermal detachment as it progresses involving less than 10% body surface area. Ocular involvement includes conjunctival and corneal blisters, erosions, and corneal perforation. SJS is in the same disease spectrum as toxic epidermal necrolysis, but covering less body surface area.

Note: Stevens-Johnson syndrome, toxic epidermal necrolysis (TEN), and their overlap syndrome progress into skin sloughing from the body. Use an additional code to identify the percentage of skin exfoliation.

L51.2 Toxic epidermal necrolysis [Lyell]

Toxic epidermal necrolysis (TEN) is further along the same disease spectrum as Stevens-Johnson syndrome, involving significant sloughing of skin over 30% of the body surface area, resembling the skin loss that occurs with a severe burn. The treatment is also undertaken in a burn unit. There may also be mucositis and mucosal erosions.

Note: Stevens-Johnson syndrome, toxic epidermal necrolysis, and their overlap syndrome progress into skin sloughing from the body.

Note: Use an additional code to identify the percentage of skin exfoliation.

L51.3 Stevens-Johnson syndrome-toxic epidermal necrolysis overlap syndrome

This overlap syndrome is a clinically recognized condition between SJS and TEN that presents with an intermediate percentage of body surface area affected by epidermal detachment or skin sloughing (between 10 and 30

percent), also with related mucositis and mucosal erosion. SJS and TEN often result from adverse drug reactions.

Note: Use an additional code to identify the percentage of skin exfoliation.

L51.9 Erythema multiforme, unspecified

Erythema multiforme (EM) is an acute, self-limiting eruption marked by a distinctive, classical, target-appearing lesion. The presenting severity covers a wide spectrum. EM minor is a localized eruption with minimal or no mucosal involvement. It usually presents with mildly itchy, symmetrical, pink-red blotches with a ring around a pale center, starting on the extremities. Resolution happens within 10 days. EM major is a severe form that may be life-threatening. It involves mucous membrane erosions plus typical or raised target type lesions on the extremities and/or face, with epidermal detachment of less than 10% body surface. The etiology is not really known. A predisposing infection, particularly herpes simplex, but also bacterial and fungal infections, as well as drug reactions, commonly to sulfa and penicillin, have been implicated.

L52 Erythema nodosum

Erythema nodosum is an inflammatory skin disorder that involves flat, firm, warm, red, tender or painful nodules about an inch across under the skin. After a few days, the lesions turn purple, and then fade to brown after several weeks. The nodules commonly appear on the front of the lower legs but also on other areas such as the buttocks, thighs, calves, and ankles. Erythema nodosum usually resolves in about 6 weeks. The exact etiology is unknown, but is associated with many types of infections, common medicament sensitivities such as penicillins, and some underlying conditions such as leukemia, lymphoma, rheumatic fever, and ulcerative colitis.

L53 Other erythematous conditions

This category is used to report erythematous conditions, in which the skin becomes red due to the congestion of blood in the capillaries.

L53.0 Toxic erythema

Toxic erythema is a generalized eruption of the skin spread over a wide area of the body with redness, swelling, warmth, and /or blotchy red macules, papules, or pustules caused by an active systemic reaction to a toxic agent such as a drug, bacterial toxin, or other toxins that may be associated with a systemic disease. This pathologic reaction may occur in response to vasodilator or neurogenic chemicals associated with the toxin that precipitate dilation of blood vessels and increased blood flow. This condition usually occurs with a fever.

L53.1 Erythema annulare centrifugum

Erythema annulare centrifugum is a chronic, red, ring-shaped eruption of the skin that occurs at any age, most commonly on the upper and lower legs, and sometimes on the face, trunk, or arms. It usually begins as small, raised, pink spots that slowly enlarge into a ring-shaped lesion with a central area that flattens out and clears. The annular lesions enlarge a few millimeters a day and reach about 6-8 cm in diameter, although they may not form complete rings and be irregular shaped instead. Erythema annulare centrifugum has no specific cause and the lesions rarely cause any symptoms, but it is sometimes associated with an underlying disease or other factor such as bacterial, viral, or fungal infections, drugs like penicillin, chloroquine, and amitriptyline, chronic appendicitis, Grave's disease, obstructed bile ducts, and eating certain foods such as blue cheese. In these related cases, the rash usually resolves when the underlying disease is treated or ingestion of the offending food or drug is stopped. Histological findings that show perivascular lymphocytic infiltration help to diagnose erythema annulare centrifugum. The outbreak can last weeks to months and usually goes away on its own. There is no curative treatment, although topical corticosteroids can help relieve any itching, redness, and swelling.

Note: The classification of figurate, or gyrate, erythemas remains controversial with much ambiguity in medical literature. Erythema annulare centrifugum (EAC) is considered one of the figurate, or gyrate, erythemas but has grown to include several different histological and clinical variants.

L53.2   Erythema marginatum

Erythema marginatum is an uncommon skin rash occurring on the trunk and limbs that appears as slightly raised macular rings 0.5 cm -2.0 cm in diameter with a pale center, eventually becoming red or pink over time. The rash is superficial, nonpruritic, painless, and blanches under pressure. The rash can last minutes, hours, or weeks, and can recur frequently over many months in erythema marginatum perstans. The face, soles of the feet, and palms of the hands usually remain unaffected. This condition affects people of all ages and is generally considered to be a symptom indicating the presence of another underlying medical condition. Causes often linked with erythema marginatum include allergic reactions to drugs such as penicillin and chloroquine, pregnancy, bradykinin action and hereditary angioedema, malignancies like leukemia and lymphoma, glomerulonephritis, sepsis, and infections such as Candida albicans, E. coli, and Streptococcus pyogenes. Since erythema marginatum is not a disease in its own sense and usually remains rather asymptomatic, treatment mainly depends on diagnosing the patient and managing or curing the underlying disease or condition.

Note: The erythema marginatum rash is most often seen as a clinical feature indicating acute rheumatic fever. The presence of the rash, known as erythema marginatum rheumaticum, is used as a criterion for diagnosing rheumatic fever, and is also linked with myocarditis, polyarthritis, subcutaneous nodules, and Sydenham's chorea. In cases of erythema marginatum in (or due to) acute rheumatic fever, the condition itself is not coded, and rheumatic fever, code I00, is reported.

L53.3   Other chronic figurate erythema

Chronic figurate or gyrate erythemas are a group of skin disorders characterized by the erythematous eruption of ring-like or curved , pruritic or nonpruritic lesions that may be scaling or nonscaling with intense lymphohistiocytic behaviors and often unknown etiology. Their classification as to specifically identified types and inclusive types remains controversial with much ambiguity and controversy in medical literature. One other identified type of chronic figurate erythema is known as erythema gyratum repens. The circular rash spreads in bands over the body like waves, and has been likened to the striping of a zebra. The lesions spread very fast at nearly 1 cm per day with pronounced desquamation and itching. Lesions usually appear only on the trunk and extremities, although in a few cases hyperkeratosis of the palms has been noted. In a high percentage of cases, the rash is linked to an underlying malignancy, most frequently breast, lung, and esophageal cancers. Other cases have been associated with pregnancy, CREST syndrome, drug hypersensitivity, and tuberculosis while others are idiopathic. Histopathologic findings of perivascular lymphocytic infiltration in the deeper dermis aids in distinguishing erythema gyratum repens from other differential diagnoses. Treatment is aimed at the underlying condition and amelioration of intense pruritis.

L53.9   Erythematous condition, unspecified

Erythroderma that is not otherwise specified refers to what is usually an intense and widespread outbreak of an inflammatory skin disease with redness, swelling, and often scaling or peeling that involves a great percentage of skin surface area. The condition may be idiopathic erythroderma, also known as 'Red man syndrome'; a sign or symptom of another underlying condition or systemic disease; or it may occur as a widespread extension of some other pre-existing skin disorder. Erythroderma usually affects those over 40 years old and can develop rapidly with varying degrees of itching. There may be concomitant oozing and thick scaling that affects the scalp or palms of the hands and soles of the feet with keratoderma. The course of unspecified erythroderma, especially of unknown etiology, is unpredictable. Appropriate treatment of the skin condition itself may clear the skin, or it may persist for long periods and undergo times of acute exacerbation. Treating, removing, or correcting any known cause of an unspecified type of erythroderma may cure the skin disease.

L55   Sunburn

A sunburn is skin damage resulting from overexposure to the sun's ultraviolet rays. Skin type and age affect how easily a person will burn and how the skin reacts to sunlight. Individuals with fair or freckled skin, blue eyes, and red or blonde hair typically burn easily. Children under 6 and adults over 60 are also much more sensitive to solar radiation. Burns are classified based on the severity and level of cellular damage that has occurred.

L55.0   Sunburn of first degree

A sunburn is skin damage resulting from overexposure to the sun's ultraviolet rays. Most sunburns are first degree burns that produce skin redness, possible minor inflammation, and mild pain or discomfort, especially when touched, but do not produce blisters. First degree burns become dry and the skin peels as the burn heals, which usually takes about a week. They are superficial burns and affect only the outer layer of skin, the epidermis. First degree burns are treated with home care such as soaking the burned area in cold water, applying aloe vera gels or creams to soothe the skin, and taking ibuprofen or acetaminophen for pain relief.

L55.1   Sunburn of second degree

A sunburn is skin damage resulting from overexposure to the sun's ultraviolet rays. Second degree sunburns are marked by skin that is red and painful with inflammation and the eruption of fluid-filled blisters. The blisters may pop and ooze fluid onto the burn, giving it a wet appearance and exposing the burned area to an increased risk of infection. These burns are more serious than superficial burns as cellular damage extends beyond the top layer into the deeper skin layers, affecting nerve endings. Second degree burns may be treated with home care such as soaking the burned area in cold water, applying antibiotic creams, and taking over the counter pain medication. The open, weeping blisters may also require frequent bandaging to prevent infection. Second degree burns usually heal within three weeks; however, the worse the blistering appears, the longer the burn may take to heal. Burns that cover a large area may necessitate emergency medical care.

L55.2   Sunburn of third degree

A sunburn is skin damage resulting from overexposure to the sun's ultraviolet rays. Third degree sunburns are the worst with extensive damage. The usual signs of severely sunburned skin are extreme pain, redness, swelling, and severe blistering accompanied by symptoms of sun poisoning, which include nausea, chills, rapid heart rate, rapid breathing, and even dehydration and shock. Third degree burns associated with heat exhaustion or dehydration are a medical emergency. Treatment may consist of intravenous fluids with electrolytes, oral or intravenous antibiotics, wound dressing with antibiotic creams or ointments, pain medications, and possible skin grafting.

L56   Other acute skin changes due to ultraviolet radiation

This condition occurs when the patient has a hypersensitivity to sunlight. Acute skin changes range in severity. Some highly sensitive patients may experience symptoms after just seconds of sun exposure. Some skin products may aggravate this condition.

L56.0   Drug phototoxic response

Drug phototoxic response is an acute cutaneous disease that manifests as the result of combining a chemical with light. The chemical could be in a systemic medication taken orally or in a topically applied compound. Use of the chemical itself, or light exposure by itself, will not induce a reaction. The photoactivation of the chemical produces the skin condition. A drug phototoxic response can be difficult to distinguish from a drug photoallergic response, but it generally appears as an exaggerated sunburn with edema only on areas of skin that have been exposed to the sun. Vesicles and bullae often develop in severe cases, and sometimes pigment changes are noted. Phototoxicity often requires a larger amount of the chemical agent than an allergic response, and can appear within a few minutes of only one exposure with sufficient amounts of light and drug. A phototoxic reaction occurs because the photoactivated chemical compound induces direct damage to cell membranes and tissues, and sometimes even DNA. This is essentially an inflammatory response to reactive oxidative damage that appears as a sunburn. Symptom relief measures and avoidance of the causative agent is the recommended treatment.

L56.1 **Drug photoallergic response**

Drug photoallergic response is an acute cutaneous disease that manifests as the result of combining a chemical with light. The chemical could be in a systemic medication taken orally or in a topically applied compound. Use of the chemical itself, or light exposure by itself, will not induce a reaction. The photoactivation of the chemical produces the skin condition. A drug photoallergic response can be difficult to distinguish from a drug phototoxic response, but it generally appears as allergic contact dermatitis on sun-exposed skin, spreading into unexposed areas. In the acute phase, the reaction usually manifests as a pruritic eczematous eruption with vesicles, turning into redness, scaling, and lichenification with chronic exposure. Photoallergic responses develop only in a minority of people exposed to the compound and light, are less prevalent than phototoxic responses, and require a much smaller amount of the chemical agent. Photoallergic responses usually require more than one exposure to the agent and the response is often delayed 24-72 hours after sufficient exposure due to the fact that this is a cell-mediated immune response to the light-activated drug when it becomes a complete antigen after developing a metabolite that binds to certain proteins in the skin. Symptom relief measures and avoidance of the causative agent as well as any sun exposure is the recommended treatment.

L56.2 **Photocontact dermatitis**

Photocontact dermatitis is an uncommon, acute, cutaneous reaction that occurs when the active ingredients in cosmetics or other products such as sunscreen, fragrances, coal tar, insecticides, or disinfectants are applied to the skin and exposed to sunlight. The induced skin condition may be either phototoxic, causing direct damage to cells, tissue, and even DNA; or the skin reaction may be photoallergic, causing a cell-mediated immune response to the light-activated photosensitizing agent as an antigen. The clinical presentation of photocontact dermatitis varies depending upon the agent and the type of reaction—a toxic type generally appears rather quickly after exposure as a bad sunburn, while an allergic type generally appears within 24-48 hours as eczema in the exposed area. Another photosensitizing agent is found in some plants, such as lemons and bergamot lime. Contact with the plant, its juice or oil, followed by sun exposure causes a phototoxic reaction with blistering, swelling, and streaks of hyperpigmentation that later leave dark marks on the skin. Berloque dermatitis is named for this type of reaction that occurs with the application of eau de cologne containing oil of bergamot (with its phototoxic component, bergapten), followed by sunbathing. Symptom relief measures and avoidance of the causative agent and sun exposure is the recommended treatment.

L56.2 **Polymorphous light eruption**

Polymorphous light eruption is a type of itchy rash that appears with clusters of raised, tiny, red bumps in rough patches in those with a developed sensitivity to sunlight. The rash appears more often in spring and summer when an individual's sunlight exposure increases and tends to be in areas that are commonly covered throughout the winter and exposed in good weather, such as the arms, neck, and upper chest. Although the outbreaks lessen through the summer, hydrocortisone cream may need to be applied to manage disruptive outbreaks, or controlled light therapy may be used as treatment. Sunlight avoidance and/or liberal use of sunscreen is recommended. Polymorphic light eruption generally recurs every year after the sensitivity is developed once the rash appears.

L56.3 **Solar urticaria**

Solar urticaria is a rare type of benign, but persistent photodermatosis that produces wheals, or hives, with redness, stinging, and itching after a brief period of exposure to ultraviolet light or visible light with the appropriate wavelength. The condition can appear suddenly on both exposed skin and areas covered by light clothing, and may be accompanied by other symptoms such as nausea, vomiting, headaches, and respiratory spasms. The condition may disappear within a few hours if sun exposure is avoided. The condition is thought to be an immunoglobulin E hypersensitivity reaction to photoallergens. Treatment is unpredictable and involves the use of oral antihistamines to stop the outbreak of hives, and specific phototherapy or photochemotherapy for longer lasting tolerance to sunlight. The best management is avoidance of sun exposure.

L56.5 **Disseminated superficial actinic porokeratosis (DSAP)**

Disseminated superficial actinic porokeratosis (DSAP) is an inherited skin condition seen in people of European descent during the summer that causes dry patches of characteristic lesions on the skin due to solar radiation. The lesions typically begin as a small, colored papule around a hair follicle with a plug and then expand to a raised, well-defined, keratotic ring that spreads out with a thinned center and darkened ridge. The center may become very red or covered with a thick scale. The lesions most often appear on the lower arms and legs. Many patients with this condition have high levels of sun exposure and are at an elevated risk for developing actinic keratoses and other types of skin cancer. Various creams, oral medications, and phototherapies have been used without long-term efficacy. Cryotherapy may be applied to individual lesions with the use of moisturizer and the restriction of sun exposure.

L57.0 **Actinic keratosis**

Actinic keratosis, also known as solar keratosis and senile keratosis, is a type of pre-cancerous growth that appears as a rough, scaly, thick, or crusted patch of skin that may vary in reddish color and feel like a hard, warty surface. Actinic keratosis lesions usually develop in areas with years of sun exposure, most commonly on the face, ears, scalp, neck, and back of the hand in older adults. Early treatment can eliminate the lesion and prevent its progression into squamous cell carcinoma. Treatment consists of medications to be applied topically, such as fluorouracil and imiquimod cream, or ingenol or diclofenac gel, and photodynamic therapy in which the damaged skin cells are made sensitive to light with the application of a photosensitizing agent followed by exposure to intense laser light. Surgical removal with curettage or cryotherapy may also be done. Limiting time in the sun, using sunscreen, and wearing coverings such as broad brimmed hats and tight weave clothing is the best defense.

L57.1 **Actinic reticuloid**

Actinic reticuloid, also known as chronic actinic dermatitis, is actually considered a type of sun-induced pseudolymphoma from severe hypersensitivity to UVA and UVB radiation, and sometimes even artificial light. Actinic reticuloid most often affects middle-aged and elderly males. This is a severe, chronic, lymphocytic skin disease that resembles malignant T-cell lymphomas with spontaneously regressing changes. Actinic reticuloid appears with clinical variation, but usually as an eczematous, pruritic eruption on exposed areas like the head and neck. The eruption is often severely inflamed, itchy, red, and thickened or crusty, and can be provoked in as little as 30 seconds, even from sunlight coming through glass or light from fluorescent lamps. The lesions may spread to areas normally covered from light exposure. Non-cutaneous T-cell lymphoma has been documented as developing in the course of actinic reticuloid syndrome. Lifestyle changes for avoiding sunlight as well as contact allergens are necessary. Topical creams, oral immune suppressants, and even hospitalization in a dark room may be used. In some cases, the disease has resolved spontaneously, but usually remains a lifelong condition for most.

L57.2 **Cutis rhomboidalis nuchae**

Cutis rhomboidalis nuchae is a cutaneous condition affecting the back of the neck in which the skin becomes leathery and deeply wrinkled, or furrowed. The condition occurs with long-term, prolonged sun exposure that thickens the epidermis, or outermost layer of skin, while causing abnormalities in the dermis, or middle layer of skin. Cutis rhomboidalis nuchae does not require treatment, but is a sign of severe, long-term sun damage. Preventive measures are best and consist of using sunscreen, wearing a hat and other protective clothing, and avoiding intense, midday sun exposure.

L57.3 **Poikiloderma of Civatte**

Poikiloderma of Civatte is a benign condition mainly affecting the skin on the sides of the neck in women but sparing the shaded areas. Poikiloderma refers to skin changes composed of thinning, discoloration, and blood vessel dilation. The affected skin is reddish brown in a rash-like appearance with prominent hair follicles. The etiology is unclear, but it is known to occur with fair skin and cumulative exposure, as well as use of cosmetics with photosensitizing agents, and hormonal factors. There is no specific medical treatment.

L57.4   Cutis laxa senilis

Cutis laxa senilis, also known as elastosis senilis and elastolysis, is a rare connective tissue disease that causes the skin to lose its natural elasticity and hang in loose, pendulous folds. The elastic fibers in the skin degenerate and the skin then sags and stretches with no elastic recoil. The underlying molecular changes causing this are unknown; however, it has been linked to copper deficiency, both from defective utilization and low serum levels. The enzyme, lysyl oxidase, indispensible in the production of elastin and collagen, is copper dependent. Some inflammatory cells also release elastases which may damage the elastic fibers. Half of acquired cases are preceded by an eruption resembling eczema, erythema multiforme, urticaria, or reactions to penicillin. Intense skin inflammation and plaques recur in episodes with characteristic skin laxity following in the affected areas. Fever and malaise may accompany the inflammatory outbreaks. The face and neck are commonly involved first with downward progression of the disease. Since elastin is critical to lung function, pulmonary manifestation also typically occurs in the form of emphysema, which is the most common cause of death with the acquired form.

L57.5   Actinic granuloma

Actinic granuloma, also known as O'Brien granuloma, is a rare connective tissue disorder in which asymptomatic, ring-shaped plaques develop in areas of abnormal skin where the connective tissue has been broken down through long-term sun and heat exposure. This usually occurs in fair-skinned, middle aged adults. The plaques begin as pink papules or nodules that persist for years and slowly enlarge, merging together into larger, thickened, ring-shaped plaques from 1-10 cm in diameter. The lesions usually have a raised border and a pale, thinned center and are thought to be an inflammatory and repair response. Histopathology findings help in diagnosing actinic granuloma, which is difficult to distinguish from other granulomas and often confused with necrobiosis lipoidica, sarcoidosis, or granuloma annulare. Microscopic findings show infiltrates of foreign body giant cells such as macrophages in the process of engulfing and digesting the abnormal elastic fibers. There is still debate over classification of actinic granuloma as a specific condition or whether it is a variant of granuloma annulare located in sun-exposed areas.

L57.9   Skin changes due to chronic exposure to nonionizing radiation, unspecified

These skin changes usually occur in light-skinned people due to extensive exposure to the sun. Patients with this condition are at an elevated risk of developing skin cancer.

L58.0   Acute radiodermatitis

Acute radiodermatitis is acute skin damage occurring as a result of radiation exposure and experienced by up to 95% of radiation oncology patients. Injury to the skin includes localized erythema, edema, dry or moist desquamation or shedding with epilation (hair loss), and ulceration. Acute skin changes occur within 90 days of therapy due to DNA damage and cytokine-mediated inflammation, although erythema and swelling may be apparent within a few hours of treatment. Dry desquamation is associated with mild cases and is marked by blanchable erythema, epilation, scaling, pruritis, and pigment changes. It usually occurs within a few days or a week from damage to hair follicles and sebaceous glands, and typically resolves after a couple of weeks. Moist desquamation usually occurs after 4-5 weeks of therapy and is associated with moderate cases; it is marked by serous oozing from red, exposed skin in skin folds and is often painful with the presence of bullae. This occurs as basal cells are destroyed and dermis integrity is compromised, putting the patient at risk for staph infection. Severe cases spread to other areas of the skin and include painful ulcers, hemorrhaging, and even necrosis. Acute radiodermatitis often resolves within a few weeks of therapy, but requires careful monitoring for prevention of infection and help in healing. Treatment is based on the severity of symptoms, patient comfort, and the promotion of wound healing.

Note: Both The Radiation Therapy Oncology Group and The National Cancer Institute have established assessment tools for classifying acute radiodermatitis by severity using specific grade levels 1-4.

L58.1   Chronic radiodermatitis

Chronic radiodermatitis is long-term skin changes experienced by radiation oncology patients as a result of radiation exposure that develops months or years after treatment. Chronic radiodermatitis is due to permanent damage to the dermal layer. This is marked by fibrosis, epilation, telangiectasia, and atrophy in varying degrees. Severe, chronic radiodermatitis also involves ulceration. Treatment is based on the severity of symptoms, patient comfort, and the promotion of wound healing. There is widespread discrepancy in nursing interventions, prevention, and management of radiodermatitis as the efficacy of many treatments lacks sufficient evidence for standardized recommendations or protocols.

Note: Both The Radiation Therapy Oncology Group and The National Cancer Institute have established assessment tools for classifying chronic radiodermatitis by degrees of atrophy, telangiectasia, and presence of concomitant conditions using grade levels 1-4.

L59.0   Erythema ab igne [dermatitis ab igne]

Erythema ab igne is a skin condition marked by localized areas of redness in an interlacing or net-like pattern with hypermelanosis caused by prolonged, repeated exposure to heat lower than that which would cause a thermal burn. The lesion is seen on areas where heat sources such as hot water bottles, heating pads, and hot packs are repeatedly applied. Repeated exposure to heated car seats, infrared lamps, stoves, space heaters, open ovens, or fires will also produce dermatitis ab igne. Cases known as 'laptop thigh' occur in those who continually set the computer directly on their legs. Other cases appear when heat is repeatedly applied to lessen pain, which may be the only visible sign of an underlying condition such as splenomegaly, pancreatic cancer, or gastric disorders. Mild, blanchable erythema is initially present in a wide, lattice-like pattern. The classic reticulated pattern becomes fixed and nonblanchable with dusky, discolored skin that may be purple, brown, or blue with repeated exposure. The entire lesion usually approximates the size and shape of the heat source. Older lesions may become atrophic over the discoloration, or hyperkeratotic with bullae. Some patients experience mild itching and burning, but dermatitis ab igne normally remains asymptomatic. The duration of heat exposure necessary to cause cumulative damage to the skin can vary from months to years. Long-term risks include the development of squamous cell or Merkel cell carcinomas and reactive angiomatosis. No definitive therapy is in place. Eliminating exposure to the heat source in early cases may resolve the lesion.

L60.0   Ingrowing nail

An ingrown nail occurs when the sharp edge of a nail (usually a toenail) grows into the skin of the nail fold, causing pain and possible infection.

L63   Alopecia areata

Alopecia areata occurs when some of the hair on the head or body is lost in patches. The scalp may become inflamed. This condition usually goes away on its own, and the hair will grow back.

L65.0   Telogen effluvium

Telogen effluvium is a disorder in which hair loss is caused by stress, shock, surgery, or other psychically traumatic events. The hair usually grows back.

L68.0   Hirsutism

Hirsutism is generally defined as the abnormal growth of hair or excessive hairiness; however, the common clinical usage of the term refers to unwanted hair in a male pattern of growth on a female. Hirsutism causes excessive hair growth with stiff, pigmented hairs appearing on body areas where men typically grow hair—on the face, chest, and/or back. This may be a family trait with no identifiable cause as seen in some Mediterranean and Middle Eastern populations, or it may be due to a hormone imbalance when a higher than normal proportion of androgens is produced in a female. This can occur in conditions such as Cushing's syndrome, polycystic ovarian syndrome, and congenital adrenal hyperplasia. Medications have also been known to cause hirsutism, such as danazol used in treating endometriosis. Hirsutism can be more than a cosmetic problem, inducing mental and emotional anguish. Diagnosis aims at determining etiology to rule out any significant underlying disease. Idiopathic hirsutism and cases caused by less serious underlying conditions generally begin at puberty. Hirsutism that begins later in life, or accelerates rapidly may be a sign of an adrenal or ovarian tumor. Diagnostic evaluation also includes quantitating the disorder based on the amount of terminal hair in androgen-sensitive body areas such as the upper lip, chin, chest, thigh, forearm, upper back, and upper abdomen. Terminal hair is course, curly, and pigmented and is dependent on the production of androgen. Quantitating terminal hair as well as other signs of hyperandrogenism gives an idea of the amount of overproduction occurring and the degree of concern for other, more serious conditions. Intervention is aimed at the underlying disorder. Systemic therapies may be used to decrease ovarian or adrenal hormone production, or inhibit the action of androgen in the skin. In some cases, cosmetic measures alone are sufficient, such as plucking, waxing, bleaching, or laser hair removal.

L68.1 Acquired hypertrichosis lanuginosa

Acquired hypertrichosis lanuginosa is a rare, cutaneous, paraneoplastic disease marked by rapid growth of long, fine, unpigmented lanugo-type hair, particularly on the face. This type of hair growth is also known as 'malignant down.' The name derives from lanugo hairs present in the 3rd month of fetal life to the end of gestation that are shed before birth. This condition is a marker for internal malignancy, such as breast, lung, uterine, colon, or bladder cancer, often occurring later in the course of the cancer, as with metastatic progression of the disease. The mechanism is unknown, but it is thought to be a response to substances released by the tumor. Acquired hypertrichosis lanuginosa is also associated with other signs and symptoms like glossitis with a burning sensation and papillary hypertrophy, lymphadenopathy, diarrhea, weight loss, and disturbances in taste and smell. It will often disappear with removal or regression of the primary tumor and reappear with local or metastatic recurrence. Treatment is directed at the underlying malignancy, but in these cases, acquired hypertrichosis lanuginosa is associated with a poor prognosis.

L68.2 Localized hypertrichosis

Localized hypertrichosis is an excess of vellus hair within a specific body area. Vellus hair is fine, soft, and lightly pigmented and its growth is not dependent upon the production of the male hormone, androgen. Hypertrichosis is usually idiopathic but is also caused by metabolic disorders such as anorexia nervosa, hyperthyroidism, and porphyria. Medications such as glucocorticoids, cyclosporine, phenytoin, minoxidil, diazoxide, and hexachlorobenzene have also been associated with hypertrichosis. Acquired localized hypertrichosis (ALH) is associated with reflex sympathetic dystrophy cases following trauma or surgery such as fracture fixation, and is also found to result from friction, chronic irritation, inflammation, and particularly with occlusion as the application of plaster casts. This is thought to correlate with vasodilation and increased blood supply with its concomitant abundance in oxygen and nutrients to the area involved, which stimulates hair growth. ALH is benign and usually transient, clearly up spontaneously.

L70 Acne

Acne is a common skin condition that occurs when hair follicles become clogged with oil and dead skin cells. Non-inflammatory acne lesions are called comedones and may appear black or white. Inflammatory acne lesions include papules, pustules, or pimples (small, red, pus filled bumps), nodules (large solid lumps), and cysts (large, painful, pus filled lumps).

L70.2 Acne varioliformis

Acne varioliformis is a rare form of acne that causes the formation of lesions on the brow and scalp. These lesions can leave scars.

L71.9 Rosacea, unspecified

Rosacea is a chronic skin condition that affects the middle third of the face. The skin reddens as the capillaries in the face dilate, and pimples often appear as well.

L72.11 Pilar cyst

Pilar cysts are a common type of epidermal cyst with an outer wall of keratinizing epithelium derived from the outer hair root sheath, or trichilemma, of the follicle. The squamous epithelium undergoes rapid keratinization to form the cyst wall. More than 90% occur on the scalp where the densest population of hair follicles is and they are the second most common type appearing on the scalp and neck. They appear more often in women in middle age. Pilar cysts are benign and can occur sporadically or as inherited. They are solitary 30% of the time. Pilar cysts present as smooth, asymptomatic swellings that move, sometimes with overlying hair loss, and the contents, which contain keratin and the byproducts of its breakdown, can ooze out to form a soft, cutaneous layer. In 2% of pilar cysts, a proliferating group of cells leads to tumors, called trichilemmal proliferating cysts.

L72.12 Trichodermal cyst

Trichodermal or trichilemmal proliferating cysts arise out of pilar cysts becoming proliferating tumors that grow very rapidly. They may also arise as the first occurrence of these type of cysts, which are derived from the outer root sheath of the deeper parts of a hair follicle forming a keratinized epidermal wall enclosing semi-solid hair keratin. They become aggressive locally, proliferating and becoming large and ulcerated, even though they are most often benign. They rarely become malignant. They can rupture, exacerbating local inflammation, and discharge may occur. Treatment is with surgical excision.

L74.0 Miliaria rubra

Also called prickly heat, miliaria rubra is an inflammatory skin condition caused by obstruction of the sweat glands. The resultant rash resembles a small cluster of red pimples on the skin. Also known as heat rash, this disorder occurs most often in hot, humid climates.

L74.4 Anhidrosis

Anhidrosis is a condition in which the body lacks the ability to sweat, which results in overheating in high temperatures or during exertion.

L75.2 Apocrine miliaria

Fox-Fordyce disease is a disorder of the sweat ducts which causes small blisters to form around the pubic area, nipples, chest, and armpits. This condition is chronic, and occurs chiefly in women.

L82 Seborrheic keratosis

A common form of noncancerous skin lesion found in older adults and with long term exposure to sun. The color ranges from dark brown or black to pale tan. The growths are almost barnacle-like with a slightly raised appearance, rounded or oval in shape, and a scaly or flaky surface. Seborrheic keratosis can look like melanomas or warts, but they only involve the top layer of epidermis and there is no viral involvement. They most commonly appear on areas with the greatest sun exposure, such as the head, face, and neck, but also on the shoulders, chest, and back. The lesions are normally painless and require no treatment, but may be removed for cosmetic reasons.

Note: This includes Leser-Trelat disease or sign, which is the eruption of multiple seborrheic keratoses in association with an internal malignancy, which is most usually noted with an adenocarcinoma of the digestive tract.

L82.0 Inflamed seborrheic keratosis

Seborrheic keratosis growths are normally painless and asymptomatic, but the growths may itch, rub or catch on clothing, or otherwise become irritated and inflamed, and even bleed.

L82.1 Other seborrheic keratosis

A very common type of noncancerous skin lesion affecting older adults and caused by long periods of exposure to the sun. The lesions are almost barnacle-like, having a black, brown, or pale appearance that is slightly elevated with a waxy, crusty, or scaly top, turning into hard granular crusts in later stages.

L83 Acanthosis nigricans

Acquired acanthosis nigricans is a condition in which the skin thickens abnormally and dark, wart-like skin patches develop in the body folds. This condition is typically benign in children, but can be a sign of one or more malignant tumors in adults.

L84   Corns and callosities

Corns are horny thickened patches of skin of the feet and toes due to friction with footwear. They may become inflamed. Callosities (more commonly called calluses) are overgrowths of the thick layer of skin on the soles of the feet or palms of the hands, etc., due to friction.

L85.8   Other specified epidermal thickening

Other specified epidermal thickening includes conditions such as cornu cutaneum, keratosis pilaris, dyskeratosis, arsenical keratosis, and keratoacanthoma. Keratosis pilaris is a common skin condition affecting any age, but most often those under 30. Rough, dry patches with small, red or white bumps form on the upper arms, thighs, buttocks, or cheeks. The rough areas may be itchy and tend to worsen in winter. Some cases are only individual, sandpaper-like bumps similar to goose flesh. Keratosis pilaris usually resolves on its own and requires no treatment although the bumps may become inflamed. Cornu cutaneum, or a cutaneous horn, is an uncommon type of tumor in the unusual shape of a horn or a cone protruding from the skin surface. The growth is composed of keratin and appears on sun-exposed skin in the elderly. Different underlying processes cause the lesion growth, most of which are benign, but may also be premalignant or malignant in nature due to an actinic keratosis or squamous cell carcinoma base. Most can be removed by shaving technique with electrodesiccation of the base. Keratoacanthoma is a common, low-grade skin cancer erupting at an injury site in sun damaged skin containing hair follicles. It resembles a small volcano and may begin like a small boil with a solid keratin-filled core. Keratoacanthoma grows rapidly and may shrink and resolve by itself after a couple of months, although most are removed surgically as it can be difficult to discern from more serious forms of cancer.

L88   Pyoderma gangrenosum

Pyoderma gangenosum is a rare type of ulcerating skin disease that is connected with another underlying systemic disease such as rheumatoid arthritis, inflammatory bowel disease, and hematological disorders in at least half of patients afflicted. The etiology is unclear, but appears to be related to immune system misregulation that alters neutrophilic chemotaxis and causes the skin to become infiltrated by sterile neutrophils. The initial lesion presents similar to a spider bite with a small, red pustule that turns into an ulcerative lesion. Other organs and tissues, particularly the lungs, may also manifest with neutrophilic infiltration. The disease occurs in both sexes of all ages, although predominantly in adults between 40-60 years of age. Treatment consists of antibiotics, anti-inflammatories like corticosteroids and immunosuppressive agents, other biologic agents, and narcotics for pain. Most patients improve with immunosuppressive therapy. Others require multiple therapies and long term care. The disease has the tendency to recur at sites of skin trauma and can make wound healing after surgical care difficult.

L89   Pressure ulcer

A decubitus ulcer, commonly known as a bedsore or pressure ulcer, is a type of ulcer that typically occurs over the bony projections in a patient who is bedridden for a significant length of time due to lack of circulation and oxygenation to the affected tissue. Pressure ulcers occurs particularly at the hips, heels, shoulders, and similar areas where there is not much cushioning. Bedsores frequently affect more than one body part at a time, grow quickly, and can easily become infected.

The depth of the lesion is directly related to healing, burden of care, risk of severe ulcer onset, and the amount of suffering. The staging of ulcers follows descriptive guidelines of the lesion: An unstageable ulcer may be due to the fact that dressings cannot be removed or due to the presence of a sterile blister or eschar that makes the ulcer inaccessible at present for staging.

Stage I is considered a superficial lesion with discoloration of the skin, but the lesion is not actually an ulcer at this point. It presents as a non-blanching reddened area on the skin. Stage I indicates a higher risk for

serious pressure ulcer but does not cause much suffering or increased treatment burden.

Stage II is a superficial injury presenting as a blister, abrasion, shallow open crater, or some type of partial thickness skin loss that does not extend through the skin. Detection at this stage is reliable, the treatment level is moderate, and direct suffering is limited.

Stage III is the level of serious pressure ulcers with full thickness skin loss and damage or necrosis that extends into subcutaneous soft tissues. Extensive treatment and direct suffering are involved at this stage.

Stage IV involves full thickness skin loss, also with necrosis, as in stage III, but extending through the soft tissue into underlying muscle, tendon, or bone.

Note: Code any gangrene that is presently associated with the ulcer first.

L89.15   Pressure ulcer of sacral region

Note: The sacral region includes the coccyx, or tailbone area.

L90.6   Striae atrophicae

Striae atrophicae are stretch marks in the skin that occur during pregnancy, obesity, or rapid growth during puberty.

L92.3   Foreign body granuloma of the skin and subcutaneous tissue

A foreign body becomes lodged in the skin, leading to the formation of a granuloma, which is comprised of tumorous cells surrounded by a mass of white blood cells called lymphocytes, forming one or more small nodules.

L93   Lupus erythematosus

Lupus erythematosus constitutes a group of autoimmune disorders that target the body's connective tissue. The patient will typically present with a scaly rash on the face and head, as well as a fever.

L94.6   Ainhum

Ainhum is the spontaneous amputation of a digit, usually the fifth toe. Typically, this occurs to males living in tropical climates who do not wear shoes.

L97   Non-pressure chronic ulcer of lower limb, not elsewhere classified

This category is used to report other types of chronic, nonhealing ulcers of the skin of the lower limb besides decubitus or pressure ulcers. Other types of nonhealing chronic ulcers may occur due to circulatory disorders, atherosclerosis, and diabetic complications.

Note: The associated underlying condition must be coded before the ulcer, such as atherosclerosis of the lower extremity, postphlebitic or postthrombotic syndrome, diabetes ulcers, gangrene, chronic hypertension, and varicose ulcers.

L98.1   Factitial dermatitis

Dermatitis factitia are self-inflected skin lesions, typically caused by scratching.

M00   Pyogenic arthritis

Pyogenic arthritis, sometimes called septic arthritis, is caused by a bacterial infection that invades one particular joint, or spreads throughout the body, affecting multiple joints. In some cases, septic arthritis will be due to an injection or wound infection in close proximity to a joint. Pyogenic arthritis normally affects only one joint, most commonly the knee or hip. It presents with severe pain and swelling in the affected joint, which may be warm to the touch and accompanied by chills and fever. Children often experience vomiting. It can usually be treated with antibiotics and arthrocentesis.

Diseases of the Musculoskeletal System and Connective Tissue | M00-M99

M00.00 Staphylococcal arthritis, unspecified joint

Staphylococcal arthritis is the most common caused of septic, or pyogenic, arthritis, as staphylococcal bacteria can be found even on healthy skin. Since the synovial lining of joints cannot defend well from invading microorganisms, the joint's reaction to a staphylococcal infection produces inflammation, swelling, and effusion that increases pressure within the affected joint while reducing blood flow at the same time. Staphylococcal septic arthritis causes extreme pain and difficulty moving the affected joint. Arthrocentesis and rapid antibiotic treatment are necessary to prevent permanent joint damage and degeneration of joint tissue.

M00.01 Staphylococcal arthritis, shoulder

Staphylococcal arthritis is the most common caused of septic, or pyogenic, arthritis, as staphylococcal bacteria can be found even on healthy skin. Since the synovial lining of joints cannot defend well from invading microorganisms, the joint's reaction to a staphylococcal infection produces inflammation, swelling, and effusion that increases pressure within the affected joint while reducing blood flow at the same time. Staphylococcal septic arthritis of the shoulder causes extreme pain and difficulty when moving the shoulder. Arthrocentesis and rapid antibiotic treatment are necessary to prevent permanent joint damage and degeneration of joint tissue.

M00.02 Staphylococcal arthritis, elbow

Staphylococcal arthritis is the most common caused of septic, or pyogenic, arthritis, as staphylococcal bacteria can be found even on healthy skin. Since the synovial lining of joints cannot defend well from invading microorganisms, the joint's reaction to a staphylococcal infection produces inflammation, swelling, and effusion that increases pressure within the affected joint while reducing blood flow at the same time. Staphylococcal septic arthritis of the elbow causes extreme pain and difficulty when moving the elbow. Arthrocentesis and rapid antibiotic treatment are necessary to prevent permanent joint damage and degeneration of joint tissue.

M00.03 Staphylococcal arthritis, wrist

Staphylococcal arthritis is the most common caused of septic, or pyogenic, arthritis, as staphylococcal bacteria can be found even on healthy skin. Since the synovial lining of joints cannot defend well from invading microorganisms, the joint's reaction to a staphylococcal infection produces inflammation, swelling, and effusion that increases pressure within the affected joint while reducing blood flow at the same time. Staphylococcal septic arthritis of the wrist causes extreme pain and difficulty when moving the wrist. Arthrocentesis and rapid antibiotic treatment are necessary to prevent permanent joint damage and degeneration of joint tissue.

M00.04 Staphylococcal arthritis, hand

Staphylococcal arthritis is the most common caused of septic, or pyogenic, arthritis, as staphylococcal bacteria can be found even on healthy skin. Since the synovial lining of joints cannot defend well from invading microorganisms, the joint's reaction to a staphylococcal infection produces inflammation, swelling, and effusion that increases pressure within the affected joint while reducing blood flow at the same time. Staphylococcal septic arthritis of the hand causes extreme pain and difficulty when moving the hand. Arthrocentesis and rapid antibiotic treatment are necessary to prevent permanent joint damage and degeneration of joint tissue.

M00.05 Staphylococcal arthritis, hip

Staphylococcal arthritis is the most common caused of septic, or pyogenic, arthritis, as staphylococcal bacteria can be found even on healthy skin. Since the synovial lining of joints cannot defend well from invading microorganisms, the joint's reaction to a staphylococcal infection produces inflammation, swelling, and effusion that increases pressure within the affected joint while reducing blood flow at the same time. Staphylococcal septic arthritis of the hip causes extreme pain and difficulty when moving the hip. Arthrocentesis and rapid antibiotic treatment are necessary to prevent permanent joint damage and degeneration of joint tissue.

M00.06 Staphylococcal arthritis, knee

Staphylococcal arthritis is the most common caused of septic, or pyogenic, arthritis, as staphylococcal bacteria can be found even on healthy skin. Since the synovial lining of joints cannot defend well from invading microorganisms, the joint's reaction to a staphylococcal infection produces inflammation, swelling, and effusion that increases pressure within the affected joint while reducing blood flow at the same time. Staphylococcal septic arthritis of the knee causes extreme pain and difficulty when moving the knee. Arthrocentesis and rapid antibiotic treatment are necessary to prevent permanent joint damage and degeneration of joint tissue.

M00.07 Staphylococcal arthritis, ankle and foot

Staphylococcal arthritis is the most common caused of septic, or pyogenic, arthritis, as staphylococcal bacteria can be found even on healthy skin. Since the synovial lining of joints cannot defend well from invading microorganisms, the joint's reaction to a staphylococcal infection produces inflammation, swelling, and effusion that increases pressure within the affected joint while reducing blood flow at the same time. Staphylococcal septic arthritis of the ankle or foot causes extreme pain and difficulty when moving the ankle or foot. Arthrocentesis and rapid antibiotic treatment are necessary to prevent permanent joint damage and degeneration of joint tissue.

M00.08 Staphylococcal arthritis, vertebrae

Staphylococcal arthritis is the most common caused of septic, or pyogenic, arthritis, as staphylococcal bacteria can be found even on healthy skin. Since the synovial lining of joints cannot defend well from invading microorganisms, the joint's reaction to a staphylococcal infection produces inflammation, swelling, and effusion that increases pressure within the affected joint while reducing blood flow at the same time. Staphylococcal septic arthritis of the vertebrae causes extreme pain and difficult movement in the back. Arthrocentesis and rapid antibiotic treatment are necessary to prevent permanent joint damage and degeneration of joint tissue.

M00.09 Staphylococcal polyarthritis

Staphylococcal polyarthritis is the most common caused of septic, or pyogenic, polyarthritis as staphylococcal bacteria can be found even on healthy skin. Since the synovial lining of joints cannot defend well from invading microorganisms, the joints' reaction to a staphylococcal infection produces inflammation, swelling, and effusion that increases pressure within the affected joints while reducing blood flow at the same time. Staphylococcal septic polyarthritis causes extreme pain and difficult movement in multiple joints at the same time, usually from an internal infection that spreads throughout the body. Arthrocentesis and rapid antibiotic treatment are necessary to prevent permanent joint damage and degeneration of joint tissue.

M00.10 Pneumococcal arthritis, unspecified joint

Pneumococcal arthritis is caused by the bacterium *Streptococcus pneumoniae*. This is a less common type of pyogenic arthritis. Most patients also have some type of underlying medical condition or risk factor, such as rheumatoid arthritis or extra-articular pneumococcal infection, such as pneumonia. Since the synovial lining of joints cannot defend well from invading microorganisms, the joint's reaction to a pneumococcal infection produces inflammation, swelling, and effusion that increases pressure within the affected joint while reducing blood flow at the same time. This can lead to permanent joint damage and degeneration. Pneumoococcal septic arthritis causes extreme pain and difficulty moving the affected joint. Uncomplicated cases can often be treated with arthrocentesis and many weeks of antibiotic treatment.

M00.11 Pneumococcal arthritis, shoulder

Pneumococcal arthritis is caused by the bacterium *Streptococcus pneumoniae*. This is a less common type of pyogenic arthritis. Most patients also have some type of underlying medical condition or risk factor, such as rheumatoid arthritis or extra-articular pneumococcal infection, such as pneumonia. Since the synovial lining of joints cannot defend well from invading microorganisms, the joint's reaction to a pneumococcal infection produces inflammation, swelling, and effusion that increases pressure within the affected joint while reducing blood flow at the same time. This can lead to permanent joint damage and degeneration. Pneumoococcal septic arthritis of the shoulder causes extreme pain and difficulty moving the shoulder. Uncomplicated cases can often be treated with arthrocentesis and many weeks of antibiotic treatment.

M00.12 Pneumococcal arthritis, elbow

Pneumococcal arthritis is caused by the bacterium *Streptococcus pneumoniae*. This is a less common type of pyogenic arthritis. Most patients also have some type of underlying medical condition or risk factor, such as rheumatoid arthritis or extra-articular pneumococcal infection, such as pneumonia. Since the synovial lining of joints cannot defend well from invading microorganisms, the joint's reaction to a pneumococcal infection produces inflammation, swelling, and effusion that increases pressure within the affected joint while reducing blood flow at the same time. This can lead to permanent joint damage and degeneration. Pneumoococcal septic arthritis of the elbow causes extreme pain and difficulty moving elbow. Uncomplicated cases can often be treated with arthrocentesis and many weeks of antibiotic treatment.

M00.13 Pneumococcal arthritis, wrist

Pneumococcal arthritis is caused by the bacterium *Streptococcus pneumoniae*. This is a less common type of pyogenic arthritis. Most patients also have some type of underlying medical condition or risk factor, such as rheumatoid arthritis or extra-articular pneumococcal infection, such as pneumonia. Since the synovial lining of joints cannot defend well from invading microorganisms, the joint's reaction to a pneumococcal infection produces inflammation, swelling, and effusion that increases pressure within the affected joint while reducing blood flow at the same time. This can lead to permanent joint damage and degeneration. Pneumoococcal septic arthritis of the wrist causes extreme pain and difficulty moving the wrist. Uncomplicated cases can often be treated with arthrocentesis and many weeks of antibiotic treatment.

M00.14 Pneumococcal arthritis, hand

Pneumococcal arthritis is caused by the bacterium *Streptococcus pneumoniae*. This is a less common type of pyogenic arthritis. Most patients also have some type of underlying medical condition or risk factor, such as rheumatoid arthritis or extra-articular pneumococcal infection, such as pneumonia. Since the synovial lining of joints cannot defend well from invading microorganisms, the joint's reaction to a pneumococcal infection produces inflammation, swelling, and effusion that increases pressure within the affected joint while reducing blood flow at the same time. This can lead to permanent joint damage and degeneration. Pneumoococcal septic arthritis of the hand causes extreme pain and difficulty moving the hand. Uncomplicated cases can often be treated with arthrocentesis and many weeks of antibiotic treatment.

M00.15 Pneumococcal arthritis, hip

Pneumococcal arthritis is caused by the bacterium *Streptococcus pneumoniae*. This is a less common type of pyogenic arthritis. Most patients also have some type of underlying medical condition or risk factor, such as rheumatoid arthritis or extra-articular pneumococcal infection, such as pneumonia. Since the synovial lining of joints cannot defend well from invading microorganisms, the joint's reaction to a pneumococcal infection produces inflammation, swelling, and effusion that increases pressure within the affected joint while reducing blood flow at the same time. This

can lead to permanent joint damage and degeneration. Pneumoococcal septic arthritis of the hip causes extreme pain and difficulty moving the hip. Uncomplicated cases can often be treated with arthrocentesis and many weeks of antibiotic treatment.

M00.16 Pneumococcal arthritis, knee

Pneumococcal arthritis is caused by the bacterium *Streptococcus pneumoniae*. This is a less common type of pyogenic arthritis. Most patients also have some type of underlying medical condition or risk factor, such as rheumatoid arthritis or extra-articular pneumococcal infection, such as pneumonia. Since the synovial lining of joints cannot defend well from invading microorganisms, the joint's reaction to a pneumococcal infection produces inflammation, swelling, and effusion that increases pressure within the affected joint while reducing blood flow at the same time. This can lead to permanent joint damage and degeneration. Pneumoococcal septic arthritis of the knee causes extreme pain and difficulty moving the knee. Uncomplicated cases can often be treated with arthrocentesis and many weeks of antibiotic treatment.

M00.17 Pneumococcal arthritis, ankle and foot

Pneumococcal arthritis is caused by the bacterium *Streptococcus pneumoniae*. This is a less common type of pyogenic arthritis. Most patients also have some type of underlying medical condition or risk factor, such as rheumatoid arthritis or extra-articular pneumococcal infection, such as pneumonia. Since the synovial lining of joints cannot defend well from invading microorganisms, the joint's reaction to a pneumococcal infection produces inflammation, swelling, and effusion that increases pressure within the affected joint while reducing blood flow at the same time. This can lead to permanent joint damage and degeneration. Pneumoococcal septic arthritis of the ankle or foot causes extreme pain and difficulty moving the ankle or foot. Uncomplicated cases can often be treated with arthrocentesis and many weeks of antibiotic treatment.

M00.18 Pneumococcal arthritis, vertebrae

Pneumococcal arthritis is caused by the bacterium *Streptococcus pneumoniae*. This is a less common type of pyogenic arthritis. Most patients also have some type of underlying medical condition or risk factor, such as rheumatoid arthritis or extra-articular pneumococcal infection, such as pneumonia. Since the synovial lining of joints cannot defend well from invading microorganisms, the joint's reaction to a pneumococcal infection produces inflammation, swelling, and effusion that increases pressure within the affected joint while reducing blood flow at the same time. This can lead to permanent joint damage and degeneration. Pneumoococcal septic arthritis of the vertebrae causes extreme pain and difficulty in moving the back. Uncomplicated cases can often be treated with arthrocentesis and many weeks of antibiotic treatment.

M00.19 Pneumococcal polyarthritis

Pneumococcal polyarthritis is caused by the bacterium *Streptococcus pneumoniae*. This is a less common type of pyogenic polyarthritis with most patients having some type of underlying medical condition or risk factor, such as rheumatoid arthritis, or other pneumococcal infection, like pneumonia or bacteremia. Since the synovial lining of joints cannot defend well from invading microorganisms, the joints' reaction to a pneumococcal infection produces inflammation, swelling, and effusion that increases pressure within the affected joints and reduces blood flow. Pneumoococcal polyarthritis causes extreme pain and difficult movement in multiple joints at the same time and can lead to permanent joint damage and degeneration without prompt treatment. Over half the cases of pneumococcal polyarthritis will have involvement of at least one knee.

M00.20 Other streptococcal arthritis, unspecified joint

Other streptococcal arthritis includes cases of pyogenic arthritis caused by streptococcal bacteria other than *Streptococcus pneumoniae*, such as group A, group B, and enterococcus. Most patients also have some type of underlying comorbidity or risk factor, such as rheumatoid arthritis, diabetes, or carcinoma, or are receiving immunosuppressive therapy. Since the synovial lining of joints cannot defend well from invading microorganisms, the joint's reaction to a streptococcal infection produces inflammation, swelling, and effusion that increases pressure and reduces blood flow within the affected joint. This causes extreme pain and difficulty moving the joint and can lead to permanent joint damage and degeneration. Group B streptococcal arthritis in particular, can be devastating and must be treated promptly with arthrocentesis and antibiotics. Delaying treatment even for a few days can result in significant morbidity risk.

M00.21   Other streptococcal arthritis, shoulder

Other streptococcal arthritis includes cases of pyogenic arthritis caused by streptococcal bacteria other than *Streptococcus pneumoniae*, such as group A, group B, and enterococcus. Most patients also have some type of underlying comorbidity or risk factor, such as rheumatoid arthritis, diabetes, or carcinoma, or are receiving immunosuppressive therapy. Since the synovial lining of joints cannot defend well from invading microorganisms, the joint's reaction to a streptococcal infection produces inflammation, swelling, and effusion that increases pressure and reduces blood flow at the same time. This can lead to permanent joint damage and degeneration. Septic streptococcal arthritis of the shoulder causes extreme pain and difficulty moving the shoulder. Group B streptococcal arthritis in particular, can be devastating and must be treated promptly with arthrocentesis and antibiotics. Delaying treatment even for a few days can result in significant morbidity risk.

M00.22   Other streptococcal arthritis, elbow

Other streptococcal arthritis includes cases of pyogenic arthritis caused by streptococcal bacteria other than *Streptococcus pneumoniae*, such as group A, group B, and enterococcus. Most patients also have some type of underlying comorbidity or risk factor, such as rheumatoid arthritis, diabetes, or carcinoma, or are receiving immunosuppressive therapy. Since the synovial lining of joints cannot defend well from invading microorganisms, the joint's reaction to a streptococcal infection produces inflammation, swelling, and effusion that increases pressure and reduces blood flow at the same time. This can lead to permanent joint damage and degeneration. Septic streptococcal arthritis of the elbow causes extreme pain and difficulty moving the elbow. Group B streptococcal arthritis in particular, can be devastating and must be treated promptly with arthrocentesis and antibiotics. Delaying treatment even for a few days can result in significant morbidity risk.

M00.23   Other streptococcal arthritis, wrist

Other streptococcal arthritis includes cases of pyogenic arthritis caused by streptococcal bacteria other than *Streptococcus pneumoniae*, such as group A, group B, and enterococcus. Most patients also have some type of underlying comorbidity or risk factor, such as rheumatoid arthritis, diabetes, or carcinoma, or are receiving immunosuppressive therapy. Since the synovial lining of joints cannot defend well from invading microorganisms, the joint's reaction to a streptococcal infection produces inflammation, swelling, and effusion that increases pressure and reduces blood flow at the same time. This can lead to permanent joint damage and degeneration. Septic streptococcal arthritis of the wrist causes extreme pain and difficulty moving the wrist. Group B streptococcal arthritis in particular, can be devastating and must be treated promptly with arthrocentesis and antibiotics. Delaying treatment even for a few days can result in significant morbidity risk.

M00.24   Other streptococcal arthritis, hand

Other streptococcal arthritis includes cases of pyogenic arthritis caused by streptococcal bacteria other than *Streptococcus pneumoniae*, such as group A, group B, and enterococcus. Most patients also have some type of underlying comorbidity or risk factor, such as rheumatoid arthritis, diabetes, or carcinoma, or are receiving immunosuppressive therapy. Since the synovial lining of joints cannot defend well from invading microorganisms, the joint's reaction to a streptococcal infection produces inflammation, swelling, and effusion that increases pressure and reduces blood flow at the same time. This can lead to permanent joint damage and degeneration. Septic streptococcal arthritis of the hand causes extreme pain and difficulty moving the hand. Group B streptococcal arthritis in particular, can be devastating and must be treated promptly with arthrocentesis and antibiotics. Delaying treatment even for a few days can result in significant morbidity risk.

M00.25   Other streptococcal arthritis, hip

Other streptococcal arthritis includes cases of pyogenic arthritis caused by streptococcal bacteria other than *Streptococcus pneumoniae*, such as group A, group B, and enterococcus. Most patients also have some type of underlying comorbidity or risk factor, such as rheumatoid arthritis, diabetes, or carcinoma, or are receiving immunosuppressive therapy. Since the synovial lining of joints cannot defend well from invading microorganisms, the joint's reaction to a streptococcal infection produces inflammation, swelling, and effusion that increases pressure and reduces blood flow at the same time. This can lead to permanent joint damage and degeneration. Septic streptococcal arthritis of the hip causes extreme pain and difficulty moving the hip. Group B streptococcal arthritis in particular, can be devastating and must be treated promptly with arthrocentesis and antibiotics. Delaying treatment even for a few days can result in significant morbidity risk.

M00.26   Other streptococcal arthritis, knee

Other streptococcal arthritis includes cases of pyogenic arthritis caused by streptococcal bacteria other than *Streptococcus pneumoniae*, such as group A, group B, and enterococcus. Most patients also have some type of underlying comorbidity or risk factor, such as rheumatoid arthritis, diabetes, or carcinoma, or are receiving immunosuppressive therapy. Since the synovial lining of joints cannot defend well from invading microorganisms, the joint's reaction to a streptococcal infection produces inflammation, swelling, and effusion that increases pressure and reduces blood flow at the same time. This can lead to permanent joint damage and degeneration. Septic streptococcal arthritis of the knee causes extreme pain and difficulty moving the knee. Group B streptococcal arthritis in particular, can be devastating and must be treated promptly with arthrocentesis and antibiotics. Delaying treatment even for a few days can result in significant morbidity risk.

M00.27   Other streptococcal arthritis, ankle and foot

Other streptococcal arthritis includes cases of pyogenic arthritis caused by streptococcal bacteria other than *Streptococcus pneumoniae*, such as group A, group B, and enterococcus. Most patients also have some type of underlying comorbidity or risk factor, such as rheumatoid arthritis, diabetes, or carcinoma, or are receiving immunosuppressive therapy. Since the synovial lining of joints cannot defend well from invading microorganisms, the joint's reaction to a streptococcal infection produces inflammation, swelling, and effusion that increases pressure and reduces blood flow at the same time. This can lead to permanent joint damage and degeneration. Septic streptococcal arthritis of the ankle or foot causes extreme pain and difficulty moving the ankle or foot. Group B streptococcal arthritis in particular, can be devastating and must be treated promptly with arthrocentesis and antibiotics. Delaying treatment even for a few days can result in significant morbidity risk.

M00.28   Other streptococcal arthritis, vertebrae

Other streptococcal arthritis includes cases of pyogenic arthritis caused by streptococcal bacteria other than *Streptococcus pneumoniae*, such as group A, group B, and enterococcus. Most patients also have some type of underlying comorbidity or risk factor, such as rheumatoid arthritis, diabetes, or carcinoma, or are receiving immunosuppressive therapy. Since the synovial lining of joints cannot defend well from invading microorganisms, the joint's reaction to a streptococcal infection produces inflammation, swelling, and effusion that increases pressure and reduces blood flow at the same time. This can lead to permanent joint damage and degeneration. Septic streptococcal arthritis of the vertebrae causes extreme pain and difficulty moving the back. Group B streptococcal arthritis in particular, can be devastating and must be treated promptly with arthrocentesis and antibiotics. Delaying treatment even for a few days can result in significant morbidity risk.

M00.29   Other streptococcal polyarthritis

Other streptococcal polyarthritis includes cases of pyogenic arthritis affecting more than one joint caused by streptococcal bacteria other than *Streptococcus pneumoniae*, such as group A, group B, and enterococcus. Most patients also have some type of underlying comorbidity or risk factor, such as rheumatoid arthritis, diabetes, or carcinoma, or are receiving immunosuppressive therapy. Since the synovial lining of joints cannot defend well from invading microorganisms, the joints' reaction to a streptococcal infection produces inflammation, swelling, and effusion that increases pressure and reduces blood flow at the same time. This can lead to permanent joint damage and degeneration. Septic streptococcal polyarthritis causes extreme pain and difficulty moving multiple joints. Group B streptococcal arthritis in particular, can be devastating and must be treated promptly with arthrocentesis and antibiotics. Delaying treatment even for a few days can result in significant morbidity risk.

M00.80 Arthritis due to other bacteria, unspecified joint

Pyogenic arthritis due to other bacteria includes cases of septic arthritis caused by causative agents such as *Mycoplasma pneumoniae, Klebsiella pneumoniae, E.coli, H. influenzae, Proteus mirabilis,* pseudomonas, or *Clostridium perfringens.* Since the synovial lining of joints cannot defend well from invading microorganisms, the joint's reaction to a bacterial infection produces inflammation, swelling, and effusion that increases pressure within the affected joint while reducing blood flow at the same time. Pyogenic arthritis causes extreme pain and difficulty moving the affected joint. Arthrocentesis and rapid antibiotic treatment are necessary to prevent permanent joint damage and degeneration of joint tissue.

M00.81 Arthritis due to other bacteria, shoulder

Pyogenic arthritis due to other bacteria includes cases of septic arthritis caused by causative agents such as *Mycoplasma pneumoniae, Klebsiella pneumoniae, E.coli, H. influenzae, Proteus mirabilis,* pseudomonas, or *Clostridium perfringens.* Since the synovial lining of joints cannot defend well from invading microorganisms, the joint's reaction to a bacterial infection produces inflammation, swelling, and effusion that increases pressure within the affected joint while reducing blood flow at the same time. Pyogenic arthritis of the shoulder causes extreme pain and difficulty moving the shoulder. Arthrocentesis and rapid antibiotic treatment are necessary to prevent permanent joint damage and degeneration of joint tissue.

M00.82 Arthritis due to other bacteria, elbow

Pyogenic arthritis due to other bacteria includes cases of septic arthritis caused by causative agents such as *Mycoplasma pneumoniae, Klebsiella pneumoniae, E.coli, H. influenzae, Proteus mirabilis,* pseudomonas, or *Clostridium perfringens.* Since the synovial lining of joints cannot defend well from invading microorganisms, the joint's reaction to a bacterial infection produces inflammation, swelling, and effusion that increases pressure within the affected joint while reducing blood flow at the same time. Pyogenic arthritis of the elbow causes extreme pain and difficulty moving the elbow. Arthrocentesis and rapid antibiotic treatment are necessary to prevent permanent joint damage and degeneration of joint tissue.

M00.83 Arthritis due to other bacteria, wrist

Pyogenic arthritis due to other bacteria includes cases of septic arthritis caused by causative agents such as *Mycoplasma pneumoniae, Klebsiella pneumoniae, E.coli, H. influenzae, Proteus mirabilis,* pseudomonas, or *Clostridium perfringens.* Since the synovial lining of joints cannot defend well from invading microorganisms, the joint's reaction to a bacterial infection produces inflammation, swelling, and effusion that increases pressure within the affected joint while reducing blood flow at the same time. Pyogenic arthritis of the wrist causes extreme pain and difficulty moving the wrist. Arthrocentesis and rapid antibiotic treatment are necessary to prevent permanent joint damage and degeneration of joint tissue.

M00.84 Arthritis due to other bacteria, hand

Pyogenic arthritis due to other bacteria includes cases of septic arthritis caused by causative agents such as *Mycoplasma pneumoniae, Klebsiella pneumoniae, E.coli, H. influenzae, Proteus mirabilis,* pseudomonas, or *Clostridium perfringens.* Since the synovial lining of joints cannot defend well from invading microorganisms, the joint's reaction to a bacterial infection produces inflammation, swelling, and effusion that increases pressure within the affected joint while reducing blood flow at the same time. Pyogenic arthritis of the hand causes extreme pain and difficulty

moving the hand. Arthrocentesis and rapid antibiotic treatment are necessary to prevent permanent joint damage and degeneration of joint tissue.

M00.85 Arthritis due to other bacteria, hip

Pyogenic arthritis due to other bacteria includes cases of septic arthritis caused by causative agents such as *Mycoplasma pneumoniae, Klebsiella pneumoniae, E.coli, H. influenzae, Proteus mirabilis,* pseudomonas, or *Clostridium perfringens.* Since the synovial lining of joints cannot defend well from invading microorganisms, the joint's reaction to a bacterial infection produces inflammation, swelling, and effusion that increases pressure within the affected joint while reducing blood flow at the same time. Pyogenic arthritis of the hip causes extreme pain and difficulty moving the hip. Arthrocentesis and rapid antibiotic treatment are necessary to prevent permanent joint damage and degeneration of joint tissue.

M00.861 Arthritis due to other bacteria, right knee

Pyogenic arthritis due to other bacteria includes cases of septic arthritis caused by causative agents such as *Mycoplasma pneumoniae, Klebsiella pneumoniae, E.coli, H. influenzae, Proteus mirabilis,* pseudomonas, or *Clostridium perfringens.* Since the synovial lining of joints cannot defend well from invading microorganisms, the joint's reaction to a bacterial infection produces inflammation, swelling, and effusion that increases pressure within the affected joint while reducing blood flow at the same time. Pyogenic arthritis of the knee causes extreme pain and difficulty moving the knee. Arthrocentesis and rapid antibiotic treatment are necessary to prevent permanent joint damage and degeneration of joint tissue.

M00.87 Arthritis due to other bacteria, ankle and foot

Pyogenic arthritis due to other bacteria includes cases of septic arthritis caused by causative agents such as *Mycoplasma pneumoniae, Klebsiella pneumoniae, E.coli, H. influenzae, Proteus mirabilis,* pseudomonas, or *Clostridium perfringens.* Since the synovial lining of joints cannot defend well from invading microorganisms, the joint's reaction to a bacterial infection produces inflammation, swelling, and effusion that increases pressure within the affected joint while reducing blood flow at the same time. Pyogenic arthritis of the ankle or foot causes extreme pain and difficulty moving the ankle or foot. Arthrocentesis and rapid antibiotic treatment are necessary to prevent permanent joint damage and degeneration of joint tissue.

M00.88 Arthritis due to other bacteria, vertebrae

Pyogenic arthritis due to other bacteria includes cases of septic arthritis caused by causative agents such as *Mycoplasma pneumoniae, Klebsiella pneumoniae, E.coli, H. influenzae, Proteus mirabilis,* pseudomonas, or *Clostridium perfringens.* Since the synovial lining of joints cannot defend well from invading microorganisms, the joint's reaction to a bacterial infection produces inflammation, swelling, and effusion that increases pressure within the affected joint while reducing blood flow at the same time. Pyogenic arthritis of the vertebrae causes extreme pain and difficulty moving the back. Arthrocentesis and rapid antibiotic treatment are necessary to prevent permanent joint damage and degeneration of joint tissue.

M00.89 Polyarthritis due to other bacteria

Pyogenic polyarthritis due to other bacteria includes causative agents such as *Mycoplasma pneumoniae, Klebsiella pneumoniae, E.coli, H. influenzae, Proteus mirabilis,* pseudomonas, or *Clostridium perfringens.* Since the synovial lining of joints cannot defend well from invading microorganisms, the joints' reaction to a bacterial infection produces inflammation, swelling, and effusion that increases pressure within multiple affected joints while reducing blood flow at the same time. Pyogenic polyarthritis causes extreme pain and difficult movement in multiple joints. Arthrocentesis and rapid antibiotic treatment are necessary to prevent permanent joint damage and degeneration of joint tissue.

M02.3 Reiter's disease

Reiter's disease is actually a syndrome of inflammatory reactions occurring in genetically susceptible people after infection of the genitourinary

2016 Plain English Descriptions for ICD-10-CM | Chapter 13 Diseases of the Musculoskeletal System and Connective Tissue | M05 – M12.8

Diseases of the Musculoskeletal System | M05 – M12.8

tract, most commonly by *Chlamydia trachomatis,* especially in bisexual or homosexual males, ages 20-40 with an STD, or those with an affected family member. It can also occur after infection of the digestive tract. This disease is known as reactive arthritis, but it affects the eyes and the genitourinary tract with specific symptoms, as well as the joints. Women may have milder symptoms than men. There is no cure. Treatment is intended to slow or stop progression of the disease and lessen symptoms. Most people recover from the initial episode in a few months, but have recurring bouts.

M05 Rheumatoid arthritis with rheumatoid factor

Rhematoid arthritis (RA) is an autoimmune, systemic, inflammatory disease mainly affecting the synovial lining of joints and progressing in three stages-first with swelling, pain, warmth, and stiffness around the joint, followed by a rapid division of new cells, causing the synovium to thicken, and then the release of enzymes that digest bone and cartilage, leading to pain, joint deformity and instability, and loss of function. RA commonly begins in the small joints of the hands and wrists and is often symmetrical, affecting the same joints on both sides. RA is accompanied by other physical symptoms including morning pain and stiffness or pain with prolonged sitting; flu-like low grade fever and muscle ache; disease flare-ups followed by remission; and sometimes rheumatoid nodules under the skin, particularly over the elbows. Cartilage, bone, and ligament damage occurs in advanced stages. RA can also affect other organs of the body. RA normally occurs between the ages of 30 and 50. It also afflicts children and men, who are often more severely affected. A particular genetic marker in white blood cells, HLA-DR4, puts certain people at increased risk for RA. The immune system in people with RA mistakes the body's own healthy tissue for foreign invaders and attacks it. Some people also have an increase in rheumatoid factor antibody that helps direct the production of normal antibodies. It is also believed that RA may be triggered by an abnormal response to some kind of infection. Many researchers are in debate over whether RA is one disease or actually a complex of several different related diseases.

M05.0 Felty's syndrome

Felty's syndrome is an atypical form of rheumatoid arthritis that also presents with fever, an enlarged spleen, recurring infections, and a decreased white blood count. Treatment includes the same medications as are used for rheumatoid arthritis, and in some cases the spleen may be removed to promote the production of white blood cells and decrease the recurring infections.

M05.1 Rheumatoid lung disease with rheumatoid arthritis

Rheumatoid lung is a type of lung disease due to rheumatoid arthritis. It may present with symptoms ranging from no symptoms at all to coughing and shortness of breath, chest pain, and fever in addition to the usual symptoms of the arthritis.

M08.0 Unspecified juvenile rheumatoid arthritis

Juvenile chronic polyarthritis, more commonly called juvenile rheumatoid arthritis or JRA, presents with all the symptoms of normal rheumatoid arthritis in addition to fever, a reddish rash, weight loss, eye pain that grows worse when looking at a light, and swollen glands. JRA is rarely life-threatening, and often improves or goes into remission at puberty.

M08.1 Juvenile ankylosing spondylitis

Also known as Marie-Struempell disease, rheumatoid spondylitis, and Bechterew's syndrome, ankylosing spondylitis is a chronic, progressive, autoimmune arthropathy that affects the spine and sacroiliac joints, eventually leading to spinal fusion and rigidity. Almost all of the autoimmune spondylarthropathies share a common genetic marker, HLA-B27, although the cause is still unknown. The disease appears in some predisposed people after exposure to bowel or urinary tract infections. The most common patient is a young male, aged 15-30, as it affects men about three times more than women. Swelling occurs in the intervertebral discs and in the joints between the spine and pelvis. Patients have persistent buttock and low back pain and stiffness alleviated with exercise. Over time, the vertebrae may become fused together, progressing

up the spine and affecting other organs. The disease is related to other inflammatory conditions in the body such as iridocyclitis, inflammatory bowel disease, psoriasis, Reiter's disease, and heart valve involvement in extreme cases. Prodromal rheumatism-like symptoms may occur at a very young age. Diagnosis is made before visible changes on x-ray appear by using tomography and MRI of the sacroiliac joints. Over the long term, progressed cases show spinal osteopenia with compression fractures and a hump back, and the visible formation of abnormal bony outgrowths, called syndesmophytes, on the spine.

M10 Gout

Gout is a disease in which uric acid builds up in the body and forms crystals in one or more joints or other organs. This in turn causes sudden episodes of severe pain and inflammation, usually in one joint at a time and often in the big toe. These episodes may be initiated or made worse by drinking too much alcohol, eating too much or too little, surgery, illness, joint injury, and/or chemotherapy. It usually develops in men over the age of forty and post-menopausal women and is treated by diet, medication, and in rare instances, surgery.

M10.0 Idiopathic gout

Gout is a urate metabolism disorder in which monosodium urate crystals deposit in the joints and soft tissues, such as the bursae and tendons, causing accompanying pain, inflammation, and degeneration of bones and joints. There is generally an excessive level of uric acid in the blood, or hyperuricemia, that leads to gout. Acute primary gout is also known as gout attacks or flares, idiopathic gout, or gouty bursitis. This stage is a symptomatic inflammation from urate crystals in one or more joints. Acute attacks are intermittent and unpredictable, very painful, and often debilitating. The first metatarsophalangeal joint of the big toe is almost always affected. Other joints include the ankle, midfoot, knee, fingers, and elbow.

M12.0 Chronic postrheumatic arthropathy [Jaccoud]

Chronic postrheumatic arthropathy is a condition of the hands and/or feet that may occur after repeated rheumatic attacks. Over time, the hands or feet take on a gnarled, twisted appearance, losing functionality.

M12.1 Kaschin-Beck disease

Kaschin-Beck disease is a degenerative disorder of the spine that is rare in the United States, but common in the Far East. It presents with enlarged joints, shortened fingers and toes, and in some cases with severe dwarfism. It is thought to be caused either by a selenium and vitamin E nutritional deficiency or by a fungal infection.

M12.2 Villonodular synovitis (pigmented)

Villonodular synovitis, often called pigmented villonodular synovitis or PVS, is a condition in which the lining of a joint, most often the knee, becomes swollen, retains fluid, and grows. This growth causes pain to the bone. It is most often treated by removing the lining surgically or through radiation therapy.

M12.3 Palindromic rheumatism

Palindromic rheumatism is a rare type of inflammatory arthritis in which the patient experiences repeated episodes of pain, swelling, heat, and stiffness of the joints. It usually affects 1-3 joints at a time. An episode builds over the course of several hours and then lasts several days or weeks before subsiding for a period of weeks or months. While this disorder can recur over many years, it fortunately does not cause any permanent damage to the joints. Episodes are typically treated with anti-inflammatory medication.

M12.8 Other specific arthropathies, not elsewhere classified

Other specific arthropathies includes transient arthropathy. Transient arthropathy indicates that the joint pain and swelling is short-lived and temporary, rather than being long-term as with most forms of arthritis. In most cases, such short-lived joint pain is associated with an infection or injury.

M13.8 Other specified arthritis

Other specified arthritis includes allergic and climacteric arthritis. Allergic arthritis is caused by a hypersensitivity reaction to a specific allergen. Climacteric arthritis appears with the onset of menopause, and is thought to be due to the hormonal imbalance that occurs during that period. Hormone replacement therapy to ease the symptoms of menopause will usually help to decrease the symptoms of the arthritis, too.

M15 Polyosteoarthritis

Polyosteoarthritis is a degenerative disease affecting multiple joints including articular cartilage and subchondral bone. The condition is characterized by pain, stiffness, immobility, and swelling and can affect any joint but is most common in the weight bearing joints of the hip and knee. Additional problems usually related to decreased movement include regional muscle atropy and ligament laxity.

M1A Chronic gout

This chronic disorder of urate metabolism causes monosodium urate crystals to deposit in the joints and soft tissues, such as bursae and tendons. Following recurrent acute attacks, the disease then progresses past the intercritical times, known as the flare-free periods of the disease, to a chronic form of gout marked by persistent pain and stiffness. Tophi may be present which are aggregates of uric acid crystals that form in and around joints and soft tissues, even in other organs. Tophi can be seen clinically as obvious bumps and deformities and on x-ray as bony destruction or erosion in some cases.

M20 Acquired deformities of fingers and toes

Acquired deformities of the toes are those which develop over time due to abnormal growth, injury, disorder, or another disease process, rather than being present from birth. Most acquired deformities of the toes affect the great toe.

M20.01 Mallet finger

Mallet finger is a condition in which the distal joint of a finger bends (flexes), but will not fully straighten by itself. This usually occurs as a result of damage to the extensor tendon running along the backside of the finger which exerts the pulling force that straightens it.

M20.02 Boutonnière deformity

Boutonniere deformity is a condition in which the tendon responsible for extending the finger becomes detached from the top of the bone in the middle of the finger and slips to one side. This prevents the patient from straightening the finger and causes the bone to become prominent at the site of the injury. If not treated quickly, the tendon loses its elasticity and the condition becomes permanent.

M20.03 Swan-neck deformity

Swan-neck deformity causes the finger to become hyperextended (to bend backwards instead of becoming straight) and difficult or impossible to fully flex, so that the patient cannot completely close a fist.

M20.1 Hallux valgus (acquired)

Hallux valgus, more commonly known as a bunion, is a displacement of the joint in the big toe that causes it to twist towards the smaller toes, sometimes completely overlapping the second toe. It is more common in women than in men due to women wearing tighter fitting shoes. In addition to the obvious deformity, it presents with redness, swelling, and pain. A bunion may be treated conservatively with special footwear and rest, or it may require surgical intervention to treat.

M20.2 Hallux rigidus

Hallux rigidus indicates an inflexible, or stiff, big toe, usually due to arthritis or other damage to the cartilage of the toe. This causes pain and swelling in the joint of the big toe and limited motion at the metatarsophalangeal joint.

M20.3 Hallux varus (acquired)

Hallux varus is a displacement of the joint of the big toe in which it turns away from the rest of the toes. In addition to the obvious deformity, it presents with redness, swelling, and pain. Hallux varus may be treated conservatively with special footwear and rest, but it more often requires surgical intervention.

M20.4 Other hammer toe(s) (acquired)

Hammertoe (on a toe other than the big toe) causes the metatarsal joint of the affected toe to displace upwards rather than to one side or the other. This causes the affected toe to be flexed and pulled downward, giving the toe a hammer-like appearance. As with other acquired deformities, this causes pain and swelling at the joint.

M20.5 Other deformities of toe(s) (acquired)

Other deformities of the toes include a clawtoe that is contracted at the PIP and DIP joints (middle and end joints) in the toe, leading to severe pressure and pain. Ligaments and tendons that have tightened cause the toe's joints to curl downwards. Claw toes may occur in any toe, except the big toe.

M21 Other acquired deformities of limbs

Other acquired deformities develop over time due to abnormal growth, injury, disorder, or other disease process, rather than being present at birth.

M21.02 Valgus deformity, not elsewhere classified, elbow

This subcategory includes cubitus valgus, a common deformity in which the elbow and forearm are angled away from the body to a much greater degree than normal when the arm is fully extended. It is most often caused by an improperly-healed fracture of the lateral condyle, which is the bulb of the humerus that connects to the elbow which is further away from the body.

M21.05 Valgus deformity, not elsewhere classified, hip

Coxa valga is a deformity of the hip joint in which the angle between the femoral head and neck and the femoral shaft is increased, usually beyond 135 degrees. This causes pain and limping and leads to lateral subluxation or dislocation of the femoral head. It is usually seen in patients with neuromuscular disease such as poliomyelitis or cerebral palsy, or skeletal dysplasias and juvenile idiopathic arthritis. For instance, if the hip adductor and extensor muscles are weakened or overpowered by the adductor muscles, it can cause this type of deformity and impaired ambulation. Nonsurgical treatment measures include physical therapy to strengthen weaker muscles, orthotic devices or casts, and surgical therapies.

M21.06 Valgus deformity, not elsewhere classified, knee

This subcategory includes genu valgum or 'knock knee,' a deformity in which the knees are angled in and touch each other with the ankles apart and not touching whenever the legs are straightened. This causes the legs to angle inward. Most young children will have a certain degree of genu valgum until the legs straighten. Knock knee that occurs in adulthood may be caused by a lack of vitamin D, obesity, osteomyelitis and injury to the lower leg.

M21.12 Varus deformity, not elsewhere classified, elbow

This subcategory includes cubitus varus, a deformity in which the elbow and forearm deviate inwards toward the midline of the body whenever the arm is fully extended. The most common cause is a prior supracondylar humeral fracture with crooked healing, after which the deformity can be noticed only with the arm in full extension. This is sometimes known as a 'gunstock' deformity and can be corrected when causing functional problems using a corrective osteotomy of the humerus with fixation until healed.

M21.15 Varus deformity, not elsewhere classified, hip

Coxa vara is a deformity of the hip in which the angle of the femoral head and neck and the femoral shaft decreases to less than 120 degrees causing an inward curvature of the hip. Pain, stiffness, a limping gait, and a difference in leg length can result. Acquired coxa vara often occurs from a fracture or other type of traumatic injury. Surgery is usually needed to correct the femoral neck-shaft angle and restore a normal and balanced skeletal structure.

2016 Plain English Descriptions for ICD-10-CM   Chapter 13 Diseases of the Musculoskeletal System and Connective Tissue | M21.16 – M24.7

Diseases of the Musculoskeletal System   M21.16 – M24.7

M21.16 Varus deformity, not elsewhere classified, knee

This subcategory includes genu varum or 'bow leg,' a deformity in which the legs bow outward away from each other and the knees stay far apart when the person stands with the feet and ankles together. A certain degree of varus is considered normal in young children. Genu varum is diagnosed when both legs continue to bow beyond age three, but treatment is not usually undertaken unless the bowing is extreme. Casts, braces, or special shoes may be used to help correct the deformity. Surgery may be needed for older children in severe cases.

M21.33 Wrist drop (acquired)

Wrist drop is a condition in which the hand hangs down at the wrist and remains in a flexed position because of muscle paresis. The patient is unable to extend or raise the hand. This often occurs as a result of injury or dysfunction of the radial nerve. This may correct itself when after a few days if caused by the hand being held in the same position too long. Other conditions causing wrist drop include Guillain-Barre syndrome, lead poisoning, multiple sclerosis, and myasthenia gravis.

M21.37 Foot drop (acquired)

Foot drop is an abnormal dropping of the forefoot that may be temporary or permanent, due to weakness or paralysis of the anterior muscles in the foot, usually caused by damage to the peroneal nerve. The patient is unable to lift the front of the foot, resulting in an abnormal gait as the front of the foot is dragged while walking. The patient may raise the entire leg from the thigh like going up stairs while walking. Foot drop is not a disorder in itself, but rather a symptom of a greater problem such as nerve or muscle injury or damage, or disease process that affects the brain and spinal cord.

M21.4 Flat foot [pes planus] (acquired)

Flat foot is a condition in which the arch of the foot does not develop in childhood, which affects about one out of five people. Flat foot doesn't cause any complications as long as the feet are supple and the Achilles tendon isn't tight. However, as the foot becomes more rigid in age, or if the foot is not supple for other reasons, pain, callouses, redness, and other difficulties such as plantar fasciitis can result.

M21.51 Acquired clawhand

Claw hand is a condition in which one or more fingers become curved or bent, giving the hand the appearance of a claw (similar to hammertoe). It can result from damage to the nerves, muscles, or tendons in the hand.

M21.52 Acquired clubhand

Clubhand is more often a congenital condition, but this code refers only to clubhand that is acquired later in life. Clubhand usually results from damage to the nerves of the hand, causing the fingers and wrist to curl inward.

M21.53 Acquired clawfoot

Claw foot is a deformity with a high arch and the toes flexed upwards so that only the ball and possibly the heel of the foot can touch the ground.

M21.54 Acquired clubfoot

Acquired clubfoot is a condition in which the patient's foot looks as if it has been turned inward at the ankle, with the bottom of the foot facing the other leg, forcing the person to walk on the outer side of the foot or the ankle. The acquired form is often the result of injury or neuromuscular causes such as paralysis in early childhood.

M21.86 Other specified acquired deformities of lower leg

Other specified aquired deformities of the lower limb includes genu recurvatum, a condition in which one or both knees are hyperextended, bending backwards rather than remaining straight, when locked. This causes pain and difficulty in walking and makes the knees much more prone to injuires such as dislocation.

M22.4 Chondromalacia patellae

Chondromalacia of the patella literally means softening of the cartilage of the knee-cap. When the cartilage softens, it may break down, causing pain when the patient is engaged in activity that is strenuous on the knees,

such as sports. If caught early, it can be treated successfully in about 85% of patients with specialized exercises and anti-inflammatory medication.

M23.2 Derangement of meniscus due to old tear or injury

A derangement of the meniscus of the knee is a condition in which the connective tissue (cartilage) becomes torn or damaged due to an old injury. There are two cartilages in the knee. The medial meniscus is the cartilage that cushions the knee joint closer to the inside of the leg, while the lateral meniscus cushions the knee joint closer to the exterior side of the leg. These cartilages are shaped roughly like a crescent moon or kidney bean. The "tips" of the crescent shape are known as "horns," which are pointed towards the other cartilage.

M23.20 Derangement of unspecified meniscus due to old tear or injury

In a bucket-handle tear of the medial or lateral meniscus, the cartilage tears in the interior curve, but not completely, so that the separated part of the cartilage resembles a handle attached at both ends to the rest of the cartilage.

M24.0 Loose body in joint

A loose body in the joint occurs when a loose fragment of bone or cartilage becomes lodged in the joint. This acts like a pebble in a gear, and will impair movement as it grinds and damages the joint. Treatment requires surgical removal of the fragment.

M24.1 Other articular cartilage disorders

An articular cartilage disorder is a condition in which the cartilage responsible for movement within joints becomes torn or damaged due to an old injury.

M24.2 Disorder of ligament

This include ligamentous laxity and instability secondary to an old injury. Laxity of a ligament indicates that the ligament has been stretched, usually by a previous injury such as a dislocation of that joint, making future dislocations far more likely. In some cases, surgical intervention is required to tighten the ligament.

M24.3 Pathological dislocation of joint, not elsewhere classified

Pathological dislocation is the dislocation of a joint that is not due to injury, but to an underlying disease of that particular joint, such as tuberculosis. The hip joint is the most common location of pathological dislocation.

M24.4 Recurrent dislocation of joint

Recurrent dislocation of a joint occurs when the patient previously suffered a dislocation of the affected joint which resulted in permanent stretching or tearing of the ligaments. This causes the joint to rest very loosely in its socket, making it easy to dislocate again. Surgical tightening of the ligaments is often required to correct this disorder.

M24.5 Contracture of joint

Contracture of a joint occurs when scar tissue from a pre-existing injury or disease tightens a joint, preventing it from moving through its normal full range of motion. Surgical intervention is usually needed to remove the excess scar tissue and release the contracture.

M24.6 Ankylosis of joint

Ankylosis of a joint occurs when a disease or injury results in fibrous (scar) tissue forming across a joint, causing severe stiffening or even complete immobility of the joint.

M24.7 Protrusio acetabuli

The acetabulum is the cup-shaped depression in the hipbone in which the ball-and-socket of the femur rests. An unspecified intrapelvic protrusion of the acetabulum is a disorder in which the cup-shaped depression sinks outward, in effect filling it in, resulting in the ball of the femur being pushed out of place and possibly dislocating.

M25.0   **Hemarthrosis**

Hemarthosis is a condition in which the joint fills with blood, presenting with swelling, immobility, and pain. Treatment may include draining the excess blood through a needle.

M26.01   **Maxillary hyperplasia**

Maxillary hyperplasia is an overgrowth in the size of the upper jaw due to an abnormal increase or proliferation of cells.

M26.02   **Maxillary hypoplasia**

Maxillary hypoplasia is underdevelopment of the upper jaw.

M26.03   **Mandibular hyperplasia**

Mandibular hyperplasia is an overgrowth in the size of the lower jaw due to an abnormal increase or proliferation of cells.

M26.04   **Mandibular hypoplasia**

Mandibular hypoplasia is underdevelopment of the lower jaw.

M26.05   **Macrogenia**

Macrogenia is a condition in which the patient has an abnormally large chin that is out of proportion with the rest of his or her facial features.

M26.06   **Microgenia**

Microgenia is a condition in which the patient has an abnormally small chin that is out of proportion with the rest of his or her facial features.

M26.07   **Excessive tuberosity of jaw**

The tuberosity of the jaw is the rounded, bony protrusion behind the last molar on either side of both jaws. An excessive tuberosity of the jaw indicates that these protrusions are large enough to cause discomfort or crowd the teeth. In some cases, this condition may not be noticed until the patient is being fitted for dentures.

M26.11   **Maxillary asymmetry**

In maxillary asymmetry, the upper jaw bone does not have the same dimensions on the right side as it does on the left. This prevents the lower jaw bone from lining up correctly.

M26.21   **Malocclusion, Angle's class**

Malocclusion is a poor biting position in which the teeth are misaligned. There is an incorrect relationship between the teeth of the two dental arches. This causes problems of varying degree due to the way in which the opposing teeth in the upper and lower jaw meet when biting or chewing. The term is accredited to Edward Angle, considered the father of modern orthodontics. The Angle classification is based upon the relative position of the maxillary first molar.

M26.211   **Malocclusion, Angle's class I**

Angle class I is a neutrocclusion in which a normal molar occlusion is seen as described for the upper first molar. Although the back molars of both jaws line up correctly with each other, the other teeth may have spacing, crowding, or even eruption problems.

M26.212   **Malocclusion, Angle's class II**

Angle class II is a distocclusion indicating that the first maxillary molar does not align with the first lower molar in its normal groove, but rests anteriorly, or in front of it, between the first mandibular molar and the second premolar. This causes a case of retrognathism, or overjet, in the bite.

M26.213   **Malocclusion, Angle's class III**

Angle Class III is a mesiocclusion which means that the first maxillary molar rests posteriorly, or behind, the buccal groove of the first mandibular molar. This causes a case of prognathism, or negative overjet, in which the lower jaw protrudes forward beyond the upper.

M26.220   **Open anterior occlusal relationship**

An open anterior occlusal relationship indicates that the back molars touch when the jaws are closed but that the front teeth do not.

M26.221   **Open posterior occlusal relationship**

An open posterior occlusal relationship indicates that the front teeth touch when the mouth closes, but that the rear molars do not.

M26.23   **Excessive horizontal overlap**

Excessive horizontal overlap is caused when a narrow angle between the ramus (the vertical part of the lower jaw) and the body (the almost horizontal part) of the mandible causes the appearance of an overbite.

M26.24   **Reverse articulation**

Reverse articulation includes both anterior and posterior crossbite. This is a type of malocclusion in which a tooth has a more buccal or lingual position in relation to its corresponding antagonist tooth in the other jaw. Normally, the cusps of the maxillary teeth match into the grooves of the mandibular teeth in a specific way. A crossbite arises when this relationship is reversed. An anterior crossbite affects the front teeth when one or more of the upper front teeth close behind the front bottom teeth. A posterior crossbite affects the teeth on the sides and occurs whenever one or more upper molars meet the inner cupst of the bottom molars, closing behind the bottom molars. Reverse articulation may be a result of a hereditary narrow maxilla, delayed loss of baby teeth, and tooth shifting from prolonged thumb-sucking, pacifier use, and even mouth breathing.

M26.33   **Horizontal displacement of fully erupted tooth or teeth**

Horizontal displacement of one or more teeth results in a "tipped over" appearance of the affected tooth or teeth.

M26.34   **Vertical displacement of fully erupted tooth or teeth**

Vertical displacement of the alveolus and teeth indicates that one or more teeth as well as their sockets have been separated from the bone of the jaw, usually by trauma to the face. Vertical displacement gives affected teeth the appearance of being too long or too short.

M26.35   **Rotation of fully erupted tooth or teeth**

When a tooth is rotated from its normal position, the edge of the affected tooth may be facing forward and is openly visible rather than the normal, flat surface that should face forward.

M26.36   **Insufficient interocclusal distance of fully erupted teeth (ridge)**

The interocclusal distance of the teeth is the distance between the teeth in the upper and lower jaw when the jaw is in its "at rest" position. Insufficient distance can lead to tooth grinding and excessive wear-and-tear.

M26.37   **Excessive interocclusal distance of fully erupted teeth**

The interocclusal distance of the teeth is the distance between the teeth in the upper and lower jaw when the jaw is in its "at rest" position. Excessive interocclusal distance of the teeth leaves a gap between the teeth when the jaw is at rest.

M26.4   **Malocclusion, unspecified**

Malocclusion is a poor biting position in which the teeth are misaligned. There is an incorrect relationship between the teeth of the two dental arches. This causes problems of varying degree due to the way in which the opposing teeth in the upper and lower jaw meet when biting or chewing.

M26.52   **Limited mandibular range of motion**

Limited mandibular range of motion indicates that the patient is unable to either completely open or completely close his or her mouth with restricted lateral, or side to side movement of the lower jaw.

M26.53   **Deviation in opening and closing of the mandible**

Deviation in opening and closing of the mandible indicates that the jaw moves from side-to-side as the patient opens and closes his or her mouth.

2016 Plain English Descriptions for ICD-10-CM   Chapter 13 Diseases of the Musculoskeletal System and Connective Tissue | M26.54 – M27.61

Diseases of the Musculoskeletal System   M26.54 – M27.61

M26.54   Insufficient anterior guidance

Insufficient anterior guidance is insufficient muscle control over the movement of the front teeth that can result in excessive wear-and-tear or damage to the front teeth due to repeatedly clipping them too hard on food or each other.

M26.55   Centric occlusion maximum intercuspation discrepancy

The teeth normally develop in such a way that when the jaw is closed, the protrusions of one tooth settle comfortably into the pits of its companion tooth on the opposite jaw; this is called intercuspation. Centric occlusion maximum intercuspation discrepancy indicates that due to a misalignment of the teeth, when the jaw is closed, it must slide into an unnatural position in order for the teeth to interlock properly.

M26.56   Non-working side interference

Non-working side interference occurs in some cases where the muscles on one of the hinges of the jaw are not doing their job properly, causing the muscles of the other hinge to take the load, and actually interfering with the function of the jaw. This usually manifests as the jaw being pulled to one side.

M26.57   Lack of posterior occlusal support

Lack of posterior occlusal support indicates that due to malformations in one or both jaws, the muscles are not able to affect full force in closing the mandible.

M26.61   Adhesions and ankylosis of temporomandibular joint

In adhesions and/or ankylosis of the temporomandibular joint (TMJ), it becomes stiff or fused with the temporal bone via the growth of abnormal bone or a fibrous, tough, and ligament-like tissue forming across the space of the joint, preventing ease of movement.

M26.63   Articular disc disorder of temporomandibular joint

Articular disc disorder affects the cartilage that cushions the TMJ, in most cases, by displacing the disc and stretching it out. This can result in the disc slipping out of place, locking the jaw, or in it becoming folded over itself, causing pain and swelling.

M26.69   Other specified disorders of temporomandibular joint

This code reports sounds in the temporomandibular joint, such as popping and clicking, as the patient opens and closes the jaw.

M27.1   Giant cell granuloma, central

A granuloma is a group of cells surrounded by a "cuff" of lymphocytes, or white blood cells, which can appear as a part of the body's response to infection. A central giant cell granuloma in the jaw presents as a swollen sphere of tissue, usually in the gum, which is inflamed and painful to the touch. These are most common in patients over the age of sixty and usually require surgical removal.

M27.2   Inflammatory conditions of jaws

This includes osteonecrosis of the jaw bone (ONJ) or 'dead jaw,' in addition to osteitis, osteomyelitis, periostitis, and sequestrum inflammatory conditions affecting the jaw. Osteonecrosis is a disfiguring and disabling condition marked by the literal death of jaw bone tissue that generally develops whenever the jaw fails to heal from minor trauma, such as a tooth extraction that exposes the bone. The condition can remain asymptomatic for many weeks or months and may manifest with pain, swelling, or infection in the gums or jaw; gums that won't heal; teeth becoming loose; a feeling of heaviness in the jaw; and exposed bone. This can occur in cancer patients who have received bisphosphonates for chemotherapy or oral bisphosphonates for osteoporosis. The disease is very difficult to treat and requires vigilant medical and oral monitoring care.

Note: Osteonecrosis caused by radiation therapy to the jaw region requires an additional code to identify the type of radiation.

M27.3   Alveolitis of jaws

Alveolitis of the jaw is a painful inflammation, usually due to infection, of the sockets in the gum and jaw from which the teeth grow and that hold the tooth roots in place. This can put the teeth at risk of being lost.

M27.5   Periradicular pathology associated with previous endodontic treatment

Conditions in this subcategory address disease processes occurring around the root of a tooth. These problems have been caused by prior treatment involving the dental pulp, the tooth root, and the structures surrounding and supporting the apex of the tooth's root.

M27.51   Perforation of root canal space due to endodontic treatment

The center of a tooth within the crown is a hollow area that houses the pulp, or living soft tissue of the tooth. The pulp is connected to the tip of the root(s) of the tooth through very thin, hollow canals running down through the center of the root(s). Blood vessels and nerves that supply the tooth run through these canals. An infection in the pulp material requires a procedure to scrape it out and seal up the space with an inert material in order to save the tooth. Perforation of a root canal space happens when an endodontic instrument the dentist is using accidentally goes through the root of the tooth or the floor of the pulp chamber within the crown. Repair material can sometimes be placed in the perforated area and the surrounding bone will heal, or it may result in mechanical failure from a leaking root canal system.

M27.52   Endodontic overfill

Endodontic overfill is a complication of a root canal procedure that occurs when the root is not properly filled after removal of the pulp tissue and too much inert material is placed into the prepared space. Overfill of gutta-percha (the purified, inert, latex material made from the sap of the percha tree used to fill root canals) or extruding sealant act as chronic irritants. Too great of an overfill places the gutta percha and root canal cement in contact with bone. Overfill prevents healing of the initial problem and can cause a breakdown of the root tip and more apical pathology such as periapical lesions.

M27.53   Endodontic underfill

Endodontic underfill is also a complication of a root canal procedure that occurs when the prepared root space is not properly filled with enough inert material. This results in an inability to fully treat the tooth to the end of the root and can leave the tooth open to continued lesion formation and pathological activity.

M27.6   Endosseous dental implant failure

A dental implant is a type of tooth replacement consisting of an artificial tooth root that holds a prosthetic tooth or bridge. An endosseous implant is seated within the jaw bone and requires adequate bone to support the implant as well as conscientious and diligent oral health care and maintenance. There are, however, a certain number of implants that fail either pre- or post-osseointegration.

M27.61   Osseointegration failure of dental implant

This type of dental implant failure is sometimes considered a pre-osseointegration failure that arises from early complications of implant placement, such as hemorrhagic problems, or pre-existing conditions such as poor bone quality. The complications prevent the implant from integrating with the surrounding bone and soft tissue. This code also includes iatrogenic causes of implant failure.

M27.62 Post-osseointegration biological failure of dental implant

Biological post-osseointegration dental implant failure can be caused by any number of complications that may arise after placement and integration of the implant and include periodontal inflammation or infection around the implant; lack of oral hygiene; unattached gingiva; and occlusal trauma on the implant from the forces acting on it due to weakened bone, bruxism, or other problems.

M27.63 Post-osseointegration mechanical failure of dental implant

Mechanical post-osseointegration dental implant failure can be caused by any failure of the prosthesis itself, such as a fracture of the implant body, causing loss of the implant.

Note: Fractured dental restorative material or a fracture of teeth themselves are not coded here.

M27.8 Other specified diseases of jaws

Other specified diseases of jaw includes exostosis of the jaw -- a ridge of cartilage that forms along the jaw, usually just below the teeth, which typically begins to develop in early adulthood. This disorder is painless and rarely presents a problem or requires correction, but in some cases may grow to several centimeters in size and can contribute to periodontal disease (disease of the roots of the teeth) by forcing food towards the teeth instead of away from them. In these cases, surgical removal of the excess cartilage may be advisable. Other conditions included here are fibrous dysplasia of the jaw, and unilateral condylar hypoplasia and hyperplasia.

M30.0 Polyarteritis nodosa

Polyarteritis nodosa is an autoimmune disease in which the body's immune system mistakenly attacks small and medium-sized blood vessels, resulting in the death of the tissue these vessels supply with blood. The most commonly affected tissues are the kidneys, bowels, heart, and skin. Typical symptoms include fever, weight loss, muscle and joint aches, weakness, and fatigue. A definitive diagnosis requires biopsies of the affected tissue.

M30.3 Mucocutaneous lymph node syndrome [Kawasaki]

Acute febrile mucocutaneous lymph node syndrome, also known as MCLS or Kawasaki disease, is a rare fever disease of children which features conjunctivitis, red, swollen lips and gums, and swollen lymph nodes in the neck as the primary symptoms. Ulcers of the gums and a bright red rash are also present. The cause of this disease is not known, and it usually resolves without serious complications, although meningitis and arthritis have been known to occur.

M31.0 Hypersensitivity angiitis

Hypersensitivity angiitis is a condition in which small blood vessels, usually located near the skin, become inflamed. Other organs can be affected, usually the gastrointestinal tract or the kidneys. This disease can be acute or chronic. The most common symptoms are itching and burning of the skin, as well as the formation of small lesions. This includes Goodpasture's syndrome, a rare autoimmune disease in which the patient's immune system attacks the Goodpasture antigen in the kidneys and the lungs, resulting in the destruction of the kidneys and bleeding from the lungs.

M31.2 Lethal midline granuloma

A lethal midline granuloma is a severe tumor associated with infection that appears in the nose or sinuses and may be fatal if not diagnosed and treated in time.

M31.3 Wegener's granulomatosis

Wegener's granulomatosis is an autoimmune disorder in which the patient's immune system mistakenly attacks small blood vessels. The affected vessels provide blood to the skin, kidneys, and lungs, although other organs may be affected. Skin lesions are common, as is arthritis and renal failure.

M31.4 Aortic arch syndrome [Takayasu]

Takayasu's disease is an inflammatory disease of the aorta that leads to poor blood supply to bodily tissues. The most common symptom is coolness or pain in the extremities, as well as headache and diffuse pain in the chest and abdomen. Dizziness, fatigue, and weight loss are also common.

M31.5 Giant cell arteritis with polymyalgia rheumatica

Giant cell arteritis is a condition that most often occurs in the elderly in which abnormally large cells block the passage of blood through the retinal, temporal, or intracerebral arteries. Common symptoms are fever, headache, vision problems, and tenderness of the scalp.

M32 Systemic lupus erythematosus (SLE)

Systemic lupus erythematosus is an autoimmune disorder that affects numerous parts of the body, including the joints, skin, kidneys, heart and blood vessels, lungs, and brain. It can present with varying symptoms but the most common are extreme fatigue, painful and/or swollen joints (i.e., arthritis), fever, kidney problems, and a skin rash that can give the patient's face a wolf-like appearance (giving the disease its name). These symptoms appear in episodes known as "flares" and then go into remission. There is no cure for lupus, but medication can reduce symptoms and allow the patient to live a normal, healthy life.

M33 Dermatopolymyositis

Dermato(poly)myositis is an inflammatory disease which presents with a sudden, severe, bluish-purple rash on the face, neck, shoulders, upper chest, elbows, knees, knuckles, and back which either accompanies or precedes an equally severe onset of muscle weakness that affects the muscles closest to the trunk (e.g., the shoulders and hips) more than those further out (e.g., the elbows, hands, and fingers). In some patients, calcium deposits may form under the skin, which appear as hard bumps. Most cases respond well to therapy, which may include steroid drugs and physical rehabilitation.

M33.2 Polymyositis

Polymyositis is another inflammatory disease which like dermatomyositis presents with weakness in the muscles, especially those closest to the trunk. It does not, however, present with dermatopolymyositis' characteristic rash. It often presents in combination with other illnesses with similar or overlapping symptoms, making diagnosis more difficult.

M34 Systemic sclerosis [scleroderma]

Systemic sclerosis, sometimes called scleroderma, is a diffuse connective tissue disease that affects the skin, blood vessels, skeletal muscles, and internal organs by causing the build-up of scar tissue (fibrosis). It presents with whitening, blueness, or redness in the fingers and/or toes, pain and stiffness in the joints, thickening and hardening of the skin which causes a mask-like facial expression, heartburn, difficulty swallowing, etc.

M35.0 Sicca syndrome [Sjögren]

Sicca syndrome, also known as Sjögren syndrome, is an autoimmune disorder that most often presents with dry eyes and mouth, rheumatoid arthritis, or another similar disease of the connective tissue, and chronic inflammatory diseases (e.g., lupus) which are usually especially noticible in the glands. About 90% of sicca syndrome patients are middle age or older women.

M35.2 Behçet's disease

Behçet's syndrome is characterized by recurring crops of painful ulcers of the mouth, skin, and genitals, as well as severe inflammation of the uvea of the eye, retinal vasculitis, and optic atrophy. Arthritis and digestive system involvement often accompanies these symptoms. The cause of the disease is not known, but is not suspected to be contagious.

M35.3 Polymyalgia rheumatica

Polymyalgia rheumatica is an inflammatory disorder in which the patient feels perpetually stiff and sore, as if having done strenuous exercise for a long while. The cause of this disorder is not known, but it is suspected to be an autoimmune disorder, in which the body's own immune system attacks

2016 Plain English Descriptions for ICD-10-CM   Chapter 13 Diseases of the Musculoskeletal System and Connective Tissue | M35.7 – M43.1

Diseases of the Musculoskeletal System   M35.7 – M43.1

one or more of its systems. There is no cure for this disease, but it normally vanishes in one or two years on its own.

M35.7   Hypermobility syndrome

Hypermobility syndrome is a chronic condition in which the patient's joints are laxer and more fragile than in the average person. The term "double jointed" is often used to describe these patients. The joints of those suffering from hypermobility are often painful and need extra protection during exercise; e.g., knee braces for running or jogging. In some cases, surgical intervention to tighten loose joints may be advised.

M35.8   Other specified systemic involvement of connective tissue

Other specified systemic involvement of connective tissue includes eosinophilia myalgia syndrome, also called EMS, first diagnosed in 1989 and associated with taking L-tryptophan, a health food supplement that was sold as a sleep aid. It is an inflammatory disease of the skin, muscles, nerves, heart, blood vessels, and lungs and initially presents with acute pain and muscle cramps, tremors, numbness or a tingling or burning sensation, and tenderness and swelling of the extremities. In its later stages, it can present with short term memory loss, difficulty concentrating, heart and liver disease, high blood pressure, the buildup of fibrous (scar) tissue, chronic fatigue, sleeping disorders, and symptoms similar to post-traumatic stress disorder. There is no cure, and treatment targets reducing the inflammation.

M36.0   Dermato(poly)myositis in neoplastic disease

Dermato(poly)myositis is an inflammatory disease which presents with a sudden, severe, bluish-purple rash on the face, neck, shoulders, upper chest, elbows, knees, knuckles, and back which either accompanies or precedes an equally severe onset of muscle weakness that affects the muscles closest to the trunk (e.g., the shoulders and hips) more than those further out (e.g., the elbows, hands, and fingers). When this disorder is caused by neoplastic disease, report the underlying, causative neoplasm first.

M36.1   Arthropathy in neoplastic disease

Arthropathy indicates pain and swelling of the joints that is occurring due to a neoplasm as the underlying cause, such as leukemia, multiple myeloma, and malignant histiocytosis, which must be coded first.

M40   Kyphosis and lordosis

The spine is normally straight from side-to-side, but has a gentle outward curve at the thoracic (chest-level) of the spine and a gentle inward curve at the lumbar spine. Kyphosis is an abnormal degree of outward curvature in the thoracic vertebrae, giving the back a rounded or hunchback appearance. Lordosis is an abnormal inward curvature in the lumbar vertebrae that gives the back a swayback appearance. This may be caused by spondylolisthesis and achondroplasia.

M40.0   Postural kyphosis

Postural kyphosis is a common type of abnormal curvature of the spine that is mainly due to slouching.

M40.1   Other secondary kyphosis

Other types of secondary kyphosis may be caused by developmental problems, degenerative disease, osteoporosis, compression fractures, and trauma.

M40.3   Flatback syndrome

Flatback syndrome is a disorder resulting in a postural defect in which the person is unable to stand upright due to a loss of the normal inward sway or curvature of the lumbar spine. Some patients may even begin to have reverse outward curving, or lumbar kyphosis, of the lower back. Flatback can occur in patients with thoracolumbar kyphosis, in which the aggravated outward curvature of the spine just above the lumbar area causes flattening of the normal lumbar curve. This condition is more likely to occur in older adults who have had scoliosis surgery, particularly those who have had distraction instrumentation used down to the sacral area, such as a

Harrington rod. The use of segmental instrumentation in spine surgery has now lessened the occurrence of flatback.

M41   Scoliosis

Scoliosis is an abnormal side-to-side curvature of the spine. This most often gives the spine an S-shape appearance (with two curves), although C-shaped scoliosis can occur. Other symptoms caused by scoliosis include uneven hips and shoulders, backaches, and tiredness in the spine after sitting or standing for a while. Scoliosis most often affects girls and is more prone to worsening during growth spurts. Treatment depends on the type of scoliosis, how much growing is yet to occur, where the curve is located, and how severe the presentation is. Physical therapy and back braces are used to prevent further curving and can be adjusted as the patient grows. This treatment works best on those over 10 years old. Surgery may be needed using metal rods held with hooks and screws to correct the curve.

Note: This category includes kyphoscoliosis, which presents with both the side-to-side curve in addition to an exaggerated outward thoracic curve.

M41.0   Infantile idiopathic scoliosis

Infantile idiopathic scoliosis is abnormal side-to-side curvature of the spine without known cause that occurs in children age three and under. Resolving infantile idiopathic scoliosis is a type of scoliosis which is present from birth or a very young age, but which diminishes or vanishes altogether as the child grows. Progressive infantile idiopathic scoliosis likewise appears at birth or shortly thereafter, but grows worse rather than better as the child grows.

M41.11   Juvenile idiopathic scoliosis

Juvenile idiopathic scoliosis is abnormal side-to-side curvature of the spine without known cause that occurs in children aged 4-10.

M41.12   Adolescent scoliosis

Adolescent idiopathic scoliosis is abnormal side-to-side curvature of the spine without known cause that occurs in children age 11-18.

M41.4   Neuromuscular scoliosis

Neuromuscular scoliosis is an abnormal side-to-side curvature of the spine caused by a disorder of the nervous system that affects the muscles, such as poliomyelitis, spina bifida, cerebral palsy, muscular dystrophy, and Friedriech's ataxia.

M42.0   Juvenile osteochondrosis of spine

Juvenile osteochondrosis is an inflammation of the immature spine which includes the epiphysis, a growth plate area of cartilage that normally transforms into bone as the skeleton matures. The disease is characterized by an initial process of degeneration or aseptic necrosis, which can lead to fractures and malformations of the skeleton, followed by regeneration and recalcification. Juvenile osteochondrosis of the spine is usually marked by kyphosis (hunchback) and degeneration of the discs as well.

M43.0   Spondylolysis

Spondylolysis is a defect of the pars interarticularis in the vertebrae which predisposes them to fracture. There may be a genetic link to the condition or it may result from trauma or overuse in certain sports, such as gymnastics and football. The condition occurs most commonly in the lumbar region (specifically L5) during adolescence. Symptoms can include low back pain and/or pain in the legs, hamstring tightness, changes in posture and gait.

M43.1   Spondylolisthesis

Acquired spondylolisthesis is a condition in which one of the vertebrae slips out of its proper place onto the bone below it. This can result in increased curvature of the spine and some of the nerves of the spinal cord becoming compressed. Symptoms include lower back pain; muscle tightness in the hamstring area; and pain, tingling, numbness, or weakness in the legs and buttocks, although symptoms can range from mild to severe.

Note: Spondylolisthesis is a common sports injury in adolescents and the acute traumatic cases are reported in the injuries chapter.

M43.6 Torticollis

Torticollis, sometimes called wry-neck, is a condition in which the patient has spasmodic contractions of the neck muscles on one side, limiting neck motion and causing the head to be held consistently to that side, as if cocking an ear to listen to something. This condition may be treated with gentle stretching exercises or, in some cases, surgery.

M45 Ankylosing spondylitis

Also known as Marie-Struempell disease, rheumatoid spondylitis, and Bechterew's syndrome, ankylosing spondylitis is a chronic, progressive, autoimmune arthropathy that affects the spine and sacroiliac joints, eventually leading to spinal fusion and rigidity. Almost all of the autoimmune spondylarthropathies share a common genetic marker, HLA-B27, although the cause is still unknown. The disease appears in some predisposed people after exposure to bowel or urinary tract infections. The most common patient is a young male, aged 15-30, as it affects men about three times more than women. Swelling occurs in the intervertebral discs and in the joints between the spine and pelvis. Patients have persistent buttock and low back pain and stiffness alleviated with exercise. Over time, the vertebrae may become fused together, progressing up the spine and affecting other organs. The disease is related to other inflammatory conditions in the body such as iridocyclitis, inflammatory bowel disease, psoriasis, Reiter's disease, and heart valve involvement in extreme cases. Prodromal rheumatism-like symptoms occur at a very young age. Diagnosis is made before visible changes on x-ray appear by using tomography and MRI of the sacroiliac joints. Over the long term, progressed cases show spinal osteopenia with compression fractures and a hump back, and the visible formation of abnormal bony outgrowths, called syndesmophytes, on the spine.

M46.0 Spinal enthesopathy

Spinal enthesopathy is a general term referring to a disorder of the sites where the muscular tendons and ligaments attach to the spine and can include inflammatory and degenerative disorders.

M46.1 Sacroiliitis, not elsewhere classified

Sacroiliitis is an inflammation of the sacroiliac joint, which connects the spine and the pelvis. It is often associated with ankylosing spondylitis, and can cause skeletal changes in the long term, such as irregular bony ridges on the pelvis.

M47 Spondylosis

Spondylosis is a term describing degeneration of the spinal (facet) joints, usually due to aging and loss of fluid of the intervertebral discs, also known as arthrosis or osteoarthritis of the spine. It may or may not present with myelopathy or radiculopathy, or cause compression syndromes of the anterior spinal or vertebral arteries.

M47.1 Other spondylosis with myelopathy

Spondylosis is a medical term for degeneration of the spinal (facet) joints, usually due to aging of the intervertebral discs, also known as arthrosis or osteoarthritis of the spine. Myelopathy is a disorder of the spinal cord itself caused by spondylogenic compression of the cord, causing pain, numbness, muscle weakness, or even paralysis below the level of the affected nerves.

M47.2 Other spondylosis with radiculopathy

Spondylosis is a medical term for degeneration of the spinal (facet) joints, usually due to aging of the intervertebral discs, also known as arthrosis or osteoarthritis of the spine. Radiculopathy is a disease of the spinal nerves and nerve roots caused by irritation due to damage or deformity of intervertebral discs and osteoarthritic changes in the vertebrae, resulting in pain radiating from the spine, weakness, numbness, and difficulty with certain muscle movements.

M48.0 Spinal stenosis

Spinal (caudal) stenosis is a narrowing of the spinal canal, which contains and protects the spinal cord and the nerve roots that branch from it. Severe stenosis may compress the spinal cord or nerve roots and become symptomatic. It often causes severe back pain and may also cause numbness and muscle weakness in the lower body and/or leave the patient very susceptible to herniated discs. It may be caused by aging, a congenital condition (i.e., the spinal canal is too narrow at birth), or another disease or injury. Treatment may range from conservative approaches, such as bed rest, changing posture, and medication, to surgical correction.

M48.1 Ankylosing hyperostosis [Forestier]

Ankylosing vertebral hyperostosis, also called diffuse idiopathic skeletal hyperostosis (DISH) and Forestier's disease, is a type of unique spondyloarthropathy in which calcification moves along the sides of contiguous vertebrae of the spine in association with inflamed tendons that calcify at their attachment points to the spine. This creates the formation of bone spurs with accompanying pain and stiffness in the areas of bony change.

M48.2 Kissing spine

Kissing spine, also called Baastrup's syndrome or disease, is a common form of spinal degeneration seen in the elderly. In kissing spine, the spinous processes, the parts of the vertebrae that project outward and onto which the muscles attach, grow until they are very close together or actually in contact with each other, causing pain, inflammation, and immobility.

M48.3 Traumatic spondylopathy

Traumatic spondylopathy, also called Kummell's disease, is a compression fracture of one or more vertebrae, often after spinal surgery. It presents with pain in the spine and may affect the patient's motor coordination of the legs.

M48.8 Other specified spondylopathies

Other specified spondylopathies includes ossification of the posterior longitudinal ligament. Ossification is a condition in which other tissues are transformed into bone. Ossification of the posterior longitudinal ligament in the cervical region often causes stenosis (see above) and compression of the spinal cord (myelopathy) and presents with pain, numbness, and/or muscle weakness throughout the body as a result. This is a progressive disorder and surgical treatment is usually required to relieve symptoms.

M49 Spondylopathies in diseases classified elsewhere

This category includes spinal curvature or deformities, kyphosis or scoliosis, and other spondylopathies occuring in diseases classified elsewhere.

Note: Some specific infectious diseases known to cause spondylitis or spondylopathy as well as curvature of the spine, such as tuberculosis, have a more specific code that must be assigned.

M50 Cervical disc disorders

The intervertebral discs are soft, gel-like cushions that support the spine and keep the vertebrae from resting directly on each other and grinding together. Each disc has a strong outer ring called the annulus, which actually serves as a ligament to connect each vertebra to the next. The soft interior of the disc contains a large volume of fluid and serves as a shock absorber for the spine.

M50.0 Cervical disc disorder with myelopathy

Myelopathy is a disorder of the spinal cord itself caused by compression of the cord, due to damage or deformity of the (cervical) intervertebral discs. This causes pain, numbness, muscle weakness, or even paralysis below the level of the affected nerves.

Note: Cervical disc degeneration or displacement stated as occuring with cervicalgia or spinal cord compression is reported here.

M50.1 Cervical disc disorder with radiculopathy

Radiculopathy is a disease of the spinal nerves and nerve roots caused by irritation due to damage or deformity of (cervical) intervertebral discs, resulting in pain radiating from the spine, weakness, numbness, and difficulty with certain muscle movements.

Note: Cervical disc degeneration or displacement stated as occuring with neuritis or radiculitis of the spinal nerves or nerve roots is reported here.

M50.2   Other cervical disc displacement

A disc displacement, or "slipped disc," occurs when the soft interior of the disc bulges through a rupture in the surrounding annulus. In many instances, there are no noticeable symptoms of having a slipped disc, but it is associated with pain, particularly if the prolapsed (bulging) disc tissue presses on the spinal cord or the nerve roots, causing pain, numbness, and/or muscle weakness.

Note: If the disc displacement is specified as presenting with cervicalgia or compression of the cord, report the appropriate level code from subcategory M50.0 for cervical disc disorder with myelopathy.

Note: If the disc displacement is noted as occurring with neuritis ar radiculitis, report the appropriate level code from subcategory M50.1 for cervical disc disorder with radiculopathy.

M50.3   Other cervical disc degeneration

Degeneration of a cervical vertebral disc occurs over time as the soft part of the disc dehydrates, altering the disc height as it becomes harder and loses its cushioning effect. This adversely affects the mechanics of the spinal column and the function of other structures, such as muscles and ligaments. Many patients do not exhibit any severe symptoms and many even be asymptomatic; however, the condition can become quite painful and is associated with neck pain. Disc degeneration is a precursor to disc herniation and can lead to spinal stenosis in the long term.

Note: If the disc degeneration is specified as presenting with cervicalgia or compression of the cord, report the appropriate level code from subcategory M50.0 for cervical disc disorder with myelopathy.

Note: If the disc degeneration is noted as occurring with neuritis ar radiculitis, report the appropriate level code from subcategory M50.1 for cervical disc disorder with radiculopathy.

M51   Thoracic, thoracolumbar, and lumbosacral intervertebral disc disorders

The intervertebral discs are soft, gel-like cushions that support the spine and keep the vertebrae from resting directly on each other and grinding together. Each disc has a strong outer ring called the annulus, which actually serves as a ligament to connect each vertebra to the next. The soft interior of the disc contains a large volume of fluid and serves as a shock absorber for the spine.

M51.0   Thoracic, thoracolumbar and lumbosacral intervertebral disc disorders with myelopathy

Myelopathy is a disorder of the spinal cord itself caused by compression of the cord, due to damage or deformity of the (thoracic, lumbar, or lumbosacral) intervertebral discs, causing pain, numbness, muscle weakness, or even paralysis below the level of the affected nerves.

Note: Thoracic, thoracolumbar, and lumbosacral disc degeneration or disc displacement stated as occuring with spinal cord compression is reported here.

M51.1   Thoracic, thoracolumbar and lumbosacral intervertebral disc disorders with radiculopathy

Radiculopathy is a disease of the spinal nerves and nerve roots caused by irritation due to damaged or deformed intervertebral discs, resulting in pain radiating from the spine, weakness, numbness, and difficulty with certain muscle movements.

Note: Thoracolumbar and lumbosacral disc degeneration or disc displacement stated as occuring with sciatica, neuritis, or radiculitis is reported here.

M51.2   Other thoracic, thoracolumbar and lumbosacral intervertebral disc displacement

A disc displacement, or "slipped disc," occurs when the soft interior of the disc bulges through a rupture in the surrounding annulus. In many instances, there are no noticeable symptoms of having a slipped disc, but it is associated with lower back pain, known as lumbago. If the prolapsed (bulging) disc tissue actually presses on the spinal cord or the nerve roots, it can cause severe pain, numbness, and/or muscle weakness.

Note: If the disc displacement is specified as presenting with compression of the cord or spinal cord involvement, report the appropriate level code from subcategory M51.0 for thoracic, thoracolumbar, and lumbosacral disc disorder with myelopathy.

Note: If the disc displacement is noted as occurring with sciatica, neuritis, or radiculitis, report the appropriate level code from subcategory M51.1 for disc disorder with radiculopathy.

M51.3   Other thoracic, thoracolumbar and lumbosacral intervertebral disc degeneration

Degeneration of a thoracic, thoracolumbar, or lumbosacral vertebral disc occurs over time as the soft part of the disc dehydrates, altering the disc height as it becomes harder and loses its cushioning effect. This adversely affects the mechanics of the spinal column and the function of other structures, such as muscles and ligaments. Many patients do not exhibit any severe symptoms and many even be asymptomatic; however, the condition can become quite painful and is associated with back pain. Disc degeneration is a precursor to disc herniation and can lead to spinal stenosis in the long term.

Note: If the disc degeneration is specified as presenting with compression of the cord or spinal cord involvement, report the appropriate level code from subcategory M51.0 for thoracic, thoracolumbar and lumbosacral disc disorder with myelopathy.

Note: If the disc degeneration is noted as occurring with sciatica, or radiculitis, report the appropriate level code from subcategory M51.1 for thoracic, thoracolumbar and lumbosacral disc disorder with radiculopathy.

M51.4   Schmorl's nodes

Schmorl's nodes are an unusual defect in which the soft center of the disc pushes (herniates) into a pocket or cavity in the bone of the vertebra. These cavities are usually the result of previous trauma to the spine through disease or injury. This condition usually presents with back pain, most often in the mid- to lower spine, and is most common in patients of 14–18 years of age.

M53.0   Cervicocranial syndrome

Cervicocranial syndrome is a condition that often results from whiplash injuries to the nerves of the upper spine and neck just below the brain. It presents with vertigo, dizziness, double-vision (diplopia), partial loss or clouding of one or more senses, a stuffy feeling in the ears, and headache.

M53.1   Cervicobrachial syndrome

Cervicobrachial syndrome (diffuse) is a term used to indicate a collection of symptoms that arise due to the anterior neck muscles compressing the nerve root known as the brachial plexus, which controls movement of and sensation from the nerves of the shoulder and arm. This disorder presents with pain that radiates from the shoulder to the arm and/or the back of the neck, and may also present with muscle weakness in the arm.

M53.2X8 Spinal instabilities, sacral and sacrococcygeal region

The sacrum is the part of the spinal column that forms part of the pelvis, which is formed by the fusion of five originally separate vertebrae in the lower back. This code should be used to report hypermobility of the coccyx, which is caused when the four vertebrae do not fuse correctly during early childhood.

M54.0   Panniculitis affecting regions of neck and back

Panniculitis is a rare inflammation of the subcutaneous fat, which can present with painful lumps or nodules beneath the skin that may appear pink, red, or even black and blue, on the surface. Occasional fever, pain, and severe fatigue are also common. This is often a chronic condition with no direct cure.

M54.1 Radiculopathy

This includes neuritis of specified general areas, such as brachial, thoracic, lumbar, and lumbosacral neuritis, and radiculitis that is not otherwise specified. Radiculitis is the swelling or inflammation of nerve roots at their connection to the spinal column, causing pain to radiate along the whole dermatome, or sensory distribution of the affected nerve. Brachial neuritis, for instance is a condition that presents with severe pain in one or both shoulders, which worsens when the patient moves the shoulder. The cause of brachial neuritis is not known but is suspected to be due to an autoimmune dysfunction; that is, the body's own immune system attacks the affected nerves. Lumbaosacral neuritis is severe pain in the lower back and possibly one or both legs. This is followed by swelling and abnormal sensations such as burning, tingling, pricking, or tickling. Symptoms of neuritis or radiculitis may fade on their own within weeks, though low-grade pain may persist long term.

M54.2 Cervicalgia

Cervicalgia indicates pain in the neck which does not radiate outward to other areas of the body. It is usually due to constant tension in the neck muscles and is usually treated with ice and a neck collar to allow the neck muscles to rest.

M54.3 Sciatica

Sciatica is a condition in which the patient suffers from severe pain in the sciatic nerve that runs from the lower back down through the back of each leg. Sciatica is a set of symptoms characterized by shooting pain in the back and in the rear of the leg, parasthesia, burning and tingling sensations, and/or weakness in the low back, buttocks, or lower extremities. Usually only one side is affected. Symptoms result from compression of one or more spinal nerves (L1, L2, L3, S1, S2, S3) that form the sciatic nerve (right and left branches). Causes can include herniated discs, spinal stenosis, pregnancy, injury or tumors.

M54.4 Lumbago with sciatica

Lumbago is an unspecified source or type of low back pain, which can occur together with sciatica, which is severe pain of the sciatic nerve running from the lower back down through the back of the leg.

M60.0 Infective myositis

Infective myositis is an inflammation of muscle tissue that occurs due to a bacterial, viral, or parasitic infection. It presents with pain, swelling, and muscle weakness that resolve once the infection is treated. This category includes tropical pyomyositis, more often called simply infective pyomyositis because the disease has spread beyond its original home in the tropical regions. Streptococcus bacteria are the most common source of infection. It presents as an infected, pus-filled pocket (or abscess) in the muscle, most commonly afflicting the muscles of the legs. Initial symptoms are stiffness and pain in the affected area. The infection is treated with antibiotics, but if left untreated, it will usually spread, causing septic shock and possibly death.

M60.2 Foreign body granuloma of soft tissue, not elsewhere classified

A foreign body becomes lodged in the muscle or other soft tissue and causes the formation of a granuloma, a hard, nodular (knob-like) inflammation surrounded by a mass of lymphocytes, that occurs as an immune response to the presence of the foreign body, such as a splinter.

M61 Calcification and ossification of muscle

Muscular calcification and ossification are related conditions that occur when calcium deposits build up in the muscles, causing them to harden. As the process continues, the muscle become more like bone (ossifying), which results in a loss of mobility.

M61.0 Myositis ossificans traumatica

Traumatic myositis ossificans is a condition in which the body reacts to an injury to a muscle (usually blunt trauma rather than an open wound) by attempting to repair it in the manner that bone is repaired. This results in a calcium buildup and the formation of bony tissue in the joints close to the site of the injury, reducing the range-of-motion in those joints.

Note: This type of ossification has also been noted in cases of paralysis due to spinal injury. When quadriplegia or paralegia is associated with myositis ossificans, report with subcategory M61.2

M61.1 Myositis ossificans progressiva

Progressive myositis ossificans is a genetic disorder that causes ongoing ossification, or hardening, of muscle tissue from an early age, disabling and ultimately resulting in the death of the patient.

M61.10 Myositis ossificans progressiva, unspecified site

Progressive myositis ossificans is a progressive, genetic disorder that causes ossification, or hardening, of the muscle from an early age, disabling and ultimately resulting in the death of the patient.

M61.4 Other calcification of muscle

Postoperative heterotopic calcification occurs as a reaction of the body to surgery, usually affecting the muscle and tissue at the site of the surgical incision.

M62.0 Separation of muscle (nontraumatic)

Separation of a muscle, also called diastasis of a muscle, is a condition in which a muscle separates along the grain of the muscle fibers, as opposed to a rupture, which occurs across the grain of the muscle fibers. This most commonly occurs in sphincter muscles, such as those in the anus or the abdominal muscle wall.

M62.1 Other rupture of muscle (nontraumatic)

A nontraumatic rupture of the muscle is a tear in the muscle that occurs due to weakening by disease or an undetermined cause. Such ruptures are more common in older patients and are often due to wear-and-tear on the muscle tissue as it loses its ability to repair itself as quickly.

M62.4 Contracture of muscle

Contracture is a shortening of the muscle and/or tendon sheath which prevents normal movement and flexibility. A muscle spasm can vary in intensity and duration, as well as the root cause. Causes for muscle spasms, or contractions, can include prolonged immobilization, reduced blood supply, scarring from trauma or burns, and degenerative diseases affecting the muscles.

M62.82 Rhabdomyolysis

Rhabdomyolysis is a disease characterized by severe muscle destruction throughout the body, often as a result of trauma or exposure to drugs or toxins. It presents with acute muscle pain and weakness; myoglobin (a type of muscle protein) in the urine, giving it a dark red color; and kidney failure. The severity of the disease and the prognosis depends on the underlying cause.

M62.83 Muscle spasm

A muscle spasm is a sudden, painful, involuntary contracture of a muscle(s). It can vary in intensity and duration, as well as in root cause. Causes include abnormal or malfunctioning nerve signals, muscle fatigue (overuse, exertion), dehydration, electrolyte imbalance, decreased blood supply and certain medications.

M65.2 Calcific tendinitis

Calcium deposits in the tendon can cause friction and wear-and-tear on the soft tissue, resulting in pain, inflammation, and loss of mobility. The pain often comes in waves of sudden, shooting pain, and if left untreated, lasting damage to the tendon can result. Surgical removal of the calcium deposits is often required.

M65.3 Trigger finger

Trigger finger occurs when the sheaths of the tendons that help bend the fingers and thumb become inflamed (tenosynovitis), compressing the tendon. This causes pain and a popping sensation as the patient bends and straightens his or her fingers. In some cases, the finger may become stuck in a bent position. Surgery may be required to correct this condition.

M65.4   Radial styloid tenosynovitis [de Quervain]

Radial styloid tenosynovitis, also called de Quervain's disease or de Quervain's tenosynovitis, is a similar condition to trigger finger, but affects the thumb and wrist rather than the fingers, causing pain and stiffness that is usually most prominent in the wrist just behind the thumb.

M65.8   Other synovitis and tenosynovitis

Synovitis is an inflammation of the synovium, a thin layer of tissue that lines the space between the joints. The synovium serves to keep foreign matter out of the joints and produces joint fluid to lubricate the interior. Tenosynovitis is an inflammation of the tendons and the synovial sheath, which protects and lubricates the tendon.

M66   Spontaneous rupture of synovium and tendon

Spontaneous, or nontraumatic, rupture is a tear that occurs due to an old injury or underlying condition and not from an acute accident or trauma. A cyst is the most common cause for spontaneous rupture of a tendon or the synovium, the thin layer of tissue that lines the space between the jointed ends and produces fluid for interior lubrication.

M67.4   Ganglion

A ganglion, or ganglion cyst, is a fluid-filled pocket that forms around a joint, putting pressure on the tendons and ligaments and possibly causing pain and loss of the joint's normal range of motion. Ganglions may recede on their own or require aspiration or surgical drainage to remove.

Note: A synovial cyst is a pocket of fluid that forms in the protective sheath of the tendon and is coded elsewhere.

M67.5   Plica syndrome

A plica is a thin wall of fibrous tissue that is an extension of the synovia of the knee. Most of the time, this presents no problem to the patient. Plica syndrome occurs when the synovium becomes inflamed, causing the plica to become thicker. The thickened plica catches on the femur (thigh bone) as the knee moves, causing more inflammation, which in turn results in the plica becoming even thicker in a cycle that can only be broken by anti-inflammatory medication, and in some cases, by surgery.

M70   Soft tissue disorders related to use, overuse and pressure

This category includes bursitis cases and other soft tissue problems related to occupational posture, and originating from repetitive movements that use, overuse, and strain soft tissue of specific joints. Bursitis is inflammation of the small, fluid-filled lubricating sac of a joint that cushions movement of the tendons. A bursitide, or bursitis, is most often due to occupational reasons. For example, plumbers and roofers, who spend a large amount of time working on their knees, often contract bursitis of the knee. These typically have informal names such as miner's elbow, housemaid's knee, and weaver's bottom.

M70.2   Olecranon bursitis

Olecranon bursitis, also known as bursitis of the elbow, is a disorder of pain, redness, and swelling of the elbow joint caused by inflammation of the bursal sac. The bursa is a thin, small sac of lubricating fluid that acts as a cushion between bones and soft tissue and allows for smooth movement of the tendons around the bony point of the elbow joint. When fluid collects and the bursa becomes inflamed, the patient experiences pain and noticeable swelling. In most cases, treatment consists of draining the excess fluid.

M70.4   Prepatellar bursitis

Prepatellar bursitis is an inflammation that causes excess fluid to accumulate in the bursa, the small sac of lubricating fluid that cushions the kneecap from the soft tissue and tendons and promotes smooth movement on the knee. The inflammation can cause pain, loss of mobility, and damage to the knee when significant amounts of friction continue for longer periods. It is most prominent in plumbers, carpet layers, roofers, and others who spend a lot of time on their knees, or in athletes in high-contact sports.

M71.4   Calcium deposit in bursa

Calcium deposits in bursae, the small sacs of lubricating fluid that act as cushions between bones and soft tissue, allowing for smooth movement of tendons, results in painful friction and wear-and-tear on the joint, resulting in inflammation and loss of mobility in which lasting damage to the joint can result. Surgical removal of the calcium deposits is often required.

M72.0   Palmar fascial fibromatosis [Dupuytren]

The palmar fascia is a thin, triangular sheet of connective tissue that covers the tendons of the palm of the hand and holds them in place. Contracture of the palmar fascia, also called Dupuytren's contracture, is a disorder, thought to be inherited, that causes the palmar fascia to thicken and compress the tendons, making it more difficult to fully extend the fingers. This condition may be treated surgically.

M72.2   Plantar fascial fibromatosis

Plantar fascial fibromatosis is the growth of soft-tissue tumors in the soles of the feet that put pressure on the ligaments and can cause the toes to contract. Fibromatoses are rarely malignant, but frequently disfiguring, and cause malfunction in the surrounding tissues due to the pressure that they exert.

Note: Plantar fasciitis is included here. This is inflammation of the thick sheet of tissue on the bottom of the foot that connects the heel bone to the toes and creates the arch of the foot. This inflammation usually occurs with overstretching and overuse and is the most common orthopedic complaint of the foot, especially among runners and those with flat feet or high arches. It causes pain and stiffness in the bottom of the heel.

M72.6   Necrotizing fasciitis

Necrotizing fasciitis is the result of a bacterial infection which attacks the fascia, the tissue that connects the skin and the muscle. The bacteria usually enters the body through a wound near the site where the necrotizing fasciitis first appears. This disease is often referred to as "flesh-eating bacteria." The dead tissue must be surgically removed from the body in order to halt infection and save the life of the patient. In more advanced cases, the affected limb often needs to be amputated entirely.

M72.8   Other fibroblastic disorders

Other fibroblastic disorders includes unspecified fasciitis, infective fasciitis, and abscesses of fascia not listed elsewhere. Fascia is the strong fibrous sheet or band of connective tissue that envelops and isolates muscles of the body, providing protection and structural support.

M72.9   Fibroblastic disorder, unspecified

This includes fibromatosis that is not otherwise specified. Fibromatosis is the formation of soft tissue tumors that are rarely malignant, but frequently become disfiguring. They can cause malfunction in surrounding tissue exerting pressure on the ligaments and other nearby structures around it.

M75.0   Adhesive capsulitis of shoulder

Adhesive capsulitis of the shoulder, also sometimes referred to as "frozen shoulder," is a disorder of unknown origin that causes pain and loss of range of motion in the shoulder joint. This condition progresses in three distinct stages. In the "freezing" stage, which lasts between 10 and 36 weeks, the patient experiences the most severe pain and a gradual loss of range of motion. In the "frozen" stage, which lasts between 4 and 12 months, the pain decreases gradually, but the patient does not regain full motion of the joint. In the "thawing" stage, which can last between one and several years, the patient gradually regains nearly full motion of the limb. Treatment of this disorder concentrates on pain management and resting the joint.

M75.1   Rotator cuff tear or rupture, not specified as traumatic

The rotator cuff is a very powerful collection of muscles and tendons that control movement in the shoulder. In rotator cuff syndrome, the tendons and/or their sheaths become swollen or otherwise immobile, causing stiffness and pain when the shoulder is worked.

M75.11 Incomplete rotator cuff tear or rupture not specified as traumatic

The rotator cuff is actually a network of four muscles and many tendons that form a protective cover over the head of the humerus and hold the upper arm bone in place in the shoulder joint while allowing it to rotate. Most tears occur in people over 40 as a result of overuse, particularly from overhead repetitive motions such as with tennis, weight-lifting, rowing, and construction work. In a partial or incomplete tear, some of the tendons in one area of the cuff are damaged without the tear going all the way through the tendons. This may or may not require surgery along with physical therapy. An arthroscopy is usually done to view the tear and determine if surgical repair is needed, particularly when more conservative treatment is not alleviating the symptoms.

M75.2 Bicipital tendinitis

Bicipital tendinitis or tenosynovitis is the inflammation of the biceps tendon, which connects the bicep muscle to the shoulder.

M76 Enthesopathies, lower limb, excluding foot

Enthesopathy is a disorder that affects the sites where muscle tendons and ligaments insert and anchor themselves into the bones of the lower limb. This may include bursitis, tendinitis, spurs, and periarthritis, a chronic inflammation of the joint that is usually due to cold, trauma, or chronic strain.

M77.3 Calcaneal spur

A calcaneal spur is a small bony projection that can grow from the heel bone, usually as a result of the patient putting too much pressure on the soles of the feet over a long period of time. This causes the tendons of the foot to become damaged. The body then tries to repair the damage by overgrowing the tendons with bone, causing the spur.

M79.0 Rheumatism, unspecified

Unspecified rheumatism describes a general set of symptoms rather than a specific disease. Rheumatism is a condition in which the joints, muscles, and ligaments become inflamed and painful. Only one or a few joints may be affected, or the patient may experience the inflammation throughout the body. He or she may also experience generalized fatigue.

M79.1 Myalgia

Myalgia is muscle pain. This code includes myofascial pain syndrome which manifests with deep, aching, persistent, or even worsening pain in a muscle that does not go away despite rest, massage, or other self medicating measures.

M79.3 Panniculitis, unspecified

Panniculitis is a rare inflammation of the subcutaneous fat which can present with painful lumps or nodules beneath the skin, and may appear pink or red or even black and blue on the surface. Occasional fever, pain, and severe fatigue are also common. This is often a chronic condition, and there is no direct cure.

M79.5 Residual foreign body in soft tissue

A residual foreign body, such as a splinter or bullet, still remains where it penetrated the body's soft tissue, such as muscle, at some earlier time due to previous trauma and was never removed. This code does not apply to new injuries.

M79.81 Nontraumatic hematoma of soft tissue

An abnormal collection of blood that is localized and partially clotted within a soft tissue space, such as muscle. The hematoma arises from a break in a blood vessel wall. Spontaneous cases may arise from an aneurysm. Treatment involves drainage of the accumulated blood.

M79.A Nontraumatic compartment syndrome

Compartment syndrome is an increase is tissue pressure within a fixed compartment bounded by muscle, fascia, and bone. This can occur from both traumatic and nontraumatic events. Nontraumatic events usually include medical misadventure and significant systemic problems.

Compartment syndrome patients will have some kind of injury related to edema because edema and hemorrhage are the factors that quickly elevate compartment pressures high enough to cause ischemia in the muscles and nerves. When the pressure within the compartment exceeds the perfusion pressure of the arterioles, it causes muscle ischemia and tissue death. Symptoms of compartment syndrome include pain out of proportion with the injury that is not relieved by analgesics, edema, pain on flexion or extension, very painful passive motions, usually good capillary refill, paresthesia, weakness, and sometimes paralysis. Early recognition with fasciotomy often yields good results.

Note: Code any associated postprocedural complication first, if applicable.

M79.A1 Nontraumatic compartment syndrome of upper extremity

Nontraumatic compartment syndrome of the upper extremity can arise from a state of prolonged direct pressure and abnormal limb positioning that might occur with patients in an altered mental state, coma, drug overdose, or carbon monoxide poisoning. Certain intraoperative positions during lengthy medical procedures can put the patient at risk for both upper and lower limb compartment syndrome when the pressure is finally relieved and the patient is resuscitated, the reperfusion to the limb causes the local tissue to swell. Upper limb nontraumatic compartment syndrome may also arise without injury in patients taking anticoagulants and as an unusual complication of blood sampling procedures in patients with underlying coagulation disorders, particularly hemophilia, in which large hematomas or severe ecchymosis develop and subsequent swelling and increased pressure arise.

M79.A2 Nontraumatic compartment syndrome of lower extremity

Nontraumatic compartment syndrome of the lower extremity can arise from a state of prolonged direct pressure and abnormal limb positioning that might occur with patients in an altered mental state, coma, drug overdose, or carbon monoxide poisoning. In lower extremities, as well as upper extremities, nontraumatic compartment syndrome can also arise from certain intraoperative positions maintained during lengthy medical procedures. When the pressure is finally relieved, reperfusion to the limb causes the local tissue to swell after the patient is resuscitated. Lower limb nontraumatic compartment syndrome may occur with knee joint arthroscopy when there is a capsular tear. The infusion of fluid pumped into the joint extravasates to the surrounding leg compartments and causes compartment syndrome. Both upper and lower extremities may suffer compartment syndrome related to illness such as postviral rhabdomyolysis or hemorrhaging from coagulation disorders.

M79.A3 Nontraumatic compartment syndrome of abdomen

Nontraumatic compartment syndrome can occur in the abdomen, anywhere that soft tissue is affected within a fixed compartment bounded by muscle and fascia, when spontaneous hemorrhaging in patients with hemophilia or other coagulation disorders occurs. Patients who take anticoagulants are at increased risk for compartment syndrome arising from hemorrhaging and subsequent swelling. Abdominal compartment syndrome is also caused by intra-abdominal hypertension and leads to organ dysfunction that may arise in the form of respiratory insufficiency from reduced tidal volume or decreased urine output from decreased renal perfusion.

M80 Osteoporosis with current pathological fracture

Osteoporosis is a disease primarily affecting women over the age of 50, in which the bones lose calcium and therefore density and hardness. This causes an increased susceptibility to fractures, especially in the hip, spine, and wrist. Pathological fractures occur without any apparent trauma to the bone. In this case, the break occurs in the bone spontaneously due to weakening by the osteoporotic disease process.

M80.0   Age-related osteoporosis with current pathological fracture

Age-related osteoporosis is also known as senile, post-menopausal, or involutional osteoporosis and is reported whenever osteoporosis that is not otherwise specified is documented.

M80.8   Other osteoporosis with current pathological fracture

Other types of osteoporosis that are not related to age or post-menopausal bone changes include drug-induced osteoporosis, postsurgical malabsorption type, post-traumatic type, post-oophorectomy type, disuse osteoporosis, and even idiopathic osteoporosis with no known cause. Pathological fractures occur without any apparent trauma to the bone. In this case, the break occurs in the bone spontaneously due to weakening by the osteoporotic disease process.

M81   Osteoporosis without current pathological fracture

Osteoporosis is a disease primarily affecting women over the age of 50, in which the bones lose calcium and therefore density and hardness. This causes an increased susceptibility to fractures, especially in the hip, spine, and wrist. It is called a silent disease because most who have it exhibit no symptoms until a spontaneous fracture occurs without any apparent trauma. A bone mineral density test (BMD) is often used to detect the disease early and diagnose the risk for future fractures before any pathological break has occured.

M81.0   Age-related osteoporosis without current pathological fracture

Age-related osteoporosis is also known as senile, post-menopausal, or involutional osteoporosis and is reported whenever osteoporosis that is not otherwise specified is documented.

M81.8   Other osteoporosis without current pathological fracture

Other types of osteoporosis that are not related to age or post-menopausal bone changes include drug-induced osteoporosis, postsurgical malabsorption type, post-traumatic type, post-oophorectomy type, disuse osteoporosis, and even idiopathic osteoporosis with no apparent cause.

M83   Adult osteomalacia

Osteomalacia is a softening of bone tissue due to inadequate intake or absorption of vitamin D, calcium, and/or phosphorus (phosphate). The bone building process is affected in osteomalacia and symptoms such as muscle weakness and bone pain may be present. Causes include inadequate dietary intake of vitamin D, calcium and/or phosphorus, medical conditions that affect the absorption of nutrients including gastric surgery, celiac disease, kidney and liver disease, hyperparathyroidism, and certain drugs such as dilantin and phenobarbital.

M83.9   Adult osteomalacia, unspecified

Osteomalacia is a term that simply means soft bones. It may be termed "adult rickets" since the symptoms are the same, when the softening of the bones takes place in adulthood rather than in childhood.

M84.3   Stress fracture

A stress fracture is a small crack or several cracks that appear in the surface of a bone due to repeated stress over time from unusual or repetative overuse or force on a particular area, most commonly the lower legs and feet. Symptoms include generalized pain and tenderness with weight bearing. The pain may be more pronounced at the beginning of exercise, decrease during the activity, and increase again at the end of the workout. The patient may not experience pain or swelling until the fractures are already well established. Rest and physical therapy are usually the treatment of choice.

M84.4   Pathological fracture, not elsewhere classified

Pathologic bone fractures result from metastatic or widespread lesions that invade and destroy normal bone mass causing the bone to weaken and break.

M85.2   Hyperostosis of skull

Hyperostosis is an excessive overgrowth of bone. Hyperostosis of the skull is particularly dangerous because it can compress the brain and nerves, causing permanent damage, coma, and even death in some cases.

M85.3   Osteitis condensans

Osteitis condensans is a disorder that results in increased bone density in the iliac bone, which is part of the pelvis. In most cases, the patient experiences no symptoms, but in some cases, an inflammation of the sacral joint, where the spine joins with the pelvis, can occur, causing low back pain. The exact cause of this disorder is not known, but it occurs most often in women who have been pregnant.

M85.4   Solitary bone cyst

A cyst is a fluid-filled pocket that can form within the tissues of the body. When a solitary cyst forms inside of a bone, it can weaken the bone, leading to a pathologic fracture, as well as to an infection. A solitary bone cyst is also called a unicameral bone cyst.

M85.5   Aneurysmal bone cyst

An aneurysmal bone cyst is a blood-filled cyst that expands the bone, giving it a "blow-out" appearance similar to that of a blood vessel with an aneurysm. This type of bone cyst is considered to be a benign tumor, and like other bone cysts, increases the risk of fracture due to weakening of the bone.

M86   Osteomyelitis

Osteomyelitis is an acute or chronic bone infection, usually caused by bacteria introduced into the bone. Invading microorganisms can invade the bone in three ways: the infection may have started in another part of the body before migrating to the skeleton through the bloodstream; the bacteria may be inoculated directly into the bone through trauma or surgery; and bacteria may come from a localized infection contiguous with the bone. In children, the long bones of the arms and legs are the most commonly affected, while adults see osteomyelitis more often in the spine and pelvis. In addition to pain and swelling in and around the affected bone, osteomyelitis presents with fever, nausea, fatigue, and other general symptoms of infection.

M86.0   Acute hematogenous osteomyelitis

In hematogenous osteomyelitis, the infecting microorganisms introduced to the bone are delivered through the bloodstream. Acute cases are a sudden and severe inflammatory process as pyogenic organisms infect bone. Symptoms include bone pain, swelling, redness, and warmth of the affected area, fever, chills, and excessive sweating. More than one antibiotic may need to be given, often intravenously. This type of osteomyelitis is seen primarily in children with 85% of cases occurring in patients under 17 years old. Adult cases account for about 20% of bone infections; patients are usually over 50, and are more often male. Hematogenous osteomyelitis is associated with risk factors for bacteremia, such as intravenous drug use, the placement of central lines and urinary catheters, dialysis, sicle cell disease, and UTIs. In children, the long bones of the appendicular skeleton, such as the humerus, femur, and tibia, are the most frequent sites of infection. In adults, the flat bones of the axial skeleton, such as the pelvis, clavicle, vertebrae, and scapula are more often invaded.

M86.1   Other acute osteomyelitis

Other types of acute bone infection are due to direct inoculation of the bone by an infecting microorganism, such as trauma whenever a bone is broken, particularly in open fractures, and through surgical procedures performed on bone. Osteomyelitis through direct inoculation is seen more often in adults. Acute cases are a sudden and severe inflammatory process as pyogenic organisms infect bone. Symptoms include bone pain, swelling, redness, and warmth of the affected area, fever, chills, and excessive sweating. More than one antibiotic may need to be given, often intravenously. Any surgical implants, such as metal plates may need to be removed and the space filled with bone graft. The outcome for acute cases is often good with treatment.

M86.6 Other chronic osteomyelitis

Other types of chronic bone infection are due to direct inoculation of the bone by an infecting microorganism, or migration from localized infections next to the bone. This can occur with trauma, and through surgical procedures performed on bone or the neighboring joint--particularly those that place a permanent implant or prosthesis, such as rods, plates, screws, or joint replacement prostheses. Chronic cases are a long-term inflammatory process that can result in bone destruction over time. Symptoms may come and go for years, even following surgery to remove the infected tissue, the replaced joint, or any metal plates, rods, or screws. Symptoms include bone pain, swelling, redness, and warmth of the affected area, generalized malaise and uneasiness, and fever. More than one antibiotic may need to be given, often intravenously. Any surgical implants, particularly replaced joints, may need to be removed. The outlook is worse for chronic, long-term cases. Prognosis depends on the type of invading organism, whether or not the prosthesis can be safely removed, and the patient's overall health. In diabetics or those with poor circulation, amputation may be necessary.

M86.9 Osteomyelitis, unspecified

Unspecified osteomyelitis includes perisostitis without osteomyelitis, which is an infection of the protective, dense membrane around the bone that protects it without the invading microorganism reaching the bone tissue.

M87 Osteonecrosis

Osteonecrosis, also known as aseptic or avascular necrosis of the bone, is a condition in which one or more bones do not receive an adequate blood supply and begin to die. The dead areas of bone tissue are highly susceptible to fracturing, and do not heal normally once a fracture has taken place. A common site for this disorder is in the scaphoid bone in the wrist (just behind the bone). When this bone becomes fractured, its blood-supply is often interrupted, causing the bone to die rather than heal. This type of necrosis is called aseptic because, unlike gangrene, it is not caused by infection and does not introduce or spread infection to the bloodstream.

M87.08 Idiopathic aseptic necrosis of bone, other site

Aseptic or avascular necrosis of the jaw, also called osteonecrosis of the jaw (ONJ) or 'dead jaw' is a disfiguring and disabling condition marked by the literal death of jaw bone tissue that generally develops whenever the jaw fails to heal from minor trauma, such as a tooth extraction that exposes the bone. The condition can remain asymptomatic for many weeks or months and may manifest with pain, swelling, or infection in the gums or jaw; gums that won't heal; teeth becoming loose; a feeling of heaviness in the jaw; and exposed bone. This can occur in cancer patients who have received bisphosphonates for chemotherapy or oral bisphosphonates for osteoporosis. The disease is very difficult to treat and requires vigilant medical and oral monitoring care.

Note: The American Association of Oral and Maxillofacial Surgeons has defined osteonecrosis of the jaw as exposed bone in the maxillofacial area occurring spontaneously or following dental surgery that has no evidence of healing for more than 3-6 weeks following appropriate care in a patient who has not had radiation therapy to the oral cavity or neck.

M88 Osteitis deformans [Paget's disease of bone]

Osteitis deformans is a chronic bone disorder which is characterized by succeeding waves of bone loss followed by excessive repair attempts by the body. This cycle eventually results in malformed, flat bones and joints subject to pain, arthritis, and fractures. When osteitis deformans occurs without mention of a bone tumor as the cause, it is known as Paget's disease. Paget's disease is thought to be genetic, but rarely appears in anyone under the age of 40. In addition to the bone pain and malformation, it presents with headaches and hearing loss as it affects the skull, pressure on the nerves that cause pain, numbness, and/or muscle weakness, and hip pain.

M88.0 Osteitis deformans of skull

When osteitis deformans occurs without mention of a bone tumor as the cause, it is known as Paget's disease. Paget's disease is thought to be genetic, but rarely appears in anyone under the age of 40. In addition to the bone pain and malformation, it presents with headaches and hearing loss as it affects the skull, pressure on the nerves that cause pain, numbness, and/or muscle weakness, and hip pain.

M89.0 Algoneurodystrophy

Algoneurodystrophy, also known as Sudeck's syndrome or atrophy, is a disorder in which the patient experiences an acute atrophy (wasting away) of one or more bones following a relatively minor injury, such as a sprain or minor fracture. This atrophy presents with a burning pain that increases when the patient is under stress. This disease is most common in the elderly and women.

M89.1 Physeal arrest

Arrest of bone development, also known as epiphyseal arrest, means that the physeal growth plates in one or more bones in a young patient's body are not growing with the rest, causing a deformity, such as a short limb.

M89.4 Other hypertrophic osteoarthropathy

Hypertrophic pulmonary osteoarthropathy is a disorder that results in severe clubbing (rapid growth in thickness) of the fingers and toes. Most instances of this disease are seen in patients with cancer or another chronic disease of the lungs or airway.

M89.7 Major osseous defect

Major osseous defects are the consequence of extensive amounts of bone loss. This kind of significant bone loss most commonly results from the breakdown of bone around a previous prosthetic joint replacement, necessitating revision surgery. Bone loss, or osteolysis, also occurs from osteomyelitis, osteonecrosis, neoplastic growth, severe osteoporosis, and pathological fractures, with or without previous joint replacement. Major osseous defects caused by these factors are clinically significant because the bone into which a joint implant must be placed to repair the defect is too weak to support the prosthesis without structural bone repair. Knowledge of these bone defects and contributing factors help determine diagnosis and treatment as well as predict surgical outcomes. Primary or revision joint replacement must often be done together with morcelized or structural bone grafting and additional mechanical support for the graft such as wires, cables, cages, wedges, screws, etc. The most common area affected is the hip joint, followed by the knee.

Note: Code the underlying disease or disorder first, when it is known to have caused the major osseous defects.

M93.2 Osteochondritis dissecans

Osteochondritis dissecans is a disorder where a loose piece of bone and cartilage separates from the end of the bone due to a loss of blood supply, making the joint unstable.

M94.0 Chondrocostal junction syndrome [Tietze]

Tietze's disease, sometimes called costochondritis, affects the cartilage of the ribs, causing pain and inflammation in the rib cage that sometimes spreads to the arm. The symptoms are similar to that of a heart attack. The cause of this disease is unknown, but it is not normally a chronic disorder and the pain normally disappears on its own after a short period of time.

M94.2 Chondromalacia

Chondromalacia is a condition in which the cartilage of a joint softens and degenerates, causing tenderness, pain, and a grinding sensation at the joint. It is usually connected to the overuse of, or previous injury to, the joint in question. In most cases, this disorder can be treated by resting the joint in question, followed by physical therapy, though in some cases surgery is necessary.

M95.1   Cauliflower ear

Cauliflower ear is a condition which can occur as a result of repeated blows to the ear. The cartilage of the ear becomes partially torn from the skin, deformed, or dies as a result of interrupted blood flow, giving the ear a bumpy and lumpy appearance. Proper care after receiving an injury to the ear can usually prevent permanent deformity.

M96.1   Postlaminectomy syndrome, not elsewhere classified

Postlaminectomy syndrome is a complication that occurs due to laminectomy surgery, a procedure in which part of the bony ridge of the spine that protects the spinal cord is removed to relieve pressure on the cord. This procedure is also called open decompression. Postlaminectomy syndrome is diagnosed when the growth of scar tissue is stated to be the cause of chronic back pain after a laminectomy.

N00 **Acute nephritic syndrome**

Acute nephritic syndrome covers acute glomerular disease, acute nephritis, and acute glomerulonephritis. This is a clinical disorder of the kidneys characterized by swelling and/or inflammation and scarring of the glomeruli. The filtering system of the kidneys loses the ability to remove waste from the blood and allows protein and red blood cells to filter into the urine in the presence of hypertension. Decreased urine production is also part of the syndrome. Causes can include autoimmune disorders, post-streptococcal infections, vasculitis, hepatitis B or C, abdominal abscesses, and viral diseases. Severe damage can occur before symptoms arise, which include high blood pressure, fatigue, and swelling in limbs, in addition to blood and protein in the urine.

N00.0 **Acute nephritic syndrome with minor glomerular abnormality**

Acute nephritic syndrome is a clinical disorder of the kidneys characterized by swelling and/or inflammation and scarring of the glomeruli. The filtering system of the kidneys loses the ability to remove waste from the blood and allows protein and red blood cells to filter into the urine in the presence of hypertension. Minor morphological abnormalities are present in the glomeruli, which may be considered as nonspecific changes or minimal lesions, such as a breakdown or wrinkling in the capillaries and may consist of adaptational changes from glomerular response to toxic substances. Further, careful evaluation of morphological change is often necessary in conjunction with treatment.

N00.1 **Acute nephritic syndrome with focal and segmental glomerular lesions**

Acute nephritic syndrome is a clinical disorder of the kidneys characterized by swelling and/or inflammation and scarring of the glomeruli. The filtering system of the kidneys loses the ability to remove waste from the blood and allows protein and red blood cells to filter into the urine in the presence of hypertension. Focal segmental lesions are present as sclerosis, or scarring of the glomeruli. Focal lesions are seen as scarring affecting some of the thousands of glomeruli present in each kidney, while others remain normal. Segmental lesions appear as damage to one section of an individual, affected glomerulus.

N00.2 **Acute nephritic syndrome with diffuse membranous glomerulonephritis**

Acute nephritic syndrome is a clinical disorder of the kidneys characterized by swelling and/or inflammation and scarring of the glomeruli. The filtering system of the kidneys loses the ability to remove waste from the blood and allows protein and red blood cells to filter into the urine in the presence of hypertension. Diffuse membranous glomerulonephritis is a slowly progressing disease involving thickening of the glomerular basement membrane, due to the formation of immune complexes. Antibodies bind to antigens that are either a part of the membrane or deposited there from the circulation. The immune complex deposits trigger an attack response on the basement membrane, which cannot function normally and allows large amounts of protein to be lost in the urine.

N00.3 **Acute nephritic syndrome with diffuse mesangial proliferative glomerulonephritis**

Acute nephritic syndrome is a clinical disorder of the kidneys characterized by swelling and/or inflammation and scarring of the glomeruli. The filtering system of the kidneys loses the ability to remove waste from the blood and allows protein and red blood cells to filter into the urine in the presence of hypertension. Diffuse mesangial proliferative glomerulonephritis is a progressive disease involving mainly the mesangium with diffuse deposits of immunoglobulin, particularly IgM. The mesangial cells of the glomeruli are responsible for taking up and breaking down circulating immunoglobulins. Diffuse amounts of IgM containing immune deposits in the mesangial areas stimulates mesangial cell and matrix proliferation within the glomeruli. This may be a nonspecific type of response to glomerular injury often suspected with various kinds of systemic inflammatory diseases, autoimmune disorders, and infections.

N00.4 **Acute nephritic syndrome with diffuse endocapillary proliferative glomerulonephritis**

Acute nephritic syndrome is a clinical disorder of the kidneys characterized by swelling and/or inflammation and scarring of the glomeruli. The filtering system of the kidneys loses the ability to remove waste from the blood and allows protein and red blood cells to filter into the urine in the presence of hypertension. Diffuse endocapillary proliferative glomerulonephritis involves the deposition of immune complexes in the capillaries, triggering complement activation, and the infiltration of neutrophils and other inflammatory cells. This results in occlusion of the capillary lumens from the influx of proliferating cells and edema of the endothelial cells, producing diffuse endocapillary lesions. This is known to occur as a postinfectious process, particularly related to *Streptococcus pyogenes infection*.

N00.5 **Acute nephritic syndrome with diffuse mesangiocapillary glomerulonephritis**

Acute nephritic syndrome is a clinical disorder of the kidneys characterized by swelling and/or inflammation and scarring of the glomeruli. The filtering system of the kidneys loses the ability to remove waste from the blood and allows protein and red blood cells to filter into the urine in the presence of hypertension. Diffuse mesangiocapillary glomerulonephritis involves both the mesangium and the capillaries of the glomeruli. Immune complex deposits trigger a proliferation of mesangial cells, which take in and break down immunoglobuins. Deposits also trigger complement activation, and the infiltration of neutrophils and other inflammatory cells into the capillary walls. This results in an increase in mesangial cells and matrix as well as occlusion of the capillary lumens from the influx of inflammatory cells and concomitant edema of endothelial cells. This produces diffuse lesions in both the mesangium and capillaries of the glomeruli.

N00.6 **Acute nephritic syndrome with dense deposit disease**

Acute nephritic syndrome is a clinical disorder of the kidneys characterized by swelling and/or inflammation and scarring of the glomeruli. The filtering system of the kidneys loses the ability to remove waste from the blood and allows protein and red blood cells to filter into the urine in the presence of hypertension. Dense deposit disease is a rare condition associated with genetic risk factors or mutations regarding instructions for making proteins involved with the complement system of the body's immune response. It results in uncontrolled activation of the complement system, causing immune complex debris to build up in the glomeruli of the kidneys. Kidney function affected by this disorder tends to worsen, and half of patients end up with end stage renal disease within about 10 years of symptom onset.

Note: Dense deposit disease was previously known as membranoproliferative glomerulonephritis (MPGN) type 2, but recent discoveries suggest it is not a true form of MPGN.

N00.7 **Acute nephritic syndrome with diffuse crescentic glomerulonephritis**

Acute nephritic syndrome is a clinical disorder of the kidneys characterized by swelling and/or inflammation and scarring of the glomeruli. The filtering system of the kidneys loses the ability to remove waste from the blood and allows protein and red blood cells to filter into the urine in the presence of hypertension. Diffuse crescentic glomerulonephritis, or extracapillary glomerulonephritis is a more rare histological lesion manifesting with severe glomerular damage. It involves fibrous and cellular proliferation occurring outside the capillary, forming epithelial crescents, the presence of two or more layers of cells, which partially or totally fill the Bowman's space and may obliterate capillary loops. This results in rapid loss of kidney function within weeks or months and leads to acute renal failure. Extracapillary, or crescentic, glomerulonephritis is due to the deposition of immune complexes and/or the presence of anti-glomerular antibodies.

N00.8 Acute nephritic syndrome with other morphologic changes

Acute nephritic syndrome with other morphologic changes is a clinical disorder of the kidneys characterized by swelling and/or inflammation and scarring of the glomeruli. The filtering system of the kidneys loses the ability to remove waste from the blood and allows protein and red blood cells to filter into the urine in the presence of hypertension. Other morphological changes includes the presence of proliferative glomerulonephritis lesions in the kidney(s) that are not otherwise specified. Proliferative glomerulonephritis is caused by a range of immune-mediated and inflammatory mechanisms that result in lesions characterized by an increased number of cells in the glomeruli.

N01 Rapidly progressive nephritic syndrome

Rapidly progressive nephritic syndrome covers rapidly progressive glomerular disease, nephritis, and glomerulonephritis. This is nephritic syndrome that presents with progressive, rapid deterioration in kidney function and has a poor prognosis. Nephritic syndrome is characterized by swelling and/or inflammation and scarring of the glomeruli. Damage to the glomerular cells from inflammation causes the filtering system of the kidneys to lose the ability to remove waste from the blood, allowing protein and red blood cells to filter into the urine, along with a decreased production of urine in the presence of hypertension. Causes can include immune disorders, post-streptococcal infections, and viral diseases. Severe damage can occur from high blood pressure and inflammation before symptoms arise.

N01.0 Rapidly progressive nephritic syndrome with minor glomerular abnormality

This is nephritic syndrome that presents with progressive, rapid deterioration in kidney function and has a poor prognosis. Nephritic syndrome is characterized by swelling and/or inflammation and scarring of the glomeruli. Damage to glomerular cells from inflammation causes the kidneys to lose their ability to filter waste from blood, allowing protein and red blood cells to filter into urine along with decreased production of urine and hypertension. Minor morphological abnormalities are also present in the glomeruli, which may be considered nonspecific changes or minimal lesions, such as a breakdown or wrinkling in the capillaries, and may consist of adaptational changes in response to toxic substances. Further, careful evaluation of morphological changes is often necessary in conjunction with treatment.

N01.1 Rapidly progressive nephritic syndrome with focal and segmental glomerular lesions

This is nephritic syndrome that presents with progressive, rapid deterioration in kidney function and has a poor prognosis. Nephritic syndrome is characterized by swelling and/or inflammation and scarring of the glomeruli. Damage to glomerular cells from inflammation causes the kidneys to lose their ability to filter waste from blood, allowing protein and red blood cells to filter into urine along with decreased production of urine and hypertension. Focal segmental lesions are present as sclerosis, or scarring of the glomeruli. Focal lesions are seen as scarring affecting some of the thousands of glomeruli present in each kidney, while others remain normal. Segmental lesions appear as damage to one section of an individual, affected glomerulus.

N01.2 Rapidly progressive nephritic syndrome with diffuse membranous glomerulonephritis

This is nephritic syndrome that presents with progressive, rapid deterioration in kidney function and has a poor prognosis. Nephritic

syndrome is characterized by swelling and/or inflammation and scarring of the glomeruli. Damage to glomerular cells from inflammation causes the kidneys to lose their ability to filter waste from blood, allowing protein and red blood cells to filter into urine along with decreased production of urine and hypertension. Diffuse membranous glomerulonephritis is a slowly progressing disease involving thickening of the glomerular basement membrane, due to the formation of immune complexes. Antibodies bind to antigens that are either a part of the membrane or deposited there from the circulation. The immune complex deposits trigger an attack response on the basement membrane, which cannot function normally and allows large amounts of protein to be lost in the urine.

N01.3 Rapidly progressive nephritic syndrome with diffuse mesangial proliferative glomerulonephritis

This is nephritic syndrome that presents with progressive, rapid deterioration in kidney function and has a poor prognosis. Nephritic syndrome is characterized by swelling and/or inflammation and scarring of the glomeruli. Damage to glomerular cells from inflammation causes the kidneys to lose their ability to filter waste from blood, allowing protein and red blood cells to filter into urine along with decreased production of urine and hypertension. Diffuse mesangial proliferative glomerulonephritis is a progressive disease involving mainly the mesangium with diffuse deposits of immunoglobulin, particularly IgM. The mesangial cells of the glomeruli are responsible for taking up and breaking down circulating immunoglobulins. Diffuse amounts of IgM-containing immune deposits in the mesangial areas stimulates mesangial cell and matrix proliferation within the glomeruli. This may be a nonspecific type of response to glomerular injury often suspected with various kinds of systemic inflammatory diseases, autoimmune disorders, and infections.

N01.4 Rapidly progressive nephritic syndrome with diffuse endocapillary proliferative glomerulonephritis

This is nephritic syndrome that presents with progressive, rapid deterioration in kidney function and has a poor prognosis. Nephritic syndrome is characterized by swelling and/or inflammation and scarring of the glomeruli. Damage to glomerular cells from inflammation causes the kidneys to lose their ability to filter waste from blood, allowing protein and red blood cells to filter into urine along with decreased production of urine and hypertension. Diffuse endocapillary proliferative glomerulonephritis involves the deposition of immune complexes in the capillaries, triggering complement activation, and the infiltration of neutrophils and other inflammatory cells. This results in occlusion of the capillary lumens from the influx of proliferating cells and edema of the endothelial cells, producing diffuse endocapillary lesions. This is known to occur as a postinfectious process, particularly related to *Streptococcus pyogenes infection*.

N01.5 Rapidly progressive nephritic syndrome with diffuse mesangiocapillary glomerulonephritis

This is nephritic syndrome that presents with progressive, rapid deterioration in kidney function and has a poor prognosis. Nephritic syndrome is characterized by swelling and/or inflammation and scarring of the glomeruli. Damage to glomerular cells from inflammation causes the kidneys to lose their ability to filter waste from blood, allowing protein and red blood cells to filter into urine along with decreased production of urine and hypertension. Diffuse mesangiocapillary glomerulonephritis involves both the mesangium and the capillaries of the glomeruli. Immune complex deposits trigger a proliferation of mesangial cells, which take in and break down immunoglobuins. Deposits also trigger complement activation, and the infiltration of neutrophils and other inflammatory cells into the capillary walls. This results in an increase in mesangial cells and matrix as well as occlusion of the capillary lumens from the influx of inflammatory cells and concomitant edema of endothelial cells. This produces diffuse lesions in both the mesangium and capillaries of the glomeruli.

N01.6 Rapidly progressive nephritic syndrome with dense deposit disease

This is nephritic syndrome that presents with progressive, rapid deterioration in kidney function and has a poor prognosis. Nephritic syndrome is characterized by swelling and/or inflammation and scarring of the glomeruli. Damage to glomerular cells from inflammation causes the kidneys to lose their ability to filter waste from blood, allowing protein and red blood cells to filter into urine along with decreased production of urine and hypertension. Dense deposit disease is a rare condition associated with genetic risk factors or mutations regarding instructions for making proteins involved with the complement system of the body's immune response. It results in uncontrolled activation of the complement system, causing immune complex debris to build up in the glomeruli of the kidneys. Kidney function affected by this disorder tends to worsen, and half of patients end up with end stage renal disease within about 10 years of symptom onset.

Note: Dense deposit disease was previously known as membranoproliferative glomerulonephritis (MPGN) type 2, but recent discoveries suggest it is not a true form of MPGN.

N01.7 Rapidly progressive nephritic syndrome with diffuse crescentic glomerulonephritis

This is nephritic syndrome that presents with progressive, rapid deterioration in kidney function and has a poor prognosis. Nephritic syndrome is characterized by swelling and/or inflammation and scarring of the glomeruli. Damage to glomerular cells from inflammation causes the kidneys to lose their ability to filter waste from blood, allowing protein and red blood cells to filter into urine along with decreased production of urine and hypertension. Diffuse crescentic glomerulonephritis, or extracapillary glomerulonephritis, is a more rare histological lesion manifesting with severe glomerular damage. It involves fibrous and cellular proliferation occurring outside the capillary, forming epithelial crescents, the presence of two or more layers of cells, which partially or totally fill the Bowman's space and may obliterate capillary loops. This results in rapid loss of kidney function within weeks or months and leads to acute renal failure. Extracapillary, or crescentic, glomerulonephritis is due to the deposition of immune complexes and/or the presence of anti-glomerular antibodies.

N01.8 Rapidly progressive nephritic syndrome with other morphologic changes

This is nephritic syndrome that presents with progressive, rapid deterioration in kidney function and has a poor prognosis. Nephritic syndrome is characterized by swelling and/or inflammation and scarring of the glomeruli. Damage to glomerular cells from inflammation causes the kidneys to lose their ability to filter waste from blood, allowing protein and red blood cells to filter into urine along with decreased production of urine and hypertension. Other morphological changes includes the presence of proliferative glomerulonephritis lesions in the kidney(s) that are not otherwise specified. Proliferative glomerulonephritis is caused by a range of immune-mediated and inflammatory mechanisms that result in lesions characterized by an increased number of cells in the glomeruli.

N02 Recurrent and persistent hematuria

Recurrent and persistent hematuria is the presence of an excessive number of red blood cells (RBCs) in the urine on a continuing basis. Gross hematuria is visible as overtly dark, smoky, or bloody colored urine. Microscopic hematuria is only detectable by laboratory analysis of urine specimens. Persistent hematuria in this category is associated with histological lesions or disease of the glomeruli in the kidney(s); it is normally painless and presents as brown colored urine with misshapen, deformed, or fragmented RBCs or casts present.

N02.0 Recurrent and persistent hematuria with minor glomerular abnormality

Recurrent and persistent hematuria is the presence of an excessive number of red blood cells (RBCs) in the urine on a continuing basis. The hematuria is associated with histological or morphological lesions in the glomeruli of the kidney(s) and is normally painless, presenting as brown colored urine with misshapen, deformed, or fragmented RBCs or casts present. Minor morphological abnormalities are present in the glomeruli, which may be considered as nonspecific changes or minimal lesions, such as a breakdown or wrinkling in the capillaries and may consist of adaptational changes from glomerular response to toxic substances. Further, careful evaluation of morphological changes is often necessary in conjunction with treatment.

N02.1 Recurrent and persistent hematuria with focal and segmental glomerular lesions

Recurrent and persistent hematuria is the presence of an excessive number of red blood cells (RBCs) in the urine on a continuing basis. The hematuria is associated with histological or morphological lesions in the glomeruli of the kidney(s) and is normally painless, presenting as brown colored urine with misshapen, deformed, or fragmented RBCs or casts present. Focal segmental lesions are present as sclerosis, or scarring of the glomeruli. Focal lesions are seen as scarring affecting some of the thousands of glomeruli present in each kidney, while others remain normal. Segmental lesions appear as damage to one section of an individual, affected glomerulus.

N02.2 Recurrent and persistent hematuria with diffuse membranous glomerulonephritis

Recurrent and persistent hematuria is the presence of an excessive number of red blood cells (RBCs) in the urine on a continuing basis. The hematuria is associated with histological or morphological lesions or disease in the glomeruli of the kidney(s) and is normally painless, presenting as brown colored urine with misshapen, deformed, or fragmented RBCs or casts present. Diffuse membranous glomerulonephritis is a slowly progressing disease involving thickening of the glomerular basement membrane, due to the formation of immune complexes. Antibodies bind to antigens that are either a part of the membrane or deposited there from the circulation. The immune complex deposits trigger an attack response on the basement membrane, which cannot function normally and allows large amounts of protein to be lost in the urine.

N02.3 Recurrent and persistent hematuria with diffuse mesangial proliferative glomerulonephritis

Recurrent and persistent hematuria is the presence of an excessive number of red blood cells (RBCs) in the urine on a continuing basis. The hematuria is associated with histological or morphological lesions or disease in the glomeruli of the kidney(s) and is normally painless, presenting as brown colored urine with misshapen, deformed, or fragmented RBCs or casts present. Diffuse mesangial proliferative glomerulonephritis is a progressive disease involving mainly the mesangium with diffuse deposits of immunoglobulin, particularly IgM. The mesangial cells of the glomeruli are responsible for taking up and breaking down circulating immunoglobulins. Diffuse amounts of IgM-containing immune deposits in the mesangial areas stimulates mesangial cell and matrix proliferation within the glomeruli. This may be a nonspecific type of response to glomerular injury often suspected with various kinds of systemic inflammatory diseases, autoimmune disorders, and infections.

N02.4 Recurrent and persistent hematuria with diffuse endocapillary proliferative glomerulonephritis

Recurrent and persistent hematuria is the presence of an excessive number of red blood cells (RBCs) in the urine on a continuing basis. The hematuria is associated with histological or morphological lesions or disease in the glomeruli of the kidney(s) and is normally painless, presenting as brown colored urine with misshapen, deformed, or fragmented RBCs or casts present. Diffuse endocapillary proliferative glomerulonephritis involves the deposition of immune complexes in the capillaries, triggering complement activation, and the infiltration of neutrophils and other inflammatory cells. This results in occlusion of the capillary lumens from the influx of proliferating cells and edema of the endothelial cells, producing diffuse endocapillary lesions. This is known to occur as a postinfectious process, particularly related to *Streptococcus pyogenes infection*.

N02.5 Recurrent and persistent hematuria with diffuse mesangiocapillary glomerulonephritis

Recurrent and persistent hematuria is the presence of an excessive number of red blood cells (RBCs) in the urine on a continuing basis. The hematuria is associated with histological or morphological lesions or disease in the glomeruli of the kidney(s) and is normally painless, presenting as brown colored urine with misshapen, deformed, or fragmented RBCs or casts present. Diffuse mesangiocapillary glomerulonephritis involves both the mesangium and the capillaries of the glomeruli. Immune complex deposits trigger a proliferation of mesangial cells, which take in and break down immunoglobuins. Deposits also trigger complement activation, and the infiltration of neutrophils and other inflammatory cells into the capillary walls. This results in an increase in mesangial cells and matrix as well as occlusion of the capillary lumens from the influx of inflammatory cells and concomitant edema of endothelial cells. This produces diffuse lesions in both the mesangium and capillaries of the glomeruli.

N02.6 Recurrent and persistent hematuria with dense deposit disease

Recurrent and persistent hematuria is the presence of an excessive number of red blood cells (RBCs) in the urine on a continuing basis. The hematuria is associated with histological or morphological lesions or disease in the glomeruli of the kidney(s) and is normally painless, presenting as brown colored urine with misshapen, deformed, or fragmented RBCs or casts present. Dense deposit disease is a rare condition associated with genetic risk factors or mutations regarding instructions for making proteins involved with the complement system of the body's immune response. It results in uncontrolled activation of the complement system, causing immune complex debris to build up in the glomeruli of the kidneys. Kidney function affected by this disorder tends to worsen, and half of patients end up with end stage renal disease within about 10 years of symptom onset.

Note: Dense deposit disease was previously known as membranoproliferative glomerulonephritis (MPGN) type 2, but recent discoveries suggest it is not a true form of MPGN.

N02.7 Recurrent and persistent hematuria with diffuse crescentic glomerulonephritis

Recurrent and persistent hematuria is the presence of an excessive number of red blood cells (RBCs) in the urine on a continuing basis. The hematuria is associated with histological or morphological lesions or disease in the glomeruli of the kidney(s) and is normally painless, presenting as brown colored urine with misshapen, deformed, or fragmented RBCs or casts present. Diffuse crescentic glomerulonephritis, or extracapillary glomerulonephritis, is a more rare histological lesion manifesting with severe glomerular damage. It involves fibrous and cellular proliferation occurring outside the capillary, forming epithelial crescents, the presence of two or more layers of cells, which partially or totally fill the Bowman's space and may obliterate capillary loops. This results in rapid loss of kidney function within weeks or months and leads to acute renal failure. Extracapillary, or crescentic glomerulonephritis is due to the deposition of immune complexes and/or the presence of anti-glomerular antibodies.

N02.8 Recurrent and persistent hematuria with other morphologic changes

Recurrent and persistent hematuria is the presence of an excessive number of red blood cells (RBCs) in the urine on a continuing basis. The hematuria is associated with histological or morphological lesions in the glomeruli of the kidney(s) and is normally painless, presenting as brown colored urine with misshapen, deformed, or fragmented RBCs or casts present. Other morphological changes includes the presence of proliferative glomerulonephritis lesions in the kidney(s) that are not otherwise specified. Proliferative glomerulonephritis is caused by a range of immune-mediated and inflammatory mechanisms that result in lesions characterized by an increased number of cells in the glomerulus.

N03 Chronic nephritic syndrome

Chronic nephritic syndrome covers chronic cases of nephritis, glomerular disease, and glomerulonephritis. Chronic glomerulonephritis is an advanced stage of progressive kidney disease in which constant, continuous swelling and/or inflammation is causing destruction and scarring of the renal glomeruli. Damage to the glomerular cells from chronic inflammation causes the kidneys to lose their ability to filter waste from blood, allowing protein and red blood cells to filter into urine, along with decreased urine

production and hypertension. Causes can include autoimmune disorders, post-streptococcal infections, vasculitis, hepatitis B or C, abdominal abscesses, and viral diseases. Long-term damage can occur from chronic high blood pressure and inflammation even before severe symptoms appear.

N03.0 Chronic nephritic syndrome with minor glomerular abnormality

Chronic glomerulonephritis is an advanced stage of progressive kidney disease in which constant, continuous swelling and/or inflammation is causing destruction and scarring of the renal glomeruli. Damage to the glomerular cells from chronic inflammation causes the kidneys to lose their ability to filter waste from blood, allowing protein and red blood cells to filter into urine, along with decreased urine production and hypertension. Minor morphological abnormalities are present in the glomeruli, which may be considered as nonspecific changes or minimal lesions, such as a breakdown or wrinkling in the capillaries and may consist of adaptational changes from glomerular response to toxic substances. Further, careful evaluation of morphological changes is often necessary in conjunction with treatment.

N03.1 Chronic nephritic syndrome with focal and segmental glomerular lesions

Chronic glomerulonephritis is an advanced stage of progressive kidney disease in which constant, continuous swelling and/or inflammation is causing destruction and scarring of the renal glomeruli. Damage to the glomerular cells from chronic inflammation causes the kidneys to lose their ability to filter waste from blood, allowing protein and red blood cells to filter into urine, along with decreased urine production and hypertension. Focal segmental lesions are present as sclerosis, or scarring of the glomeruli. Focal lesions are seen as scarring affecting some of the thousands of glomeruli present in each kidney, while others remain normal. Segmental lesions appear as damage to one section of an individual, affected glomerulus.

N03.2 Chronic nephritic syndrome with diffuse membranous glomerulonephritis

Chronic glomerulonephritis is an advanced stage of progressive kidney disease in which constant, continuous swelling and/or inflammation is causing destruction and scarring of the renal glomeruli. Damage to the glomerular cells from chronic inflammation causes the kidneys to lose their ability to filter waste from blood, allowing protein and red blood cells to filter into urine, along with decreased urine production and hypertension. Diffuse membranous glomerulonephritis is a slowly progressing disease involving thickening of the glomerular basement membrane, due to the formation of immune complexes. Antibodies bind to antigens that are either a part of the membrane or deposited there from the circulation. The immune complex deposits trigger an attack response on the basement membrane, which cannot function normally and allows large amounts of protein to be lost in the urine.

N03.3 Chronic nephritic syndrome with diffuse mesangial proliferative glomerulonephritis

Chronic glomerulonephritis is an advanced stage of progressive kidney disease in which constant, continuous swelling and/or inflammation is causing destruction and scarring of the renal glomeruli. Damage to the glomerular cells from chronic inflammation causes the kidneys to lose their ability to filter waste from blood, allowing protein and red blood cells to filter into urine, along with decreased urine production and hypertension. Diffuse mesangial proliferative glomerulonephritis is a progressive disease involving mainly the mesangium with diffuse deposits of immunoglobulin, particularly IgM. The mesangial cells of the glomeruli are responsible for taking up and breaking down circulating immunoglobulins. Diffuse amounts of IgM-containing immune deposits in the mesangial areas stimulates mesangial cell and matrix proliferation within the glomeruli. This may be a nonspecific type of response to glomerular injury often suspected with various kinds of systemic inflammatory diseases, autoimmune disorders, and infections.

N03.4 Chronic nephritic syndrome with diffuse endocapillary proliferative glomerulonephritis

Chronic glomerulonephritis is an advanced stage of progressive kidney disease in which constant, continuous swelling and/or inflammation is causing destruction and scarring of the renal glomeruli. Damage to the glomerular cells from chronic inflammation causes the kidneys to lose their ability to filter waste from blood, allowing protein and red blood cells to filter into urine, along with decreased urine production and hypertension. Diffuse endocapillary proliferative glomerulonephritis involves the deposition of immune complexes in the capillaries, triggering complement activation, and the infiltration of neutrophils and other inflammatory cells. This results in occlusion of the capillary lumens from the influx of proliferating cells and edema of the endothelial cells, producing diffuse endocapillary lesions. This is known to occur as a postinfectious process, particularly related to *Streptococcus pyogenes infection.*

N03.5 Chronic nephritic syndrome with diffuse mesangiocapillary glomerulonephritis

Chronic glomerulonephritis is an advanced stage of progressive kidney disease in which constant, continuous swelling and/or inflammation is causing destruction and scarring of the renal glomeruli. Damage to the glomerular cells from chronic inflammation causes the kidneys to lose their ability to filter waste from blood, allowing protein and red blood cells to filter into urine, along with decreased urine production and hypertension. Diffuse mesangiocapillary glomerulonephritis involves both the mesangium and the capillaries of the glomeruli. Immune complex deposits trigger a proliferation of mesangial cells, which take in and break down immunoglobuins. Deposits also trigger complement activation, and the infiltration of neutrophils and other inflammatory cells into the capillary walls. This results in an increase in mesangial cells and matrix as well as occlusion of the capillary lumens from the influx of inflammatory cells and concomitant edema of endothelial cells. This produces diffuse lesions in both the mesangium and capillaries of the glomeruli.

N03.6 Chronic nephritic syndrome with dense deposit disease

Chronic glomerulonephritis is an advanced stage of progressive kidney disease in which constant, continuous swelling and/or inflammation is causing destruction and scarring of the renal glomeruli. Damage to the glomerular cells from chronic inflammation causes the kidneys to lose their ability to filter waste from blood, allowing protein and red blood cells to filter into urine, along with decreased urine production and hypertension. Dense deposit disease is a rare condition associated with genetic risk factors or mutations regarding instructions for making proteins involved with the complement system of the body's immune response. It results in uncontrolled activation of the complement system, causing immune complex debris to build up in the glomeruli of the kidneys. Kidney function affected by this disorder tends to worsen, and half of patients end up with end stage renal disease within about 10 years of symptom onset.

Note: Dense deposit disease was previously known as membranoproliferative glomerulonephritis (MPGN) type 2, but recent discoveries suggest it is not a true form of MPGN.

N03.7 Chronic nephritic syndrome with diffuse crescentic glomerulonephritis

Chronic glomerulonephritis is an advanced stage of progressive kidney disease in which constant, continuous swelling and/or inflammation is causing destruction and scarring of the renal glomeruli. Damage to the glomerular cells from chronic inflammation causes the kidneys to lose their ability to filter waste from blood, allowing protein and red blood cells to filter into urine, along with decreased urine production and hypertension. Diffuse crescentic glomerulonephritis, or extracapillary glomerulonephritis, is a more rare histological lesion manifesting with severe glomerular damage. It involves fibrous and cellular proliferation occurring outside the capillary, forming epithelial crescents, the presence of two or more layers of cells, which partially or totally fill the Bowman's space and may obliterate capillary loops. This results in rapid loss of kidney function within weeks or months and leads to acute renal failure. Extracapillary, or crescentic glomerulonephritis, is due to the deposition of immune complexes and/or the presence of anti-glomerular antibodies.

N03.8 Chronic nephritic syndrome with other morphologic changes

Chronic glomerulonephritis is an advanced stage of progressive kidney disease in which constant, continuous swelling and/or inflammation is causing destruction and scarring of the renal glomeruli. Damage to the glomerular cells from chronic inflammation causes the kidneys to lose their ability to filter waste from blood, allowing protein and red blood cells to filter into urine, along with decreased urine production and hypertension. Other morphological changes includes the presence of proliferative glomerulonephritis lesions in the kidney(s) that are not otherwise specified. Proliferative glomerulonephritis is caused by a range of immune-mediated and inflammatory mechanisms that results in lesions characterized by an increased number of cells in the glomeruli.

N04 Nephrotic syndrome

Nephrotic syndrome is a condition in which the cells surrounding the clusters of tiny blood vessels, the glomeruli, have become damaged in the presence of edema. The damage allows the leakage of protein from blood into the urine, causing a decreased amount of protein in blood, and increased blood lipid levels. With decreased blood protein, there is a decrease in the oncotic pressure of blood, but not in tissue. This in turn leads to sodium and water retention. Symptoms of nephrotic syndrome include weight gain from water retention, swollen ankles and feet, edema around the eyes, and foamy urine from the excess protein. Nephrotic syndrome can be a primary problem confined to the kidney or a secondary problem with involvement of the kidney and other body organs. Causative factors include infection, autoimmune disorders, drugs, hypertension, and diabetes. The disease is usually confirmed by testing the urine for high levels of protein.

N04.0 Nephrotic syndrome with minor glomerular abnormality

Nephrotic syndrome is a condition in which the cells surrounding the clusters of tiny blood vessels, the glomeruli, have become damaged in the presence of edema. The damage allows the leakage of protein from blood into the urine, causing a decreased amount of protein in blood, and increased blood lipid levels. With decreased blood protein, there is a decrease in the oncotic pressure of blood, but not in tissue. This in turn leads to edema from water retention. Symptoms include weight gain from water retention, swollen ankles and feet, edema around the eyes, and foamy urine from the excess protein. Minor morphological abnormalities are also present in the glomeruli, which may be considered nonspecific changes or minimal lesions, such as a breakdown or wrinkling in the capillaries, and may consist of adaptational changes in response to toxic substances. Further, careful evaluation of morphological changes is often necessary in conjunction with treatment.

N04.1 Nephrotic syndrome with focal and segmental glomerular lesions

Nephrotic syndrome is a condition in which the cells surrounding the clusters of tiny blood vessels, the glomeruli, have become damaged in the presence of edema. The damage allows the leakage of protein from blood into the urine, causing a decreased amount of protein in blood, and increased blood lipid levels. With decreased blood protein, there is a decrease in the oncotic pressure of blood, but not in tissue. This in turn leads to edema from water retention. Symptoms include weight gain from water retention, swollen ankles and feet, edema around the eyes, and foamy urine from the excess protein. Focal segmental lesions are present as sclerosis, or scarring of the glomeruli. Focal lesions are seen as scarring affecting some of the thousands of glomeruli present in each kidney, while others remain normal. Segmental lesions appear as damage to one section of an individual, affected glomerulus.

N04.2 Nephrotic syndrome with diffuse membranous glomerulonephritis

Nephrotic syndrome is a condition in which the cells surrounding the clusters of tiny blood vessels, the glomeruli, have become damaged in the presence of edema. The damage allows the leakage of protein from blood into the urine, causing a decreased amount of protein in blood, and increased blood lipid levels. With decreased blood protein, there is a decrease in the oncotic pressure of blood, but not in tissue. This in turn leads to edema from water retention. Symptoms include weight gain from water retention, swollen ankles and feet, edema around the eyes, and foamy urine from the excess protein. Diffuse membranous glomerulonephritis is a slowly progressing disease involving thickening of the glomerular basement membrane, due to the formation of immune complexes. Antibodies bind to antigens that are either a part of the membrane or deposited there from the circulation. The immune complex deposits trigger an attack response on the basement membrane, which cannot function normally and allows large amounts of protein to be lost in the urine.

N04.3 Nephrotic syndrome with diffuse mesangial proliferative glomerulonephritis

Nephrotic syndrome is a condition in which the cells surrounding the clusters of tiny blood vessels, the glomeruli, have become damaged in the presence of edema. The damage allows the leakage of protein from blood into the urine, causing a decreased amount of protein in blood, and increased blood lipid levels. With decreased blood protein, there is a decrease in the oncotic pressure of blood, but not in tissue. This in turn leads to edema from water retention. Symptoms include weight gain from water retention, swollen ankles and feet, edema around the eyes, and foamy urine from the excess protein. Diffuse mesangial proliferative glomerulonephritis is a progressive disease involving mainly the mesangium with diffuse deposits of immunoglobulin, particularly IgM. The mesangial cells of the glomeruli are responsible for taking up and breaking down circulating immunoglobulins. Diffuse amounts of IgM-containing immune deposits in the mesangial areas stimulates mesangial cell and matrix proliferation within the glomeruli. This may be a nonspecific type of response to glomerular injury often suspected with various kinds of systemic inflammatory diseases, autoimmune disorders, and infections.

N04.4 Nephrotic syndrome with diffuse endocapillary proliferative glomerulonephritis

Nephrotic syndrome is a condition in which the cells surrounding the clusters of tiny blood vessels, the glomeruli, have become damaged in the presence of edema. The damage allows the leakage of protein from blood into the urine, causing a decreased amount of protein in blood, and increased blood lipid levels. With decreased blood protein, there is a decrease in the oncotic pressure of blood, but not in tissue. This in turn leads to edema from water retention. Symptoms include weight gain from water retention, swollen ankles and feet, edema around the eyes, and foamy urine from the excess protein. Diffuse endocapillary proliferative glomerulonephritis involves the deposition of immune complexes in the capillaries, triggering complement activation, and the infiltration of neutrophils and other inflammatory cells. This results in occlusion of the capillary lumens from the influx of proliferating cells and edema of the endothelial cells, producing diffuse endocapillary lesions. This is known to occur as a postinfectious process, particularly related to *Streptococcus pyogenes infection*.

N04.5 Nephrotic syndrome with diffuse mesangiocapillary glomerulonephritis

Nephrotic syndrome is a condition in which the cells surrounding the clusters of tiny blood vessels, the glomeruli, have become damaged in the presence of edema. The damage allows the leakage of protein from blood into the urine, causing a decreased amount of protein in blood, and increased blood lipid levels. With decreased blood protein, there is a decrease in the oncotic pressure of blood, but not in tissue. This in turn leads to edema from water retention. Symptoms include weight gain from water retention, swollen ankles and feet, edema around the eyes, and foamy urine from the excess protein. Diffuse mesangiocapillary glomerulonephritis involves both the mesangium and the capillaries of the glomeruli. Immune complex deposits trigger a proliferation of mesangial cells, which take in and break down immunoglobuins. Deposits also trigger complement activation, and the infiltration of neutrophils and other inflammatory cells into the capillary walls. This results in an increase in mesangial cells

and matrix as well as occlusion of the capillary lumens from the influx of inflammatory cells and concomitant edema of endothelial cells. This produces diffuse lesions in both the mesangium and capillaries of the glomeruli.

N04.6 Nephrotic syndrome with dense deposit disease

Nephrotic syndrome is a condition in which the cells surrounding the clusters of tiny blood vessels, the glomeruli, have become damaged in the presence of edema. The damage allows the leakage of protein from blood into the urine, causing a decreased amount of protein in blood, and increased blood lipid levels. With decreased blood protein, there is a decrease in the oncotic pressure of blood, but not in tissue. This in turn leads to edema from water retention. Symptoms include weight gain from water retention, swollen ankles and feet, edema around the eyes, and foamy urine from the excess protein. Dense deposit disease is a rare condition associated with genetic risk factors or mutations regarding instructions for making proteins involved with the complement system of the body's immune response. It results in uncontrolled activation of the complement system, causing immune complex debris to build up in the glomeruli of the kidneys. Kidney function affected by this disorder tends to worsen, and half of patients end up with end stage renal disease within about 10 years of symptom onset.

Note: Dense deposit disease was previously known as membranoproliferative glomerulonephritis (MPGN) type 2, but recent discoveries suggest it is not a true form of MPGN.

N04.7 Nephrotic syndrome with diffuse crescentic glomerulonephritis

Nephrotic syndrome is a condition in which the cells surrounding the clusters of tiny blood vessels, the glomeruli, have become damaged in the presence of edema. The damage allows the leakage of protein from blood into the urine, causing a decreased amount of protein in blood, and increased blood lipid levels. With decreased blood protein, there is a decrease in the oncotic pressure of blood, but not in tissue. This in turn leads to edema from water retention. Symptoms include weight gain from water retention, swollen ankles and feet, edema around the eyes, and foamy urine from the excess protein. Diffuse crescentic glomerulonephritis, or extracapillary glomerulonephritis is a more rare histological lesion manifesting with severe glomerular damage. It involves fibrous and cellular proliferation occurring outside the capillary, forming epithelial crescents, the presence of two or more layers of cells, which partially or totally fill the Bowman's space and may obliterate capillary loops. This results in rapid loss of kidney function within weeks or months and leads to acute renal failure. Extracapillary, or crescentic, glomerulonephritis is due to the deposition of immune complexes and/or the presence of anti-glomerular antibodies.

N04.8 Nephrotic syndrome with other morphologic changes

Nephrotic syndrome is a condition in which the cells surrounding the clusters of tiny blood vessels, the glomeruli, have become damaged in the presence of edema. The damage allows the leakage of protein from blood into the urine, causing a decreased amount of protein in blood, and increased blood lipid levels. With decreased blood protein, there is a decrease in the oncotic pressure of blood, but not in tissue. This in turn leads to edema from water retention. Symptoms include weight gain from water retention, swollen ankles and feet, edema around the eyes, and foamy urine from the excess protein. Other morphological changes includes the presence of proliferative glomerulonephritis lesions in the kidney(s) that are not otherwise specified. Proliferative glomerulonephritis is caused by a range of immune-mediated and inflammatory mechanisms that result in lesions characterized by an increased number of cells in the glomeruli.

N13.3 Other and unspecified hydronephrosis

Hydronephrosis is kidney dilation or distention that results from urine overload, usually caused by an obstruction or stenosis in the ureter, bladder, or urethra. The condition can have an acute onset or be a chronic problem;

it may be unilateral or bilateral and the obstruction may be partial or complete.

Note: When the cause is known to be ureteral stricture or calculous obstruction, report with N13.1-N13.2, unless it is also accompanied by an infection, in which case hydronephrosis is reported with N13.6 as obstructive uropathy with infection.

N13.30   Unspecified hydronephrosis

Hydronephrosis is a condition in which urine backs up in the kidney due to a blockage in the flow of urine leaving the kidneys, often in the ureter, causing a distended and dilated renal calyx and pelvis. The most common symptom is pain on the afflicted side of the body. The increased pressure from fluid build-up decreases the filtration ability, and can cause permanent structural damage to renal cells.

N13.4   Hydroureter

Hydroureter is a condition in which the ureter becomes distended with urine or water due to a blockage which prevents the free flow of urine.

N13.6   Pyonephrosis

Pyonephrosis is an infection of the renal collecting system in which pus accumulates in the renal pelvis, causing distentions, complications of obstruction, and suppurative destruction of renal parenchyma, leading to kidney failure. Surgical drainage is required.

N13.7   Vesicoureteral-reflux

Vesicoureteral reflux is a disorder in which urine flows backwards from the bladder into the ureters or kidneys. This is most often diagnosed in children who may have been born with a defect in the valve preventing the retrograde flow of urine, causing infection and possibly leading to kidney damage. Vesicoureteral reflux is also diagnosed in those whose urinary tract is malfunctioning, often due to an infection. A UTI is the most common symptom with frequent urge to urinate, burning with urination, hematuria, fever, and flank pain.

N13.70   Vesicoureteral-reflux, unspecified

Vesicoureteral reflux (VUR) is most common in infants and young children but can occur at any age. The condition is characterized by a backflow of urine from the bladder to the ureters and sometimes into the kidneys that may cause progressive, long-term damage. When VUR is caused by a faulty valve at the junction of the bladder and ureter the condition is frequently unilateral and may resolve spontaneously as a child grows. VUR caused by a urethral problem is more likely to cause bilateral ureteral reflux and treatment may be required to correct the problem.

N17   Acute kidney failure

Acute kidney failure is a condition in which more than half of a patient's kidney function is lost in a period of days or hours. As a result, nitrogenous waste products begin to accumulate in the body instead of being expelled in the urine as they normally would. While there is no classic set of symptoms, most patients with acute kidney failure will notice a decrease in urine output.

N17.0   Acute kidney failure with tubular necrosis

Acute tubular necrosis is a renal disorder that involves the death of cells that form the tubules of the kidney. The tubules transport urine to the ureters while reabsorbing 99% of the water. Acute tubular necrosis is the most common cause of acute kidney failure. Necrosis of the tubules may be caused by nephrotoxic chemical exposure, including medicaments like penicillins, tetracycline, and sulfonamides, radiographic dye, and heavy metals. Tubular damage resulting in cell death may also be caused by severe dehydration or ischemia from circulatory collapse.

N17.1   Acute kidney failure with acute cortical necrosis

Acute cortical necrosis is a rare form of acute kidney failure caused by ischemic necrosis of the renal cortex. Lesions of necrotic glomeruli are usually caused by diminished blood supply perfusing the renal arteries due to vascular spasm or injury. In more advanced cases, larger necrotic lesions

or patches involving more of the cortex are marked by thrombi of the glomeruli or widespread arterial thrombosis.

N17.2   Acute kidney failure with medullary necrosis

Acute medullary [papillary] necrosis is kidney failure involving the death of the renal papillae--the area where the openings of the collecting ducts enter the kidney. This is where urine flows into the ureters. Death of this area of the kidney results in the inability to concentrate urine. Papillae necrosis is most often caused by analgesic overdose, or poisoning, but can also be caused by kidney infection, a blockage of the urinary tract, diabetes, sickle cell anemia, and transplant. Symptoms include back or flank pain, discolored urine, tissue in the urine, fever, chills, urination problems including pain, frequency, hesitancy, incontinence, and excretion of large volumes of urine.

N18   Chronic kidney disease (CKD)

Chronic kidney disease is a progressive loss of kidney function. The kidneys gradually decrease in size and experience progressive scarring. Initial symptoms include fatigue, headache, generalized itching, and weight loss. Later, decreased urine output, seizures, easy bleeding or bruising, and other symptoms that are not usually experienced until most kidney function is lost. There are five stages of the disease, with stage I being the mildest and stage V being the most severe, with the kidneys barely functioning at all. End stage renal disease indicates that the kidneys are not able to function in any meaningful capacity. Patients in stage I and II of the disease may be nearly asymptomatic, and the condition may be indicated only by urine tests, which reveal elevated levels of creatine and protein in the urine. As the disease progresses, the patient will typically experience anemia and bone loss as the kidneys lose their ability to filter the blood. Dialysis usually begins at stage IV.

N18.1   Chronic kidney disease, stage 1

This is the mildest form of chronic kidney disease. Symptoms at this stage are typically nonexistent, and the condition may only be indicated by urine tests, which reveal elevated levels of creatine and protein in the urine.

N18.2   Chronic kidney disease, stage 2 (mild)

Patients with stage II kidney disease may still be asymptomatic, or begin to experience only mild symptoms. The condition may be indicated only by urine tests, as for stage I, in which elevated levels of creatine and protein appear in the urine.

N18.3   Chronic kidney disease, stage 3 (moderate)

Stage III patients will typically begin to see symptoms and experience anemia and bone loss.

N18.4   Chronic kidney disease, stage 4 (severe)

In stage IV, anemia, bone loss, and other symptoms become more pronounced as the kidneys begin to cease functioning.

N18.5   Chronic kidney disease, stage 5

Stage V kidney disease causes severe symptoms, and the patient will be in grave danger without intensive treatment. Typically, patients at this stage of the disease will begin dialysis treatment.

Note: Chronic kidney disease, stage V now excludes stage V patients who are specified as on chronic dialysis. Stage V patients who require chronic dialysis are classified with end stage renal disease (N18.6). Stage V is the time in which the patient is coming toward the need for life-sustaining dialysis and is preparing to receive the procedure.

N18.6   End stage renal disease

At this stage, the patient's kidneys have ceased functioning in any useful capacity and the patient is past stage V chronic kidney disease and is receiving life-sustaining dialysis treatment on a required, regular basis.

N20   Calculus of kidney and ureter

Use the codes in this category to report the abnormal deposit of hardened minerals, called a calculus, or stone, within the kidney and ureter.

Diseases of the Genitourinary System

N13.30 – N20

N20.0 Calculus of kidney

A kidney stone, renal calculus, or nephrolithiasis is a hard, crystalized concretion of mineral salts that collects within the kidney. Symptoms include severe flank pain and hematuria. Dietary factors, hereditary factors, dehydration, and other conditions, such as gout, are major risk factors for the development of a kidney stone. If the stone does not or cannot pass through the urinary tract on its own, intervention such as lithotripsy to break up the stone into smaller pieces, or surgical extraction is necessary.

N21.0 Calculus in bladder

A calculus is a hard, crystalized concretion of mineral salts within the bladder. A bladder calculus or bladder stone may cause cystitis and other complications if a blockage in the flow of urine leaving the bladder results.

N25.0 Renal osteodystrophy

Renal osteodystrophy is a condition in which the bones soften and develop cysts due to an increase in toxins in the body that would normally be filtered out by the kidneys.

N25.81 Secondary hyperparathyroidism of renal origin

A condition in which kidney problems cause excessive secretion of parathyroid hormone, resulting in abnormal calcium levels in the bloodstream.

N26.1 Atrophy of kidney (terminal)

In terminal cases of atrophy, the kidneys begin to harden and develop fibrous tissue deposits, resulting in a continued decline of kidney function.

N28.85 Pyeloureteritis cystica

Pyeloureteritis cystica is a condition in which inflammation and small cysts develop in the kidney, the tissue around the kidney, and the ureter.

N30 Cystitis

Cystitis is an infection or inflammation of the urinary bladder. This condition primarily effects young and post-menopausal women. The most common cause of cystitis is a bacterial infection that makes its way up the urethra. The culprit is usually coliform bacteria, which are found in the rectum and can migrate from the anus to the end of the urethra. Typical symptoms are burning during urination, possible blood in the urine, and fever. The different types of cystitis are coded as with or without hematuria, or blood appearing in the urine.

N30.0 Acute cystitis

Acute cystitis is a sudden or severe inflammation of the urinary bladder. The most common cause is a bacterial infection (UTI) but a reaction to certain drugs, irritation from radiation therapy, an indwelling catheter or chemicals (spermicides, soaps) can also produce symptoms. The condition is characterized by urinary urgency, frequency, and pain. There may also be pelvic discomfort and pressure, blood and/or pus in the urine, and fever.

N30.1 Interstitial cystitis (chronic)

Chronic interstitial cystitis is long-term inflammation of the bladder that is not caused by bacteria. It is more common in women but may occur in men and children. The condition is characterized by a persistent urge to urinate, passing small amounts of urine frequently, suprapubic pain (in women), perineal pain (in men), chronic pelvic pain, and often pain with intercourse. A patient with this condition will wake frequently during the night to urinate, and may have a distended bladder.

N30.3 Trigonitis

Trigonitis is a nonkeratinizing, squamous metaplastic change that takes place in the triangular area of the bladder called the trigone. This area extends from the internal urethral sphincter at the bottom of the bladder to the two ureteral orifices. The condition is believed to result from chronic irritation, inflammation, or infection and may also be influenced by changes in certain hormone levels (estrogen, progesterone).

N30.4 Irradiation cystitis

Irradiation cystitis is an inflammation of the bladder due to exposure to radiation, usually occurring as a side effect of radiotherapy used as treatment for cancer.

N30.8 Other cystitis

An abscess of the bladder is coded here, in which there is an infected pocket of tissue containing pus and other cellular debris that has collected within the bladder. Cystitis cystica, or bullous cystitis, is another form of bladder inflammation occurring with the formation of cysts on the interior bladder wall.

N31.9 Neuromuscular dysfunction of bladder, unspecified

Neuromuscular dysfunction of the bladder is a non-specific condition caused by a lesion of the nervous system which affects the transmission of impulses to the bladder. This condition can cause kidney failure if urine cannot be expelled.

N32.0 Bladder-neck obstruction

This disorder occurs when the opening between the bladder and the urethra becomes blocked. Possible causes of this condition include injury, infection, blood clots, stricture, calculus buildup, or a number of other conditions. A patient with this condition will experience decreased urine output and a distended bladder.

N32.1 Vesicointestinal fistula

An intestionvesical fistula is an abnormal duct or passage that forms between the bladder and the intestines.

N32.3 Diverticulum of bladder

Diverticulum of the bladder is an abnormal outpouching, or balloon-like sac occurring within the bladder walls. Bladder diverticulum are usually small, harmless pouches in an area of weakness in the bladder wall through which the lining protrudes. They typically occur as a result of obstruction in the bladder outlet such as an enlarged prostate or scarring obstructing the urethra. Diverticula do not normally have direct symptoms, but are often discovered while looking for other causes of urinary problems during cystography or cystoscopy. If the diverticula are causing obstruction or are associated with chronic infection, retrograde flow of urine, or bladder stones, surgical treatment may be necessary.

N32.81 Overactive bladder

An overactive bladder, caused by hypertonicity of the bladder muscle, occurs when the bladder fails to relax sufficiently to accomodate the normal function of storing urine. This condition is marked by urinary urgency, possibly with incontinence, urinary frequency, and nocturia.

N32.89 Other specified disorders of bladder

Other specified disorders of the bladder may include bladder hypertrophy, calcified bladder, contracted bladder, or hemorrhaging. Bladder hypertrophy is an increased mass of the bladder wall as a consequence of bladder outlet obstruction. The smooth muscle cells of the bladder become hyperplastic, but relief of the obstruction normally reverses the increased bladder mass. Bladder wall calcification typically presents like laminating layers of heavily calcified materials. It can be caused by schistosomiasis, cancer, some types of cystitis, and tuberculosis.

N34.3 Urethral syndrome, unspecified

Urethral syndrome is a group of symptoms including painful urination, urethral discharge, lower back pain, and frequent urination that have no known cause.

N35 Urethral stricture

Use this category to report the different classified types of urethral stricture, or an abnormal narrowing of the urethra. This condition often causes pain or a burning sensation during urination.

N35.01 Post-traumatic urethral stricture, male

Post-traumatic urethral stricture is an abnormal narrowing of the urethra as the result of an injury. Strictures are more common in men due to the longer length of the urethra. Symptoms can include painful urination, decreased urine flow, and the inability to fully empty the bladder.

N36.0 Urethral fistula

A urethra fistula is an abnormal duct or passage connecting the urethra to another structure or external site of the body, such as the perineum, the rectum, or another urinary organ.

N36.1 Urethral diverticulum

A sac-like outpouching within the urethral wall.

N36.2 Urethral caruncle

A fleshy polyp-like outgrowth within the urethra, often growing from the mucous membrane.

N36.41 Hypermobility of urethra

Urethral hypermobility is a condition in which the urethra fails to close, resulting in urinary incontinence.

N36.42 Intrinsic sphincter deficiency (ISD)

Intrinsic (urethral) sphincter deficiency (ISD) is a less common type of stress incontinence caused by a weakening of the urethral sphincter muscles. It can be caused by genetics, but more often occurs following pelvic surgery, prostatectomy, another incontinence surgery, even vaginal birth, or nerve damage from another neurological problem. The sphincter muscle of the urethra malfunctions and does not remain tightly closed, allowing urine to leak because the pressure in the bladder is greater when the urethral sphincter muscle remains open.

N36.44 Muscular disorders of urethra

Use this code to report detrusor sphincter dyssynergia, a condition in which the sphincter muscle that controls the release of urine from the bladder malfunctions.

N36.5 Urethral false passage

An abnormal opening into the urethra caused by a disease, injury, or surgical procedure.

N36.8 Other specified disorders of urethra

Other specified disorders of the urethra include prolapsed urethral mucosa in which the muscles that hold the urethra in place weaken, allowing the urethra to press into the vaginal canal. This condition can lead to incontinence and urinary infection, and is often associated with pregnancy or pelvic surgery.

N39.41 Urge incontinence

The inability to control urination once the urge to urinate occurs.

N39.43 Post-void dribbling

Post-void dribbling is diagnosed when urine continues to leak from the bladder following normal urination.

N40 Enlarged prostate

Enlarged prostate includes benign (adenofibromatous) prostatic hypertrophy or hyperplasia (BPH), nodular prostate, and polyp of the prostate. The prostate is a walnut-sized gland that surrounds the urethra, the tube that carries urine from the bladder out of the body. The prostate is located just below the bladder and in front of the rectum. It has two lobes and is composed of glands and stroma. The glands are lined by two cell layers and are separated by the fibromuscular stroma between them, which accounts for about half the prostate's volume. The prostate is surrounded by a thin, outer layer of encapsulating connective tissue. The prostate continues to grow during most of a man's life and commonly becomes enlarged as a male ages. Enlargement of the prostate gland is commonly called benign prostatic hyperplasia or benign prostatic hypertrophy (BPH). The cause of BPH is not really understood, but the main factors considered to play an important role are aging, normal testicular function, a changing

balance in hormones, and the accumulation of dihydrotestosterone in the prostate that signals the growth of cells. Although the terms 'benign prostatic hyperplasia' and 'benign prostatic hypertrophy' are often used interchangeably, hyperplasia is an abnormal proliferation or increase in the number of normal cells, while hypertrophy is an overgrowth of the gland due to an abnormal increase in the size of its constituent cells. Prostate growth can occur in different types of cells and in different ways, causing different effects and requiring varied treatments. Most common symptoms arise when the gland begins to press against the urethra like a clamp on a garden hose as cells multiply and the prostate enlarges.

Prostatic enlargement does not necessarily cause problems and many men with enlarged prostates have only minor symptoms, which are rarely seen before age 40. More than 50% of men will be affected by BPH after age 60, and as many as 90% of men in their seventies and eighties will have some symptoms of BPH.

Diagnostic tests include digital rectal exam, rectal ultrasound, prostate biopsy, cystoscopy, urine flow or volume studies, and blood tests to check for prostate specific antigen. Treatments include medications to reduce hormone levels, shrink the prostate, and relax the smooth muscle in the prostate and bladder neck; minimally invasive thermotherapy procedures to destroy or ablate excess prostatic tissue using microwave generated heat, low-level radiofrequency energy, or heated water; and more invasive surgical procedures such as transurethral resection of the prostate (TURP) and open prostatectomy. Laser treatment of prostate tissue is also used in cystoscopic surgery, photoselective vaporization, and interstitial coagulation.

N40.1 Enlarged prostate with lower urinary tract symptoms

Symptoms of an enlarged prostate include a weak, slow, or delayed urinary stream; straining or pain upon urination; bloody urine; a strong, sudden urge to urinate; the need to urinate multiple times at night; incomplete bladder emptying; and urinary retention, obstruction, and incontinence.

N40.2 Nodular prostate without lower urinary tract symptoms

The normal prostate weighs about 25g, but nodular prostates can weigh from 50g-100g, feel entirely hard or firm, and have multiple nodules affecting more than one lobe. The hyperplasia begins in the inner zone of the prostate and expands to lobular involvement. Microscopically, a nodular prostate consists of nodules of glandular proliferation with some intervening increased stromal cells that may sometimes predominate, but rarely.

Note: Because a discrete, solid, hard nodule on the prostate identified by digital rectal exam is indicative of prostate cancer, these codes may be confused with a nodule on the prostate representing cancer, but malignant neoplasm of the prostate is not coded here. This code is used for asymptomatic nodular hyperplasia of the prostate.

N40.3 Nodular prostate with lower urinary tract symptoms

Symptoms of an enlarged nodular prostate include a weak, slow, or delayed urinary stream; straining or pain upon urination; bloody urine; a strong, sudden urge to urinate; the need to urinate multiple times a night; incomplete bladder emptying; and urinary retention, obstruction, and incontinence.

N41 Inflammatory diseases of prostate

This category reports cases of prostatitis, abscess, and other inflammatory conditions of the prostate. This encompasses different kinds of inflammatory conditions, many caused by bacterial agents, although evidence of an infecting organism is not always found. A prostate that is infected or inflamed can cause pain upon urination and ejaculation, and other voiding symptoms, which may turn to more serious complications if left untreated. Prostatitis can affect men of any age and estimates predict that half of all men will experience it sometime during their life. It is the most common urological disorder in men over 50.

Note: Use an additional code(s) from categories B95-B97 to identify any infecting organism(s), such as staphylococcus or streptococcus.

N41.0 Acute prostatitis

Acute bacterial prostatitis (ABP) is not a very common condition and occurs much less frequently than chronic prostatitis, but is easier to identify due to its uniform presentation. ABP is associated with certain risk factors that allow bacterial colonization, including benign prostatic hyperplasia causing urinary outlet obstruction, UTI, phimosis, unprotected intercourse, and reflux of infected urine into the intraprostatic ducts. An acute infection of the prostate usually is caused by the same bacterial agents responsible for urinary tract infections, most commonly *E. coli*, and also *Proteus mirabilis*, *Klebsiella*, *Enterobacter* species, *Pseudomonas aeruginosa*, and *Serratia* species. *Staph aureus* infection is more likely to occur in the hospital with catheterization. Other occasional infections include *Mycobacterium tuberculosis* and *Salmonella* species as well as the sexually transmitted bacteria, *Neisseria gonorrheae*. Acute bacterial prostatitis occurs more frequently in men under 35 years old. Symptoms present as acute illness with fever, low back and perineal pain, urinary urgency and frequency, dysuria, and nocturia. Sometimes myalgia, malaise, and joint pain are also present. Palpation will reveal an exquisitely tender and swollen prostate. Treatment is necessary to avoid more serious complications.

N41.1 Chronic prostatitis

Chronic prostatitis now has several different classifications, although it is still an uncertain disease process that is not well understood and does not have clear or uniformly distinguished clinical features. Chronic bacterial prostatitis is a recurrent or long standing inflammation that may follow cases of acute prostatitis or recurrent urinary tract infection. Sometimes the bacterial agents are those identified as causing urinary tract infections. In some cases, the condition may be related to *Chlamydia* or *N. gonorrheae*. Lymphocytes, plasma cells, and macrophages appear in the stroma. Symptoms may be less severe than those of acute bacterial prostatitis. Chronic bacterial prostatitis primarily affects men between 40 and 70. Chronic prostatitis that is not due to an identifiable bacterial infection is a much more common condition affecting men of all ages and ethnic backgrounds. Chronic nonbacterial prostatitis causes pelvic pain for at least three months, low back pain, dysuria, and other variable urinary and sexual symptoms without any demonstrative infective agent. Sexual dysfunction and/or pain with ejaculation are symptoms of chronic prostatitis. Another category of chronic abacterial prostatitis causes chronic pelvic pain syndrome with white blood cells present in semen and secretions expressed from the prostate. Asymptomatic inflammatory prostatitis may produce evidence of inflammation on biopsy and in semen or other secretions, but no symptoms.

N41.2 Abscess of prostate

An abscess of the prostate is an infrequent complication of acute bacterial prostatitis. A prostatic abscess is often not amenable to medical management and requires other intervention. Transrectal or perineal aspiration of the abscess is preferred, but if symptoms do not improve, surgery such as transurethral resection with drainage of the cavity may be necessary. An abscess presents a higher potential for bacteria to infect the bloodstream, cause sepsis, and spread to other parts of the body.

N41.3 Prostatocystitis

Prostatocystitis is an inflammation of the prostate gland and the bladder, including the bladder neck and prostatic urethra. This inflammation may be due to different causes such as bacterial infection or external beam radiation therapy.

N42.0 Calculus of prostate

Calculus of the prostate occurs when mineral deposits form a hard, crystalized buildup or stone in the prostate gland, which can lead to pain and trouble with urination.

N42.1 Congestion and hemorrhage of prostate

Congestion of the prostate occurs when fluids collect in the prostate, causing it to become swollen, which can interfere with urination.

N42.3 Dysplasia of prostate

Dysplasia of the prostate is a condition in which the cells of the prostate begin to multiply for no apparent cause. While not dangerous on its own, this condition is known to be a precursor of prostate cancer. This code includes prostatic intraepithelial neoplasia I and II (PIN I and II). When this neoplasia is diagnosed as level III (PIN III), it is considered carcinoma in situ of the prostate and is coded to D07.5.

N42.81 Prostatodynia syndrome

Painful prostate syndrome.

N42.83 Cyst of prostate

Prostatic cysts can usually be felt on digital rectal exam or are diagnosed by transrectal ultrasound when patients are evaluated. Prostatic cysts may be asymptomatic or they can cause urinary outlet obstruction, or voiding and prostatitis-like symptoms, as well as infertility problems. In some cases, penile discharge may occur when fluid is expressed from the cyst upon abdominal straining, such as with weight-lifting or bowel movement. Cysts may form because the ejaculatory ducts running though the prostate have become obstructed and fill with fluid, forming a cyst. Cysts may also arise from an intraprostatic ectopic ureter, or from one of the lateral lobes, even projecting into the urethra.

Note: Most cysts arise from the medial portion of the prostate. Midline cysts located posteriorly at the base of the prostate floor and arising from the utricle or Muellerian duct are not coded here. The Muellerian duct cyst is a remnant of the fused ends of the embryological duct structure that normally regresses in utero. They are rare, occurring as an isolated entity, and the aspirated fluid never contains sperm. Muellerian duct cysts in the male are considered to be congenital malformations/lesions of the periprostatic region and are coded to Q55.29. Utricular cysts are also of embryological origin and are associated with other urinary tract abnormalities. Although a prostatic utricular cyst is confined to the base of the prostate and communicates with the prostatic urethra, this type of cyst is coded to Q55.4.

N42.89 Other specified disorders of prostate

This code includes prostatic atrophy when the gland shrinks in size from tissue wasting.

N43.0 Encysted hydrocele

A hydrocele is an accumulation of serous, or lymph, fluid on the spermatic cord inside the scrotum. They are not usually dangerous, and are typically only removed if they threaten the blood supply to the testicle, or if they become uncomfortably large. An encysted hydrocele is the typical presentation.

N43.1 Infected hydrocele

Infected hydroceles can occur if an attempt is made to drain fluid from it. An infected hydrocele is dangerous and is usually removed immediately.

N43.2 Other hydrocele

Hydrocele testis is an accumulation of serous fluid in the scrotum, usually in a remnant piece of peritoneum called the tunica vaginalis that wraps around the testicle. The condition is usually painless and benign. Causes can include scarring due to cancer, trauma, hernia, infection, or an obstruction in the inguinal lymph system. The condition may also present itself in infants who are on peritoneal dialysis.

N43.3 Hydrocele, unspecified

A hydrocele is an accumulation of serous fluid, or lymph, on the spermatic cord, testes, or tunica vaginalis inside the scrotum. They can occur due to acute local injury, infection, radiotherapy, or gradual fluid accumulation and are not usually dangerous. They are typically only removed if they threaten the blood supply to the testicle, or if they become uncomfortably large.

N43.4 Spermatocele of epididymis

A spermatocele is a fluid filled cyst that may contain spermatozoa and is located in a tubule at the head of the epididyis. The condition may occur singularly or in multiples. Causes can include infection, inflammation, and trauma. Spermatoceles are common, rarely symptomatic, and usually do not affect male fertility.

N44.00 Torsion of testis, unspecified

In torsion of the testis, the testicle becomes twisted inside the scrotum, cutting off or reducing the blood supply, and endangering viability of the organ. A torsed testicle requires immediate surgery to prevent organ death. Symptoms include sudden, severe pain in the scrotum, nausea, and vomiting.

N44.01 Extravaginal torsion of spermatic cord

Extravaginal torsion occurs in the fetus developing in the womb and in neonates, in the time when the testicle is often still undescended and may delay the diagnosis of torsed testicle. In extravaginal torsion, the testicle, epididymis, and tunica vaginalis twist on the spermatic cord.

N44.02 Intravaginal torsion of spermatic cord

Intravaginal torsion is a specific type of testicle torsion that happens in connection with a congenital anomaly called bell-clapper deformity, in which the tunica vaginalis, the membrane that normally covers the sides and front of the testicle and epididymis, forms completely around the testis without the usual posterior anchoring in back. This allows the testicle to twist freely. This kind of torsion appears most often around the age of puberty.

N44.03 Torsion of appendix testis

An appendix testis is a vestige of the developing tissue, remaining in a high percentage of testes, as an appendage usually located at the superior pole in the groove between the testicle and the epididymis. The vestigial remnants of tissue are most often pedunculated, or attached by a stalk-like structure that predisposes the appendage to torsion. Resulting ischemia and infarction can cause necrosis of the appendix with pain and inflammation in the surrounding structures. Torsion of the appendix testis is often accompanied by a hydrocele and a thickened scrotal wall. A torsed appendix testis is one of the most common causes of acute scrotal pain, but the condition does not normally have any permanent consequences for the testicle's viability.

N44.04 Torsion of appendix epididymis

An appendix epididymis is a vestige of the developing wolffian duct that remains in about 23% of testes as an appendage that usually projects from the head of the epididymis on a stalk-like structure. Torsion of the epididymal appendage causes infarction and necrosis with resulting pain. Torsion of testicular appendages are usually benign conditions as the necrotic tissue is reabsorbed without sequelae.

N44.1 Cyst of tunica albuginea testis

This cyst occurs when chyle, a milky fluid comprised of lymph rich in digested nutrients, becomes trapped in the membrane which covers the blood vessels that feed the testes.

N45 Orchitis and epididymitis

This category is used to report orchitis (inflammation of the testes) and epididymitis (inflammation of the epididymis). These conditions are characterized by pain and swelling in the scrotum.

N46.0 Azoospermia

A condition in which the semen has an absent or immeasurable level of sperm present. Testicular causes are present in 49-93% of cases in which spermatogenesis fails due to absent or abnormal testes.

N46.02 Azoospermia due to extratesticular causes

A condition in which the semen has an absent or immeasurable level of sperm present. The condition may arise from extratesticular causes in which the testes and genital tract are normal but a physical obstruction limits the release of sperm during ejaculation; or drug therapy, infection, or radiation may affect hormone levels or normal sperm production processes.

N46.1 Oligospermia

Oligospermia is a low level of sperm (<15 million sperm/ml) present in semen associated with male infertility.

N46.12 Oligospermia due to extratesticular causes

Oligospermia is a condition in which the amount of sperm in semen is insufficient to achieve conception. The condtion may be transient or permanent. Extratesticular causes can include drug/alcohol/tobacco use; strenuous bicycle or horseback riding; use of androgen medications; radiation exposure for cancer treatment; or trauma, injury, or infection that obstructs the efferent ducts.

N47.0 Adherent prepuce, newborn

In adherent prepuce, the foreskin extends past the head of the penis and cannot be retracted back to expose the glans. This is a normal occurance in most newborn males. The condition usually resolves without intervention by the age of 3 years.

N47.1 Phimosis

Phimosis, or redundant prepuce, is a condition in which the head of the penis is covered in excess foreskin with the inability of the prepuce to be retracted behind the glans penis in an uncircumcised male. The condition may be present at birth and resolve without intervention or it may be due to scarring from infection and require circumcision. This excess foreskin is prone to infection and is typically removed via surgery.

N47.2 Paraphimosis

Paraphimosis is the retraction of the prepuce (foreskin) behind the head of the penis that decreases blood flow to the glans causing a tight, swollen band of tissue to form. The swelling makes it difficult, sometimes impossible, to move the foreskin back over the glans.

N47.6 Balanoposthitis

Balanoposthitis is inflammation of the head of the penis and the foreskin. This condition usually occurs in uncircumcised males when the area under the foreskin traps bacteria.

N48.0 Leukoplakia of penis

A rare type of dermatological lesion of the penis marked by circumscribed areas of thickened, white, atrophic patches that may be rough or smooth appearing on the foreskin and glans. This includes balanitis xerotica obliterans, which is a chronic, progressively sclerosing, inflammatory dermatosis affecting the male genitalia causing hardened, indurated, or sclerosed tissue formation.

N48.1 Balanitis

Balanitis is inflammation or swelling of the head of the penis, normally caused by lack of personal hygiene in uncircumcised males from lack of aeration combined with the irritation of smegma buildup.

N48.3 Priapism

Priapism is a persistent, prolonged, and painful erection lasting four hours or more and is a true urological emergency. The unwanted erection does not result from sexual desire or occurs when the penis does not return to its normal flaccid state in the absence of physical or psychological stimulation. Priapism occurs when changes in normal blood flow occur, due to changes affecting the blood itself, the blood vessels, or the related nerves. Ischemic priapism is caused by a lack of blood flow out of the penis, while non-ischemic priapism occurs when too much blood flows into the penis. Causes may be other diseases such as sickle cell anemia and leukemia; the use of drugs such as antidepressants, antipsychotics, and blood thinners; illegal drug use and drinking too much alcohol; and injury or trauma such as blood clotting, venomous bites, and spinal cord injury.

Note: The underlying cause should be coded first.

N48.6   Induration penis plastica

Induration penis plastica, also known as Peyronie's disease, is a connective tissue disorder of unknown etiology that causes the formation of fibrous tissue plaques or nodules inside the soft tissue of the penis. This results in a painful bending or deformity in the erect penis. The disease affects the tunica albuginea layer of the penis and is also known as chronic inflammation of the tunica albuginea. Calcification usually occurs in the end stage of the disease when deformity does not worsen any further. Mild cases are self-limiting and benign and require no intervention. Treatment is aimed at relieving pain and halting the fibrotic progression using oral, topical, and infectable medications, x-ray, electrical and ultrasonic therapy, and surgery in more extreme cases.

N49.0   Inflammatory disorders of seminal vesicle

Inflammation of the seminal vesicle; the most common cause of this condition is a bacterial infection, and is marked by painless, bloody ejaculate.

N49.3   Fournier gangrene

A complication of cell death or necrosis affecting the perineal, genital, or perianal regions, fournier gangrene is characterized by tissue decay that becomes black and malodorous. It is caused by infection or ischemia, and is often the result of an insufficient, or cut-off blood supply.

N50.0   Atrophy of testis

A wasting of testicular tissue, causing a descrease in size, often for no apparent reason.

N50.1   Vascular disorders of male genital organs

Vascular disorders of male genital organs includes thrombosis or bleeding of the scrotum, seminal vesicle, spermatic cord, testes, tunica vaginalis, and vas deferens; or a hematocele, a pocket or collection of blood, in the male gential organs, usually occuring in the tunica vaginalis around the testicle.

N50.8   Other specified disorders of male genital organs

Use this code to report a stricture, or abnormal narrowing, of the spermatic cord, tunica vaginalis, and vas deferens; hypertrophy or ulcer of the scrotum, seminal vesicle, spermatic cord, testes, tunica vaginalis, and vas deferens; a urethroscrotal fistula in which an abnormal connection passes from the urethra out to the scrotal tissue; edema of male genital organs in which fluid builds up inside the tissue, causing swelling and distention; atrophy of any male genital organs besides the testes in which the tissue wastes away and shrinks in size; and chylocele (nonfilarial) of the tunica vaginalis: a cyst-like lesion resulting from the escape of chyle, a milky fluid consisting of lymph and emulsified fat, into the tunica vaginalis of the testes.

N52   Male erectile dysfunction

Male erectile dysfunction, or impotence, is the inability to form or maintain an erection firm enough for sexual intercourse. The condition may be transient or permanent. Causes include stress and psychological disorders, cardiovascular disease (atherosclerosis, elevated cholesterol, hypertension), diabetes, obesity, certain medications, neurological diseases (Parkinson's, multiple sclerosis), low testosterone levels, prostate or bladder surgery, spinal cord injury, and drug/alcohol/tobacco use.

N53.14   Retrograde ejaculation

Retrograde ejaculation occurs when the bladder neck remains open during ejaculation, causing semen to flow backward into the bladder.

N60   Benign mammary dysplasia

Use this category to report non-cancerous growths like cysts and fibroadenomatous or fibrosclerotic disease in mammary tissue.

N60.0   Solitary cyst of breast

A single, benign, fluid-filled sac encapsulated in breast tissue. Cysts may appear as round or oval-shaped lumps with distinct edges and may feel firm or like a miniature water or gel-filled balloon. These are not usually removed unless they become painful or uncomfortable and they are most common in women before menopause.

N60.1   Diffuse cystic mastopathy

Diffuse cystic mastopathy, also known as fibrocystic breast disease, occurs when several benign cysts, or fluid-filled sacs, form in the breast tissue. This condition rarely harms the patient. The most common symptoms are tenderness and changes in the shape of the breast.

N60.2   Fibroadenosis of breast

Fibroadenosis is a benign breast disease that causes the formation of lumps made of fibrous and glandular tissue. The lumps are painless, mobile, and slow-growing individualized nodules that appear in breast tissue of women in child-bearing years.

N60.4   Mammary duct ectasia

Mammary duct ectasia is a condition which affects women mostly of the age approaching menopause. A dilated milk duct becomes clogged with a thick, sticky substance causing discharge and inflammation as well as pain and tenderness in the breast.

N62   Hypertrophy of breast

Hypertrophy of the breast is an abnormal largeness of breasts that typically occurs in adolescent females whose breast tissue is particularly sensitive to hormones circulated throughout the body during puberty. Back problems can occur from carrying the weight of the breast tissue, and skin problems are also possible if the dermis is forced to stretch too rapidly.

Note: Gynecomastia is also coded here, which is the abnormal enlargement of breasts in males, that can be caused by an imbalance between the hormones estrogen and testosterone.

N64.0   Fissure and fistula of nipple

A fissure is a crack in the skin of the nipple and a fistula is an abnormal connection running between the nipple and another internal tissue structure or another location on the skin.

N64.1   Fat necrosis of breast

Fat necrosis of the breast occurs when fatty tissue in the breast dies, usually as a result of traumatic injury. The dead tissue forms hard deposits which can be felt on the surface of the breast.

N64.2   Atrophy of breast

Atrophy is a shrinking and wasting of the breast tissue.

N64.3   Galactorrhea not associated with childbirth

Galactorrhea is the inappropriate discharge of milk from the breast.

N64.4   Mastodynia

Pain in the breast.

N64.53   Retraction of nipple

Retracted nipples are those that lie flat or flush with the rest of the breast when they are not being stimulated. Although retracted nipples are often called inverted nipples, inverted nipples are generally considered those that are indented into the areola and sink or turn inward instead of protruding, often as a normal variant, and that will pop out when stimulated in most cases. Retracted nipples pull flat or lie flush with surrounding breast tissue without turning inward and are most often brought about as a change in nipple position that started out as raised, and began to pull flat or fold into a narrow crease They may not return to normal position, even with stimulation. Retracted nipples may be caused by pregnancy, breastfeeding, aging, duct ectasia, and some cancers.

Note: Retracted nipples acquired in association with pregnancy, lactation, or the puerperium, are coded to subcategory O92.0.

N64.59   Other signs and symptoms in the breast

Other signs and symptoms of the breast includes bleeding from the nipple, engorgement or congestion of the breast, and acquired inverted or invaginated nipples. Inverted nipples are those that actually sink or turn inward, appearing indented. They can occur in both men and women and are most often simply a normal anatomical variance, although they can cause breast asymmetry and interfere with breastfeeding. Acquired cases may result from infection or trauma, fibrotic scar tissue, rapid weight loss, normal aging changes in breast tissue density, and diseases such as inflammatory breast cancer and Paget's disease. Inversion that develops later in life can sometimes signal a potential problem as there are forms of cancer that can cause inverted nipples. Nipple inversion is usually classified as level I, II, or III based on how easily the nipple can be coaxed out, the degree of fibrosis, and the amount of milk duct damage or impairment. Level I is characterized by protraction induced with massage, cold exposure, or tactile stimulation. There is no milk duct compression, minimal or no fibrosis, and no soft tissue defects. Level II is characterized by protraction induced using strong suction with quick nipple retraction. Milk duct compression may be present and there is usually moderate fibrosis with mildly retracted lactiferous ducts. In Level III, the nipple rarely protracts, milk duct constriction is present along with marked or severe fibrosis, and severely retracted lactiferous ducts, often with insufficient soft tissue in the nipple. Plastic surgery may be used to correct inverted nipples and maintain protraction.

N64.81 Ptosis of breast

Ptosis is a falling, drooping, or sagging of the breast tissue, which can occur naturally or following pregnancy or weight gain and loss. Age and size are also a contributing factor as skin elasticity decreases with age and the weight of breast tissue increases with size. The levels of ptosis are graded by the relationship of the nipple to the inframammary fold or crease at the bottom of the breast: Grade 1: the nipple is in front of the crease; Grade 2: the nipple falls 1-2 cm below the crease; Grade 3: the nipple points straight downward. The grade determines the type of procedure used for correction.

N64.82 Hypoplasia of breast

Hypoplasia of breast, also called micromastia, is a very small or almost absent development of the breast.

Note: Congenital absence of the entire breast is reported with Q83.0.

N64.89 Other specified disorders of breast

Other specified disorders include a galactocele, which is a cyst that contains milk encapsulated in the breast tissue.

N65 Deformity and disproportion of reconstructed breast

Breast reconstruction after mastectomy can take months or years. Even after a breast has been reconstructed, it may need additional plastic surgery to achieve a final desired result because of irregularities that need to be corrected or unacceptable aesthetic appearance in comparison with the native breast.

N65.0 Deformity of reconstructed breast

Deformities include contour irregularities, misshapen reconstructed breast(s), or excess tissue in the breast.

N65.1 Disproportion of reconstructed breast

Disproportion of a reconstructed breast is by comparison to the native breast, such as when asymmetry occurs from one to the other.

N70 Salpingitis and oophoritis

Salpingitis and oophoritis is an infection and/or inflammation of the fallopian tubes and ovaries. This category includes abscess of the tubes and/or ovaries and pyosalpinx, an accumulation of pus in the fallopian tube leading to blockage and dilation of the tube, which is usually bilateral and associated with acute pelvic inflammatory disease (PID) and tubovarian abscess.

N70.0 Acute salpingitis and oophoritis

Acute salpingitis is the sudden or severe inflammation of a fallopian tube, and oophoritis is the inflammation of one or both ovaries. These conditions usually occur as the result of an infection that begins in the lower urinary tract and is left untreated.

N70.1 Chronic salpingitis and oophoritis

Chronic salpingitis is a long-term or recurring infection or inflammation of a fallopian tube, and oophoritis is the infection or inflammation of one or both ovaries that is not as severe as acute cases. These conditions usually occur as the result of a recurring bacterial infection that begins in the lower urinary tract and is left untreated. This also includes hydrosalpinx, an accumulation of serous fluid in the fallopian tube leading to blockage and dilation of the tube. This condition may be unilateral or bilateral and is often associated with infertility.

N73.0 Acute parametritis and pelvic cellulitis

Acute parametritis is a sudden, severe inflammation of the connective tissue which is attached to the uterus.

N75.0 Cyst of Bartholin's gland

A fluid-filled, encapsulated sac of the glands that sit on either side within the vaginal orifice and secrete a lubricating substance.

N75.1 Abscess of Bartholin's gland

A pus-filled sac of infective material and cellular debris of the glands that sit on either side within the vaginal orifice and secrete a lubricating substance.

N76.0 Acute vaginitis

Acute vaginitis includes acute and unspecified vulvovaginitis. This is a sudden or severe inflammation of the vagina, or inflammation of the vagina along with the external female genital organs. Common symptoms are swelling, itching, and a burning sensation of the afflicted tissues. The most common cause of infection is a yeast infection, followed by other types of bacterial infections.

Note: Vulvar vestibulitis is coded to N94.810.

N76.1 Subacute and chronic vaginitis

Vaginitis is an inflammation of the female vagina usually due to irritation or infection (bacterial vaginosis, candidiasis, trichomoniasis) and may be subacute or chronic, lasting for a longer duration or less severe than an acute infection. Symptoms can include itching, burning, discharge (often foul smelling) and pain with intercourse. The condition is often associated with irritation or infection of the vulva (labia, clitoris, and vestibule of the vagina) that has reached the vagina.

N76.2 Acute vulvitis

A sudden or severe infection and inflammatory reaction of the female external genitalia, including the labia, clitoris, and vestibule of the vagina.

N76.4 Abscess of vulva

Pus-filled sacs appearing on the external female genitalia.

N76.5 Ulceration of vagina

The condition of an open wound(s) or festering sore(s) within the wall of the birth canal.

N76.6 Ulceration of vulva

A condition of an open wound(s) or festering sore(s) on the external female genitalia.

N76.81 Mucositis (ulcerative) of vagina and vulva

Mucositis appearing in the genital tract is a common complication of cancer treatment, such as radiation therapy to the pelvis for uterine or cevical cancer. Muscositis causes inflammation and ulcerative sores in the soft tissues of the mucous membranes in the cervix, vagina, and vulva. This is a painful condition that hampers the patient's ability to continue with the therapeutic doses of treatment.

N77.0 Ulceration of vulva in diseases classified elsewhere

An ulcer on the external female genitalia as an aspect of another primary disease or condition, which should be coded first.

N80 Endometriosis

Endometriosis is a condition in which tissue that lines the uterus migrates and begins to proliferate outside the uterine cavity, most often on the peritoneum, a membrane that lines the abdominal cavity. Endometrial cells react to hormone stimulation during the menstrual cycle causing them to thicken and bleed. This can lead to irritation, development of scar tissue and adhesions, pain, and often problems with infertility. This occurs mostly among women of child-bearing age. The most common symptom is pain in the lower abdomen, lower back, and pelvic area. Pain can also occur during urination or defecation, as well as during sexual intercourse. Some women may experience heavy menstrual periods or spotting between periods.

N80.0 Endometriosis of uterus

Abnormal uterine tissue growth contained within the uterus.

N80.1 Endometriosis of ovary

The abnormal growth of uterine tissue outside the uterus around the ovary(ies), causing inflammation, irritation, and pain, as well as possible infertility.

N80.2 Endometriosis of fallopian tube

The abnormal growth of uterine tissue outside the uterus affecting the fallopian tube(s), causing inflammation, irritation, and pain, as well as possible infertility.

N80.3 Endometriosis of pelvic peritoneum

The abnormal growth of uterine tissue outside the uterus affecting the membrane that lines the tissue of the pelvis, causing inflammation, irritation, and pain, as well as possible infertility.

N80.4 Endometriosis of rectovaginal septum and vagina

The abnormal growth of uterine tissue outside the uterus affecting the membranous partition separating the vagina from the rectum and/or the vagina itself, causing inflammation, irritation, and pain.

N80.5 Endometriosis of intestine

The abnormal growth of uterine tissue outside the uterus around the intestine(s), causing inflammation, irritation, and pain, and often mimicking the symptoms of irritable bowel syndrome.

N81 Female genital prolapse

This category is used to report incidences of genital prolapse, in which structures in the pelvis fall downward from their normal position and often push through the vaginal wall. Genital prolapse can be mild, in which the patient may not even realize it has occurred, or severe to the point that the prolapsed structure protrudes out of the vaginal opening. The most common symptoms of genital prolapse are pain while walking and a feeling of pressure in the pelvis. Urination may be difficult. Women who have had multiple pregnancies are at higher risk of experiencing genital prolapse.

N81.0 Urethrocele

The urethra protrudes through the vaginal wall.

Note: When this occurs with a cystocele, code to the type of cystocele.

N81.11 Cystocele, midline

The bladder pushes through the middle of the vaginal wall.

N81.12 Cystocele, lateral

The bladder pushes through the side wall of the vagina.

N81.2 Incomplete uterovaginal prolapse

Incomplete uterovaginal prolapse, which occurs when only part of the uterus travels downward into the vaginal canal.

N81.3 Complete uterovaginal prolapse

Complete uterovaginal prolapse is a disorder in which the uterus travels downward into the vaginal canal to the extent that it protrudes out of the vaginal opening.

N81.5 Vaginal enterocele

A vaginal enterocele is a condition in which a loop of the small intestine protrudes through the abdominal muscles into the vagina.

N81.6 Rectocele

A condition in which the rectum protrudes through the vaginal wall.

N81.81 Perineocele

A perineocele is a rare type of herniated defect of the posterior perineum that can occur between the vagina and rectum without diffuse vaginal prolapse. Signs and symptoms include perineal pressure, severe constipation, a convex shape to the perineum, the necessity of manual reduction to facilitate defecation, and a much increased distance from the posterior fourchette to the anus. The perineal herniation results from defects in the posterior levator muscles, and separation of the transverse perineal and anal sphincter muscles. Repair involves reapproximating the structures to repair the anatomical defect.

N81.82 Incompetence or weakening of pubocervical tissue

Incompetence or weakening of pubocervical tissue occurs when the muscles which support the cervix are no longer able to hold it in its proper position.

N81.83 Incompetence or weakening of rectovaginal tissue

Incompetence or weakening of the rectovaginal tissue occurs when the muscles that hold the rectum and vaginal canal in their proper places begin to weaken and are no longer able to support them.

N81.84 Pelvic muscle wasting

This condition occurs when the muscles and connective tissue of the pelvis waste away, often leading to urinary and fecal incontinence as well as genital prolapse.

N81.85 Cervical stump prolapse

The cervix is left in place when a partial or subtotal hysterectomy (also called a supracervical hysterectomy) is performed. The cervix is preserved although the uterus has been removed. The cervical stump that remains may develop a later complication if the connective tissue and pelvic support structures around it lose integrity. The cervix begins to slide or fall from its normal position down into the vagina. Cervical stump prolapse may require a trachelectomy to remove it surgically.

N82 Fistulae involving female genital tract

A fistula is an abnormal tube-like passage connecting one part of the body with another or with the external surface.

N82.0 Vesicovaginal fistula

An abnormal, tube-like passage connecting the bladder and the vagina.

N82.1 Other female urinary-genital tract fistulae

Other urinary-female genital tract fistulae include abnormal tracts between the cervix and the bladder (cervicovesical), the urethra and the vagina (urethrovaginal), a ureter and the vagina (ureterovaginal), and the uterus and the bladder (uterovesical), or the uterus and the ureter of the left or right kidney (uteroureteral).

N82.3 Fistula of vagina to large intestine

This includes a fistula communicating between the rectum and the vagina.

N82.5 Female genital tract-skin fistulae

Fistulae running from an organ within the female genital tract out to the skin surface include those connecting the uterus and the skin on the abdominal wall, and the vagina and the skin somewhere on the perineal surface.

N83.0 Follicular cyst of ovary

A fluid-filled sac on the ovary caused by larger than normal growth of a follicle which then does not rupture to release the egg.

N83.1 Corpus luteum cyst

The corpus luteum is a structure that forms after an ovarian follicle releases a fertilized egg, and secretes the hormone progesterone. A fluid-filled cyst or blood-filled sac can form on this structure.

N83.20 Unspecified ovarian cysts

Symptoms of an ovarian cyst include lower abdominal pain, bloating, painful sexual intercourse, spotting, and irregular periods.

N83.3 Acquired atrophy of ovary and fallopian tube

This is an acquired disease or condition which causes the tissue of an ovary and fallopian tube to waste away and shrink in size.

N83.4 Prolapse and hernia of ovary and fallopian tube

A prolapse of the ovary and its associated fallopian tube occurs when these structures slip out of their proper position inside the body and fall downward, or protrude through a weakened muscle wall or other structure.

N83.5 Torsion of ovary, ovarian pedicle and fallopian tube

Torsion occurs when any of these structures, or a combination of these structures, become twisted and turn over on themselves, prohibiting proper function, closing off patency of the fallopian tube, and possibly even cutting off blood supply to the tissues.

N83.6 Hematosalpinx

Hematosalpinx is an accumulation of blood in the fallopian tube leading to blockage and dilation of the tube. The condition is usually unilateral and is often associated with ectopic pregnancy.

N83.7 Hematoma of broad ligament

A cyst or tumor-like structure filled with blood on the fold of the peritoneum that anchors the side of the uterus to the pelvic wall.

N85.0 Endometrial hyperplasia

Endometrial hyperplasia is an excessive proliferation of the endometrial cells that line the uterus, causing a thickening of the uterine lining. The excessive cell reproduction is not a cancer, but is monitored as a possible precursor to endometrial carcinoma. Classification is based on pathologic mechanisms and cancer risks, necessary for determining appropriate treatment. Molecular studies show that bona fide premalignant lesions are neoplasms with monoclonal mutations. Computerized analysis has been able to define histologic features used for accurate diagnoses.

N85.01 Benign endometrial hyperplasia

Benign polyclonal proliferations of the endometrial cells occurring in response to unopposed estrogen are defined as benign endometrial hyperplasia. This is an overgrowth and thickening of the cells lining the uterus. The diagnosis is made by the pathologist after examining a sample of tissue that has been removed. The cellular overgrowth is caused by proliferation of cells in response to an abnormal, continuous hormonal stimulus from estrogen unopposed by progesterone. This can happen with polycystic ovarian disease or in adolescence and before menopause when several cycles may occur without ovulation, causing continuous estrogen activity. Some types of hyperplasia may progress to endometrial cancer in some women.

Note: Non-invasive, monoclonal proliferation of uterine endometrial cells is diagnosed as endometrial intraepithelial neoplasia (EIN) (N85.02).

N85.02 Endometrial intraepithelial neoplasia [EIN]

Endometrial intraepithelial neoplasia is a premalignant, non-invasive, mutation-bearing monoclonal neoplasm of the uterus. The neoplasm is composed of abnormal endometrial cells arising out of glands of the uterine lining and predisposes to the most common form of uterine cancer--endometrioid adenocarcinoma. The risk or timeframe for any progression toward cancer is not

consistent and each case is individually treated. Predisposing risk factors for EIN include exposure to continual estrogen stimulus without progestins, obesity, diabetes, and certain hereditary conditions.

N85.2 Hypertrophy of uterus

An abnormal increase in the size of the consitituent cells of the uterus, causing a bulky, enlarged, or 'overgrown' uterus.

N85.4 Malposition of uterus

Malposition of the uterus is a condition in which the uterus is not positioned correctly in relation to the other reproductive organs. This condition may or may not render the patient unable to conceive and carry a fetus to term. Malpositioning of the uterus includes anteversion, retroversion, and retroflexion.

N85.5 Inversion of uterus

A condition in which the uterus is upside-down in the body cavity.

N85.6 Intrauterine synechiae

A condition in which abnormal bonds or adhesions form within the uterus connecting or binding parts of the uterus together.

N85.7 Hematometra

Hematometra is a condition in which blood accumulates in the uterus.

N86 Erosion and ectropion of cervix uteri

Erosion and ectropion of the cervix is diagnosed when one or more open wounds, or ulcers form on the cervix, or it becomes everted and turns outward.

N87 Dysplasia of cervix uteri

This condition results in abnormal cell structures appearing in the cervix. No symptoms usually present with this condition; it is detected by a pap smear of cervical cells. While the dysplasia itself is not harmful, it is considered a precancerous condition, and is monitored carefully.

Note: HGSIL of cervix is coded to R87.613.

Note: CIN I and II are considered mild and moderate forms of cervical dysplasia, respectively; CIN III, or severe dysplasia of the cervix, is considered a carcinoma in situ and is coded to D06.-.

N87.0 Mild cervical dysplasia

Cervical intraepithelial neoplasia I [CIN I] is abnormal cell growth that is usually self-limiting and corrects on its own.

N87.1 Moderate cervical dysplasia

Cervical intraepithelial neoplasia II [CIN II].

N87.9 Dysplasia of cervix uteri, unspecified

Cervical anaplasia and atypism is coded as unspecified cervical dysplasia.

N88.0 Leukoplakia of cervix uteri

Leukoplakia of the cervix is marked by circumscribed lesions of thickened, white, dysplastic patches forming on the mucous membranes of the cervix.

N88.4 Hypertrophic elongation of cervix uteri

Hypertrophic elongation of the cervix is a condition in which the cervix begins to grow downward into the vaginal canal.

N89 Other noninflammatory disorders of vagina

Dysplasia of the vagina is a condition in which abnormal cell structure is found in the vaginal cells. While not harmful in and of itself, this condition is often a precursor to cancer and is monitored for increased severity in dysplastic cellular changes.

Note: Dysplasia of the vagina includes vaginal intraepithelial neoplasia I and II [VAIN I and II] but VAIN III, or severe vaginal dysplasia, is considered a carcinoma in situ and is coded to D07.2.

N89.0 Mild vaginal dysplasia

Vaginal intraepithelial neoplasia I [VAIN I].

N89.1 Moderate vaginal dysplasia

Vaginal intraepithelial neoplasia II [VAIN II].

N89.4 Leukoplakia of vagina

Leukoplakia of the vagina occurs when circumscribed lesions of thickened, white, dysplastic patches form on the mucous membrane which lines the inside of the vagina.

N89.5 Stricture and atresia of vagina

This abnormality occurs when the vaginal canal becomes abnormally narrow or stenosed. This includes vaginal adhesions that form within the canal, making abnormal connections between the sides of the vaginal wall than can cause contraction and pulling inward.

N89.6 Tight hymenal ring

The hymenal ring is a membrane that partially covers the opening to the vaginal canal. Tightness of this ring can make it difficult for the body to discharge menstrual blood.

N90 Other noninflammatory disorders of vulva and perineum

This category includes dysplasia of the external female genitalia. This is an abnormal growth of cells on the surface of the skin, most often in the outer vaginal labia, considered to be a precancerous condition also known as vulvar intraepithelial neoplasia [VIN]. The chronic skin changes are classified into three progressive stages and may continue growing slowly for years. This abnormal cell growth is associated with herpes simplex and human papilloma viruses as well as granulomatous STDs. Up to 80-90 percent of VIN cases have been shown to have DNA of the human papilloma virus present.

Note: VIN III, or severe dysplasia of the vulva, is considered a carcinoma in situ and is coded in the neoplasm chapter. The level of classification is based upon the degree of dysplasia found within individual cells and how far below the surface layer of epithelium it reaches.

N90.0 Mild vulvar dysplasia

Vulvar intraepithelial neoplasia I [VIN I] is the first degree of dysplastic cells in the vulva, or mild dysplasia. Biopsy is used to diagnose the abnormal skin cell changes. VIN I is diagnosed when only about a third of the epithelial lining has dystophic changes. Chronic itching, burning, or inflammation may be present.

N90.1 Moderate vulvar dysplasia

Vulvar intraepithelial neoplasia II [VIN II] is moderate dysplasia of the female external genitalia, diagnosed when about half the thickness of the epithelium is affected. Besides itching, burning, or inflammation that may have persisted for a long while with many topical cream treatments attempted, raised skin lesions may be red, pink, white, or gray. Some lesions appear hyperpigmented like a mole or freckle. Treatment is always a preventative measure to stop the progression to VIN III and cancer. Affected tissue is removed with a margin of normal tissue. Multiple lesions are sometimes removed with laser ablation to destroy the abnormal cells without affecting the deeper, normal tissue.

N90.4 Leukoplakia of vulva

This code includes leukoplakia, dystrophy, and kraurosis of the vulva. Leukoplakia is the development of thickened, whitish, dyplastic lesions on the external female genitalia that may be considered precancerous and are of unknown origin, but possibly associated with chronic irritation. Kraurosis is also often a precancerous lesion that resembles atrophic wasting or shriveling of the skin of the vulva.

N90.5 Atrophy of vulva

A condition in which there is significant wasting away of the tissue in the external female genitalia.

N90.6 Hypertrophy of vulva

Abnormal enlargement of the constituent cells making up the two folds of tissue on either side of the vaginal opening.

N90.811 Female genital mutilation Type I status

Type I female genital mutilation, in which the clitoris is removed.

N90.812 Female genital mutilation Type II status

Type II female genital mutilation, in which the clitoris and labia minora are removed.

N90.813 Female genital mutilation Type III status

Type III female genital mutilation, in which the entire vulva is removed.

N90.818 Other female genital mutilation status

Other female genital mutilation status, or Type IV status, includes any other form of genital mutilation or cutting, burning, application of chemicals, or stretching that may be encountered when treating immigrant populations where such practices are still done.

N90.89 Other specified noninflammatory disorders of vulva and perineum

Other specified noninflammatory disorders of the vulva and perineum include an overgrowth of the clitoral cells causing an enlarged, or hypertrophic clitoris, and adhesions that form between different areas of the vulva.

N91.0 Primary amenorrhea

Amenorrhea is the absence of menstruation in a woman of reproductive age. Primary amenorrhea is no menarche by age 16.

N91.1 Secondary amenorrhea

Amenorrhea is the absence of menstruation in a woman of reproductive age. Secondary amenorrhea is the cessation of menstruation for 3 months in a woman with previously regular periods or 9 months in a woman with previously irregular periods. Causes can include lactation, stress, low body weight, and excessive exercise.

N91.3 Primary oligomenorrhea

Scanty or infrequent menstruation in which menstruation does not occur on a typical monthly schedule (cycle >35 days or 4-9 periods per year) in a woman with previously regular periods.

N91.4 Secondary oligomenorrhea

Scanty or infrequent menstruation in which menstruation does not occur on a typical monthly schedule (cycle >35 days or 4-9 periods per year) due to other underlying conditions, such as eating disorders and polycystic ovarian syndrome (PCOS).

N92.0 Excessive and frequent menstruation with regular cycle

This code applies when regular menstrual periods occurring in a normal 21-35 day cycle are heavy, expelling excessive amounts of tissue, or heavy as well as prolonged. This also also includes polymenorrhea, in which menstrual bleeding occurs at regular intervals, but in a cycle that is less than 21 days apart.

N92.1 Excessive and frequent menstruation with irregular cycle

This includes metrorrhagia, irregular bleeding from the uterus that is not associated with the normal menstrual cycle; menometrorrhagia, prolonged and excessive menstrual bleeding that occurs at irregular intervals; menstrual bleeding that occurs at irregular, shortened periods; and irregular intermenstrual bleeding.

N92.2 Excessive menstruation at puberty

Excessive menstruation at puberty is heavy bleeding signalling the onset of menstrual periods, or irregular bleeding not associated with a regular menstrual cycle(menorrhagia) occuring at puberty.

N92.3   Ovulation bleeding

Bleeding that occurs between menstrual periods during ovulation when an egg is released from the follicle.

N93.0   Postcoital and contact bleeding

Abnormal bleeding that occurs after sexual intercourse.

N94.0   Mittelschmerz

Mittelschmerz consists of lower abdominal or pelvic pain that occurs between menstrual periods, accompanying ovulation and usually midway between normal periods. The pain may be unilateral or bilateral. Possible causes include surface pressure on the ovary from follicle growth, and stretching and/or irritation of the abdominal lining from the blood and fluid that is released with follicle rupture.

N94.1   Dyspareunia

Dyspareunia is recurrent or persistent pain associated with sexual intercourse. Causes may be physical or emotional, generalized or situational, acquired or congenital and can include thickened hymen, hypoplasia of the introitus, endometriosis, ovarian cysts, infection, prolapsed uterus, retroverted uterus, scarring from surgical procedures, vaginal dryness, uterine fibroid tumors, and interstitial cystitis.

N94.2   Vaginismus

Vaginismus is a sudden tension or severe, painful spasm of vaginal muscles making vaginal penetration painful or impossible. The pubococcygeus muscle is primarily involved but reflex of the bulbocavernosum muscle at the introitus to the vagina and the puborectalis muscle in the midvagina may also contribute to the problem.

N94.3   Premenstrual tension syndrome

Premenstrual tension syndrome (PMS) is a condition associated with the menstrual cycle. PMS is characterized by a consistent pattern of physical and/or emotional symptoms that typically begin after release of the ovum, as the follicle forms the corpus luteum and secretes progesterone in the luteal phase. Symptoms can include irritability, tension, unhappiness (dysphoria), anxiety, insomnia, fatigue, breast tenderness, bloating, abdominal cramping, and muscle and joint pain.

This code also includes **premenstrual dysphoric disorder** (PMDD), a severe form of premenstrual syndrome (PMS). PMDD is characterized by depression, anxiety, tension and irritability that typically begins after release of the ovum. There may be a genetic predisposition due to a varient in the estrogen receptor alpha gene and/or Catechol-O-methyl transferase (COMT) gene. Low levels of the brain neurotransmitter serotonin may also be present in women who experience PMDD.

N94.4   Primary dysmenorrhea

Primary dysmenorrhea describes painful cramping of the lower abdomen caused by uterine contractions that occur just before or during menstruation. This condition usually peaks with adolescence or in the early 20s and is a very common problem, often severe enough to interfere with daily activities.

N94.5   Secondary dysmenorrhea

Secondary dysmenorrhea describes painful cramping before or during menstruation that is attributable to another underlying disease, condition, or structural abnormality such as endometriosis, uterine fibroids (leiomyomas), ovarian cysts, or infections.

N94.6   Dysmenorrhea, unspecified

Painful cramping that occurs before or during menstruation.

N94.81   Vulvodynia

Pain in the female external genitalia that is often described as burning, itching, stinging, or raw. It is more common in caucasians and may start suddenly and last for months, even years.

N94.810 Vulvar vestibulitis

Vulvar vestibulitis is considered a subtype of vulvodynia appearing with tenderness and redness in the vestibule area from an unknown cause.

N94.818 Other vulvodynia

Vulvodynia is a pain syndrome causing physical and psychological disability with limitation of daily activities and sexual dysfunction. The cause of the pain is not demonstrated to be connected to human papilloma virus, sexually transmitted diseases, or malignancy, and is distinct from other forms of vulvar pain known to be brought on by yeast infections.

N95.0   Postmenopausal bleeding

Uterine bleeding occuring after the time of menopause and periods have ceased.

N95.2   Postmenopausal atrophic vaginitis

Postmenopausal atrophic vaginitis is thinning of the vaginal epithelium due to decreased estrogen levels occuring after menopause.

N96   Recurrent pregnancy loss

The status of a woman's past pregnancy history has resulted in the body's aborting the fetus in an habitual pattern. The status of recurrent pregnancy loss may necessitate genetic testing of the patient or her male partner to determine a cause.

Note: This code is used in a nonpregnant patient. For recurrent pregnancy loss with a current pregnancy, report O26.2-.

N99.511 Cystostomy infection

A cystostomy is a surgically created connection from the bladder out to the skin that is done in cases when normal urine flow is blocked, such as from traumatic urethral damage, congenital defects, swollen prostate, cancer, kidney stones, or spinal cord injury. The initial stoma catheter remains in place while the tissue around the tract heals, then the catheter is replaced periodically to help prevent infections. The duration that a catheter remains in place is the leading risk factor for developing cystostomy infection, although some catheter-associated bacteriuria may be asymptomatic. *E. coli* is the prevalent infecting microorganism. Cystostomy infections cause fever, expulsion of the catheter, redness, swelling, colored discharge, bad smell, and bleeding.

N99.512 Cystostomy malfunction

Mechanical complication of cystostomy includes any type of malfunction due to the stoma itself. Malfunction may include narrowing or stricture that may require minor surgery to repair.

N99.518 Other cystostomy complication

Other complications of cystostomy include prolapse or herniation of the stoma, or the development of a fistula or sinus tract--any problem not directly related to the mechanical functioning of the stoma or an infection.

O00.0 Abdominal pregnancy

An abdominal pregnancy is a very rare type of ectopic pregnancy, occurring in about 1% of ectopic cases, in which the fertilized ovum implants itself somewhere within the peritoneal cavity, but outside of the fallopian tube, the ovary, the uterus, or the broad ligament. Location sites for implantation include the bowel, the mesentery, the omentum, the mesosalpinx, the Douglas pouch, the pelvic wall, and the abdominal wall. This is thought to be associated with sexually transmitted disease. Symptoms can include abdominal pain, bleeding, and gastrointestinal symptoms. Major internal bleeding can cause hemorrhagic shock. Toxemia and pulmonary embolism can also be fatal complications. There is a high mortality rate for both baby and mother associated with abdominal pregnancy. Ultrasound and MRI may be used for diagnosis, and termination of the pregnancy is the standard treatment. In rare cases of a viable fetus, continuous monitoring and medical support are required with laparotomy to deliver the fetus, as no labor will occur.

O00.1 Tubal pregnancy

A tubal pregnancy is a type of ectopic pregnancy that occurs in about 1 out of every 50 pregnancies, in which the fertilized ovum implants itself within the fallopian tube instead of descending the normal route into the uterine lining. Risk factors include previous pelvic surgery, particularly with scarring, tubal ligation or reversal, endometriosis, the use of an IUD or fertility drugs, in vitro fertilization procedures, sexually transmitted diseases, being over age 35, and previous pelvic inflammatory disease or a prior ectopic pregnancy. The fallopian tube will eventually rupture as the embryo grows and the pregnancy must be terminated. Early detection is often not made as it happens in the earliest weeks of pregnancy. Emergency treatment is needed for a rupture or imminent rupture. Symptoms of a tubal pregnancy include lower abdominal pain on one side, sharp cramping, nausea and vomiting, dizziness, and vaginal bleeding. When a tube ruptures, severe pain and bleeding can cause the patient to become unconscious. Pelvic exam and ultrasound is used for confirmation and surgical or medical termination is then undertaken.

O00.2 Ovarian pregnancy

An ovarian pregnancy is a rare type of ectopic pregnancy, occurring in about 2-3% of ectopic cases, in which the fertilized ovum implants itself within the ovary. This usually occurs when the egg is not released during ovulation and becomes fertilized within the ovary, where it remains. Causative risk factors include endometriosis, the use of an IUD, prior pelvic infection, and reproductive procedures. The fallopian tube remains normal in an ovarian pregnancy. Other decisive factors for a diagnosis of ovarian pregnancy include the gestational sac being located within the ovary, connection to the uterine ovarian ligament, and the presence of placental tissue in the ovary. Ultrasound is often used, as well as laparoscopy. Exploratory laparotomy may also be done due to the fact that ovarian pregnancies are often misdiagnosed as a corpus luteum cyst. Surgical treatment usually consists of complete oophorectomy, although wedge resection may also be used.

O00.8 Other ectopic pregnancy

Other types of ectopic pregnancy include cervical, cornual, and intraligamentous pregnancy. A cervical pregnancy is a very rare type of ectopic pregnancy in which the fertilized ovum implants itself within the lining of the endocervical canal. This occurs in less than 1% of all ectopic pregnancies. Profuse vaginal bleeding tends to occur, often without pain. Some women may experience lower abdominal pain and cramping. Early detection is necessary for conservative treatment to preserve fertility and includes systemic chemotherapy combined with mechanical disruption and evacuation, and hemostatic measures such as balloon tamponade, cerclage, or uterine ligation. A cornual pregnancy is also known as an interstitial or mural pregnancy, in which the fertilized ovum implants itself in the segment of the fallopian tube that enters the uterus and is within the muscular wall of the uterus. The surrounding myometrial tissue will allow the pregnancy to proceed to the second trimester; however, rupture will eventually occur if not diagnosed earlier, with a high mortality risk from hemorrhaging. Hysterectomy or cornual resection may be necessary with uterine damage. Conservative medical treatment with methotrexate may be used when diagnosed early.

O00.9 Ectopic pregnancy, unspecified

Unspecified ectopic pregnancy occurs when a fertilized ovum implants itself anywhere other than the uterus, but the location is not specified.

O01 Hydatidiform mole

A hydatidiform mole is a disorder of pregnancy that occurs after conception when cells proliferate abnormally, resulting in the growth of a mass of cells resembling a bunch of grapes. The body will produce hormones that can produce a false positive on a pregnancy test, but an ultrasound will reveal the absence of a fetal skeleton. Most women who experience a hydatidiform mole will suspect that they are pregnant, and may experience vaginal spotting or bleeding, a larger than normal uterus, nausea, vomiting, and passing tissue. Thyroid problems can also occur along with pre-eclampsia, a type of hypertension that can occur during pregnancy.

O01.0 Classical hydatidiform mole

A classical, or complete, hydatidiform mole combines 1 reduplicating or 2 sperm cells with an egg cell that does not contain maternal DNA, creating a 46XX or 46XY cell with only paternal DNA. This type of mole has no embryonic tissue, contains only chorionic tissue, and increases the risk for choriocarcinoma, as the cells proliferate, which is a malignancy of trophoblastic cells.

O01.1 Incomplete and partial hydatidiform mole

A partial hydatidiform mole combines an egg cell containing maternal DNA and either 1 reduplicating or 2 sperm cells yielding a 69XXX, 69XXY, or greater cell with both maternal and paternal DNA. This type of mole may contain both embryonic and chorionic tissue. If molar pregnancy is recurrent, a mutation of the gene NLRP7 may be responsible.

O01.9 Hydatidiform mole, unspecified

A hydatidiform mole is a disorder of pregnancy that occurs after conception when cells proliferate abnormally, resulting in the growth of a mass of cells resembling a bunch of grapes, but without a viable embryo or the formation of a skeleton. The body will produce hormones that can produce a false positive on a pregnancy test, but an ultrasound rest will reveal the absence of a fetus, also known as trophoblastic disease or vesicular mole that is not otherwise specified.

O02 Other abnormal products of conception

This category reports conditions that occur when a fertilized egg develops in an aberrant manner.

O02.0 Blighted ovum and nonhydatidiform mole

Blighted ovum is a type of early pregnancy loss. This occurs when a fertilized ovum develops a placenta and a membrane, but no embryo in the first few weeks of pregnancy, even before the woman is aware of it. Ultrasound shows an empty gestational sac. Some patients wait for natural miscarriage while others may take a medicinal catalyst to trigger the miscarriage. Sometimes, a D&C is necessary to remove the tissues. A nonhydatidiform mole occurs when a fertilized ovum that normally becomes a fetus is non-viable and implants itself into the uterus, becoming an abnormal growth. The normal pregnancy processes become pathological, because growth is still triggered, even though there is no embryo. The molar pregnancy needs to be treated right away as it can cause serious problems. A mole may be caused by fertilization of an egg that has lost its DNA, a single egg fertilized by two sperm, or by one sperm that completely reduplicated itself.

O02.1 Missed abortion

A missed abortion occurs when a fetus dies in the womb before 20 completed weeks of gestation and the dead fetal tissue is not expelled. The dead fetus must be removed before it turns septic.

O02.81 Inappropriate change in quantitative human chorionic gonadotropin (hCG) in early pregnancy

Human chorionic gonadotropin (hCG) is a hormone produced by pregnancy that can be detected in the blood or urine before the first missed period is even known. This hormone is what is being detected in pregnancy tests. It is first detectable in blood as early as 7-8 days following ovulation by sensitive assays, and in 10-11 days in normal pregnancy tests. The hCG level doubles about every 3 days and peaks around 8-10 wks and then declines and remains lower for the rest of the pregnancy. Ectopic or tubal pregnancies and those that are destined to miscarry early show lower levels at an early decline. When there is no uterine fetus after a positive blood pregnancy test, this is known as a chemical or biochemical pregnancy, or false positive pregnancy. An ectopic or tubal pregnancy is ruled out first, and an early miscarriage is confirmed.

O03 Spontaneous abortion

Spontaneous abortion, also known as a miscarriage, is a condition usually caused by the death of the fetus due to genetic abnormalities, at which point the body expels the contents of the uterus. An incomplete stage of abortion has some tissue remaining in the uterus after spontaneous abortion. A complete abortion has expelled all tissue from the uterus with miscarriage. Miscarriage can also be caused by other problems, such as infection, an immune response, or diseases experienced by the mother.

Note: The proper selection of codes in this category is not only dependent upon the stage as complete or incomplete spontaneous abortion, but includes the specific type of complication occurring with the miscarriage, such as infection of the genital or urinary tract, hemorrhage, embolism, shock, renal failure, metabolic disorder, damage to pelvic organs, cardiac arrest, and sepsis.

O03.0 Genital tract and pelvic infection following incomplete spontaneous abortion

This code reports spontaneous abortion, or miscarriage, with some products of conception still remaining in the uterus that is complicated by an infection of the genital tract or pelvis. Genital tract and pelvic infection may consist of an infection of the ovary(ies) or fallopian tube(s), or both, endometritis, parametritis, or pelvic peritonitis. Endometritis is inflammation and infection of the uterus usually caused by bacteria from the lower reproductive or GI tract. Salpingitis and oophoritis is an infection and/or inflammation of the fallopian tubes and ovaries and may present as a localized abscess or accumulation of pus. Parametritis is inflammation of the connective tissue attached to the uterus, and pelvic peritonitis is an inflammation of the membrane that lines the pelvis that protects and supports the internal organs. Infection usually occurs by more than one microbe and includes pathogens such as gram-positive cocci, gram negative bacteria, and anaerobes. Symptoms appear as lower abdominal pain and swelling, uterine tenderness, fever, chills, headache, or malaise. Pallor, tachycardia, and leukocytosis may also occur, but a low grade fever may be the only symptom. Treatment is usually with a broad-spectrum, IV antibiotic regimen.

O03.1 Delayed or excessive hemorrhage following incomplete spontaneous abortion

This code reports spontaneous abortion, or miscarriage, with some products of conception still remaining in the uterus, complicated by delayed or excessive hemorrhage that can consist of such conditions as afibrinogenemia, defibrination syndrome, hemolysis, or intravascular

coagulation. Afibrinogenemia is an absence or marked decrease of fibrinogen which can lead to prolonged bleeding time and the inability to form blood clots. Defibrination syndrome is a bleeding disorder characterized by an abnormal reduction in the elements used in blood clotting, resulting in profuse bleeding in later stages. Diffuse or disseminated intravascular coagulation (DIC) is a condition marked by a combination of hemorrhage and microvascular coagulation. It involves a repeating cycle of clot formation and breakdown by fibrinolysis, followed by depletion of platelets and coagulation factors, and a constant release of anticoagulants. Hemolysis is the breakdown of red blood cells.

O03.2 Embolism following incomplete spontaneous abortion

This code reports spontaneous abortion, or miscarriage, with some products of conception still remaining in the uterus, complicated by embolism. An embolism occurs when a clump of material, such as air, fat, amniotic fluid, or bacterial matter migrates away from the original site and travels through the arterial system until it reaches a vessel too small for it to pass through, where it becomes lodged and causes tissue death due to lack of blood supply. Septic embolism is a clump of infectious matter blocking an area due to the presence of bacteria. Pulmonary embolism (PE) occurs when a clump of material migrates and forms a blockage in the main artery to the lungs or arterial branches in the lungs.

O03.31 Shock following incomplete spontaneous abortion

This code reports spontaneous abortion, or miscarriage, with some products of conception still remaining in the uterus, complicated by shock. Shock is a condition in which the circulatory system suffers collapse and is unable to supply enough blood to sustain body tissue. In the case of miscarriage, shock usually occurs due to massive blood loss. This includes postprocedural shock following an incomplete spontaneous abortion.

Note: If the shock is stated as due to an infection, it is coded to O03.37 as sepsis following incomplete spontaneous abortion with additional codes to identify severe sepsis (with septic shock) and the infecting agent.

O03.32 Renal failure following incomplete spontaneous abortion

This code reports spontaneous abortion, or miscarriage, with some products of conception still remaining in the uterus, complicated by renal failure, such as acute renal failure, oliguria, or renal tubular necrosis. Acute renal failure is a condition in which more than half of a patient's kidney function is lost in a period of days or hours and nitrogenous waste products begin to accumulate in the body with oliguria, a decrease in urine output. Renal tubular necrosis is a disorder involving the death of cells that form the tubules of the kidney that transport urine to the ureters while reabsorbing 99% of the water.

O03.34 Damage to pelvic organs following incomplete spontaneous abortion

This code reports spontaneous abortion, or miscarriage, with some products of conception still remaining in the uterus, complicated by damage to a pelvic organ such as a tear, perforation, or laceration of the bladder, bowel, cervix, uterus, vagina, periurethral tissue, or uterine ligaments.

O03.36 Cardiac arrest following incomplete spontaneous abortion

This code reports spontaneous abortion, or miscarriage, with some products of conception still remaining in the uterus, complicated by cardiac arrest, which is the failure of the heart muscle to contract effectively, impeding the normal circulation of blood and preventing oxygen delivery to the body.

O03.37 Sepsis following incomplete spontaneous abortion

This code reports spontaneous abortion, or miscarriage, with some products of conception still remaining in the uterus, complicated by sepsis, a systemic infection throughout the body, circulating in the bloodstream. Sepsis causes poisoning that presents with a sudden onset of fever and chills, low blood pressure, pale or bluish limbs and lips, confusion or altered mental or emotional state, increased heart and/or respiratory rate, and rash. If not treated immediately, sepsis can lead to septic shock and death.

O03.81 Shock following complete or unspecified spontaneous abortion

Miscarriage, NOS, or miscarriage with all products of conception expelled from the uterus complicated by shock. Shock is a condition in which the circulatory system suffers collapse and is unable to supply enough blood to sustain body tissue. In the case of miscarriage, shock usually occurs due to massive blood loss. This includes postprocedural shock following a complete or unspecified spontaneous abortion.

Note: If the shock is stated as due to an infection, it is coded to O03.87 as sepsis following complete or unspecified spontaneous abortion with additional codes to identify severe sepsis (with septic shock) and the infecting agent.

O04 Complications following (induced) termination of pregnancy

These codes are used to report a legally-performed abortion, in which the contents of the uterus are removed by a physician in a surgical procedure. The most common method, performed within the first trimester of pregnancy, involves suctioning out the contents of the womb when the embryo is still quite small. Other methods involve the use of drugs to terminate the fetus, and dilation and extraction, in which a late-term fetus is removed from the uterus.

Note: The proper selection of codes in this category depends upon the specific type of complication occurring with the induced termination of the pregnancy, such as infection of the genital or urinary tract, hemorrhage, embolism, shock, renal failure, metabolic disorder, damage to pelvic organs, cardiac arrest, and sepsis.

O04.81 Shock following (induced) termination of pregnancy

Shock is a condition in which the circulatory system suffers collapse and is unable to supply enough blood to sustain body tissue. In the case of induced pregnancy termination, shock usually occurs due to massive blood loss. This includes postprocedural shock following a legally induced abortion.

Note: If the shock is stated as due to an infection, it is coded to O04.87 as sepsis following (induced) termination of pregnancy with additional codes to identify severe sepsis (with septic shock) and the infecting agent.

O07 Failed attempted termination of pregnancy

This category is used to report cases of a failed attempt to induce an elective abortion and terminate a pregnancy, in which the fetus remains alive despite attempts to remove it.

Note: This code should only be used to report a failed attempted induction of a legal abortion.

Note: The proper selection of codes in this category depends upon the specific type of complication occurring with the failed attempted induced abortion, such as infection of the genital or urinary tract, hemorrhage, embolism, shock, renal failure, metabolic disorder, damage to pelvic organs, cardiac arrest, and sepsis.

O07.31 Shock following failed attempted termination of pregnancy

Shock is a condition in which the circulatory system suffers collapse and is unable to supply enough blood to sustain body tissue. In the case of attempted pregnancy termination, shock usually occurs due to massive blood loss. This includes postprocedural shock following a failed attempted abortion or incomplete elective abortion.

Note: If the shock is stated as due to an infection, it is coded to O07.37 as sepsis following failed attempted termination of pregnancy with additional codes to identify severe sepsis (with septic shock) and the infecting agent.

O08 Complications following ectopic and molar pregnancy

This category is used to report complications from an ectopic or molar pregnancy, and should be used to report complications separately that are responsible for a later episode of care; or when they are immediate complications of ectopic or molar pregnancies used with codes in categories O00-O02.

Note: The proper selection of codes depends upon the specific type of complication occurring following ectopic and molar pregnancy, such as infection of the genital or urinary tract, hemorrhage, embolism, shock, renal failure, metabolic disorder, damage to pelvic organs, cardiac arrest, and sepsis.

O08.3 Shock following ectopic and molar pregnancy

Shock is a condition in which the circulatory system suffers collapse and is unable to supply enough blood to sustain body tissue. In the case of ectopic and molar pregnancies, shock usually occurs due to massive blood loss, including postprocedural shock following surgery for an ectopic or molar pregnancy.

Note: If the shock is stated as due to an infection, it is coded to O08.82 as sepsis following ectopic or molar pregnancy with additional codes to identify severe sepsis (with septic shock) and the infecting agent.

O09 Supervision of high risk pregnancy

Codes in this category are for use with supervision of a current pregnancy to denote a present or past condition that categorizes the pregnancy as high-risk. These high-risk conditions may be a previous hydatidiform mole, pre-term labor or other poor obstetric history, in vitro fertilization, or pregnancy with a history of in utero surgery during a previous pregnancy. The current age with the first pregnancy and even with a multiple pregnancy may also constitute high-risk. Not having any prenatal care or insufficient care while pregnant causes a high-risk condition.

O09.1 Supervision of pregnancy with history of ectopic or molar pregnancy

The history of an ectopic pregnancy is one in which the fertilized egg implanted itself in any tissue other than the uterine lining, such as in the fallopian tube, abdomen, ovary, or cervix. Approximately 95% of ectopic pregnancies occur in the fallopian tube. Having had a previous ectopic pregnancy is a major risk factor for having another ectopic, or tubal, pregnancy due to the fact that it can cause tubal damage and is known to occur at higher rates in those who have already had other causative problems, such as pelvic inflammatory disease, that can leave permanent scar tissue on the inside and/or outside of tubes and ovaries. The history of a molar pregnancy is one that produced an hydatidiform or vesicular mole--an abnormal product of conception that occurs when the cells proliferate out of control, creating a growth or mass of cell clusters that causes the body to continue producing hormones as if in pregnancy, even though there is no fetus developing. This gives a false positive pregnancy result. Molar pregnancies have the potential of developing into a cancerous growth, called choriocarinoma if left untreated.

O09.5 Supervision of elderly primigravida and multigravida

Elderly primigravida or multigravida means the age of the woman at the expected date of delivery poses a potential high-risk to the pregnancy. Elderly primigravida is the first pregnancy for a female who will be 35 years of age or older at the expected date of delivery. Elderly multigravida is the second or additional pregnancy for a female who will be 35 years of age or older at the expected date of delivery.

O09.6 Supervision of young primigravida and multigravida

Young primigravida or multigravida means the extremely young age of the woman at the expected date of delivery poses a potential high-risk to the pregnancy. Young primigravida is the first pregnancy for a female less than 16 years of age at the expected date of delivery. Young multigravida is the second or additional pregnancy for a female less than 16 years of age at the expected date of delivery.

O13 Gestational [pregnancy-induced] hypertension without significant proteinuria

Pregnancy-induced hypertension is the new onset of elevated, or high blood pressure readings reaching or exceeding 140/90 mm Hg in later pregnancy, after 20 weeks of gestation, without the presence of protein in the urine. Maternal hypertension mandates monitoring for and exclusion of pre-eclampsia as hypertensive disorders in pregnancy can cause fetal and maternal morbidity.

O14 Pre-eclampsia

Pre-eclampsia is hypertension with a blood pressure reaching 140/90 mmHg or greater after the 20th week of gestation and up to 6 weeks postpartum, with proteinuria (the presence of protein in the urine).

Note: Pre-existing hypertension with pre-eclampsia is coded in category O11.

O14.0 Mild to moderate pre-eclampsia

Mild to moderate pre-eclampsia is a condition characterized by the appearance of high blood pressure of 140/90 mm Hg or greater that was not pre-existing, accompanied by protein in the urine of 0.3 g collected in a 24 hr sample or persistent 1+ reading on the dipstick, and/or edema typically of the hands and face occurring abruptly after 20 weeks of gestation, although it can occur earlier in the pregnancy and can develop gradually. The management strategies are different for mild vs severe eclampsia and the distinction is important as it can become life-threatening. If mild or moderate pre-eclampsia is not monitored carefully and treated, it can develop into severe cases, or even eclampsia, a life-threatening occurrence of seizures in the pregnant female.

O14.1 Severe pre-eclampsia

Severe pre-eclampsia is diagnosed when the basic features of mild or moderate pre-eclampsia worsen and indicate additional problems with either the mother or the fetus. Signs of severe pre-eclampsia include central nervous system problems such as severe headaches and changes in vision, or altered mental status; the onset of liver problems such as upper abdominal pain usually on the right side with nausea and vomiting; gaining more than 2 lbs/wk; twice the normal level of certain liver enzymes in the blood; very high blood pressure that rises to 160 systolic or 110 diastolic; more than 5 g of protein in the 24 hr urine sample; decreased urine output; pulmonary edema and cyanosis; stroke; and fetal growth restriction. Management strategies are different for mild and severe eclampsia and the distinction is important as it can become life-threatening. Treatment for severe cases usually involves careful monitoring until 32-34 weeks, but delivery is the main treatment in order to prevent progression to life-threatening eclampsia.

O14.2 HELLP syndrome

HELLP syndrome is a life-threatening obstetric complication occuring in later pregnancy in women who have hemolysis (the breakdown of red blood cells), elevated liver enzymes, and low platelet count. Most cases develop before the 37th week of pregnancy. Many women are diagnosed with pre-eclampsia before being diagnosed with HELLP, which occurs in up to 20% of pregnant women with severe pre-eclampsia; however, in some cases the signs of HELLP are the first warning signs of pre-eclampsia and the symptoms parallel severe pre-eclampsia. The main treatment is to deliver the baby as soon as possible since problems with the liver and the central nervous system as well as other complications can quickly worsen and threaten the mother and child.

O15 Eclampsia

Eclampsia is an acute, life-threatening complication of pregnancy that usually appears as the final phase of severe pre-eclampsia and is extremely dangerous to the mother and child, also known as toxemia. Eclampsia is marked by hypertension with a blood pressure reading greater than 140/90 mmHg after the 20th week of gestation and up to 6 weeks postpartum with proteinuria, and tonic-clonic (motor) seizures or convulsions and

even coma. This can also be present during labor as well as occur in early postpartum.

O20 Hemorrhage in early pregnancy

Bleeding, in the early stages of pregnancy, before 20 completed weeks of gestation.

Note: Do not use codes in this category if the hemorrhage accompanies any type of abortive outcome, which is reported with the appropriate hemorrhage code from categories O00-O08. Hemorrhage specified as due to a threatened abortion is reported with O20.0.

O20.0 Threatened abortion

Threatened abortion is abnormal vaginal bleeding during the early stages of pregnancy that points to a possible spontaneous miscarriage or abortion occuring before the 20th week of gestation is completed.

O21 Excessive vomiting in pregnancy

Excessive vomiting can deprive the mother of needed nutrients during the pregnancy, and can cause malnutrition and dehydration.

O21.0 Mild hyperemesis gravidarum

Excessive vomiting during pregnancy, in which the peak of this condition is usually 8-12 weeks into the pregnancy, and normally stops around 16 weeks. The most common symptoms of this condition, besides the actual vomiting, are weight loss and dehydration. This harmful type of nausea and vomiting begins before the end of the 20th week of gestation.

O21.1 Hyperemesis gravidarum with metabolic disturbance

A condition which occurs when excessive vomiting during pregnancy results in a deficiency of one or more nutrients, carbohydrate depletion, electrolyte imbalance, or dehydration. This begins before the end of the 20th week of gestation.

O21.2 Late vomiting of pregnancy

Throwing up excessively beginning after completion of the 20th week of pregnancy.

O22.0 Varicose veins of lower extremity in pregnancy

Varicose veins are swollen, dilated veins of the lower legs. Symptoms include itching and pain in the affected area, as well as heaviness or weakness in the affected limb(s). While the cause of varicose veins in pregnancy is not fully understood, it is thought that poor circulation is caused by a defect in the valves that prevent blood from flowing backwards through the veins.

O22.2 Superficial thrombophlebitis in pregnancy

Thrombophlebitis is an inflammation of a vein, particularly in the legs, due to the presence of a blot clot which presents with pain, swelling, redness, and warmth around the affected area.

Note: Superficial cases of phlebitis, thrombosis, or thrombophlebitis of the legs in pregnancy is reported with the appropriate trimester code and an additional code from the circulatory system chapter to identify the phlebitis or thrombophlebitis of a superficial vessel in a specified lower leg.

O22.3 Deep phlebothrombosis in pregnancy

Deep phlebothrombosis or deep vein thrombosis (DVT) of the proximal or distal lower extremity is the formation of a blood clot within a major vein deep in the muscles of the leg that includes the femoral, iliac, popliteal, and tibial veins. DVT of the upper extremity is the formation of a blood clot within a vein deep in the arm and includes the paired radial and ulnar veins below the elbow forming the paired brachial veins. DVT may occur without symptoms, but the affected limb is usually painful, swollen, red, and warm. DVT in itself is not as dangerous as the life-threatening condition it can precipitate when the thrombus dislodges, creating a venous embolism, that can travel to the lungs and get lodged in one of the branches of the pulmonary artery, clogging the supply of blood to the lungs and heart.

Note: When DVT occurs in the antepartum stage of pregnancy, a code for the appropriate trimester is reported, along with the most specific additional code(s) from the circulatory chapter identifying the acute or chronic case of embolism or thrombosis affecting the specified deep vein of the upper or lower extremity as well as any current use of anticoagulants.

O24   Diabetes mellitus in pregnancy, childbirth, and the puerperium

Diabetes mellitus is a systemic, metabolic disease arising from insulin-related problems. Insulin is a hormone made by the beta cells of the pancreas and secreted into the digestive system. Insulin regulates blood sugar levels as well as the transport, storage, and use of glucose and amino acids. Without effective insulin action, blood sugar levels are difficult to control and become dangerously high. The many different complications of diabetes are related to high blood sugar. In pregnancy, high blood sugar levels can pose harmful risks to the baby, even during the first few weeks of gestation, when babies of mothers with pre-existing diabetes may develop a birth defect in the heart, brain, kidneys, or lungs as they are forming. Babies born to diabetic mothers may also be very large, weighing more than 10 pounds, making vaginal birth extremely difficult, and putting the baby at risk for birth injuries. Diabetic mothers are also more likely to suffer miscarriage or stillbirth.

Note: This category includes pre-existing diabetes in pregnancy for specified trimesters, childbirth, and postpartum stages, as well as gestational diabetes that arises in pregnancy.

O24.0   Pre-existing diabetes mellitus, type 1, in pregnancy, childbirth and the puerperium

Type 1 diabetes mellitus, sometimes referred to as juvenile onset or ketosis-prone diabetes, occurs when more than 90% of the cells in the pancreas that produce insulin have been permanently damaged or destroyed. The body produces little or no insulin on its own. This type accounts for about 10% of diabetes cases and most people affected will be diagnosed before age 30. These patients require regular injections of insulin to survive. Type 1 diabetes is linked to autoimmune processes, childhood or teenage viral infections, nutritional factors, drug overdoses--particularly antibiotics, and genetic predispositions.

Note: Reporting pre-existing diabetes mellitus, type 1, in pregnancy, childbirth and the puerperium requires the use of a code from this subcategory for the current stage of pregnancy as well as an additional code from category E10 to identify the diabetic manifestations.

O24.1   Pre-existing diabetes mellitus, type 2, in pregnancy, childbirth and the puerperium

Type 2 diabetes mellitus, formerly referred to as adult onset or non-insulin dependent diabetes, occurs when the body develops a resistance to the action of insulin. Even though the pancreas is still producing insulin, sometimes even at higher levels in response to elevated blood sugars, the body's resistance results in not enough insulin to meet the body's needs. Most type 2 patients are diagnosed in adulthood at ages older than 30, although it is now being diagnosed in children, even at a very young age, due to the increasing problems of obesity, sedentary lifestyle, and lack of exercise. Type 2 diabetes can be controlled with oral medications, diet, and exercise, but sometimes also requires insulin injections. Type 2 diabetes has several risk factors including obesity, age, some racial and cultural group risk factors, certain drugs such as corticosteroids, the presence of other diseases, and familial tendency. Of these risk factors, obesity is the major one for developing type 2 diabetes. Up to 90% of type 2 diabetics are overweight. Obese people require much larger amounts of insulin to maintain normal blood sugar.

Note: Reporting pre-existing diabetes mellitus, type 2, in pregnancy, childbirth and the puerperium requires the use of a code from this subcategory for the current stage of pregnancy as well as an additional code from category E11 to identify the diabetic manifestations, and one to identify any long-term current use of insulin.

O24.4   Gestational diabetes mellitus

Gestational diabetes mellitus develops during pregnancy and affects how the cells utilize glucose for energy, causing high blood sugar that can affect the pregnancy and the health of the baby. For many women, this does not cause significant signs or symptoms, but may cause increased urination and thirst. Blood sugar usually returns to normal after the pregnancy, but those who have had gestational diabetes are at higher risk for developing type 2 diabetes later.

O24.8   Other pre-existing diabetes mellitus in pregnancy, childbirth, and the puerperium

Other pre-existing diabetes mellitus (DM) includes secondary DM due to an underlying condition, poisoning from exposure to toxic chemicals or medicinal drugs, secondary DM due to genetic defects affecting beta cell function or insulin action, and diabetes due to pancreatectomy or other procedure. Other disease processes, or underlying conditions known to induce secondary diabetes include pancreatic disorders (pancreatitis, hemochromatosis); endocrinopathies such as Cushing's disease, acromegaly, and hyperaldosteronism; malignancy; congenital disorders such as cystic fibrosis, and congenital rubella; and affective disorders like schizophrenia. Overt diabetes is caused secondarily by pancreatic disorders or endocrinopathies causing counter-regulatory hormone production. The end metabolic effect in secondary diabetes is dependent upon the impact the underlying disorder has on insulin secretion, insulin sensitivity, and the unmasking of genetic tendencies. Drugs and chemical agents known to be associated with secondary diabetes includes diuretics, antihypertensives, hormones, psychoactive agents, anticonvulsants, antineoplastics, antiprotozoals, and antiretrovirals. Complications posed to the fetus by other types of pre-existing diabetes still pose the same risks of birth defects, large gestational size at birth, miscarriage, and stillbirth.

Note: Reporting other types of pre-existing diabetes mellitus in pregnancy, childbirth, and the puerperium requires the use of a code from this subcategory for the current stage of pregnancy as well as an additional code from either category E08, E09, or E13 to identify the diabetic manifestations, and one to identify any long-term current use of insulin.

O26.2   Pregnancy care for patient with recurrent pregnancy loss

Formerly called an habitual aborter, this status is defined as one who has previously had two, three, or even more consecutive miscarriages before the 20th week of gestation for a woman in a current state of pregnancy, receiving antepartum care.

O26.4   Herpes gestationis

Herpes gestationis, also known as pemphigoid gestationis is an autoimmune blistering skin condition generally seen in the second or third trimester and/or immediately after pregnancy and is completely different from what is commonly known as the herpes virus. The condition received the name because of its herpes-like blistering appearance, but is not associated with the virus. The condition is very symptomatic with itching associated with red blisters or patches that appear all over the body. The dermatosis can last weeks or even months, and is usually treated with cortisone.

O26.5   Maternal hypotension syndrome

Also called supine hypotension syndrome, this condition affects a pregnant woman who is at or near term while lying on her back in the supine position due to the gravid uterus obstructing the inferior vena cava. This condition is affected by the size of the gravid uterus and the exact positioning of the mother as well as the fetus. Maternal hypotension can complicate labor and delivery due to the decrease in venous blood returning to the heart, and due to the resulting fetal hypoxia that occurs when the gravid uterus also obstructs the mother's aorta, causing decreased placental perfusion.

O26.84 Uterine size-date discrepancy complicating pregnancy

A discrepancy in uterine size and dates is based on whether the size as measured by the physician is larger or smaller than normal according to the date of conception estimated by the last menstrual period. A larger than normal discrepancy could result from a mutliple gestation pregnancy, too much amniotic fluid (polyhydramnios), a molar pregnancy, or pelvic mass. A smaller than normal size date discrepancy could result from too little amniotic fluid present (oligohydramnios), abortion or fetal demise, or intrauterine growth retardation.

O26.85 Spotting complicating pregnancy

Spotting, or vaginal bleeding during any phase of pregnancy can be dangerous. Vaginal bleeding is a common complication of the first trimester, affecting about 30 percent of pregnancies. Bleeding that occurs later in pregnancy is abnormal. Bleeding within the first 20 weeks may indicate an ectopic or molar pregnancy, placenta previa, or spontaneous abortion. Bleeding in the second 20 weeks may indicate placenta previa or placental abruption. Any bleeding after the 28th week is an emergency, whether or not it is accompanied by abdominal pain. Hemorrhaging at this stage complicates about 4 percent of pregnancies and is the most common cause of maternal death in the United States.

O26.87 Cervical shortening

Sonographic evidence of a cervix shortened to 2.5 cm or less occurring within the second trimester; a warning of impending premature birth in women with a prior history of early delivery. Women having a shortened cervix by the 16th week of pregnancy are three times more likely to deliver early. Cervical cerclage is an indicated procedure in these cases to conserve the pregnancy until normal delivery. Cervical shortening present alone without a history of recurrent second or early third trimester fetal loss is not sufficient enough to diagnose classic cervical insufficiency.

O30 Multiple gestation

These codes report the status of multiple gestations and indicate the number of placentae and amniotic sacs that are present. When there is more than one fetus in the womb, the number of placentae and amniotic sacs can differ, which presents a higher risk of complication. Twins, triplets, quadruplets, and other multiple gestation pregnancies are generally at increased risk for premature birth, death, and congenital anomalies. Those sharing the same placenta with only one outer membrane (monochorionic) have an even greater risk of complications and death increased many times over those in their own placental sac.

O30.0 Twin pregnancy

Twins that arise from one fertilized egg that later splits are called monozygotic and are always identical. Depending upon when the egg splits, there may be different sacs for each fetus (dichorionic/diamniotic), or they may share the same outer sac, the placenta, and have two different inner, amniotic sacs (monochorionic/diamniotic). The fetuses may also be within the same outer and inner sacs (monochorionic/monoamniotic). Twins that arise from two different fertilized eggs are always nonidentical, dizygotic twins that lie within their own chorionic and amniotic membranes and do not share blood vessels.

O30.01 Twin pregnancy, monochorionic/monoamniotic

Monochorionic/monoamniotic identical twins lie within the same two sacs. They share the same placenta and the same amniotic sac and have one chorionic and one amniotic membrane. This occurs when a single fertilized egg divides between 8 and 14 days after fertilization. This configuration presents a greater danger because of the possibility of cords becoming entangled and due to the increased risk of twin-to-twin transfuson syndrome. Monochorionic/monoamniotic gestations are rare and make up only about 1-2% of monozygotic, identical twin pregnancies.

O30.02 Conjoined twin pregnancy

About three quarters of conjoined twins will be at least partially joined in the chest wall (mid-torso or upper abdomen) and may or may not share organs. About one quarter are joined at the lower torso, sharing hips, legs, or genitalia, and about 4 percent are connected at the head. Those having separate sets of organs have a better chance of successful separation surgery.

O30.03 Twin pregnancy, monochorionic/diamniotic

Monochorionic/diamniotic identical twins share the same placenta and lie within two different inner, amniotic sacs. This occurs when the single, fertilized egg splits between the third and eighth day after fertilization. About 60-70% of identical twins are monochorionic/diamniotic. Those sharing the same placenta are at greater risk for complications and death than those fetuses that lie within their own, separate chorionic membrane, particularly due to twin-to-twin transfusion syndrome.

O30.04 Twin pregnancy, dichorionic/diamniotic

Dichorionic/diamniotic twins do not share either a placental or amniotic sac and lie within their own chorionic and amniotic membranes. All fraternal twins are dichorionic/diamniotic. About 30-40% of identical twins are dichorionic/diamniotic, which occurs when the single fertilized egg splits before the third or fourth day after fertilization.

O30.1 Triplet pregnancy

Multiple fetuses that lie within the same outer, placental sac and/or inner amniotic sac and share chorionic or amniotic membranes are always at greater risk for complications or death many times higher than those fetuses that lie within their own placental and/or amniotic sacs.

O30.11 Triplet pregnancy with two or more monochorionic fetuses

Monochorionic fetuses share the same placenta and have one chorionic membrane.

O30.12 Triplet pregnancy with two or more monoamniotic fetuses

Monoamniotic fetuses share the same amniotic sac and lie within one amniotic membrane.

O31.0 Papyraceous fetus

A papyraceous fetus is a condition in which a fetus dies in the womb and is retained beyond natural term, causing a kind of mummification to occur. This usually happens in a twin pregnancy when one fetus dies and the other remains viable.

O31.3 Continuing pregnancy after elective fetal reduction of one fetus or more

Codes in this category are used to report a condition in which the mother has chosen to reduce the number of fetuses in the womb, with at least one remaining viable after the reduction procedure. This is usually done to protect the viability of a fetus and have a live birth when the multiple gestation puts all fetuses at risk.

O32 Maternal care for malpresentation of fetus

Category O32 is used to report malpresentation of the fetus in the womb. Presentation, or lie, refers to the manner in which the baby comes out of the birth canal, or the body part of the fetus lying over the pelvic inlet. A fetus is typically positioned upside down, with the chin tucked on the chest, facing the mother's back or right kidney, with the crown of the head facing the cervix and the limbs tucked in to ensure the easiest delivery for mother and child. Malposition occurs when the child is positioned in a different fashion in the womb, and malpresentation occurs when a different body part, besides the crown of the head, is the first to escape the womb during delivery.

Note: These codes exclude obstructed labor due to the malposition or malpresentation of the fetus (O64) and are for use for conditions that necessitate observation care, hospitalization, or other specified obstetric care, or cesarean delivery before labor begins.

O32.0 Maternal care for unstable lie

Unstable lie is the term used in late pregnancy, from 37 weeks on, for a baby that continues to change its position inside the womb.

O32.1   Maternal care for breech presentation

Breech presentation occurs when the baby presents the buttocks first. A frank breech occurs with the legs flexed at the hips and the knees extended, so the baby's feet are up by the head. In a complete breech, both of the baby's knees are bent, and the buttock and feet are closest to the birth canal.

O32.2   Maternal care for transverse and oblique lie

A transverse presentation occurs when the baby's spine lies perpendicular to the spine of the mother, and an oblique presentation occurs when the baby's spine is at an angle close to 45 degrees from the spine of the mother. The shoulder usually presents first in these cases, although the trunk or arm may present first.

O32.3   Maternal care for face, brow and chin presentation

A fetus is typically positioned upside down, with the chin tucked on the chest, facing the mother's back or right kidney, with the crown of the head facing the cervix and the limbs tucked in. Malpresentation of face, brow, or chin occurs when another part of the head other than the crown presents first, without the chin being tucked, but with the neck bent backwards instead.

O32.4   Maternal care for high head at term

High head at term means the crown of the baby's head fails to enter the upper opening of the pelvis, or pelvic brim, before birth. In high head presentation, the baby's head is either not fully engaged into the pelvis or is still high in the pelvis, 'free-floating' instead of dipping down into proper position for birth.

O32.6   Maternal care for compound presentation

Compound presentation means that one of the baby's extremities, such as a hand, arm, or foot, presents along with the presenting part. The majority of compound presentations appear as a fetal arm or hand presenting with the vertex, or breech. Compound presentations occur when the pelvis is not fully occupied by the fetus because of low birth weight; when external cephalic version is done and the hand, arm, or foot becomes 'trapped' below the fetal head; and when membranes rupture while the fetal head is still high in the pelvis.

O32.8   Maternal care for other malpresentation of fetus

Other malpresentations of the fetus include a footling presentation, in which both feet are the presenting part; and an incomplete breech presentation, in which only one of the baby's knees is bent, so that one foot and the buttock are presenting, while the other knee is extended and the other foot is up against the head.

O33   Maternal care for disproportion

Category O33 reports disproportion, in which structural abnormalities of the mother and/or fetus cause complications or conditions that necessitate observation care, hospitalization, or other specified obstetric care, or cesarean delivery before labor begins.

Note: These codes exclude obstructed labor due to the malposition or malpresentation of the fetus (O65-O66).

O33.1   Maternal care for disproportion due to generally contracted pelvis

With a generally contracted pelvis, the pelvic space is abnormally narrow.

O33.2   Maternal care for disproportion due to inlet contraction of pelvis

Inlet contraction of the pelvis is a condition in which the superior portion of the pelvis or the pelvic brim, bounded by the public bones crest and the front base of the sacrum, is narrowed.

O33.3   Maternal care for disproportion due to outlet contraction of pelvis

An outlet contraction of the pelvis is an abnormally narrow inferior portion of the pelvis, bounded by the coccyx, sacrotuberous ligaments, part of the ischium, and the pubic symphysis.

O33.5   Maternal care for disproportion due to unusually large fetus

Use this code to report a condition in which an abnormally large fetus with normal formation makes vaginal delivery difficult.

O33.6   Maternal care for disproportion due to hydrocephalic fetus

A condition in which the head of the fetus is abnormally large due to a buildup of cerebrospinal fluid in the ventricles, or cavities of the brain. Cerebrospinal fluid (CSF) is produced by the choroids plexus in the ventricles starting in the sixth week of gestation. The CSF flows through openings out into the subarachnoid space to be reabsorbed by the venous system. Fetal hydrocephaly occurs when the outflow is obstructed, usually due to congenital malformation syndromes or aqueductal stenosis, in which the passage of CSF is blocked through the aqueduct of Sylvius. This enlargement of the head is normally diagnosed in utero by ultrasound or MRI.

O33.7   Maternal care for disproportion due to other fetal deformities

Other fetal abnormalities which cause disproportion between the size of the fetus and the size of the mother's pelvis may include fetal problems such as ascites, tumor growth, or myelomeningocele.

O33.9   Maternal care for disproportion, unspecified

This includes unspecified fetopelvic or cephalopelvic disproportion, a condition in which a combination of the size of the fetus, or fetus's head, and the width of the mother's pelvis makes vaginal birth difficult, or not possible.

O34   Maternal care for abnormality of pelvic organs

Category O34 is used to report abnormalities of the organs and soft tissues of the pelvis in a pregnant woman that can obstruct the delivery of a child, or necessitate hospitalization for observation, other specific obstetric care, or cesarean delivery before the onset of labor.

Note: Any associated obstructed labor is coded first with O65.5 and the specific condition is reported with additional codes.

O34.0   Maternal care for congenital malformation of uterus

Congenital malformations of the uterus include septate, bicornuate, or unicornuate uterus.

O34.1   Maternal care for benign tumor of corpus uteri

Note: This subcategory reports maternal care necessitated by the presence of a benign tumor of the body of the uterus, and not of the cervix. A benign tumor of the cervix requiring maternal care is reported with O34.4 as other abnormalities of the cervix.

O34.3   Maternal care for cervical incompetence

Cervical incompetence is a condition in which the cervix tends to dilate early in the pregnancy, prematurely ejecting the fetus from the uterus. In order to keep the cervix closed and retain the growing fetus, a cerclage procedure is done to tighten the opening.

Note: Whenever maternity care is given for cerclage or for a Shirodkar suture in place, the appropriate trimester code is reported.

O34.4   Maternal care for other abnormalities of cervix

Note: This subcategory includes maternal care necessitated by the presence of a benign tumor of the cervix.

O34.51 Maternal care for incarceration of gravid uterus

An incarcerated uterus is uncommon, but serious. It often presents with pain and urinary retention, with a retroverted uterus, in the second or third trimester. The growing uterus that is tilted backwards becomes wedged into the pelvis, usually after the first trimester, when it normally becomes anteverted spontaneously in order to accommodate the expanding uterus into the abdominal cavity. The incarcerated uterus fails to become anteverted and the continuing pregnancy enlarges the uterus within the confines of the pelvis, filling the space, and pushing upwards on the cervix. The trapped uterus causes lower abdominal, pelvic, and even back pain, and difficulty or inability to void, because the bladder is pushed upwards and outflow is blocked.

O34.53 Maternal care for retroversion of gravid uterus

A retroverted uterus tilts backward toward the rectum instead of forward into the abdomen. In most cases, this does not interfere with pregnancy and the cervix remains below the uterus. This is a normal positioning variant during early pregnancy, that will spontaneously antevert, but if it persists, it can pose a threat of incarcerated uterus.

O35.0 Maternal care for (suspected) central nervous system malformation in fetus

Central nervous system malfunctions in the fetus include hydrocephalus, spina bifida, or anencephaly.

O35.7 Maternal care for (suspected) damage to fetus by other medical procedures

Medical procedures during pregnancy to examine or reduce anmiotic fluid, take biopsies of tissue, obtain blood samples, or remove a retained intrauterine contraceptive device can cause harm to the baby as well as actual surgical procedures that are performed on the fetus in the womb.

O36.0 Maternal care for rhesus isoimmunization

Rhesus isoimmunization occurs when an Rh negative mother develops antibodies against an Rh positive fetus. The presence of Rh antigens in the blood is another way to classify blood groups and is the second most important blood grouping system next to ABO. There are many defined Rh antigens; however only 5 are identified as the most important: D, C, c, E, and e.

O36.01 Maternal care for anti-D [Rh] antibodies

Rh factor refers to the strongest or most immunogenic of the rhesus antigens, D. Those without Rh factor present (Rh negative) do not have the D antigen on the surface of their red blood cells and will form anti-D antibodies against the Rh factor present in Rh positive blood. Most Rh incompatibility antigen-antibody responses will be caused by the D antigen. In pregnancy, when the mother is Rh negative, and the baby is Rh positive, red blood cells with the antigen cross from the unborn baby into the mother's bloodstream and her immune system treats the fetal cells as a foreign invader and makes antibodies against them. The anti-D Rh antibodies cross back through the placenta and begin destroying the baby's circulating red blood cells. This can cause hemolytic disease in the newborn and mortality, but because it takes time to develop this immune response, first-time pregnancies are not affected. Any following pregnancies; however, with an Rh positive fetus will be affected unless the mother is treated with special immune globulins called RhoGAM.

O36.09 Maternal care for other rhesus isoimmunization

Although rhesus isoimmunization generally occurs against the Rh factor that refers to the strongest or most immunogenic of the rhesus antigens, the D antigen, maternal rhesus isoimmunization can occur against other Rh antigens that are present in the blood, such as C, c, E, and e whenever the mother is negative for the rhesus antigen while the baby is positive. This creates a blood type incompatibility. The mother's immune system recognizes the baby's Rh positive RBCs as a foreign invader and begins producing antibodies against the baby's blood cells. This can lead to hemolytic disease that poses increased health risks for the baby.

O36.1 Maternal care for other isoimmunization

Other isoimmunization includes ABO blood typing, or blood group, incompatibility. These are the best known surface antigens. ABO incompatibility is an immune reaction that occurs when two different, and incompatible, major blood groups are mixed together. There are three major blood types: A, B, and O. These groups are determined by very specific molecules present on the surface of the blood cells. These molecules, or antigens, act like immune system triggers against blood of a different group, i.e. A reacts against B, B reacts against A. Everyone has a combination of two of these surface antigens (Type A = AA or AO, Type B = BB or BO, Type AB). Type O lacks any surface antigens, and is known as the universal donor, because it will not trigger an immune response. However, type O can only receive type O, as it will react against the molecules on both type A and type B.

O36.11 Maternal care for Anti-A sensitization

Anti-A sensitization occurs with the transfusion of fetal to maternal blood when a mother who does not have the A group antigen becomes sensitized against it by the baby's blood, which does have the A group antigen. Exposure causes the mother's immune system to produce IgG immune globulins against the A antigen. Anti-A IgG immune globulins can cross the placenta into the fetal circulation and attack the baby's red blood cells as foreign. This reaction causes a weakly positive direct Coombs test for the neonate and can lead to ABO hemolytic disease of the newborn (HDN). In most cases, the HDN is mild and short-lived as A surface antigens are not fully developed on red blood cells in the neonate and they also occur on many different cell types, leaving less anti-A antibodies to bind specifically to red blood cells. This is normally diagnosed when a baby develops jaundice in the first day of life. Symptomatic hemolytic disease occurs in mothers with O blood type who produce enough antibodies to cause hemolysis in the baby.

Note: When the mother receives care for isoimmunization that is not otherwise specified, it is reported here as Anti-A sensitization. This includes maternal care for hydrops fetalis that is known to be due to isoimmunization.

O36.19 Maternal care for other isoimmunization

Other isoimmunization can be maternal Anti-B sensitization that occurs with the transfusion of fetal to maternal blood when a mother who does not have the B group antigen becomes sensitized against it by the baby's blood, which does have the B group antigen. Exposure causes the mother's immune system to produce IgG immune globulins against the B antigen. Anti-B IgG immune globulins can cross the placenta into the fetal circulation and attack the baby's red blood cells as foreign. This reaction causes a weakly positive direct Coombs test for the neonate and can lead to ABO hemolytic disease of the newborn (HDN). In most cases, the HDN is mild and short-lived as B surface antigens are not fully developed on red blood cells in the neonate and they also occur on many different cell types, leaving less anti-B antibodies to bind specifically to red blood cells. This is normally diagnosed when a baby develops jaundice in the first day of life. Symptomatic hemolytic disease occurs in mothers with O blood type who produce enough antibodies to cause hemolysis in the baby.

O36.2 Maternal care for hydrops fetalis

Hydrops fetalis is a severe swelling of the fetus when excess fluid accumulates in two or more fetal compartments, causing the body to swell, usually arising from an initial overproduction of interstitial fluid, followed by inadequate lymphatic drainage. These compartments can include subcutaneous tissue, the scalp, pleural space, pericardium, and the abdomen. Symptoms of hydrops in a fetus include a thickened placenta and enlarged organs.

Note: This is normally caused by an isoimmunization reaction, however when hyrops fetalis is associated with isoimmunization, it is coded to the specific type of ABO or rhesus incompatibility, or to subcategory O36.11- when the type of isoimmunization is not specified.

O36.51 Maternal care for known or suspected placental insufficiency

The placenta is an organ that secretes hormones and provides nutrition, waste elimination, and gas exchange to the developing fetus. Placental insufficiency is a complication of pregnancy in which the fetus fails to receive adequate nutrition and/or oxygen because the placenta does not develop properly or becomes damaged during the pregnancy. Risk factors for placental insufficiency include maternal diabetes, hypertension, diseases that affect blood clotting, and smoking.

O36.7 Maternal care for viable fetus in abdominal pregnancy

Abdominal pregnancy is one type of ectopic pregnancy in which the fertilized ovum implants itself not in the lining of the uterus, but elsewhere in the abdominal cavity, outside of the fallopian tube or ovary. These type of ectopic pregnancies are very rare with a high mortality, but abdominal pregnancies can still lead to the delivery of a viable infant.

O36.81 Decreased fetal movements

Decreased fetal movement within the womb may be a sign of fetal disease or abnormality or even fetal demise, and so decreased movement from the baby is a cause for testing to determine the viability of the fetus.

O40 Polyhydramnios

Polyhydramnios is a condition in which there is an excess amount of amniotic fluid in the amniotic sac. Levels are measured by an amniotic fluid index (AFI) or deep pocket evaluation. Polyhydramnios is diagnosed with an AFI measurement greater than 25 cm or a single deep pocket measurement less than 8, or a fluid level of 2000mL or more at 32-36 weeks gestation. This condition is sometimes caused by chromosomal abnormalities, such as Down syndrome, twin to twin transfusion syndrome, maternal diabetes, and Rh factor incompatibility; however, most cases are of unknown cause. Most cases are mild, but too much fluid can cause premature membrane rupture, placental abruption, premature delivery, growth restriction with skeletal malformations, and stillbirth. It is monitored and treated with medications that can reduce the fluid level, or amniocentesis reduction.

O41.0 Oligohydramnios

Oligohydramnios is a deficiency of amniotic fluid in the amniotic sac. Fluid levels are measured by an amniotic fluid index (AFI) or deep pocket evaluation. Oligohydramnios is diagnosed with an AFI measurement less than 5 cm, or the absence of a fluid pocket 2-3 cm deep, or a fluid volume less than 500 mL at 32-36 weeks of gestation. This can be caused by birth defects, leaky membranes, placental problems, fetal kidney disease, renal agenesis and other urinary abnormalites, and maternal problems such as dehydration, hypertension, pre-eclampsia, and diabetes. In early pregnancy the fluid is produced by the mother; but by 20 weeks gestation, it is largely made up of fetal urine. Since amniotic fluid is essential for protection and normal development of the fetus, oligohydramnios can result in compression of the fetal organs, birth defects, growth restriction and deformities, premature delivery, and complications in labor such as cord compression and meconium staining. Treatment is based on gestational age. Maternal rehydration is helpful and amnioinfusion may be done during labor or through amniocentesis.

O41.12 Chorioamnionitis

Chorioamnionitis is an inflammation of the membranes around the fetus--the chorion or placental tissue, and the amnion or amniotic fluid. It is usually associated with a bacterial infection and is dangerous to both the mother and child. Chorioamnionitis can cause septicemia in the mother and lead to premature birth and serious infection in the newborn. The infecting organisms responsible are usually those normally found in the vaginal canal, such as *E. coli*, even Group B streptococcus. Chorioamnionitis often occurs when membranes are ruptured for an extended amount of time that allows the bacteria in the birth canal the opportunity to migrate upwards. Symptoms can include fever, tender uterus, increased heart rate of mother and/or fetus, and a foul odor to the amnion. Amniocentesis and laboratory testing is done for diagnosis. Antibiotics are administered as soon as the infection is diagnosed, and often continued after delivery.

O41.14 Placentitis

Placentitis is an inflammation of the placenta, an organ that secretes hormones and provides nutrition, waste elimination, and gas exchange to the developing fetus. Placentitis may cause miscarriage, preterm labor, and/or placental retention post delivery. TORCH infections are the most common cause of placentitis and include toxoplasmosis (T), other infections (O-coxsackievirus, varicella-zoster virus, HIV, parvovirus B19), rubella (R), cytomegalovirus (C), and herpes simplex-2 (H).

O42 Premature rupture of membranes

Premature rupture of membranes (PROM) reports a rupture of the amniotic sac and subsequent release of the amniotic fluids that occurs before contractions start. This is reported by the length of time between rupture and the onset of delivery as well as the weeks of gestation when the membranes rupture. Preterm premature rupture is defined as PROM before 37 completed weeks of gestation. Full-term premature rupture is defined as PROM after 37 completed weeks. Onset of labor is concomitantly reported as occurring either within 24 hours of rupture or more than 24 hours following rupture, which is also sometimes referred to as delayed delivery following PROM.

O44 Placenta previa

Placenta previa is an obstetric complication that occurs when the placenta implants and grows in the lower part of the uterus and covers all or part of the cervix opening into the birth canal. During pregnancy, the placenta grows and moves as the uterus stretches. It is common for the placenta to be low in the womb in early pregnancy, but by the third trimester the placenta should have moved to be near the top of the womb with the cervix open for delivery. Placenta previa can be marginal, next to the cervix but not covering the opening; partially covering the cervical opening; or completely covering the cervix. The main symptom is sudden vaginal bleeding often starting near the end of the second trimester or at the beginning of the third trimester. The hemorrhaging can be severe, stop on its own, or start again weeks later. Sometimes labor will begin after several days of heavy bleeding, and in other cases, hemorrhaging begins after labor starts. Severe bleeding can be life threatening to mother and baby, and delivery may be necessary before vital organs are fully formed.

O45 Premature separation of placenta [abruptio placentae]

The placenta is an organ that provides nourishment to the fetus during pregnancy and normally detaches after delivery. Placentae abruptio is the premature separation of the placenta from its attachment to the uterine wall before the baby is born and can be life threatening to both the mother and fetus. The cause may be difficult to ascertain but may occur with abdominal trauma or with a rapid loss of amniotic fluid, blood clotting disorders, and elevated maternal blood pressure. Any amount of placental separation before delivery is included and can cause back and abdominal pain, uterine contraction without relaxation, and vaginal bleeding. Treatment includes IV fluids, blood transfusion, and monitoring for signs of shock or fetal distress. Emergency cesarean section may be necessary. The most severe form of placentae abruptio can result in the baby's death, but smaller separations may be monitored without worsening.

O45.0 Premature separation of placenta with coagulation defect

A rare complication of abruptio placentae is a disruption of the blood clotting mechanisms (clotting cascade) which can lead to hemorrhage and/or microvascular coagulation.

O45.01 Premature separation of placenta with afibrinogenemia

Fibrinogen is a coagulation factor necessary for clot formation. In premature separation of the placenta occurring with afibrinogenemia, there is an absence or marked decrease of fibrinogen which can lead to prolonged bleeding time and the inability of blood to form clots.

O45.02 **Premature separation of placenta with disseminated intravascular coagulation**

Disseminated intravascular coagulation (DIC) is a rare complication of abruptio placentae with a combination of hemorrhage and microvascular coagulation. It involves a repeating cycle of clot formation and breakdown by fibrinolysis, followed by depletion of platelets and coagulation factors, and a constant release of anticoagulants.

O46 **Antepartum hemorrhage, not elsewhere classified**

Antepartum hemorrhage (APH) is vaginal bleeding after the 24th week of pregnancy not caused by placenta previa or abruptio placentae. Bleeding can be maternal in origin such as benign show of blood as the cervix softens and begins to dilate, or from a more serious cause such as uterine rupture. Bleeding that arises from the fetus can be due to vasa previa.

O46.0 **Antepartum hemorrhage with coagulation defect**

A rare complication of antepartum hemorrhage is a disruption of the blood clotting mechanisms (clotting cascade) which can lead to hemorrhage and/or microvascular coagulation.

O46.01 **Antepartum hemorrhage with afibrinogenemia**

Fibrinogen is a coagulation factor necessary for clot formation. In antepartum hemorrhage with afibrinogenemia, there is an absence or marked decrease of fibrinogen which can lead to prolonged bleeding time and the inability of blood to form clots.

O46.02 **Antepartum hemorrhage with disseminated intravascular coagulation**

Disseminated intravascular coagulation (DIC) is a rare complication of antepartum bleeding with a combination of hemorrhage and microvascular coagulation. It involves a repeating cycle of clot formation and breakdown by fibrinolysis, followed by depletion of platelets and coagulation factors, and a constant release of anticoagulants.

O47 **False labor**

False labor refers to the less painful, few, and far between Braxton Hicks contractions that are not contributing to impending labor. This is a kind of tightening or cramping in the lower abdomen similar to menstrual cramping. This type of false labor cramping can become more intense, rhythmic, and more frequent, but real diagnosis of labor must be accompanied by cervical dilation and effacement, which does not occur with Braxton Hicks.

O48.0 **Post-term pregnancy**

Post-term pregnancy is defined as pregnancy that continues after 40 completed weeks to 42 completed weeks.

O48.1 **Prolonged pregnancy**

Prolonged pregnancy is defined as pregnancy that has continued to advance beyond 42 completed weeks of gestation.

O60 **Preterm labor**

Preterm labor is defined as the onset of spontaneous labor that occurs before 37 completed weeks of gestation.

O69.0 **Labor and delivery complicated by prolapse of cord**

Umbilical cord prolapse is a serious but rare complication of childbirth that poses imminent danger for the baby and must be addressed immediately. It occurs either prior to or during labor and delivery, often as a complication of premature rupture of membranes, breech presentation in premature delivery, and with multiple births. The cord drops down through the cervical opening ino the birth canal ahead of the baby and can then become trapped against the baby's body during delivery. Prolapse causes a loss of oxygen to the fetus through the cord, which is the baby's lifeline, and can result in brain damage or mortality. If the stress on the cord cannot be relieved immediately, then emergency C-section is necessary.

O69.3 **Labor and delivery complicated by short cord**

The average length of the umbilical cord at term is 50-60 cm. A short cord at term is around 35 cm. For an infant to be delivered without complications, an untangled cord must be long enough to reach from its insertion at the placenta to the outside of the birth canal. It is believed that fetal movement in the womb creates the tension that results in cord growth, and that a short cord could be a marker for disorders causing decreased fetal movement, intrauterine constraints on the fetus, and placental abruption. Determining cord length prenatally is not possible. A short cord may make it impossible to delivery vaginally and necessitate C-section. Cord length may be measured after birth in cases of oligohydramnios, placental abruption, or breech presentation because an abnormally short cord length points toward some kind of long-term fetal condition.

O69.4 **Labor and delivery complicated by vasa previa**

Vasa previa is a rare and devastating complication of pregnancy in which unprotected fetal blood vessels (unsupported by the umbilical cord or the placenta) grow across the internal cervical os. These vessels run within the membranes, obstructing the baby's passage into the birth canal, and are at risk of rupturing along with the membranes. Vasa previa can be caused by the cord inserting directly into the membranes and leaving vessels unprotected as they run into the placenta. Other risk factors associated with vasa previa include in vitro fertilization, placenta previa, and multiple pregnancies. When these unprotected vessels rupture, bleeding occurs from the fetoplacental circulation, and results in rapid exsanguination and death of the fetus.

O70.0 **First degree perineal laceration during delivery**

First degree perineal lacerations include rupture or tear involving the fourchette, labia, skin, vagina, vulva, or any slight perineal laceration of superficial tissues occurring during delivery.

O70.1 **Second degree perineal laceration during delivery**

Second degree perineal lacerations include rupture or tear of fourchette, skin, labia, vagina, or vulva also involving the pelvic floor, perineal muscles, or vaginal muscles occurring during delivery.

O70.2 **Third degree perineal laceration during delivery**

Third degree perineal lacerations include rupture or tear of fourchette, skin, labia, vagina, or vulva involving the pelvic floor, perineal muscles, or vaginal muscles and the anal spincter or rectovaginal septum occurring during delivery.

O70.3 **Fourth degree perineal laceration during delivery**

Fourth degree perineal lacerations include rupture or tear of fourchette, skin, labia, vagina, or vulva involving the pelvic floor, perineal muscles, or vaginal muscles and the anal spincter or rectovaginal septum extending into the anal or rectal mucosa.

O75.82 **Onset (spontaneous) of labor after 37 completed weeks of gestation but before 39 completed weeks gestation, with delivery by (planned) cesarean section**

This code is used to identify deliveries done by planned C-section in cases when the patient presents after 37 completed weeks but before 39 completed weeks gestation already in labor and the physician determines that it is better to proceed with the planned C-section rather than take measures to stop the labor and wait until the 39th week. This code can only be applied for spontaneous onset of labor within the specified time frame, followed by delivery brought about by a planned cesarean section.

O80 **Encounter for full-term uncomplicated delivery**

Category O80 is used to report the normal delivery of a fetus, requiring little or no assistance with or without episotomy, and without forceps or manipulation. Use this code only to report an uncomplicated, spontaneous, vaginal delivery of a single, live, full-term infant.

O85 **Puerperal sepsis**

Puerperal sepsis, or postpartum pyemia, is a pregnancy-related toxic condition of infection and pyemia of the birth canal and uterus, usually of the placental site. It occurs as a complication following birth that could lead to obstetric shock and even death. Infection can be caused by a multitude of microbes from the lower genital or GI tract and includes pathogens such as gram-positive cocci, gram negative bacteria, and anaerobes. Puerperal sepsis infects the bloodstream and becomes widespread. It is contagious and can be spread from patient to patient by unwashed hands and is still prevalent in developing countries.

O86.12   Endometritis following delivery

Endometritis is inflammation and infection of the uterus usually caused by bacteria from the lower reproductive or GI tract. The mode of delivery, such as C-section before or after labor has begun vs. vaginal delivery, has an affect on the incidence of postpartum endometritis. Infection is usually by more than one microbe and includes pathogens such as gram-positive cocci, gram negative bacteria, and anaerobes. Symptoms appear as lower abdominal pain, uterine tenderness, fever, chills, headache, or malaise within 24-72 hours of delivery. Pallor, tachycardia, and leukocytosis usually occur, but a low grade fever may be the only symptom. Treatment is usually with a broad-spectrum, IV antibiotic regimen.

O86.81   Puerperal septic thrombophlebitis

Puerperal septic pelvic thrombophlebitis is a rare complication of postpartum infection. The inflammatory condition affects the adnexa of the pelvis and can manifest as ovarian vein thrombophlebitis (OVT) or deep septic pelvic (DSPT) thrombophlebitis. Patients with OVT usually present with fever and abdominal pain within a week of delivery or surgery. Thrombosis of the ovarian vein can be visualized radiographically. Patients with DSPT usually present with fever within a few days of delivery or surgery that continues despite antibiotics and no radiographic evidence. Uterine infection or intrapartum trauma to vascular structures causes endothelial damage. Ovarian vein dilation in pregnancy and low post-partum ovarian venous pressures result in venous stasis. The hypercoagulable state of pregnancy completes the physiological conditions for the development of thrombosis. Medical treatment consists of antibiotics and anticoagulants, although the condition does not always respond to heparin treatment. Surgical treatment may consist of pelvic vein ligation.

O98.0   Tuberculosis complicating pregnancy, childbirth and the puerperium

Tuberculosis (TB) is a disease caused by *Mycobaterium tuberculosis* and is transmitted primarily through inhalation of infected air from those already infected. The most common site of tuberculous infection is within the lungs and other parts of the respiratory system, but the tubercles can spread to other locations in the body through the lymph and blood vessels. Symptoms of TB include a cough that goes on for two or more weeks, sometimes with small amounts of blood in the phlegm, fever, night sweats, and unexplained weight loss. Other symptoms may be present depending on the location of the infection.

O98.1   Syphilis complicating pregnancy, childbirth and the puerperium

Syphilis complicating pregnancy, childbirth, and the puerperium includes congenital cases of syphilis, and early, late, and latent types of syphilis in the pregnant female. Syphilis is caused by infection with the gram negative spirochete bacterium, *Treponema pallidum*. It is a sexually transmitted disease that can be passed to the neonate through an infected mother. Syphilis can cause long-term complications and even death, when not properly treated. Complications can appear even 30 years after infection and include uncoordinated muscle movements, paralysis, progressive blindness, dementia, damage to internal organs including the brain, nerves, eyes, liver, bones, heart, and blood vessels. Babies contracting syphilis through an infected mother may have many problems. It can lead to low birth weight, prematurity, and even stillbirth. Some infected babies may be born asymptomatic but develop serious problems within a few weeks such as cataracts, deafness, or seizures.

O98.2   Gonorrhea complicating pregnancy, childbirth and the puerperium

Gonorrhea, also called blenorrhagia or blenorrhea, is a sexually transmitted disease that may also be passed from an infected mother to the neonate at birth or even later to infants of an infected mother. Symptoms of a primary infection include bacteremia, painful urethritis, burning on

urination, and a purulent discharge from the urinary tract. Females often remain asymptomatic or experience symptoms that are mild enough to be mistaken for a bladder or vaginal infection. Lesions may appear on the mouth, genitals, or anus. The eyes may also become infected. Untreated cases can cause serious and permanent problems. Women are particularly at risk for serious complications, regardless of the severity of symptoms, such as pelvic inflammatory disease which can cause abscesses, chronic pain, and permanent damage to fallopian tubes. Gonorrhea may disseminate and spread to the blood or joints and become life-threatening.

O99.21   Obesity complicating pregnancy, childbirth, and the puerperium

Obesity is a common health problem associated with serious complications that add substantial risk to pregnancy. Obese women (those with a body mass index of 30 of higher) have an increased risk of problems during pregnancy, such as hypertension, gestational diabetes, and thromboembolic or clot-related vascular accidents. Complications during labor and delivery are increased with obese women more likely to require a Caesarean section. Morbidity in the neonate is also increased. Babies born to obese mothers are more likely to be admitted to an intensive care unit and have a higher rate of neural tube defect.

O99.28   Other endocrine, nutritional and metabolic diseases complicating pregnancy, childbirth and the puerperium

Note: Diabetes mellitus, malnutrition, and postpartal thyroiditis are not reported within this category, but with specific codes for those conditions affecting pregnancy, childbirth, and the puerperium.

O99.33   Smoking (tobacco) complicating pregnancy, childbirth, and the puerperium

Smoking and the use of tobacco products while pregnant is known to cause a host of problems that complicate pregnancy. These adverse effects from tobacco include ectopic pregnancy, spontaneous abortion, premature rupture of membranes, preterm delivery, low birth weight, and stillbirth.

O99.35   Diseases of the nervous system complicating pregnancy, childbirth, and the puerperium

This includes any condition classified in the nervous system chapter from encephalitis, myelitis, and encephalomyelitis, to systemic and muscular atrophies, extrapyramidal and movement disorders, demyelinating diseases, migraines, transient ischemic attacks, neuropathies, causalgias and other nerve root and plexus disorders, hemiplegia and paraplegia, and epilepsy and seizure disorders. In the case of epilepsy complicating pregnancy, childbirth, and the puerperium, one quarter to a third of pregnant women with epilepsy will experience increased seizures despite taking anti-epileptic medication. Hormones, increased maternal plasma volume, and increased drug clearance contribute to the lessened effect of the medication. However, uncontrolled seizures, particularly tonic-clonic episodes are hazardous during pregnancy and can cause miscarriage, falls and subsequent trauma, fetal hypoxia, bradycardia, and acidosis. The risk from discontinuing medication outweighs possible adverse effects of the medication, although all common anti-epileptic drugs have been associated with congenital malformations. Pregnancy complications seen more frequently in women with epilepsy include hyperemesis gravidarum, anemia, bleeding, premature labor, and failure to progress.

O99.84   Bariatric surgery status complicating pregnancy, childbirth and the puerperium

Women of childbearing years who have had surgery for obesity are instructed that they must not become pregnant within an 18 month to 2 year minimum period following the bariatric procedure. Because gastric banding or gastric bypass causes such rapid weight loss, the nutritional deficiencies associated with this kind of surgery are very dangerous to both the mother and the developing fetus.

Certain Conditions Originating in the Perinatal Period | P00-P96

P00.0   **Newborn (suspected to be) affected by maternal hypertensive disorders**

This includes newborns affected by gestational or pre-existing hypertension, pre-eclampsia, and eclampsia. Pre-eclampsia is hypertension with a blood pressure reaching 140/90 mmHg or greater after the 20th week of gestation and up to 6 weeks postpartum, with proteinuria. Pre-eclampsia not only affects the mother's kidneys, liver, and brain, but is a disorder of placental dysfunction and is one of the leading causes of neonatal complications, causing low birth weight, fetal growth restriction, pre-mature birth, and stillbirth. Eclampsia is an acute, life-threatening complication of pregnancy that is extremely dangerous to mother and baby. It usually appears as the final phase of severe pre-eclampsia and is marked by hypertension with a blood pressure reading greater than 140/90 mmHg after the 20th week of gestation and up to 6 weeks postpartum with proteinuria, and tonic-clonic (motor) seizures or convulsions and even coma.

P00.2   **Newborn (suspected to be) affected by maternal infectious and parasitic diseases**

This includes newborns affected by infectious disease in the mother, including influenza of identified virus. Infections during pregnancy can spread to the baby, known as 'vertical transmission'. This can occur anytime during the perinatal period--in utero, during delivery, or even while breastfeeding. Congenital infections cross the placenta and lead to developmental abnormalities in the size of the baby or the fetal head, as well as defects in the heart and lungs, limbs, and abdomen. Common infections passed in utero include toxoplasmosis, rubella, hepatitis B, and viruses such as coxsackie, Epstein-Barr, varicella, and herpes simplex. Perinatal infections transmitted during labor and delivery generally include sexually transmitted diseases, and postnatal infections transmitted in breastmilk include HIV, Group B streptococcus, and cytomegalovirus.

P00.3   **Newborn (suspected to be) affected by other maternal circulatory and respiratory diseases**

This includes newborns affected by respiratory and circulatory diseases in the mother except hypertensive disorder, or identified infectious influenza. This may include rheumatic and ischemic heart diseases, cardiovascular disorders and diseases of the arteries, veins, or lymphatic vessels, and diseases of pulmonary circulation. Respiratory diseases include asthma, chronic obstructive pulmonary disease, and pneumoconioses. Pregnancy induces profound hemodynamic changes that affect the circulatory system. Heart rate increases; the blood plasma volume increases faster than a proportionate rise in red blood cells, causing a decrease in hematocrit levels; blood pressure normally decreases due to decreased systemic vascular resistance; and cardiac output increases up to 50% causing elevated pulmonary pressures as well. During delivery, heart rate, blood pressure, vascular resistance, and cardiac output all increase with each contraction, and postpartum changes also strain the circulatory system. This can be dangerous for any abnormal heart or vascular system, and strain the lungs. Fetal complications from maternal circulatory or respiratory disease include intrauterine growth restriction, formation of congenital anomalies, pre-term delivery, and perinatal death.

P00.4   **Newborn (suspected to be) affected by maternal nutritional disorders**

This includes newborns affected by maternal malnutrition, vitamin and mineral deficiencies, trace element and other nutrient deficiencies, or dietary imbalances, such as too much of any one nutritional element. This could include protein calorie malnutrition, vitamin A, B, C, D, E, or K deficiency, a lack of calcium, zinc, selenium, iron, magnesium, manganese, etc., or even a lack of essential fatty acids. The manifestation of the nutritional disorder affecting the developing fetus will depend upon the particular role that the vitamin, mineral, or trace element plays in health and proper development, or the toxic effect produced by too much of the dietary constituent.

P00.5   **Newborn (suspected to be) affected by maternal injury**

This includes newborns affected by injury, poisoning, or other consequences of external causes incurred by the mother, such as traumatic fractures, lacerations, foreign bodies, toxic effects of chemical exposure, burns, and corrosions. The developing fetus is highly sensitive to the toxic effect of chemicals, some of which can harm the fetus at levels that have no obvious effects on the mother. Common industrial chemicals in widespread use and environmental pollutants that can affect fetal brain development include household cleaners, pesticides, weed killers, chemicals used in making carpets, toys, and clothing, and byproducts of manufacturing processes, such as dioxins. Unintentional chemical exposure is absorbed through the skin and hair, from the air, and through ingesting food and drink. The harmful chemicals have a deleterious effect on the function of endocrine tissue, genes, proteins, and many other small molecules within the developing brain, and can lead to autism, dyslexia, cerebral palsy, and attention deficit disorder.

P00.6   **Newborn (suspected to be) affected by surgical procedure on mother**

This code includes newborns affected by anmiocentesis. Amniocentesis is a procedure to withdraw fluid from the uterus either for testing purposes or for treatment. The fluid surrounds and protects the baby in the womb and contains fetal cells and chemicals used to diagnose certain conditions, look for infection, or determine maturity of the baby's lungs. Some risks may occur, even if rare. Needle injury may affect the baby if an arm or leg is moved into the needle's path. Leaking amniotic fluid may lead to orthopedic problems for the infant.

Note: A newborn affected by complications of a surgical procedure done in utero is coded to subcategory P96.5.

P00.7   **Newborn (suspected to be) affected by other medical procedures on mother, not elsewhere classified**

This code includes newborns affected by radiation to the mother. Ionizing radiation is produced not only by machines that deliver radiation as a therapeutic treatment, but also by diagnostic machines that take images such as x-ray or fluoroscopy. Ionizing radiation is also used in the form of radionuclides, or radioactive isotopes, used in brachytherapy and liquid radioactive therapy administration. Most diagnostic tests will not expose the developing fetus to a dose of radiation that would increase the risk of birth defects. The level reported to increase the incidence of harmful fetal effects is above 200 mSv, and a diagnostic dose is usually around 50 mSv. The stage, or number of weeks, of the developing embryo is also a consideration for the type of damage that may be incurred. Most harmful affects on a fetus are from radiation therapy for cancer for radioactive iodine for hyperthyroidism when it is deemed to be a greater risk to the mother to wait for treatment, or the mother is not aware she is pregnant.

P00.81   **Newborn (suspected to be) affected by periodontal disease in mother**

An association between periodontal disease (PD) in pregnancy and adverse outcomes of pregnancy is increasingly being recognized in studies, leading to an understanding of the importance of good dental health. Mothers with PD are more likely to have premature labor and spontaneous pre-term birth of low birth weight babies, or spontaneous abortion than those who consume alcohol or smoke.

P00.89 Newborn (suspected to be) affected by other maternal conditions

This includes newborns affected by localized maternal infections, such as of the genital tract, complications of surgical or medical care for the mother, and maternal systemic lupus erythematosus (SLE). Lower genital tract infections, in particular, have been related to pre-term birth of low-birth-weight infants that results in a high rate of immediate complications in the neonate. In the latter case, about 20% of women with SLE will develop high blood pressure and pre-eclampsia, have premature labor and pre-term delivery, or miscarriage. Certain antibodies can also increase the tendency for the formation of blood clots, including in the arteries and veins of the placenta.

P01.0 Newborn (suspected to be) affected by incompetent cervix

Cervical incompetence is a condition in which the cervix tends to dilate early in the pregnancy, prematurely ejecting the fetus from the uterus. In order to keep the cervix closed and retain the growing fetus, a cerclage procedure is done to tighten the opening.

P01.1 Newborn (suspected to be) affected by premature rupture of membranes

Premature rupture of membranes (PROM) reports a rupture of the amniotic sac and subsequent release of the amniotic fluids that occurs before contractions start. This is reported by the length of time between rupture and the onset of delivery as well as the weeks of gestation when the membranes rupture. Preterm premature rupture is defined as PROM before 37 completed weeks of gestation. Full-term premature rupture is defined as PROM after 37 completed weeks. Onset of labor is concomitantly reported as occurring either within 24 hours of rupture or more than 24 hours following rupture, which is also sometimes referred to as delayed delivery following PROM.

P01.2 Newborn (suspected to be) affected by oligohydramnios

Oligohydramnios is a condition in which there is an insufficient amount of amniotic fluid in the womb. Fluid levels are measured by an amniotic fluid index (AFI) or deep pocket evaluation. Oligohydramnios is diagnosed with an AFI measurement less than 5 cm, or the absence of a fluid pocket 2-3 cm deep, or a fluid volume less than 500 mL at 32-36 weeks of gestation. This can be caused by leaky membranes, placental problems, and maternal problems such as dehydration, hypertension, pre-eclampsia, and diabetes. Since amniotic fluid is essential for development of the fetus, oligohydramnios can result in compression of the fetal organs, birth defects, growth restriction and deformities, premature delivery, and complications in labor such as cord compression and meconium staining.

P01.3 Newborn (suspected to be) affected by polyhydramnios

Polyhydramnios is a condition in which there is an excess amount of amniotic fluid in the amniotic sac. Levels are measured by an amniotic fluid index (AFI) or deep pocket evaluation. Polyhydramnios is diagnosed with an AFI measurement greater than 25 cm or a single deep pocket measurement less than 8, or a fluid level of 2000mL or more at 32-36 weeks gestation. Most cases are mild, but too much fluid can cause premature membrane rupture, placental abruption, premature delivery, growth restriction with skeletal malformations of the fetus, and stillbirth. It is monitored and treated with medications that can reduce the fluid level, or amniocentesis reduction.

P01.4 Newborn (suspected to be) affected by ectopic pregnancy

Ectopic pregnancy occurs when a fertilized ovum implants itself anywhere other than the uterus. This includes a newborn affected by an adominal pregnancy in which the fertilized ovum implants itself not in the lining of the uterus, but elsewhere in the abdominal cavity, outside of the fallopian

tube or ovary. These type of ectopic pregnancies are very rare with a high mortality, but abdominal pregnancies can still lead to the delivery of a viable infant.

P02.0 Newborn (suspected to be) affected by placenta previa

Placenta previa is an obstetric complication that occurs when the placenta implants and grows in the lower part of the uterus and covers all or part of the cervical opening into the birth canal. During pregnancy, the placenta grows and moves as the uterus stretches. It is common for the placenta to be low in the womb in early pregnancy; but by the third trimester, the placenta should have moved to be near the top of the womb with the cervix open for delivery. Hemorrhaging often starts near the end of the second trimester or at the beginning of the third trimester and can be severe, stop on its own, or start again weeks later. Sometimes labor will begin after several days of heavy bleeding, and in other cases, hemorrhaging begins after labor starts. Severe bleeding can be life threatening to mother and baby, and delivery may be necessary before vital organs are fully formed.

P02.1 Newborn (suspected to be) affected by other forms of placental separation and hemorrhage

This also includes newborns affected by maternal blood loss from accidental or antepartum hemorrhage, or placental damage from amniocentesis, cesarean section, or surgical induction as well as abruptio placentae. Abruptio placentae is the premature separation of the placenta from its attachment to the uterine wall before the baby is born and can be life threatening to both the mother and fetus. The cause may be difficult to ascertain but may occur with abdominal trauma or with a rapid loss of amniotic fluid, blood clotting disorders, and elevated maternal blood pressure.

P02.3 Newborn (suspected to be) affected by placental transfusion syndromes

Placental transfusion syndromes include twin to twin transfusion syndrome, the most common complication of monochorionic pregnancies causing perinatal mortality in twins. The syndrome is believed to result from an uncompensated arteriovenous anastomosis within a monochorionic placenta, which gives a greater net flow of blood to one twin at the expense of the other.

P02.4 Newborn (suspected to be) affected by prolapsed cord

Umbilical cord prolapse is a serious but rare complication of childbirth that poses imminent danger for the baby and must be addressed immediately. It occurs either prior to or during labor and delivery, often as a complication of premature rupture of membranes, breech presentation in premature delivery, and with multiple births. The cord drops down through the cervical opening ino the birth canal ahead of the baby and can then become trapped against the baby's body during delivery. Prolapse causes a loss of oxygen to the fetus through the cord, which is the baby's lifeline, and can result in brain damage or mortality.

P02.69 Newborn (suspected to be) affected by other conditions of umbilical cord

This includes newborns affected by a short umbilical cord or vasa previa. The average length of the umbilical cord at term is 50-60 cm. A short cord at term is around 35 cm. For an infant to be delivered without complications, an untangled cord must be long enough to reach from its insertion at the placenta to the outside of the birth canal. Determining cord length prenatally is not possible. A short cord may make it impossible to deliver vaginally and necessitate C-section. Cord length may be measured after birth because an abnormally short cord length points toward some kind of long-term fetal condition.

Vasa previa is a rare and devastating complication of pregnancy in which unprotected fetal blood vessels (unsupported by the umbilical cord or the placenta) grow across the internal cervical os. These vessels run within the membranes, obstructing the baby's passage into the birth canal, and are at risk of rupturing along with the membranes. Vasa previa can be caused by the cord inserting directly into the membranes and leaving vessels unprotected as they run into the placenta. When these unprotected vessel rupture, bleeding occurs from the fetoplacental circulation, and results in rapid exsanguination and death of the fetus.

P02.7 Newborn (suspected to be) affected by chorioamnionitis

Chorioamnionitis is an inflammation of the membranes around the fetus--the chorion or placental tissue, and the amnion or amniotic fluid. It is usually associated with a bacterial infection and is dangerous to both the mother and child. Chorioamnionitis can cause septicemia in the mother and lead to premature birth and serious infection in the newborn by organisms normally found in the vaginal canal, such as *E. coli*, even Group B streptococcus.

P03.0 Newborn (suspected to be) affected by breech delivery and extraction

Breech delivery occurs when the baby presents the buttocks first. A frank breech occurs with the legs flexed at the hips and the knees extended, so the baby's feet are up by the head. In a complete breech, both of the baby's knees are bent, and the buttocks and feet are closest to the birth canal. In a footling breech, one or both of the baby's feet present first and will deliver before the rest of the body. Breech extraction is a technique in which the obstetrician grabs the feet of the baby and pulls them gently into the birth canal to facilitate the vaginal breech birth. C-section may also be necessary for breech presentation, especially when twins are involved or if a baby is in fetal distress because the head would be the last body part to emerge and passage is not so easilty facilitated with a breech.

P03.1 Newborn (suspected to be) affected by other malpresentation, malposition and disproportion during labor and delivery

This includes newborns affected by a contracted pelvis of the mother, or transverse lie or oblique lie of the fetus for delivery presentation. Transverse lie occurs when the baby's spine lies perpendicular to the spine of the mother, and an oblique presentation occurs when the baby's spine is at an angle close to 45 degrees from the spine of the mother. The shoulder usually presents first in these cases, although the trunk or arm may present first.

P03.5 Newborn (suspected to be) affected by precipitate delivery

A newborn affected by labor that occurred very quickly with a rapid second stage and rapid expulsion.

P03.82 Meconium passage during delivery

This code is used to report the passage of meconium, the first fecal matter from the fetus, during delivery of the child. This substance is typically expelled from the fetus during or shortly before birth, and is not typically problematic for mother or child.

P05.0 Newborn light for gestational age

An infant who weighs less than the normal parameters for the length of time spent in the womb and who displays signs of malnutrition such as dry, peeling skin and loss of subcutaneous tissue in addition to the low birth weight.

P05.1 Newborn small for gestational age

Smaller than normal infant in relation to the amount of time the fetus was in the womb. The newborn may or may not also be light for weight in additional to being small in size for gestational age and display signs of fetal malnutrtion such as dry, peeling skin and loss of subcutaneous tissue.

P05.2 Newborn affected by fetal (intrauterine) malnutrition not light or small for gestational age

An infant showing signs of fetal malnutrition, such as dry, peeling skin, and loss of subcutaneous tissue, although still within the normal weight and size parameters for the length of gestation.

P08.0 Exceptionally large newborn baby

This code is used to report an abnormally large baby, defined as weighing 4500 grams or more at birth.

P08.21 Post-term newborn

Use this code to report a post-term infant, where the fetus gestates for a period between 40 and 42 weeks.

P08.22 Prolonged gestation of newborn

Prolonged term of gestation is longer than 42 weeks.

P22.1 Transient tachypnea of newborn

Transitory tachypnea of a newborn is a condition in which the newborn experiences a short bout of quick, shallow breathing.

P23 Congenital pneumonia

Congenital pneumonia is present at birth and may be transmitted hematogenously (from the mother via the placenta), through an ascending infection coming from the birth canal, or by aspiration of infected amniotic fluid. An infant with congenital pneumonia may have tachypnea (rapid breathing), grunting, retractions, nasal flaring, increased respiratory secretions, and cyanosis.

P23.0 Congenital pneumonia due to viral agent

Viral agents responsible for congenital pneumonia can include cytomegalovirus, herpes simplex virus, hepatitis, rubella, and mumps.

P23.1 Congenital pneumonia due to Chlamydia

Chlamydia is a bacteria frequently spread by sexual partners and is often asymptomatic in women. Chlamydia is the most frequently reported bacterial sexually transmitted disease. Many people do not know they are infected because symptoms can be mild or absent, with three quarters of infected women having no symptoms at all. Chlamydia is passed from mother to baby through vaginal childbirth to cause congenital pneumonia.

P23.2 Congenital pneumonia due to staphylococcus

Staphylococcus causes typical pneumonia symptoms with persistent fever and chills. Symptoms can worsen rapidly with severely deteriorating lung function that could be fatal. Abscesses occasionally form in the lung tissue and air-filled lung cysts may develop in children. Pus in the pleural cavity may need to be drained with a chest tube or by needle aspiration.

P23.3 Congenital pneumonia due to streptococcus, group B

Group B Streptococcus (GBS) is a common bacteria frequently associated with neonatal pneumonia, passed to the newborn during delivery. Group B Streptococcus indicates an infection by the bacterium *Streptococcus agalactiae*. This bacterium commonly resides in the gastrointestinal, urinary, and vaginal tracts of healthy women. Routine maternal screening for GBS and treatment with antibiotics prior to delivery has decreased the incidence of congenital pneumonia and systemic infections.

P23.4 Congenital pneumonia due to Escherichia coli

Escherichia coli is a bacterium commonly found in the intestines as a normal part of the flora that helps digest food. Most *E. coli* is harmless and does not cause disease in humans, but when the bacteria invade other areas of the body, such as the birth canal, and thereby infect the neonate, serious illness such as congenital pneumonia can result.

P23.5 Congenital pneumonia due to Pseudomonas

Pseudomonas is a widespread, opportunistic, gram negative bacteria with many strains resistant to antibiotics because the bacteria can exist with a biofilm coating that makes it more resistant to antibiotics. It is a common bacteria found in soil, water, and on the skin of both humans and animals and can survive in almost any moist environment. It does not usually infect healthy persons, normally only those who are immunocompromised, but it can be a lethal pulmonary pathogen when causing pneumonia. The bacterium produces the enzyme collagenase that breaks down collagen fibers. It attaches itself to mucous tissue through tiny, hair-like fimbriae. Treatment is crucial for survival.

P24.00 Meconium aspiration without respiratory symptoms

Inhalation of the first fecal matter released by the fetus during birth without causing any symptoms.

P25.1 Pneumothorax originating in the perinatal period

Pneumothorax is a collapsed lung caused by air within the pleural space between the two layers that line the outside of the lung and the inside of the chest wall. The air expands the pleural space and pushes against the lung, causing it to collapse, producing sudden chest pain on the affected side with shortness of breath.

P28.0 Primary atelectasis of newborn

Primary atelectasis is a congenital crisis in which the newborn suffers a collapsed lung due to primary failure of the terminal air sacs of the lung to open sufficiently caused by pulmonary hypoplasia or immaturity associated with a short gestation.

P28.2 Cyanotic attacks of newborn

Cyanotic attacks are a condition in which a newborn with normal skin tone suddenly begins to turn blue due to a lack of oxygen for a certain period of time before returning to normal color.

P28.81 Respiratory arrest of newborn

Respiratory arrest of the newborn is the complete cessation of all spontaneous ventilatory movement, like a prolonged apneic period. Repiratory arrest differs from respiratory failure in that the normal tidal flow and movement of the lungs is still present in respiratory failure but the lungs fail to exchange oxygen and carbon dioxide properly, while in respiratory arrest, all breathing action stops.

P29.11 Neonatal tachycardia

Abnormally fast newborn heart rate.

P29.12 Neonatal bradycardia

In neonatal bradycardia, the newborn's heartbeat is abnormally slow, usually under 60 beats per minute.

P29.3 Persistent fetal circulation

Persistent fetal circulation (PFC) is also known as persistent newborn pulmonary hypertension. This condition is relatively rare and usually occurs in sick newborns with meconium aspiration syndrome, intrauterine hypoxia and/or ischemia, birth asphyxia, respiratory distress, and severe sepsis. Severe hypoxia and acidosis result that can lead to mortality, but due to anticipation and early recognition of PFC in modern NICU facilities, as well as improved neonatal care, severe cases of PFC are rarely seen. The condition arises when the newborn's systemic and pulmonary circulation either fail to shift away from the antenatal pattern when the baby is born or convert back to a fetal pattern after birth. In the fetus, blood is shunted away from the lungs because they are not used to exchange oxygen and carbon dioxide. When the newborn first begins to breathe, this pattern of circulation changes dramatically as blood is directed to the lungs for gas exhange. The change in pulmonary pressure after birth from a high vascular resistance to a low vascular resistance is what helps to close the fetal connections for blood flow and redirect it to the lungs. With PFC, there is right to left ductal and/or atrial shunting in the presence of elevated right ventricular pressure.

P35.0 Congenital rubella syndrome

Rubella, also called German measles or three-day measles, is a highly contagious but mild disease to most patients, that can cause serious complications for a neonate when the fetus is infected from the mother. Congenital rubella syndrome can occur in an infant when the mother is infected with rubella virus shortly before conception or during the 1st and 2nd trimesters of pregnancy. When the mother contracts the virus 0-28 days prior to conception, the incidence of fetal infection is 43%; the incidence increases to 51% at 0-12 weeks gestation and decreases to 23% at 13-26 weeks gestation. Rubella syndrome typically has a triad of congenital defects including sensorineural deafness; abnormal eye development including retinopathy, cataracts, or microphthalmia; and heart defects, such as patent ductus arteriosus. Anomalies of the brain, spleen, or liver may also occur.

P35.1 Congenital cytomegalovirus infection

Cytomegalovirus (CMV) causes congenital infection in an infant that acquires it from the birth canal of the mother during delivery whenever primary infection or reactiviation of CMV occurs during the pregnancy. The virus is able to cross the placenta and has a 50% transmission rate to the fetus. Symptoms include low birth weight, microcephaly and developmental delays, seizures, hearing loss, visual impairments, and hepatosplenomegaly.

P35.2 Congenital herpesviral [herpes simplex] infection

Herpes simplex virus (HSV) will rarely cross the placenta with maternal infection, but is more commonly transmitted through infected secretions in the birth canal during labor and delivery causing congenital infection in the fetus. HSV infections can present with external lesions affecting the skin, eyes, and mouth; in internal organs such as the liver and lungs; or in the brain and central nervous system causing encephalitis or meningitis.

P35.3 Congenital viral hepatitis

Viral hepatitis is able to cross the placenta with maternal infection and cause congenital infection in the fetus. The disease is often asymptomatic but can cause acute or chronic liver inflammation leading to liver damage and an increased risk of liver cancer and cirrhosis.

P36 Bacterial sepsis of newborn

Bacterial sepsis in the newborn is a severe infection transmitted hematogenously (from the mother via the placenta), through an ascending infection from the birth canal or by aspiration of infected amniotic fluid. An infant with *Staphylococcus aureus* sepsis may appear acutely ill. Symptoms can include pallor, lethargy, poor feeding, unstable temperature, tachycardia, rapid breathing, grunting, cyanosis, and apnea.

P36.0 Sepsis of newborn due to streptococcus, group B

Group B streptococcus (GBS) is commonly found in the human gastrointestinal, reproductive, and urinary tracts. GBS is a common bacteria found in the vaginal tract of healthy women. Sepsis caused by *S. agalactiae* is most commonly seen in newborns who acquire the infection from their mothers during delivery and is a very serious pathogen that can be deadly without early treatment. An infant infected with GBS sepsis will appear acutely ill. Symptoms can include pallor, lethargy, poor feeding, unstable temperature, tachycardia (elevated heart rate), tachypnea (rapid breathing), cyanosis, and apnea (short periods without breathing). Routine maternal screening and treatment with antibiotics prior to delivery has decreased the incidence of newborn infections.

P36.4 Sepsis of newborn due to Escherichia coli

Escherichia coli is a facultative, anaerobic, gram negative bacillus that inhabits the intestinal tract as part of its normal flora that helps digest food. Most *E. coli* is harmless and does not cause disease in humans, but when the bacteria invade other areas of the body, such as the birth canal, thereby infecting the neonate, serious illness can result, such as infection of the bloodstream causing sepsis. The bacteria produce endotoxins that can lead to disseminated intravascular coagulation and death.

P36.5 Sepsis of newborn due to anaerobes

Anaerobic bacteria identified with neonatal sepsis include gram negative Bacteroides, Fusobacterium, Veillonella, and gram positive Peptostreptococcus, Clostridium, Propionibacterium, and Eubacterium.

P37.0 Congenital tuberculosis

Congenital tuberculosis (TB) is a rare, often fatal infection during the neonatal period (birth to day 28). *Mycobacterium tuberculosis* can spread from the placenta through the umbilical vein to the fetus or by aspiration/ingestion of contaminated fluid and secretions. TB infection may present as pneumonia with elevated lymphocytes in cerebral spinal fluid, fever, or hepatosplenomegaly.

P37.1　Congenital toxoplasmosis

Toxoplasmosis infection by the parasite *Toxoplasma gondii* can be transmitted from an infected mother during gestation, labor, or delivery causing congenital infection in the fetus. The condition may cause preterm labor, low birth weight, damage to the retina, hearing loss, skin rashes, seizures, developmental delays, and hepatosplenomegaly.

P37.2　Neonatal (disseminated) listeriosis

Listeria monocytogenes is a bacterium that can be transmitted from an infected mother to the fetus causing congenital listeriosis. The organism is able to cross the placenta and may also be contracted from the urogenital tract during labor and delivery. Maternal listeriosis can cause miscarriage, still birth, and preterm labor.

P37.4　Other congenital malaria

Malaria parasites can be transmitted from an infected mother to the fetus causing congenital malaria parasitemia. The parasite is able to cross the placenta on maternal erythrocytes during gestation and/or labor and delivery. Symptoms include poor feeding, fever, anemia, jaundice, and hepatosplenomegaly.

P37.5　Neonatal candidiasis

Candida fungus can be transmitted from an infected mother to the fetus causing congenital candidiasis. The route is usually stemming from the urogenital tract of the mother during labor and delivery. The condition may be cutaneous, involving just the skin and mucous membranes with an extensive macular, erythematous rash that includes a pustular, papular, or vesicular phase and ends in extensive desquamation, or sluffing of skin. Rarely, the condition presents systemically without a rash as pneumonia, meningitis, candiduria, or candidemia.

P38　Omphalitis of newborn

Omphalitis is an infection of the umbilical cord stump. Symptoms can include redness, swelling of skin around the stump, purulent drainage, fever, tachycardia, hypotension, lethary, and poor feeding. Untreated infection can lead to sepsis and necrotizing fasciitis. Omphalitis is relatively rare; however, preterm delivery, chorioamnionitis, and umbilical catheters put an infant at increased risk of developing the condition.

P39.0　Neonatal infective mastitis

Neonatal infective mastitis is an uncommon infection of breast tissue in an infant (newborn to 28 days). *Staphylococcus aureus* is the most common bacteria cultured from infected tissue followed by other staphylococcus species and streptococcus species. Symptoms can include swelling and redness of the areola and the underlying or surrounding breast tissue, abscess formation, and fluid drainage from the nipple.

P39.1　Neonatal conjunctivitis and dacryocystitis

The conjunctiva is a thin, transparent membrane which covers and protects the sclera, the white of the eye, as well as the inside of the eyelids. Conjunctivitis, sometimes called pink-eye, is an inflammation that presents with the tell-tale pink coloration of the white of the eye, swelling and irritation, and excessive tearing. Conjunctivitis caused by an infection typically begins in one eye and spreads to the other and is highly contagious. A common type of conjunctivitis in newborns is chlamydial conjunctivitis when the fetus is infected by the mother as it passes through the birth canal. The infection causes pustules and swelling on the inside of the eyelid, as well as a discharge of pus and mucus from the eye. The eye may turn red, and the cornea may become involved as well as infecting the lacrimal sac at the inner corner of the eye.

P50　Newborn affected by intrauterine (fetal) blood loss

When the fetus loses blood in the prenatal or perinatal period, anemia develops in the neonate. Since blood volume is very low in neonates, even a small amount of acute blood loss (15-20 mL) results in anemia. Fetal blood loss may occur from fetal to maternal hemorrhage, twin to twin transfusion

syndrome, umbilical cord complications, abnormalities in the placenta, diagnostic procedures, or maternal trauma. Perinatal hemorrhage may be brought on by a precipitous or rapid delivery less than 3 hours after labor has begun, causing tearing of the umbilical cord, or by obstetrical accidents during Cesarean section.

P50.0　Newborn affected by intrauterine (fetal) blood loss from vasa previa

Vasa previa is a rare and devastating complication of pregnancy in which unprotected fetal blood vessels (unsupported by the umbilical cord or the placenta) grow across the internal cervical os. These vessels run within the membranes, obstructing the baby's passage into the birth canal, and are at risk of rupturing along with the membranes. Vasa previa can be caused by the cord inserting directly into the membranes and leaving vessels unprotected as they run into the placenta. When these unprotected vessels rupture, bleeding occurs from the fetoplacental circulation, and results in rapid exsanguination and death of the fetus.

P51　Umbilical hemorrhage of newborn

Umbilical cord hemorrhage occurs infrequently but is associated with a high risk of fetal asphyxia or death. This type of hemorrhage is usually spontaneous and characterized by leakage of blood from the umbilical vein or an artery into the wharton jelly. Aneurysm of an artery or rupture of a dilation along the umbilical vein may be the underlying cause of hemorrhage.

P52.0　Intraventricular (nontraumatic) hemorrhage, grade 1, of newborn

A grade I cerebral hemorrhage is a disorder in which the bleeding occurs in a small area around the brain ventricles.

P52.1　Intraventricular (nontraumatic) hemorrhage, grade 2, of newborn

In grade II cerebral hemorrhage, bleeding occurs inside the ventricles.

P52.21　Intraventricular (nontraumatic) hemorrhage, grade 3, of newborn

A grade III cerebral hemorrhage should be reported when the affected ventricles are enlarged from profuse bleeding.

P52.22　Intraventricular (nontraumatic) hemorrhage, grade 4, of newborn

In grade IV newborn cerebral hemorrhage, blood seeps from the ventricles into the surrounding brain tissue.

P55.0　Rh isoimmunization of newborn

Hemolytic disease from isoimmunization poses increased risks to the newborn. Rh isoimmunization is an incompatibility of blood protein types between the mother and the fetus. When a woman is Rh negative, she does not have a certain protein on the surface of her red blood cells (RBCs). An Rh positive fetus does have the protein and this creates a blood type incompatibility. The mother's immune system recognizes the baby's Rh positive RBCs as a foreign invader and begins producing antibodies against the baby's blood cells. This does not usually cause a problem in the first pregnancy, but will attack subsequent pregnancies causing jaundice, anemia, retardation, and in severe cases, when hemolytic disease of the newborn develops fully, it can cause death in utero or shortly after birth.

P55.1　ABO isoimmunization of newborn

Hemolytic disease of the newborn due to ABO isoimmunization is a rarer form of the condition than that due to Rh isoimmunization and occurs when the mother's blood type (A, B, O) is incompatible with the blood type of the fetus. ABO isoimmunization is an immune reaction that occurs when two different, and incompatible, major blood groups are mixed together. The three major blood types, A, B, and O are determined by very specific molecules, or antigens, present on the surface of blood cells. These antigens act like immune system triggers against blood of a different group. Hemolytic disease in the newborn from ABO isoimmunization can be caused by maternal Anti-A or Anti-B sensitization that occurs when a mother who does not have the A or B group antigen becomes sensitized against it by the baby's blood, which does have the A or B group antigen. Exposure causes the mother's immune system to produce IgG immune globulins against the A or B antigen in the baby's blood. The immune globulins cross the placenta into the fetal circulation and attack the baby's red blood cells as foreign and leads to ABO hemolytic disease of the newborn (HDN). In most cases, the HDN is mild and short-lived as A and B surface antigens are not fully developed on red blood cells in the neonate and they also occur on many different cell types, leaving less Anti-A or Anti-B antibodies to bind specifically to red blood cells. This is normally diagnosed when a baby develops jaundice in the first day of life. Symptomatic hemolytic disease occurs when mothers with O blood type produce enough antibodies to cause hemolysis in the newborn.

P56   Hydrops fetalis due to hemolytic disease

Hydrops fetalis is an accumulation of excess fluid in two or more fetal compartments, usually arising from an initial overproduction of interstitial fluid, followed by inadequate lymphatic drainage. These compartments can include subcutaneous tissue, scalp, pleural space, pericardium, and the abdomen. Hydrops fetalis due to hemolytic disease can be caused by immune mediated destruction of the fetal red blood cells by the mother's immune system (most commonly Rh-anti D isoimmunization), twin to twin transfusion syndrome, severe anemia, and hemorrhagic disorders.

P56.0   Hydrops fetalis due to isoimmunization

Hydrops fetalis due to isoimmunization may be caused by Rh isoimmunization or an ABO blood type isoimmunization. Isoimmunization is an immune reaction that occurs when two different, and incompatible, blood types are mixed together. Rh isoimmunization is an incompatibility of specific blood protein types between the mother and the fetus. When a woman is Rh negative, she does not have a certain protein on the surface of her red blood cells (RBCs). An Rh positive fetus does have the protein and this creates a blood type incompatibility. ABO isoimmunization is more rare than that due to Rh isoimmunization and occurs when the mother's major blood type (A, B, O) is incompatible with the blood type of the fetus. In either case, the mother's immune system recognizes the baby's red blood cells as a foreign invader and begins producing antibodies against the baby's blood cells.

P57   Kernicterus

Kernicterus is a neonatal encephalopathy caused by hyperbilirubinemia. Excess bilirubin circulating in the blood can cross the blood-brain barrier and accumulate in the gray matter of the central nervous system. Bilirubin is neurotoxic, causing irreversible destruction of neurons by apoptosis and necrosis.

P57.0   Kernicterus due to isoimmunization

Kernicterus due to isoimmunization is neonatal brain dysfunction due to hyperbilirubinemia, a serious form of jaundice, caused by the destruction of the infant's red blood cells by the mother's immune system. Isoimmunization is an immune reaction that occurs when two different, and incompatible, blood types are mixed together. In this case, the mother's immune system recognizes the baby's red blood cells as a foreign invader and begins producing antibodies against the baby's blood cells, destroying them and releasing bilirubin into the blood stream. The excess bilirubin circulating in the blood crosses the blood-brain barrier and accumulates in the baby's central nervous system, becoming toxic and causing irreversible destruction of brain cells.

P59.1   Inspissated bile syndrome

Inspissated bile syndrome is an uncommon cause of jaundice in a newborn that results from the presence of intraluminal bile plugs, sludge, or gallstones blocking the bile ducts.

P59.3   Neonatal jaundice from breast milk inhibitor

Neonatal jaundice from breast milk inhibitor occurs when factors present in breast milk increase enterohepatic circulation of bilirubin. B-glucuronidase is one factor that uncouples bilirubin bound to glucuronic acid. A genetic polymorphism in coding sequences of two genes, UDPGT1A1 and OATP2, can lead to elevated bilirubin linked to breast milk inhibitors. Treatment includes interruption of breast milk feedings for 24-48 hours and phototherapy.

P59.9   Neonatal jaundice, unspecified

Jaundice (hyperbilirubinemia, neonatal icterus) is fairly common in newborns. It is characterized by a yellow discoloration of the sclera of the eye and skin, caused by elevated levels of unconjugated bilirubin. The condition can be due to the relative inactivity of an enzyme, glucuronosyltransferase, that converts unconjugated bilirubin to conjugated bilirubin, shorter life span of fetal red blood cells, and low conversion of bilirubin to urobilinogen in the intestine.

P70.0   Syndrome of infant of mother with gestational diabetes

Infants born to a mother who suffers from a persistently elevated blood sugar level are often larger than normal, making a normal vaginal birth difficult and necessitating C-section. These babies may also suffer an episode of low blood sugar shortly after birth because their own level of insulin production is high, sometimes requiring intravenous glucose solution. Severe cases of hypoglycemia can even trigger seizures in the infant. The baby may also suffer from jaundice and respiratory distress syndrome, even if they are not born prematurely; but very often, the baby needs to be delivered early, before the lungs and liver are mature enough to function properly, due to the large size and excessive weight of the baby.

P74.0   Late metabolic acidosis of newborn

Acidosis in the newborn is a decreased pH in blood and body tissues due to the accumulation of hydrogen ions and acid or a depleted amount of bicarbonate (alkaline or base content). Metabolic acidosis is a shift in the body's acid/base balance to the acidic side because of a loss of base or retention of fixed or nonvolatile acids that exist in the body other than carbonic acid.

P76.0   Meconium plug syndrome

Select this code to report meconium obstruction, in which the dark green feces that comprises a newborn's first bowel movement blocks the intestine.

P76.2   Intestinal obstruction due to inspissated milk

An intestinal obstruction in the newborn due to thickened, condensed breast milk within the digestive system.

P77   Necrotizing enterocolitis of newborn

Necrotizing enterocolitis is a condition primarily seen in premature and sick infants, in which portions or areas of the bowel suffer necrosis, or death of the tissue. In neonates, this is the most common medical and surgical emergency. It occurs when acute inflammation or infection by intestinal bacteria sets in, attacking the intestinal walls, and causing the tissue to begin to die. This condition is diagnosed in stages of severity.

P77.1   Stage 1 necrotizing enterocolitis in newborn

Stage I necrotizing enterocolitis in newborn (NEC) is suspected NEC with mild, nonspecific, systemic signs like bradycardia and apnea; intestinal signs like mild abdominal distention; and x-rays that may be normal or show mild distention. There may also be the presence of blood in the stool. Treatment is nothing by mouth with antibiotics for three days.

P77.2   Stage 2 necrotizing enterocolitis in newborn

Stage II is definite disease. All of the mild systemic signs of stage I are present plus absent bowel sounds and moderate illness such as mild levels of metabolic acidosis and thrombocytopenia. There is definite abdominal tenderness and x-rays show ileus and/or pneumatosis intestinalis and portal vein gas with or without ascites. This is often called medical NEC as infants are treated medically by stopping feedings by mouth; draining air and fluid from the stomach and intestines; giving IV fluid, nutritional replacement, and antibiotics for infection; and careful monitoring. Some infants may be back on regular feedings within 72 hours. Central venous access devices are often placed to ensure optimal, uninterrupted delivery of antibiotic and maximized nourishment.

P77.3 Stage 3 necrotizing enterocolitis in newborn

Stage III represents advanced NEC with severe illness that is progressing towards surgical intervention. In the first part of the stage, the patient has an intact bowel and all conditions of the previous stages with the addition of hypotension, respiratory failure, severe metabolic acidosis, coagulopathy, or neutropenia. There is marked abdominal distention with generalized peritonitis and definite ascites. Treatment involves NPO for two weeks, fluid resuscitation, and ventilator support with surgical consultation. When perforated bowel is observed, surgical treatment includes resecting the affected bowel with ostomy placement and later reanastomosis.

P78.2 Neonatal hematemesis and melena due to swallowed maternal blood

Use this code to report hematemesis (vomiting blood) and melena (bloody stools) due to swallowed maternal blood. These conditions occur when the newborn swallows blood during delivery.

P83.0 Sclerema neonatorum

Sclerema neonatorum is a rare condition in which the subcutaneous fat of an infant begins to harden, causing a waxy hardness of the skin to develop. This disease usually occurs in infants who are premature or already ill.

P83.1 Neonatal erythema toxicum

Neonatal erythema toxicum is a harmless, self-limiting, common rash that appears in approximately half of all infants carried to term. The rash usually appears within a couple of days of birth and consists of tiny, firm, yellowish white bumps that may be filled with fluid surrounded by a red ring. At other times, the rash may appear as splotchy redness without the tiny bumps. It can cover most of the baby's skin or be localized to one area, but rarely affects the palms or soles of the feet. Toxic erythema of the newborn is not associated with any health problems, is not contagious, and often goes away on its own in a matter of days or within a week. More severe cases may have urticarial papules appear on the back and buttocks. There is no known associated cause. No virus or bacteria have been found and the fluid within the tiny blisters contains harmless blood cells.

P83.2 Hydrops fetalis not due to hemolytic disease

Hydrops fetalis is an accumulation of excess fluid in two or more fetal compartments, usually arising from an initial overproduction of interstitial fluid, followed by inadequate lymphatic drainage. These compartments can include subcutaneous tissue, the scalp, pleural space, pericardium, and the abdomen. Nonhemolytic causes of hydrops fetalis are most commonly heart/lung diseases, genetic abnormalities, and TORCH infections-- toxoplasmosis (T), other infections (O)- coxsackievirus, varicella-zoster virus, HIV, parvovirus B19), rubella (R), cytomegalovirus (C), and herpes simplex-2 (H).

P84 Other problems with newborn

This code includes acidemia, acidosis, hypercapnia, mixed metabolic and respiratory acidosis of newborn, as well as anoxia or hypoxia, hypoxemia, and asphyxia of newborn. Hypoxemia is a state of deficient oxygenation of the blood. Hypoxia is a deficiency of oxygen reaching the tissues of the body. These conditions may be noted within the normal birth process, and are coded here when they have not led to brain damage.

P91.2 Neonatal cerebral leukomalacia

A condition in which the white matter that comprises the inner part of the brain becomes soft and damaged. This affects the transmission of neural impulses from the brain to the spinal cord. This condition can be hard to diagnose. The most common symptom seems to be problems moving the legs.

P91.6 Hypoxic ischemic encephalopathy [HIE]

Hypoxic-ischemic encephalopathy (HIE) is perinatal cerebral injury, or brain damage, causing morbidity and mortality in the neonate. The condition that causes this brain damage is ischemia resulting from hypoxemia, hypercapnia, and acidosis that have gone beyond what may occur during a normal birth process. Mild, moderate, and severe cases of HIE are determined by clinical presentation and imaging evidence.

P91.61 Mild hypoxic ischemic encephalopathy [HIE]

Mild cases of hypoxic ischemic encephalopathy [HIE] are marked by slightly increased muscle tone and brisk deep tendon reflexes during the first few days of life. Certain transient behavior abnormalities, such as irritability, excessive crying, excessive sleepiness, and poor feeding may be observed. With mild cases, after the first few days of life, the findings from a central nervous system examination return normal.

P91.62 Moderate hypoxic ischemic encephalopathy [HIE]

With moderate cases of hypoxic ischemic encephalopathy [HIE], the infant appears lethargic with diminished deep tendon reflexes and significant hypotonia. Normal reflexes such as grabbing and sucking are sluggish or absent and the infant can experience bouts of apnea. Seizures may occur within the first 24 hours. The infant may display an initial period of only mild HIE followed by a sudden deterioration, in which seizure intensity might increase. Full recovery is possible in moderate cases and the long-term outcome is better in these instances.

P91.63 Severe hypoxic ischemic encephalopathy [HIE]

With severe hypoxic ischemic encephalopathy [HIE], the infant is typically in a stupor or coma and does not respond to any physical stimulus. Respiratory support may be required as breathing is irregular. Muscles have generalized hypotonia, while deep tendon reflexes are depressed with an absence of neonatal reflexes such as sucking or grabbing. Cranial nerve evaluation shows disturbances in ocular movements, nystagmus, bobbing, or loss of conjugate gaze. Pupils are dilated or fixed and poorly reactive. Seizures are often generalized and may increase during the 48 hours after onset. The fontanelle may bulge with increasing cerebral edema, and heart rate and blood pressure are irregular. A feeding tube may be required for weeks or months. Multiple organ systems are involved, such as the heart, kidney, liver, lungs, and the hematological system. The mortality rate for severe cases has been reported up to 75%, with most deaths occurring in the first week of life. Up to 80% who survive develop serious complications, 10-20% develop moderately serious disabilities, and about 10% remain healthy.

P92.01 Bilious vomiting of newborn

Bilious vomiting in the newborn is an urgent condition that requires immediate attention. With or without abdominal distention, bilious vomiting indicates intestinal obstruction and that a surgical condition is present. A naso- or orogastric tube is placed immediately for gastric decompression. An IV line is placed for administration of fluids, nutrition, and electrolytes. When the patient is hemodynamically stable, a focused examination is done that includes plain abdominal films and contrast studies. Pediatric surgeons and neonatologists are immediately consulted for perioperative and operative management when dilated loops of bowel and air-fluid levels demonstrate intestinal obstruction. The condition is caused by duodenal or jejunoileal atresia, malrotation and volvulus, meconium ileus, and necrotizing enterocolitis.

P92.1 Regurgitation and rumination of newborn

Regurgitation (bringing up food from the stomach) and rumination (rechewing and reswallowing regurgitated food) is not uncommon in infants and children. It normally occurs within minutes of a meal and no retching or sour taste is present. Weight loss, foul smelling breath, and raw chapped lips may be symptoms of the disorder.

P92.2 Slow feeding of newborn

Slow feeding or slow milk intake of a newborn may lead to poor weight gain, as well as nutritional and growth problems. It can be due to slow flow of breastmilk or improper size or shape nipple on a bottle. It can also occur when the bottle or breast is taken away too soon because the infant is feeding slower than normal and requires more time to ingest the required amount of milk. Premature infants with an underdeveloped sucking and swallowing reflex, infants with congenital anomalies of the mouth or face, and those with neurological disorders may be slow feeders.

P92.3 Underfeeding of newborn

Underfeeding of a newborn is usually identified by poor weight gain. Underfeeding may occur when there is insufficient breast milk or formula, when an infant is sleepy or lethargic and feeds for only short periods of time, or when a congenital anomaly is present that limits the infant's ability to feed on demand.

P92.4 Overfeeding of newborn

Overfeeding of a newborn is usually identified by rapid weight gain. Overfeeding can be due to the infant suckling at the breast for extended periods of time or stimulating the infant's mouth with a nipple when bottle feeding to encourage feeding. Symptoms often include abdominal distention and vomiting.

P92.5 Neonatal difficulty in feeding at breast

Neonatal difficulty in feeding at the breast can be due to maternal factors and infant factors. A mother's breast may be too firm, too large, or the nipple may be flat or inverted. Milk let down may be too slow which requires the infant to suck excessively or it may be too fast, causing the infant to choke and gag. An infant may have a small mouth, large tongue, or a tight frenulum of the tongue.

P92.6 Failure to thrive in newborn

Failure to thrive in a newborn means delayed physical growth and weight gain failure that can cause developmental delays. Children who are undernourished in the first year of life, especially, have developmental delays. This diagnosis is given to newborns 28 days old and under who remain underweight and do not gain weight for unclear reasons. The determination is based on growth chart comparisons, thorough examination, and parental answers about the baby's health and environment. Medical disorders, such as gastrointestinal reflux, esophageal narrowing, and malabsorption, as well as minor disorders caused by cleft palate or cleft lip, such as difficulty swallowing, are often the cause of failure to thrive. Some environmental and social factors can also be responsible, such as parental neglect or abuse, parental mental health instability, or disruptive family situations.

P96.5 Complication to newborn due to (fetal) intrauterine procedure

Procedures performed on the fetus while still in utero include: vesico-amniotic shunting for urinary tract obstruction, placement of thoracic-amniotic shunt, resection of malformed pulmonary tissue, removal of sacrococcygeal teratoma, laser ablation of anastomic vessels in twin to twin transfusion syndrome, neural tube defect repair in spina bifida, and tracheal occlusion for congenital diaphragmatic hernia. Open fetal surgery carries a high risk of complications that can affect the newborn or cause loss of the fetus. Endoscopic fetal surgery is becoming available as a possible option for intervention and treatment.

P96.83 Meconium staining

A condition in which fetal fecal matter is found in the amniotic fluid.

Q00.0 Anencephaly

Anencephaly is a defect that occurs when the head end of the neural tube that forms the brain and spinal cord in the embryo fails to close during the 3rd or 4th week of pregnancy and the fetus develops without a brain in the cranial vault, or even without a skull or scalp. Most infants with anencephaly are stillborn. Babies born with this defect may have a functioning brainstem that responds with reflex actions, but die shortly after delivery.

Q00.1 Craniorachischisis

Craniorachischisis is a severe neural tube defect characterized by a total or partial fissure involving exposure of both the skull and spinal column. The condition is very rare and includes both anencephaly and spinal bifida (myelomeningocele). The cause is believed to be both genetic and environmental and most fetuses with this condition will typically miscarry.

Q00.2 Iniencephaly

Iniencephaly is a severe neural tube defect characterized by an occipital bone defect, myelomeningocele at the level of the cervical vertebrae, and retroflexion in which the fetus' head is severely bent backwards at an angle so that the face looks upward. The neck is usually absent, and other defects of the skull, chest, and gastrointestinal system are usually apparent. The condition is very rare and babies with iniencephaly seldom live longer than a few hours after delivery.

Q01 Encephalocele

An encephalocele is a defect in the neural tube that forms the brain and spinal cord in the embryo that results in the brain and its protective membranes protruding through an opening in the skull.

Q01.0 Frontal encephalocele

Frontal encephalocele is a sac-like protrusion of brain tissue, protective membrane, and/or cerebral spinal fluid through an opening in the midline, anterior area of the skull.

Q01.1 Nasofrontal encephalocele

Nasofrontal encephalocele is a sac-like protrusion of brain tissue, protective membrane, and/or cerebral spinal fluid through an opening in the area of the forehead, extending down to the nasal cavities.

Q01.2 Occipital encephalocele

Occipital encephalocele is a sac-like protrusion of brain tissue, protective membrane, and/or cerebral spinal fluid through an opening in the posterior area of the skull.

Q01.8 Encephalocele of other sites

Other sites of an encephalocele can include the nasoethmoidal (nose and ethmoid sinus) area and the naso-orbital (nose and eyes) area.

Q02 Microcephaly

Microcephalus is a condition in which the head, brain, or both are abnormally small in relation to body size, gender, and age.

Q03 Congenital hydrocephalus

Congenital hydrocephalus is a condition present at birth in which excess cerebral spinal fluid (CSF) accumulates in the brain from an abnormality in the balance between production and absorption of CSF flowing through the ventricles and exiting into the cisterns. It can be caused by infection or other influences during fetal development, trauma during the pregnancy, exposure to teratogenic substances, and defects of the spine (open neural tube defects). The excess fluid causes increased pressure inside the baby's skull with widening of the spaces or ventricles of the brain that leads to enlargement of the head, convulsions, visual problems, and mental impairment. Treatment usually involves the surgical placement of a shunt to divert the flow of CSF from the brain to another area of the body where it can be reabsorbed in the bloodstream.

Q03.0 Malformations of aqueduct of Sylvius

Stenosis or obstruction in the acqueduct between the third and fourth ventricles in the middle of the brain, known as the aqueduct of Sylvius, is one of the more common causes of noncommunicating or obstructive type of hydrocephalus. This form of hydrcephalus results when the cerebrospinal fluid is blocked along one of its narrow passageways between the ventricles of the brain.

Q03.1 Atresia of foramina of Magendie and Luschka

Atresia of the foramina of Magendie and Luschka is a congenital malformation of the 4th ventricle in the brain. The foramen Magendie is a single opening in the midline of the 4th ventricle that drains cerebrospinal fluid (CSF) into the cisterna magna. The foramina Luschka are two lateral (right and left) openings from the 4th ventricle that drain CSF into the cerebellopontine angle cistern. When these openings are absent or obstructed, CSF does not circulate properly and will cause a build up of fluid in the ventricle (hydrocephalus).

Q04.0 Congenital malformations of corpus callosum

The corpus callosum is a band of white matter that connects the two hemispheres of the brain. Malformations of this structure can include agenesis (complete or partial absence), hypogenesis (partial formation), dysgenesis (malformation), and hypoplasia (underdevelopment).

Q04.1 Arhinencephaly

Arhinencephaly is a congenital defect of the brain often occurring together with cleft lip or palate and manifesting with a spectrum of malformations related to different degrees of failed lobation of the brain hemispheres. It is usually characterized by partial or compete absence of the olfactory bulbs or nerve tracts, and parts of the hippocampus with its related commissural systems. Arhinencephaly may also be associated with external hydrocephaly.

Q04.2 Holoprosencephaly

Holoprosencephaly (HPE) is a congenital defect of the face and brain caused by an early embryonic failure of the forebrain to divide into two hemispheres. Three forms of HPE have been identified. Alobar HPE is the most severe and is characterized by almost complete failure of forebrain separation. The nose is missing and the eyes are merged into a single median structure. Semilobar HPE has some forebrain separation and facial anomalies may or may not be present. Lobar HPE may have a considerable amount of forebrain separation, rare facial anomalies, and brain function can be nearly normal. No single cause has been identified for this condition.

Q04.3 Other reduction deformities of brain

Other reduction deformities of the brain includes agenesis, hypoplasia, or aplasia of part of the brain, agyria, mircogyria, or pachygyria, lissencephaly, and hydranencephaly. Microgyria is a developmental malformation of the brain in which the normal ridges or folds on the brain surface are exceptionally small, either generally or in one focal area of the brain. Unilateral forms of microgyria in a relatively small area may cause only mild neurological problems, such as seizures. Bilateral forms of microgyria produce more serious neurological problems such as delayed development, epilepsy, muscle weakness or paralysis, and trouble swallowing. Generalized bilateral cases are most severe, causing severe intellectual and movement disabilities, and recurring seizures that cannot be controlled with medication. Agyria is an absence of ridges or folds on the brain surface and pachygyria is broad folds on the brain surface. Lissencephaly encompasses a continuous spectrum of malformations from complete to variable degrees of agyria and pachygyria, also known as 'smooth brain.' Patients with severe cases of an absence of normal folds in the cerebral cortex usually do not live beyond 10 years of age.

Q04.4   Septo-optic dysplasia of brain

Septo-optic dysplasia (SOD, de Morsier syndrome) is characterized by hypoplasia of the optic nerve and absence of a midline structure of the brain called the septum pellucidum. Hypopituitarism may also be present. The optic disc is usually small and nystagmus is present. Vision may be normal or the individual can be partially or totally blind. Seizures are frequently associated with the condition and pituitary hormones may be absent or at lower than normal levels. Growth hormone deficiency is often associated with this condition.

Q04.5   Megalencephaly

Megalencephaly (macroencephaly) is an abnormal, enlarged, heavy brain. The brain enlargement is possibly due to a disturbance in neuron proliferation and brain cell production. Symptoms include developmental delays, seizures, and corticospinal (brain cortex and spinal cord) dysfunction.

Q04.6   Congenital cerebral cysts

Congenital cerebral cysts is a rare condition characterized by the formation of cavities in the cerebral cortex of the brain. Causes include abnormal development of the brain, trauma, or localized softening of brain tissue (encephalomalacia) from hemorrhage or inflammation. Cerebral cysts can cause very minor neurological problems or be severely disabling.

Q04.8   Other specified congenital malformations of brain

Other specified congenital malformations of the brain includes macrogyria and Arnold-Chiari syndrome, type IV. Macrogyria is abnormally large folds or ridges on the surface of the cerebral cortex, caused by a reduced number of sulci in the cerebrum, and an increase in brain tissue. This can cause developmental delay with mental retardation, epilepsy, palsy, and oromotor dysfunction with an inability to coordinate the muscles of the mouth, affecting swallowing and communication. Arnold-Chiari syndrome, type IV is a rare malformation involving an incomplete, underdeveloped cerebellum, sometimes with spina bifida and exposed portions of the skull.

Q04.9   Congenital malformation of brain, unspecified

Unspecified congenital malformations of the brain include any anomaly, deformity, or otherwise unspecified disease of the brain, such as a localized lesion, that has been present from birth, whether occurring during fetal development or the birth process, by inheritance, or environmental factors.

Q05   Spina bifida

Spina bifida means cleft or split spine. This occurs whenever the neural tube of the developing embryo does not close all the way, leaving an abnormal vertebral opening at any level in the spinal column. This results in a permanently disabling birth defect, although with a wide range of severity. The manifestations of spina bifida are many, including (hydro) meningocele, myelomeningocele, syringomyelocele, and rachischisis. Meningocele is a protrusion of part of the protective covering of the spinal cord within a sac-like structure that may or may not be covered by skin, through an open spinal column defect. Spinal fluid surrounds the tissue in the protruding sac, which does not contain any neural elements, and there is usually minor disability, although some may experience paralysis and bladder and bowel dysfunction. Myelomeningocele, also called spina bifida cystica, and syringomyelocele are both a protrusion, or herniation, of the protective membrane and neuronal tissue of the spinal cord through an open defect in the spinal column. Syringomyelocele, however, is due to an increase in the cerebrospinal fluid within the syrinx, or central cavity, of the cord that expands the cord tissue into a thin-walled sac and pushes itself and neighboring membrane out through the open defect. Serious nerve damage and disabilities with partial or complete paralysis below the level of the deformity occurs even with surgical treatment within days of birth. Rachischisis is a very severe form of spina bifida, known as complete spina

bifida, in which there is a cleft or fissure through the entire vertebral column level, often from the cervical level down to the sacrum.

Q05.0   Cervical spina bifida with hydrocephalus

Cervical spina bifida occurs whenever the neural tube of the developing embryo does not close all the way, leaving an abnormal vertebral opening in the spinal column at the cervical level. The manifestations of spina bifida most likely to occur with hydrocephalus are syringomyelocele and myelomeningocele, also called spina bifida cystica. Myelomeningocele and syringomyelocele are both a protrusion, or herniation, of the protective membrane and neuronal tissue of the spinal cord through an open defect in the spinal column. Syringomyelocele, however, is due to an increase in the cerebrospinal fluid within the syrinx, or central cavity, of the cord that expands the cord tissue into a thin-walled sac and pushes itself and neighboring membrane out through the open defect. These types of spina bifida most often occur with hydrocephalus because the cerebrospinal fluid (CSF) that protects the brain and spinal cord is not able to flow and drain normally. CSF builds up, causing swelling of the head and pressure on the brain. Serious nerve damage and disabilities include partial or complete paralysis below the cervical level, even though it is treated surgically within the first three days of life.

Q05.1   Thoracic spina bifida with hydrocephalus

Thoracic spina bifida occurs whenever the neural tube of the developing embryo does not close all the way, leaving an abnormal vertebral opening in the spinal column at the thoracic level. The manifestations of spina bifida most likely to occur with hydrocephalus are syringomyelocele and myelomeningocele, also called spina bifida cystica. Myelomeningocele and syringomyelocele are both a protrusion, or herniation, of the protective membrane and neuronal tissue of the spinal cord through an open defect in the spinal column. Syringomyelocele, however, is due to an increase in the cerebrospinal fluid within the syrinx, or central cavity, of the cord that expands the cord tissue into a thin-walled sac and pushes itself and neighboring membrane out through the open defect. These types of spina bifida most often occur with hydrocephalus because the cerebrospinal fluid (CSF) that protects the brain and spinal cord is not able to flow and drain normally. CSF builds up, causing swelling of the head and pressure on the brain. Serious nerve damage and disabilities include partial or complete paralysis below the thoracic level, even though it is treated surgically within the first three days of life.

Q05.2   Lumbar spina bifida with hydrocephalus

Lumbar spina bifida occurs whenever the neural tube of the developing embryo does not close all the way, leaving an abnormal vertebral opening in the spinal column at the lumbar level. The manifestations of spina bifida most likely to occur with hydrocephalus are syringomyelocele and myelomeningocele, also called spina bifida cystica. Myelomeningocele and syringomyelocele are both a protrusion, or herniation, of the protective membrane and neuronal tissue of the spinal cord through an open defect in the spinal column. Syringomyelocele, however, is due to an increase in the cerebrospinal fluid within the syrinx, or central cavity, of the cord that expands the cord tissue into a thin-walled sac and pushes itself and neighboring membrane out through the open defect. These types of spina bifida most often occur with hydrocephalus because the cerebrospinal fluid (CSF) that protects the brain and spinal cord is not able to flow and drain normally. CSF builds up, causing swelling of the head and pressure on the brain. Serious nerve damage and disabilities include partial or complete paralysis below the lumbar level, even though it is treated surgically within the first three days of life.

Q05.3   Sacral spina bifida with hydrocephalus

Sacral spina bifida occurs whenever the neural tube of the developing embryo does not close all the way, leaving an abnormal vertebral opening in the spinal column at the sacral level. The manifestations of spina bifida most likely to occur with hydrocephalus are syringomyelocele and myelomeningocele, also called spina bifida cystica. Myelomeningocele and syringomyelocele are both a protrusion, or herniation, of the protective membrane and neuronal tissue of the spinal cord through an open defect in the spinal column. Syringomyelocele, however, is due to an increase in the cerebrospinal fluid within the syrinx, or central cavity, of the cord

Malformations/Deformations/Abnormalities

Q04.4 – Q05.3

that expands the cord tissue into a thin-walled sac and pushes itself and neighboring membrane out through the open defect. These types of spina bifida most often occur with hydrocephalus because the cerebrospinal fluid (CSF) that protects the brain and spinal cord is not able to flow and drain normally. CSF builds up, causing swelling of the head and pressure on the brain. Serious nerve damage and disabilities include partial or complete paralysis below the sacral level, even though it is treated surgically within the first three days of life.

Q05.4 Unspecified spina bifida with hydrocephalus

Spina bifida means cleft or split spine and occurs whenever the neural tube of the developing embryo does not close all the way, leaving an abnormal vertebral opening at any level in the spinal column. The manifestations of spina bifida most likely to occur with hydrocephalus are syringomyelocele and myelomeningocele, also called spina bifida cystica. Myelomeningocele and syringomyelocele are both a protrusion, or herniation, of the protective membrane and neuronal tissue of the spinal cord through an open defect in the spinal column. Syringomyelocele, however, is due to an increase in the cerebrospinal fluid within the syrinx, or central cavity, of the cord that expands the cord tissue into a thin-walled sac and pushes itself and neighboring membrane out through the open defect. These types of spina bifida most often occur with hydrocephalus because the cerebrospinal fluid (CSF) that protects the brain and spinal cord is not able to flow and drain normally. CSF builds up, causing swelling of the head and pressure on the brain. Serious nerve damage and disabilities include partial or complete paralysis below the lesion level, even though it is treated surgically within the first three days of life.

Note: Use this unspecified code when a type of spina bifida is documented with hydrocephalus, but without mention of the vertebral level where the defect occurred.

Q05.5 Cervical spina bifida without hydrocephalus

Cervical spina bifida occurs whenever the neural tube of the developing embryo does not close all the way, leaving an abnormal vertebral opening in the spinal column at the cervical level. The manifestation of spina bifida most likely to occur without hydrocephalus is meningocele. A meningocele is a protrusion of part of the protective covering of the spinal cord within a sac-like structure that may or may not be covered by skin, through an open spinal column defect. Spinal fluid surrounds the tissue in the protruding sac, which does not contain any neural elements, and there is usually minor disability, although some may experience paralysis and bladder and bowel dysfunction. With meningocele, the cerebrospinal fluid that protects the brain and spinal cord is most often still able to flow and drain normally, so it does not build up causing hydrocephalus.

Q05.6 Thoracic spina bifida without hydrocephalus

Thoracic spina bifida occurs whenever the neural tube of the developing embryo does not close all the way, leaving an abnormal vertebral opening in the spinal column at the thoracic level. The manifestation of spina bifida most likely to occur without hydrocephalus is meningocele. A meningocele is a protrusion of part of the protective covering of the spinal cord within a sac-like structure that may or may not be covered by skin, through an open spinal column defect. Spinal fluid surrounds the tissue in the protruding sac, which does not contain any neural elements, and there is usually minor disability, although some may experience paralysis and bladder and bowel dysfunction. With meningocele, the cerebrospinal fluid that protects the brain and spinal cord is most often still able to flow and drain normally, so it does not build up causing hydrocephalus.

Q05.7 Lumbar spina bifida without hydrocephalus

Lumbar spina bifida occurs whenever the neural tube of the developing embryo does not close all the way, leaving an abnormal vertebral opening in the spinal column at the lumbar level. The manifestation of spina bifida most likely to occur without hydrocephalus is meningocele. A meningocele is a protrusion of part of the protective covering of the spinal cord within a sac-like structure that may or may not be covered by skin, through an open spinal column defect. Spinal fluid surrounds the tissue in the protruding sac, which does not contain any neural elements, and there is usually minor disability, although some may experience paralysis and bladder and bowel

dysfunction. With meningocele, the cerebrospinal fluid that protects the brain and spinal cord is most often still able to flow and drain normally, so it does not build up causing hydrocephalus.

Q05.8 Sacral spina bifida without hydrocephalus

Sacral spina bifida occurs whenever the neural tube of the developing embryo does not close all the way, leaving an abnormal vertebral opening in the spinal column at the sacral level. The manifestation of spina bifida most likely to occur without hydrocephalus is meningocele. A meningocele is a protrusion of part of the protective covering of the spinal cord within a sac-like structure that may or may not be covered by skin, through an open spinal column defect. Spinal fluid surrounds the tissue in the protruding sac, which does not contain any neural elements, and there is usually minor disability, although some may experience paralysis and bladder and bowel dysfunction. With meningocele, the cerebrospinal fluid that protects the brain and spinal cord is most often still able to flow and drain normally, so it does not build up causing hydrocephalus.

Q05.9 Spina bifida, unspecified

Spina bifida means cleft or split spine and occurs whenever the neural tube of the developing embryo does not close all the way, leaving an abnormal vertebral opening at any level in the spinal column. This results in a permanently disabling birth defect, although with a wide range of severity. The manifestations of spina bifida are many, including (hydro)meningocele, myelomeningocele, syringomyelocele, and rachischisis.

Note: Use this unspecified code when a type of spina bifida other than occulta (Q76.0) is documented without any further specification as to the vertebral level of the open defect or whether or not it is occurring with or without hydrocephalus.

Q06.2 Diastematomyelia

Diastematomyelia is a condition in which the spinal cord is separated by a bony or fibrous disc. This condition often occurs in concert with spina bifida. Patients affected by this disorder commonly experience scoliosis and weakness in the lower extremities.

Q06.4 Hydromyelia

Hydromyelia occurs when an abnormal widening of the central canal of the spinal cord creates space where an excessive amount of cerebrospinal fluid can build up. As fluid accumulates, it exerts pressure on the spinal cord and may damage nerves. The widened cavity that forms in hydromyelia is connected to the 4th ventricle in the brain and is almost always associated with congenital hydrocephalus and related birth defects such as Budd-Chiari malformation and Dandy-Walker syndrome. In rare cases, hydromyelia has resoved on its own, but surgery is usually done to correct the flow of CSF.

Q10.0 Congenital ptosis

Congenital ptosis is a congenital drooping of the upper eyelid.

Q11.0 Cystic eyeball

Cystic eyeball is a deformity in which there is a cystic mass in place of the eyeball. A vestigial, non-functional eyeball may be present.

Q11.1 Other anophthalmos

Anophthalmos is the agenesis, or lack of development, of the eyes in the fetus. There may be vestigial remnants of nonfunctioning eye structures present instead of a fully formed eye.

Q11.2 Microphthalmos

Microphthalmos describes a condition in which the eyeballs are abnormally small. Defects of the cornea and lens are common with this condition, and vision is usually adversely affected or absent.

Q12.0 Congenital cataract

A congenital cataract is a partial or complete clouding over of the crystalline lens present from birth that obscures vision and causes blindness since the lens is opaque and cannot focus incoming light onto the retina. A capsular and subcapsular cataract occurs when the cataract is located both in front

Malformations/Deformations/Abnormalities

Q05.4 – Q12.0

of and behind the membrane that covers the lens of the eye. In cortical and zonular cataracts, the cataract affects the cortex of the lens of the eye, as well as the ciliary zonules that connect the capsule of the eye to the lens. A nuclear type cataract affects the nucleus at the core of the eye lens.

Q12.3 Congenital aphakia

Congenital aphakia describes the absence of the lens of the eye from birth.

Q12.4 Spherophakia

Spherophakia describes a congenital anomaly in the shape of the lens of the eye that is formed as a sphere.

Q13.0 Coloboma of iris

A coloboma is a defect in the formation of the eye that occurs before birth. It manifests as a key-hole type defect in a particular structure of the eye because pieces of tissue that form that structure are missing. This is due to the developmental choroidal gap between structures in the eye failing to close in early prenatal stages. Coloboma most often affects the iris and may occur in one or both eyes. Severity can range from those with no vision problems to blindness.

Q13.1 Absence of iris

Aniridia is a congenital defect of the eye in which the iris is underdeveloped or completely absent. This condition almost always affects both eyes.

Q13.3 Congenital corneal opacity

A congenital defect in which the cornea is opaque or cloudy, causing impaired vision in that eye.

Q14.1 Congenital malformation of retina

This code includes congenital or hereditary retinoschisis. The hereditary type of retinoschisis is much less common than the degenerative type reported in the eye chapter. The congenital type is an X-linked disorder affecting mostly males. It causes the retina to split into two layers and can affect the nerve tissue in the macula, resulting in loss of visual resolution needed for detailed viewing. This is not the same as retinal detachment, in which the retina pulls away from the choroid.

Note: This code also includes other congenital retinal disorders, such as congenital retinal aneurysm.

Q14.2 Congenital malformation of optic disc

This includes coloboma of the optic disc. Coloboma is a defect in the formation of the eye that occurs before birth. It manifests as a key-hole type defect in a particular structure of the eye because pieces of tissue that form that structure are missing. This is due to the developmental choroidal gap between structures in the eye failing to close in early prenatal stages. It may occur in one or both eyes. Coloboma of the optic disc is extremely rare and causes moderate to severe blindness. The optic disc has an excavated, funnel-shaped area where the optic nerve from the eye reaches the optic nerve from the brain.

Q15.0 Congenital glaucoma

Congenital glaucoma is a condition characterized by elevated intraocular eye pressure from an increase in intraocular fluid, causing enlargement of the entire globe (buphthalmos). Congenital cases of glaucoma may be evident at birth or diagnosed later within the first year or two of life. The condition is caused by anomalies in how the angle of the anterior chamber in the eye develops which makes it abnormally deep. The entire globe may be enlarged, the cornea opaque with rupture of Descemet's membrane, the iris atrophied, and the anterior sclera thin. Symptoms include photophobia, hyperlacrimation, and blepharospasm. Blindness occurs in untreated cases.

Q16.0 Congenital absence of (ear) auricle

This code describes a congenital defect in which the entire outer ear is missing, including the auditory canal. This defect may affect one or both ears.

Q16.3 Congenital malformation of ear ossicles

Malformations of the ossicles (small bones) of the middle ear can severely impact hearing. These small bones, known as the malleus, incus, and

stapes, may be anomalous in different ways. They way be deformed, positioned in the wrong place, or even fused together.

Q16.4 Other congenital malformations of middle ear

Use this code to report an anomaly of the middle ear, except for the ossicles (bones) in the middle ear. For example, the meatus, or auditory canal, may be abnormally narrow or completely closed.

Q17.0 Accessory auricle

An accessory auricle is a congenital condition in which there is residual, redundant tissue of the outer ear structure present. The person may have an additonal ear lobe, an appendage of tissue or a tag attached somewhere to the auricle, or even an additional outer ear present.

Q17.1 Macrotia

Macrotia is an abnormally large pinna of the ear. The pinna is the visible, external portion of the ear.

Q17.2 Microtia

Microtia is a condition in which the auricle, or the outer portion of the ear, is abnormally small.

Q18.0 Sinus, fistula and cyst of branchial cleft

A branchial cleft cyst is a lump or mass that forms during development of the embryo when the tissues that form the neck and collarbone area fail to develop normally. The cyst may appear as small pits, lumps, or skin tags on either side of the neck and may have drainage when the cyst is formed by fluid from open spaces or abnormal passages left when the branchial cleft fails to close during development. These open passages are called branchial cleft sinuses or fistulas. Both sinuses and cysts can become infected.

Q18.1 Preauricular sinus and cyst

Preauricular sinus and cyst, also called a congenital auricular fistula, are common malformations. Cysts may be a nodule or clump of skin located adjacent to the external ear. A sinus may appear as a dent or a dimple and is a tiny, tubular, abnormal communication out to the external surface in front of the ear. Preauricular cysts and sinuses may become infected, but they usually remain asymptomatic and are treated surgically if they become problematic and infected too often.

Q18.3 Webbing of neck

Webbing of the neck is a congenital condition that often occurs with other birth defects, and consists of a thick flap of skin that extends from the side of the neck to the shoulder.

Q18.4 Macrostomia

Macrostomia is an abnormally large mouth.

Q18.5 Microstomia

Microstomia is an abnormally small mouth.

Q18.6 Macrocheilia

Macrocheilia is a condition in which the lips are abnormally large.

Q18.7 Microcheilia

Microcheilia is a condition in which the lips are abnormally small.

Q20.0 Common arterial trunk

Common truncus, also called persistent truncus arteriosus, is one of the least common congenital heart defects in which there is abnormal communication between the ascending aorta and the pulmonary artery, near the semilunar valve. It occurs when the early fetal truncus vessel developing into the heart fails to divide into the two structures that make the aorta and the pulmonary artery. As a result, the baby is born with only a single common vessel coming from both the ventricles (the main pumping chambers of the heart) instead of the two normal vessels that each come from a ventricle. There is typically a hole between the two ventricles with a single valve positioned over the hole. The common truncus shares that one valve coming from both chambers. In very rare cases, the common vessel is almost completely on one ventricle instead of being positioned over both.

The pulmonary arteries taking blood to the lungs come off of this common, single vessel. Babies are blue because the blood going to the body has not all passed through the lungs to be oxygenated; there is often leakage between the ventricles; and the coronary arteries bringing oxygen to the heart are often abnormal as well. Babies can develop cardiogenic shock and congestive heart failure because of fluid overload. Major surgery is required very early in which the hole between the ventricles is closed and the common truncus vessel is formed to take blood from the left ventricle out to the body's circulation. Another conduit is created from the right ventricle and the pulmonary arteries are attached so that blood can go from the right side of the heart to the lungs to be oxygenated.

Q20.1 Double outlet right ventricle

Double outlet right ventricle is a rare congenital heart defect in which at least half of one great artery and all of the other arise from the right ventricle. Since both arteries arise from the right ventricle, there is always a ventricular septal defect (VSD) present to allow some kind of emptying outlet for blood from the left ventricle. The position of the great arteries to the VSD and the presence of any great artery obstruction determine surgical options. There are three most common subtypes of double outlet right ventricle:

1). *VSD below the aortic valve with no pulmonary stenosis* the majority of blood from the right ventricle and some from the left passing across the defect will shunt into the pulmonary artery. Oxygenated blood from the left is also still directed appropriately into the aorta. This resembles a large left to right shunt and presents with congestive heart failure and normal oxygen saturation. This is the simplest repair since the defect site sits close to the aortic valve. The VSD is closed and the aortic valve is included as part of the left ventricle, making a tunnel excluding right ventricle blood from the systemic circulation.

2). *VSD below the pulmonary artery* the oxygenated blood from the left ventricle goes back to the pulmonary artery, while deoxygenated blood from the right ventricle goes into the aorta, creating pathophysiology like that of complete transposition of great vessels, presenting with cyanosis and possible cardiogenic shock-like state. This is also called the Taussig-Bing form of double outlet right ventricle. This type may have two surgical courses for repair, depending on whether or not there is pulmonary outflow obstruction. If no aortic or pulmonary stenosis is present, the ventricular defect is closed so the left ventricle ejects into the pulmonary artery and then an arterial switch repair is performed as for complete transposition. If there is obstruction or stenosis, the arterial switch cannot be performed and a Rastelli repair is done instead, in which an intraventricular baffle is created to channel blood to the aorta and a conduit from the right ventricle to the pulmonary artery is placed.

3). *VDS below the aorta with pulmonary stenosis* this is a complex case in which many other defects also occur, such as an atrial septal defect 25% of the time, additional ventricular septal defects of the muscle wall, patent ductus arteriosus, mitral valve abnormalities, and coronary artery anomalies. These patients are similar to those with Tetralogy of Fallot and require defect closure so that blood from the left ventricle goes only into the aorta with patch augmentation of the outflow tract from the right ventricle to relieve pulmonary stenosis.

Q20.3 Discordant ventriculoarterial connection

This code reports complete transposition of the great vessels. This is a congenital heart anomaly in which the aorta, that normally carries oxygen-rich blood from the left ventricle out to the body, and the pulmonary artery, that normally carries venous, oxygen-poor blood from the right ventricle to the lungs for oxygenation, are reversed. The aorta is connected to the right ventricle causing venous blood depleted of oxygen to go back out to the body, bypassing the lungs. The pulmonary artery is attached to the left ventricle so the oxygen-rich blood is carried back to the lungs. Complete transposition results in two separate circuits of blood flow, instead of one connected circuit. Infants only survive when there is one or more other connection to allow the blood to mix together within the heart and get some oxygenated blood out to the body's circulation, such as an atrial or ventricular septal septal, or a patent ductus arteriosus in which there is a connection between the pulmonary artery and the aorta. Early surgical

repair may be one of two types of surgery: the first one creates a tunnel (called a baffle) between the atria that redirects oxygen-rich blood to the right side and out through the aorta and redirects venous blood to the left ventricle and pulmonary artery, leaving the anomalous connections as they function. This procedure is called a venous switch, intra-atrial baffle procedure, Mustard procedure, or Senning procedure. The second type of surgery is called an arterial switch operation in which the aorta and the pulmonary artery are disconnected from their anomalous positions and returned to their normal position in the correct ventricle.

Q20.4 Double inlet ventricle

This code is used to report a common or single ventricle, in which there is no septum or membrane dividing the right ventricle from the left ventricle.

Q20.5 Discordant atrioventricular connection

Congenital corrected transposition of the great vessels is reported here. This is another rare heart defect in which the left atrium is connected to the right ventricle, from which the aorta arises. Patients with isolated congenital corrected transposition may not present with symptoms until adulthood. Rhythm disturbances and tricuspid regurgitation may appear in the 40s, causing congestive heart failure later. No treatment may be required for patients who have no other associated abnormalities because their life expectancy is near normal. For those with other defects, repair may be performed to address only those defects, such as ventricular septal defect closure, relief of pulmonary stenosis, and tricuspid regurgitation, leaving the right ventricle as the systemic ventricle. This often leads later to progressive right ventricular failure. To avoid this, an anatomic repair may be done to establish the morphological left ventricle as the systemic ventricle. This can include the alternative double switch procedure using two surgical techniques combining arterial switch with a Senning or Mustard procedure.

Q21.2 Atrioventricular septal defect

An ostium primum atrial septal defect is an opening present at the anterior bottom of the atrial septum at the level of the tricuspid and mitral valves. It is also called endocardial cushion defect because it involves the endocardial cushion part of the heart where the atrial septum meets the ventricular septum and the mitral valve meets the tricuspid valve. Because of its proximity to the valves and an inadequate amount of tissue in the inferior rim of the septum, this type of defect cannot be sealed with device placement by cardiac catheterization and requires surgical repair that is usually undergone between the ages of 2 and 5.

Q21.3 Tetralogy of Fallot

The tetralogy of Fallot is a group of heart defects that occur together. A ventricular septal defect is present as a hole or gap between the two bottom ventricles of the heart, along with a narrowing just below the pulmonary valve causing pulmonary stenosis or atresia. Aortic dextroposition is also present as the aorta will be attached to the heart over the gap between the two ventricles, instead of in the left ventricle. The right ventricle is hypertrophic and more muscular than normal.

Q22.4 Congenital tricuspid stenosis

Congenital stenosis of the tricuspid valve is an abnormal narrowing of the valve that prevents blood from flowing back into the right atrium from the right ventricle.

Q22.5 Ebstein's anomaly

Ebstein's anomaly occurs when the tricuspid valve is displaced downward into the right ventricle of the heart. Heart failure and erratic heart rhythms may result.

Q23.0 Congenital stenosis of aortic valve

Congenital stenosis of the aortic valve is an abnormal narrowing of the valve that prevents blood from flowing back into the heart's left ventricle from the aorta.

Q23.1 Congenital insufficiency of aortic valve

A congenital insufficiency of the aortic valve occurs when the aortic valve fails to close properly and results in a backflow of blood from the aorta to the left ventricle.

Malformations/Deformations/Abnormalities

Q20.1 – Q23.1

Q23.2   Congenital mitral stenosis

Congenital mitral valve stenosis is a narrowed opening in the valve between the left chambers of the heart that is present from birth. Children born with mitral stenosis will often have other heart defects as well. The narrowed valve restricts the forward flow of blood through the left atrium to the left ventricle. As a result of the valve not being able to open wide enough, pressure builds up and causes the upper chamber to swell. The pooling blood backed up in the left atrium may then begin to collect within the lung tissue, resulting in pulmonary edema and difficulty breathing, and leading to congestive heart failure. In children, symptoms of a stenosed valve may be present from birth, but will almost always develop within the first two years of life. Symptoms include cough, poor feeding, sweating while feeding, difficult breathing or shortness of breath, and poor growth or failure to thrive. Tests used to diagnose the stenosed heart valve and any lung congestion include imaging with x-ray, CT scan, MRI, and echocardiogram, and the use of an electrocardiogram. A cardiac murmur may be heard through a stethoscope as a sound like a distinctive rumbling, snap, or other abnormal heart sound. Treatment depends on the severity of the condition. Some cases may be mild and the symptoms treated with medications, although children will often require surgical repair or replacement of the valve.

Q23.3   Congenital mitral insufficiency

A congenital mitral insufficiency is a deformity present at birth in which the mitral valve fails to close completely, making in incompetent and allowing blood in the left ventricle to regurgitate, or backflow into the left atrium. When blood flows backwards as the heart contracts, less blood is pumped out to the rest of the body, triggering the heart to work harder, pumping with more force. This leads to congestive heart failure.

Q23.4   Hypoplastic left heart syndrome

Hypoplastic left heart syndrome is a condition in which the entire left side of the heart fails to develop properly. The left ventricle, aorta, mitral valves, and aortic valves are absent or underformed.

Q24.0   Dextrocardia

Dextrocardia is a congenital malposition of the heart and cardiac apex within the chest cavity in which the heart is located and pointing toward the right side of the body instead of the left. The simplest form of dextrocardia occurs when the placement, shape, and structure of the heart are mirror images of a normal heart. Other cases may occur with heart wall and blood vessel defects, and defects of other abdominal organs.

Q24.1   Levocardia

Levocardia is a rare anomaly in which the heart is in the normal left-sided position, but the thoracic and abdominal organs are reversed or transposed to the wrong side of the body. This condition usually occurs with other structural defects of the heart itself.

Q24.2   Cor triatriatum

Cor triatriatum is a congenital defect in which the heart has three atrial chambers, with the left atrium being divided into two segments.

Q24.6   Congenital heart block

A congenital heart block is a deformity in which malformed tissue connecting different parts of the heart fails to conduct electrical signals properly for normal heart rhythmn.

Q25.0   Patent ductus arteriosus

Patent ductus arteriosus is a condition in which the ductus arteriosus fails to close at birth. The ductus arteriosus connects the pulmonary artery to the aortic arch in the fetus. When this remains open, the child may experience shortness of breath and irregular heart rhythms, leading to congestive heart failure if left untreated.

Q25.1   Coarctation of aorta

Coarctation of the aorta is a congenital condition in which the aorta is abnormally narrow just below the juncture where arteries branch off into the left arm. This causes high blood pressure in the heart and brain, and low blood pressure below the blockage, especially in the kidneys. This condition often produces no apparent symptoms, and may be discovered only after a blood pressure screening.

Q25.5   Atresia of pulmonary artery

Pulmonary artery atresia or agenesis is a failure of the pulmonary valve to form, with the artery's origin not connected to the heart, and is usually seen with other associated defects such as patent ductus arteriosus. The abnormal or absent valve does not allow blood to flow from the right ventricle to the lungs to get oxygenated. This manifests as soon as a baby is born.

Q25.71   Coarctation of pulmonary artery

The pulmonary artery is the large, main artery that sends oxygen poor blood returning from the circulation into the lungs to be enriched with oxygen again. Pulmonary artery coarctation is a narrowing or stenosis of the artery or its left or right branches that makes it difficult for blood to flow to the lungs and become oxygenated. This forces the heart and body to work harder than they should without enough oxygen and causes symptoms such as fatigue, shortness of breath, rapid breathing and heart rate, and swelling in the lower extremities, face, or abdomen. Increased pressure in the right ventricle of the heart that pumps blood into the pulmonary arteries can end up damaging heart muscle.

Q25.72   Congenital pulmonary arteriovenous malformation

Pulmonary arteriovenous malformation (PAVM) or aneurysm is an abnormal connection between the pulmonary artery and the pulmonary vein, which is usually congenital, although it may not manifest until adulthood when it is very small. The abnormal connection, also called a fistula, allows blood to pass through the lungs without receiving enough oxygen. Although many people have no symptoms, some may have difficulty breathing or exercising, shortness of breath with exertion, and bloody sputum or nosebleeds. It may get progressively worse and lead to hemodynamic complications related to hypoxemia, such as cyanosis and polycythemia, or other serious complications such as systemic embolization and pulmonary hemorrhage.

Note: An acquired pulmonary arteriovenous fistula, which may also be referred to as an acquired pulmonary arteriovenous malformation (PAVM) or aneurysm is coded elsewhere. Acquired PAVM can occur in a variety of conditions such as cirrhosis or other dysfunction of the liver, schistosomiasis, mitral valve stenosis, actinomycosis, and trauma. Liver disease is particularly related because of hepatopulmonary interactions.

Q25.79   Other congenital malformations of pulmonary artery

Other congenital anomalies of pulmonary artery include congenital pulmonary aneurysm, which is a bulge in the wall of the main artery that carries returning blood back to the lungs to be oxygenated. The bulging causes a weak spot that could potentially become life-threatening if this weakened area ruptures. Symptoms include weakness, difficulty with movement, and even hoarseness when the bulge presses on the laryngeal nerve. If the aneurysm starts to leak, breathing becomes difficult and as blood goes into the lungs, it causes chest pain. These symptoms can come on quickly and once it ruptures, sudden weakness followed by loss of consciousness follows due to the sudden drop in blood pressure from internal bleeding. A stent may be placed to strengthen the weakened arterial wall and emergency surgery is necessary if the aneurysm has started to leak.

Q26.2   Total anomalous pulmonary venous connection

Total anomalous pulmonary venous connection is a rare congenital heart defect in which all four pulmonary veins that normally carry oxygenated blood from the lungs to the left atrium of the heart to be pumped out to the rest of the body are malpositioned and drain into the systemic circulation. There are variants based on where the pulmonary veins are connected. In approximately half of the cases, the anomalous connection is above the heart and blood drains into the brachiocephalic, or innominate, veins, or into the superior vena cava. In cardiac connections, the pulmonary veins drain into the right atrium or coronary sinus. In subdiaphragmatic cases, the pulmonary veins are connected to the portal or hepatic veins, and a few cases may have mixed areas of anomalous connections. This condition is fatal if there is not also an atrial septal defect present, or the foramen oval remains open. Surgical correction early in infancy, usually in the first month of life, is necessary.

Q26.3 Partial anomalous pulmonary venous connection

A partial anomalous pulmonary venous connection occurs when only some of the pulmonary veins which return oxygenated blood to the left atrium of the heart to be pumped out to the rest of the body connect to the right atrium or coronary sinus instead, or elsewhere above or below the heart into the systemic venous circulation.

Q30.0 Choanal atresia

Choanal atresia is a condition in which the fetus' nasal airways are blocked or obstructed by membranous or bony tissue. After labor, the infant will be unable to breathe and nurse simultaneously, and may be cyanotic.

Q31.0 Web of larynx

A web of the larynx is membranous tissue growing between the vocal cords, interfering with speech.

Q31.5 Congenital laryngomalacia

Congenital laryngomalacia is an abnormality of the laryngeal cartilage in which the tissue above the vocal cords is soft and/or floppy. The softened, immature cartilage in the upper larynx collapses when the infant inhales and obstructs the airway. This is the most common cause of stridor in infants. In about 90% of cases, the condition simply requires time for the cartilage to mature and the noises disappear. Complicated conditions can cause some serious problems, but they are rare.

Q32.0 Congenital tracheomalacia

Congenital tracheomalacia is an abnormal condition of softened, weak, or flaccid cartilage in the walls of the trachea that has not developed properly. The supportive tissue of the windpipe is not rigid, but floppy, and causes breathing difficulties directly after birth.

Q32.2 Congenital bronchomalacia

Congenital bronchomalacia is an abnormal condition of softened, weak, or deficient cartilaginous rings in the walls of the bronchial tubes, causing noisy breathing and wheezing. It can also lead to recurrent respiratory infections, severe dyspnea, respiratory insufficiency, and atelectasis.

Q33.3 Agenesis of lung

Agenesis is the congenital absence of a lung or lobe of a lung.

Q33.4 Congenital bronchiectasis

Congenital bronchiectasis is a condition in which the muscle and elastic tissue lining the bronchial tubes are abnormally dilated. Symptoms include cough, dry or productive of sputum, shortness of breath, and fatigue.

Q33.6 Congenital hypoplasia and dysplasia of lung

Hypoplasia is an underdeveloped, small lung or lobe of a lung; dysplasia is the abnormal growth and development of a lung or lobe of a lung present from birth.

Q35 Cleft palate

Cleft palate (palatoschisis) is a failure of the lateral palatine process, nasal septum, and/or the median palatine process to fuse during fetal development. The palate of the upper mouth separating the nasal cavity from the oral cavity is not fully closed. These conditions interfere with normal speech development. Children with a cleft palate can suffer from infections if food passes into the middle ear through the Eustachian tubes, which would typically be protected by the roof of the mouth. These conditions are easily correctable with surgery and/or prosthesis.

Q35.1 Cleft hard palate

A cleft hard palate is a failure of the bony palate of the upper mouth separating the nasal cavity from the oral cavity to fuse during development,

leaving a gap in the bony hard palate or roof of the mouth. In some instances, the cleft is covered by the oral mucous membrane and may not be easily identified on physical exam.

Q35.3 Cleft soft palate

A cleft soft palate is a failure of the palate of the upper mouth separating the nasal cavity from the oral cavity to fuse during development, leaving a gap in the soft area of the roof of the mouth behind the hard palate. In some instances the cleft is covered by the oral mucous membrane and may not be easily identified on physical exam.

Q36 Cleft lip

Cleft lip (cheiloschisis) is a failure of the maxillary and/or medial nasal processes to fuse during fetal development. This causes an indentation or gap in the upper lip on one side, in the middle, or both sides that may continue into the nose. A bilateral cleft lip appears as two separate gaps on either side that completely or partially divide the upper lip. Cleft lip may be found alone or in conjunction with a cleft palate. Dental, feeding, and speech problems as well as ear infections and hearing loss may be associated with orofacial clefts.

Q36.9 Cleft lip, unilateral

A unilateral cleft lip appears as one gap to either side that completely or partially divides the upper lip.

Q37.1 Cleft hard palate with unilateral cleft lip

A hard cleft palate with unilateral cleft lip is one contiguous gap partially or completely separating the hard roof of the mouth (hard palate) and the upper lip.

Q38.1 Ankyloglossia

Ankyloglossia, or "tongue tie," is a congenitally short, thick, or tight lingual frenulum that extends too far toward the tip of the tongue, and inhibits range of motion. The frenulum is the membrane that connects the underside of the tongue to the floor of mouth. This affects feeding, speech, and oral hygiene. Ankyloglossia can vary in severity and may resolve spontaneously or require surgery in the way of frenotomy or frenuloplasty.

Q38.2 Macroglossia

Macroglossia is a disorder in which the tongue is abnormally large. The condition may lead to cosmetic and functional difficulties with speech, eating, swallowing, and sleep.

Q38.3 Other congenital malformations of tongue

Aglossia is the congenital absence of the tongue. Congenital adhesions of the tongue are reported when the tongue is stuck to other surfaces inside the mouth, or to itself. In a fissure of the tongue, the tongue is divided by a gap that may run only a short way down the tongue, or may separate it almost to its base. Microglossia is reported when the tongue is abnormally small.

Q38.4 Congenital malformations of salivary glands and ducts

The congenital absence of salivary glands can lead to dry mouth and increased risk of infections in the mouth, as well as problems with digestion. Atresia of the salivary duct means that the channel which carries saliva from the salivary gland to the mouth was formed with an abnormal blockage, stopping proper flow of the saliva. A salivary gland fistula is an abnormal passage connecting the gland and another structure or external surface. This code is also used to report an extra, or accessory salivary gland or duct.

Q39.0 Atresia of esophagus without fistula

Esophageal atresia is a condition in which the esophagus ends in a blind pouch instead of connecting to the stomach.

Q39.1 Atresia of esophagus with tracheo-esophageal fistula

Esophageal atresia with tracheo-esophageal fistula is a condition in which the esophagus ends in a blind pouch instead of connecting to the stomach and an abnormal connection between the trachea and the esophagus occurs because the tracheoesophageal ridges failed to fuse during early embryonic development. This must be repaired immediately following birth, otherwise food may end up in the respiratory system.

Q39.2 Congenital tracheo-esophageal fistula without atresia

A tracheoesophageal fistula is an abnormal passageway between the trachea and the esophagus that occurs when the tracheoesophageal ridges fail to fuse during early embryonic development. This can occur without an additional anomaly of the esophagus, such as atresia, but must still be repaired immediately following birth, otherwise food may end up in the respiratory system.

Q39.3 Congenital stenosis and stricture of esophagus

Congenital esophageal stenosis or stricture is an abnormal narrowing of an intact esophagus present from birth. This narrowing restricts the passage of anything swallowed as food, fluid, or saliva from the mouth to the stomach.

Q39.4 Esophageal web

Esophageal web is a thin membrane of normal mucosal or submucosal tissue that protrudes and obstructs the esophagus. In congenital esophageal web, the tissue is usually circumferential with a central or eccentric orifice and is located in the middle or inferior third of the esophagus. Esophageal web is a fairly common condition, often asymptomatic, but can be associated with swallowing difficulties.

Q40.0 Congenital hypertrophic pyloric stenosis

Congenital hypertrophic pyloric stenosis is a fairly common condition in infants and is characterized by thickening of the muscles that form the pylorus, the valve between the stomach and the duodenum. This thickening constricts or obstructs the opening causing delayed emptying of food from the stomach into the intestine. Symptoms can include projectile vomiting and failure to gain weight.

Q40.1 Congenital hiatus hernia

Congenital hiatal hernia is a rare condition characterized by the protrusion of all or part of the stomach though the diaphragm, the sheet of muscle that separates the chest and abdominal cavities, into the esophagus. Symptoms can include failure to thrive, epigastric distention, and projectile vomiting. Complications may include gastric volvulus, incarceration, and perforation.

Q41 Congenital absence, atresia and stenosis of small intestine

The small intestine extends from the stomach pylorus to the cecum. Congenital absence, atresia, or stenosis (narrowing) of any of the three portions of the small intestine--the duodenum, jejunum or ileum, may be caused by a vascular accident in utero, annular pancreas, or have no known cause.

Q41.0 Congenital absence, atresia and stenosis of duodenum

The duodenum is the first segment of the small intestine. It is the tubular structure that connects the stomach to the jejunum. A congenital defect of the duodenum is present at birth. There may be complete absence of the segment, complete intrinsic obstruction (atresia), or incomplete intrinsic narrowing (stenosis). With atresia, the proximal and distal segments of the duodenum end blindly with the proximal end dilated and the distal end empty. In stenosis, a stricture or perforated intraluminal diaphragm is present and causes a narrowing along the segment.

Q41.1 Congenital absence, atresia and stenosis of jejunum

The jejunum is the middle segment of the small intestine. It is a hollow tube that connects the duodenum to the ileum. A congenital defect of the jejunum is present at birth. The jejunum may be completely obliterated, or a portion may be narrowed as a result of a vascular accident in utero that leads to ischemia of the segment. A genetic disorder that results in a

missing fold of the stomach membrane may cause the jejunum to twist around the marginal artery of the colon creating a complete blockage, or atresia.

Q41.2 Congenital absence, atresia and stenosis of ileum

The ileum is the last segment of the small intestine. It is a hollow tube that connects the small intestine to the large intestine by the ileocecal valve. A congenital defect of the ileum is present at birth. The ileum may be completely obliterated, or a portion may be narrowed as a result of a vascular accident in utero that leads to ischemia of the segment. The ischemic area of the ileum may also twist around the arteries forming a mucosal web, fibrous cord, or mesenteric gap resulting in a complete blockage or atresia.

Q41.9 Congenital absence, atresia and stenosis of small intestine, part unspecified

Atresia occurs when a length of the small intestine is abnormally closed off completely, and stenosis occurs when a length of intestine is abnormally narrowed.

Q42 Congenital absence, atresia and stenosis of large intestine

The large intestine extends from the cecum to the anus. Congenital absence, atresia, or stenosis can occur in any segment of the colon--descending, transverse, ascending, or sigmoid colon, as well as in the rectum or anus.

Q42.0 Congenital absence, atresia and stenosis of rectum with fistula

The rectum is the terminal end of the large intestine that stores feces. A congenital defect in the rectum is present at birth. There is usually a normal anal opening and the rectal defect may not be diagnosed until the infant fails to pass meconium stool and/or develops abdominal distention. Atresia is a complete blockage of the rectum, while stenosis is a narrowing of a segment of the rectum. When a rectal fistula is present, the colon is usually high in the pelvis and the abnormal passageway connects the rectum to the bladder, urethra, scrotum, or vagina.

Q42.1 Congenital absence, atresia and stenosis of rectum without fistula

The rectum is the terminal end of the large intestine and stores feces. A congenital defect is present at birth. There is usually a normal anal opening and the rectal defect may not be diagnosed until the infant fails to pass meconium stool and/or develops abdominal distention. Atresia is a complete blockage of the rectum, while stenosis is a narrowing of a segment of the rectum. When there is no fistula present, the defect is usually low with the colon close to the skin.

Q42.2 Congenital absence, atresia and stenosis of anus with fistula

The anus is the opening through which feces exits the intestinal tract. A congenital defect in the anus is present at birth. The opening is either completely absent or located in an unusual place. Atresia is a complete blockage of the anal opening, while stenosis is a narrowing of the opening. When an anal fistula is present, the colon may connect to the bladder, urethra, scrotum, or vagina.

Q42.3 Congenital absence, atresia and stenosis of anus without fistula

The anus is the opening through which feces exits the intestinal tract. A congenital defect in the anus is present at birth. The opening is either completely absent or located in an unusual place. Atresia is a complete blockage of the anal opening, and stenosis is a narrowing of the opening.

Q43.0 Meckel's diverticulum (displaced) (hypertrophic)

Meckel's diverticulum is the most commonly identified congenital anomaly of the gastrointestinal tract. This defect is characterized by an abnormal pouch or sac branching off from the first segment of the small intestine. The small pouch is usually about two inches in length, located in the distal ileum, and contains embryonic tissue remnants of the jejunum, duodenum, stomach, or pancreas. Patients with this condition are usually asymptomatic, but when the cells are gastric or pancreatic in nature, they can secrete acid and enzymes that cause inflammation and erosion that may lead to rectal bleeding and abdominal pain.

Q43.1   Hirschsprung's disease

Hirschsprung's disease affects the colon and involves a congenital lack of nerves, or ganglion cells, in one or more sections of the gastrointestinal tract, particularly in the lower part. The condition causes decreased peristalsis, constipation, and possible bowel obstruction because without these nerves, the contents of the colon cannot move through the intestinal tract. This results in an abnormal enlargement of the large intestine above the section that is missing nerves. The area near the anus is the most common site affected. It occurs more often in males and may involve a genetic defect. The condition can present in a newborn when no stool is passed in the first 24-48 hours and require surgery, or manifest itself as chronic constipation and swollen abdomen in children and adults.

Q43.3   Congenital malformations of intestinal fixation

Anomalies of intestinal fixation occur when the intestines are abnormally attached or adhere to other structures in the body.

Q43.7   Persistent cloaca

Persistent cloaca is a rare, complex malformation of the female anorectal and genitourinary tracts characterized by fusion of the rectum, vagina, and urethra creating a single channel or cloaca.

Q44.0   Agenesis, aplasia and hypoplasia of gallbladder

The gallbladder is a small organ that concentrates bile produced in the liver. Agenesis of the gallbladder is a rare congenital anomaly in which the gallbladder is completely absent due to failure of the cystic bulb to develop in utero. Aplasia or hypoplasia of the gallbladder are also rare and result in underdevelopment of the gallbladder. Hypoplasia is often associated with extrahepatic biliary atresia. These conditions are usually asymptomatic because bile is being produced in the liver and secreted directly into the small intestine to digest dietary fat.

Q44.2   Atresia of bile ducts

Congenital biliary atresia is a condition present at birth and characterized by a blockage of the ducts that carry bile from the liver to the gallbladder or the common bile duct, the tube that transports bile from the liver to the small intestine. Bile ducts remove waste from the liver and contain salts that enter the small intestine in the area of the duodenum to aide in fat digestion. Symptoms can include jaundice, poor growth from malabsorbtion, vitamin deficiencies, hyperlipidemia, cirrhosis, portal hypertension, and ultimately liver failure.

Q44.3   Congenital stenosis and stricture of bile ducts

Congenital stenosis or stricture of the bile ducts is a condition present at birth and characterized by an abnormal narrowing of the ducts that carry bile from the liver to the gallbladder or the common bile duct, the tube that transports bile from the liver to the small intestine. Bile ducts remove waste from the liver and contain salts that enter the small intestine in the area of the duodenum to aide in fat digestion. Stenosis or stricture impedes the flow of bile and may present with the same symptoms and outcome as atresia, or a complete blockage. Symptoms can include jaundice, poor growth from malabsorbtion, vitamin deficiencies, hyperlipidemia, cirrhosis, portal hypertension, and ultimately liver failure.

Q44.4   Choledochal cyst

Choledochal cyst is a congenital abnormality of the bile duct that may involve the extrahepatic biliary radicles, intrahepatic biliary radicles, or both. Type I is the most common and is a saccular or fusiform dilation of all or part of the common bile duct. Type IA is saccular and involves almost the entire extrahepatic bile duct. Type IB is saccular and involves only a limited segment of the extrahepatic bile duct. Type IC is more fusiform and involves all or most of the extrahepatic bile duct. Type II appears as an isolated diverticulum protruding out from the wall of the common bile duct, sometimes connected by a stalk. Type III arises from the intraduodenal

portion of the common bile duct. Type IVA involves multiple dilations of both intrahepatic and extrahepatic bile ducts. Type IVB involves multiple dilations of only the extrahepatic bile duct. Type V (Caroli disease) involves multiple dilations of only the intrahepatic bile duct.

Q44.6   Cystic disease of liver

Cystic disease of the liver is a congenital disorder that is usually asymptomatic. There may be a single simple cyst or multiple cysts. When multiple cysts are present, it is often associated with congenital autosomal dominant polycystic kidney disease and a mutation of the PKD1 or PKD2 genes. In the absence of polycystic kidney disease, a mutation of a third gene, protein kinase C substrate 80K-H, may be responsible for cystic liver disease.

Q51   Congenital malformations of uterus and cervix

Congenital anomalies of the uterus are known as Müllerian anomalies, which also encompass all congenital anomalies of the cervix and vagina as well as the uterus. Müllerian duct anomalies all stem from the same embryonic origin when any part of the process of cellular differentiation for the formation of the female reproductive tract fails.

Note: The American Society of Reproductive Medicine recognizes seven types of uterine anomalies that follow the American Fertility Society (AFS) Classification Scheme: agenesis, unicornate, didelphus, bicornuate, septate, arcuate, and DES related anomalies from in utero exposure to diethylstilbestrol. Müllerian anomalies cause higher rates of infertility, first and second trimester spontaneous abortion, preterm labor and delivery, fetal malposition, and retained placenta. Some forms can be surgically corrected.

Q51.0   Agenesis and aplasia of uterus

Agenesis of the uterus is a congenitally absent or missing uterus caused by failure of the embryonic Müllerian ducts to develop. Uterine agenesis is most often accompanied by a concomitant congenital malformation of the cervix and upper portion of the vagina as well, usually also agenesis. Females with a missing uterus will be hormonally normal with normal ovaries as these develop from another embryonic source, namely germ cells that migrate from the primitive yolk sac into the peritoneal cavity mesenchyme. The most common form of uterine/cervical agenesis is the Mayer-Rokitansky-Kuster-Hauser syndrome, which is combined agenesis of the uterus, cervix, and upper portion of the vagina in differing presentations. Females with agenesis of the uterus will still experience puberty with the growth of secondary sex characteristics. Ovulation will still occur, but without a menstrual cycle. Agenesis of the uterus is the leading cause of primary amenorrhea and patients with this anomaly have no potential for self-reproduction outside of in vitro fertilization and surrogacy.

Q51.2   Other doubling of uterus

This code includes complete or partial septate uterus. Septate uterus is a Class V Müllerian anomaly resulting from resorption failure of the septum between the two developing horns. The remaining septal wall in the center divides the uterus into two cavities. The septum can extend for variable lengths and may be partial or complete, extending down to the cervical os. The septum can be an extension of the myometrium or composed of fibrous tissue. The fundus is typically seen as convex or flat. Septate uterus has the highest incidence of reproductive problems and is surgically corrected using transvaginal hysteroscopic resection of the septum.

Q51.3   Bicornate uterus

Bicornuate uterus is a Class IV Müllerian anomaly resulting from nonfusion of the Müllerian ducts, either partial or complete. The uterus is seen with a concave fundus, having a cleft of myometrium greater than 1 cm that extends down within the fundus, either into the body of the uterus (incomplete), or down to the level of the internal or external cervical os (complete). The distance between the distal ends of the uterine horns continuous with the fallopian tubes is greater than 4 cm. There are two uterine cavities with normal endometrium. It can be difficult to determine a bicornuate versus septate versus didelphic uterus. The concave fundus forming the cleft is the most reliable and important imaging finding. The lower uterine segment is partially fused, maintaining some degree of fusion between the 2 horns, while the upper segments remain separated. The horns of the bicornuate uterus are also smaller and not fully developed. Patients may be surgical candidates for metroplasty, usually performed abdominally.

Q51.4　Unicornate uterus

Unicornate uterus is a Class II Müllerian anomaly in the American Fertility Society classification scheme. It appears as a banana-shaped uterus without the normal rounded fundal contour or triangular appearance and is the result of a complete, or nearly complete failure of one half of the uterus to develop. Incomplete arrested development results in a rudimentary horn with or without the presence of a functioning endometrial cavity. The rudimentary horn may be communicating or noncommunicating with the body. There is no rudimentary horn with complete unilateral development failure. If a rudimentary horn with functioning endometrium is obstructed, there is no passage for menstrual blood to leave and results in a distended pelvic mass and pain. This is when the presence of a unicornate uterus may come to attention and require surgical removal of the horn. If the contralateral side is fully developed, the uterus will function normally, although the patient is at greater risk for premature delivery or breech presentation.

Q51.5　Agenesis and aplasia of cervix

Cervical agenesis is an absent or missing cervix that may or may not accompany a congenitally absent uterus and/or vagina. If cervical agenesis occurs when there is a midline uterus present, menstrual blood from periods will not be able to exit the body. As the endometrium sheds its lining, the blood goes in a retrograde direction. In these cases, the uterus can be maintained and retrograde menses suppressed with continuous use of oral contraceptives. Surgery may also be done to connect the uterus to the vagina, which is either present from birth or also surgically created.

Q51.810　Arcuate uterus

Arcuate uterus is a Class VI Müllerian anomaly with a single uterine cavity and a flat or convex outer contour of the fundus. Mild thickening of the midline fundal myometrium causes a small fundal indentation or impression in the endometrial cavity. An arcuate uterus is sometimes considered a normal variation as it is not associated with any particular increased risk of pregnancy loss or other gynecologist/obstetric complications.

Q51.811　Hypoplasia of uterus

Hypoplasia of the uterus is considered as Class I Müllerian duct anomaly together with agenesis in the American Fertility Society classification. In the Musset classification, it is considered together with DES syndrome (diethylstilbestrol exposed) uterus as it causes the same hypoplastic presentation of an irregular, T-shaped uterus with a very small endometrial cavity and a reduced intercornual distance of less than 2 cm. The intercornual distance is the distance between the distal ends of the uterine horns that are continuous with the fallopian tubes. Hypoplastic uterus may be associated with hormonal dysfunction, remaining as an infantile uterus that is very small and has poorly differentiated zones of anatomy.

Q51.820　Cervical duplication

Cervical duplication is also a form of Müllerian fusion anomaly that occurs when the two embryonic tubes, or ducts, that meet in the midline and normally fuse to form the female reproductive tract fail to fuse, leaving two cervices, as happens with duplicated uteri. Cervical duplication may or may not also occur in conjuction with complete vaginal septum. The duplicate uteri and cervices are capable of normal reproduction, although they are smaller than a normal single uterus. This puts the risk of premature labor and breech presentation higher.

Q52.0　Congenital absence of vagina

Vaginal agenesis is a congenitally absent or incomplete vagina, which usually occurs with a very small or absent uterus and cervix when the agenesis involves the upper portion of the vagina, as these structures are formed from the same embryonic source. Absence of the lower vagina may occur with a normal uterus, cervix, and upper vagina. If there is a functioning uterine structure present without the upper vagina, menstrual

blood from periods will not be able to exit the body. As the endometrium sheds its lining, the blood goes in a retrograde direction. If the lower vagina is missing, the blood creates a large pelvic mass within the upper vagina. In the latter case, surgery can be done to 'pull down' the distended upper vagina to a normal vaginal opening. Upper vaginal agenesis requires surgical creation of a functioning vagina.

Q52.11　Transverse vaginal septum

Transverse vaginal septum is a horizontal tissue barrier left from embyonic development that blocks off the vagina. The septum may occur at many levels and may have a small hole or fenestration that allows for regular, although lengthy, menstrual periods, or it may completely block the vagina. The fibrous wall of tissue may also occur with an otherwise normal vagina and hymenal opening. Surgery is ususally required to resect the fibrous barrier.

Q52.12　Longitudinal vaginal septum

Longitudinal vaginal septum is a fusion anomaly that results in a vertical wall of tissue running up the vagina and creating two vaginas. One side may be larger than the other. A complete vertical vaginal septum occurs with duplication of the rest of the reproductive tract that also forms from the same Müllerian embryonic tubes, or ducts that normally meet in the middle and fuse. When fusion fails, it creates two uteri and two cervices along with a divided vagina. The entire fibrous wall of the septum can be removed surgically to create a normal vagina.

Q52.3　Imperforate hymen

An imperforate hymen is a condition in which the membrane which protects the opening of the vaginal canal is abnormally thick.

Q53.1　Undescended testicle, unilateral

A unilateral undescended testis (cryptorchidism) is the failure of one testicle to descend from the groin or abdomen into the scrotum prior to birth. The condition is seen most often in premature infants and may resolve spontaneously or require surgical intervention.

Q53.2　Undescended testicle, bilateral

Undescended bilateral testicles is a birth anomaly in which both testes are fixed in place high in the scrotum or up near the groin and have not moved down into normal position within the scrotal sac. This is correctly surgically as undescended testicles have a higher incidence of cancer.

Q54　Hypospadias

Hypospadias is an abnormal placement of the male urinary meatus, the opening of the urethra, other than at the end of the penis.

Q54.0　Hypospadias, balanic

Hypospadias is an abnormal opening of the urethral meatus. The normal urethral opening is at the tip of the penis. In Grade I or balanic, coronal, or glandular hypospadias, the urethral opening is along the urethral groove on the underside of the penis, but still located on the glans or corona.

Q54.1　Hypospadias, penile

Hypospadias is an abnormal opening of the urethral meatus. The normal urethral opening is at the tip of the penis. In Grade II or penile hypospadias, the urethral opening is along the urethral groove on the underside of the penis below the glans and along the shaft.

Q54.2　Hypospadias, penoscrotal

Hypospadias is an abnormal opening of the urethral meatus. The normal urethral opening is at the tip of the penis. In Grade III or penoscrotal hypospadias, the urethral opening is along the urethral groove on the underside of the penile shaft at the junction of the scrotum or in the midline of the scrotum toward the perineum.

Q54.3　Hypospadias, perineal

Hypospadias is an abnormal opening of the urethral meatus. The normal urethral opening is at the tip of the penis. In Grade IV or perineal hypospadias, the urethral opening is along the urethral groove on the underside of the scrotum at the junction with the perineum or along the midline of the perineum, between the scrotum and the anus.

Q54.4   Congenital chordee

Congenital chordee is an abnormal upward or downward curvature of the penis that is present at birth. Chordee occurs at the junction of the penile glans (head) and the shaft and is most obvious with an erection. The condition may be associated with hypospadias. The condition may result from tethering of penile skin with a normal urethra and corpora; fibrosis and contracture of Bucks or dartos fascia; a large corpora with a small urethral length; or a short, fibrotic urethra.

Q54.8   Other hypospadias

Other types of hypospadias may be due to disorders of sexual development or intersex states when gender is not clearly identifiable and chromosome analysis is necessary to determine the sex of the infant.

Q55.22   Retractile testis

A retractile testicle can move from its normal position in the scrotal sac to a position that is higher up in the scrotum or in the groin. The condition usually resolves before or during puberty at which time the testicle will descend into its normal position in the scrotum and remain fixed in place.

Q55.62   Hypoplasia of penis

Hypoplasia of the penis, or micropenis, is a condition in which the penis is abnormally small. The penis is functional, and the infant will typically be treated with testosterone shots so that the organ will grow to a normal size.

Q55.64   Hidden penis

A hidden penis is one which is withdrawn into the body cavity at birth.

Q56.3   Pseudohermaphroditism, unspecified

Pseudohermaphroditism occurs when the infant has the internal sexual organs of one sex and the external sexual organs of the opposite sex.

Q60   Renal agenesis and other reduction defects of kidney

Renal agenesis is the failure of one or both kidneys to develop during gestation. Renal dysgenesis is a nonspecific term applied to any form of abnormal or underdevelopment of the kidneys. Renal hypoplasia is a congenital condition in which the one or both kidneys have a small but normal shape and retain functionality.

Q60.0   Renal agenesis, unilateral

Unilateral renal agenesis is a congenital abnormality in which one of the kidneys fails to develop during gestation. It may be associated with other abnormalities of the urinary or reproductive systems. Unilateral renal agenesis is more common than bilateral. It is usually asymptomatic, and may also be caused by a genetic defect. Women with unilateral renal agenesis often have associated Müllerian duct abnormalities that can affect fertility. Most individuals can live a normal life with only one functioning kidney.

Q60.1   Renal agenesis, bilateral

Bilateral renal agenesis is the failure of both kidneys to develop during gestation. Bilateral renal agenesis is rare and may be caused by a genetic defect. The condition often results in true Potter's syndrome and oligohydramnios--a low volume of amniotic fluid producing features that include clubbed feet, cranial anomalies, and pulmonary hypoplasia, or underdeveloped lungs.

Q60.3   Renal hypoplasia, unilateral

Unilateral renal hypoplasia is a congenital condition in which one kidney is small in size with a normal architecture, but a decreased number of nephrons.

Q60.4   Renal hypoplasia, bilateral

Bilateral renal hypoplasia is the underdevelopment of both kidneys. The organs are small in size with a normal architecture, but a decreased number of nephrons. The condition may be associated with other abnormalities of the urinary or reproductive systems. Bilateral renal hypoplasia is a leading cause of end stage renal disease in children.

Q60.6   Potter's syndrome

Potter's syndrome is the atypical appearance of a fetus or infant due to oligohydramnios, a low volume of amniotic fluid. Features include clubbed feet, cranial anomalies, and pulmonary hypoplasia, or underdeveloped lungs. True Potter's syndrome results from renal agenesis, polycystic kidney disease, or ureteral/urethral atresia although the term may also be used when oligohydramnios is caused by other factors such as amniotic rupture and uteroplacental insufficiency.

Q61.1   Polycystic kidney, infantile type

Inherited (autosomal recessive) polycystic kidney disease causes multiple cysts to form on both kidneys and progresses much faster than the dominant, or adult type, leading to kidney and liver failure in childhood or early adolescence.

Q61.2   Polycystic kidney, adult type

The most common form of inherited polycystic kidney disease, this (autosomal dominant) condition causes multiple cysts to form in both kidneys, and results in impaired function and abnormally large size of the kidneys. This condition is slowly progressive, and may not be diagnosed until late adolescence or adulthood.

Q61.3   Polycystic kidney, unspecified

Multiple cysts are present on one or both kidneys.

Q61.4   Renal dysplasia

A condition in which there is abnormal growth or development of kidney cells which may or may not impair kidney function.

Q61.5   Medullary cystic kidney

Medullary cystic kidney causes the formation of cysts in the center of the kidneys, which slowly impair their function and cause scarring. Patients with this condition typically experience frequent urination, weakness, and low sodium. While appearing at birth, this disease is progressive. Common symptoms which occur later in the disease process between the late 20's and early 50's include weight loss, pale skin, nausea, seizures, and internal bleeding. Complete kidney failure follows soon after.

Note: This code also includes sponge kidney, a condition in which the kidneys fill with pools of urine which do not flow properly to the bladder. The kidneys can become infected, and patients with this condition are at increased risk of developing kidney stones. Some patients with this disorder will never develop symptoms.

Q62.0   Congenital hydronephrosis

Congenital hydronephrosis is a condition present from birth in which urine is backed up in the kidney due to a blockage somewhere along the normal route of urine leaving the kidney. This often occurs in the ureter, causing a distended and dilated renal calyx and pelvis. The increased pressure from fluid build-up decreases the filtration ability, and can cause permanent structural damage to renal cells.

Q62.11   Congenital occlusion of ureteropelvic junction

A congenital occlusion of the ureteropelvic junction is a birth defect or malformation blocking the flow of urine at the point where the renal pelvis drains into the ureter. The renal pelvis is the funnel-shaped chamber that unites the major calices, the tubes through which urine leaves the kidneys.

Q62.12   Congenital occlusion of ureterovesical orifice

A congenital occlusion of the ureterovesical orifice is a birth defect or malformation blocking the flow of urine at the point where the ureter coming from the kidney drains into the bladder.

Q62.31   Congenital ureterocele, orthotopic

A congenital orthotopic ureterocele is diagnosed when the end of the ureter slips out of place and down into the bladder (the tube turns partially inside-out), which may impair the flow of urine.

Q62.4   Agenesis of ureter

Agenesis of the ureter is the absence of the tube leading from the kidney into the bladder due to a failure to develop in utero.

Q64.0   Epispadias

Epispadias is a rare congenital defect in which the urethra typically opens on the upper penile surface in boys, although the urethral opening may also be positioned in the abdomen.

Q64.1   Exstrophy of urinary bladder

In exstrophy of the urinary bladder, the bladder is turned inside out, and the skin which covers the lower region is missing, exposing the bladder wall to the collected urine. This condition must be surgically repaired, and is usually indicative of other birth defects affecting the genitourinary tract.

Q64.4   Malformation of urachus

The urachus is a canal that connects the bladder of a fetus to the umbilical cord. The urachus is supposed to close following birth, but if it stays open, it can be subject to infection.

Q65.81   Congenital coxa valga

Coxa valga is a deformity of the hip joint in which the angle between the femoral head and neck and the femoral shaft is increased, usually beyond 135 degrees. This angle is normally about 115 degrees. This can lead to lateral subluxation or dislocation of the femoral head. It is usually seen in patients with other birth defects such as cerebral palsy or skeletal dysplasia.

Q65.82   Congenital coxa vara

Coxa vara is a deformity of the hip in which the angle between the femoral head and neck and the femoral shaft is decreased to less than 120 degrees, causing an inward curvature of the hip. Pain, stiffness, and a difference in leg length can result. Surgery is usually needed to correct the femoral neck-shaft angle and restore a normal and balanced skeletal structure.

Q66.0   Congenital talipes equinovarus

A talipes equinovarus birth defect is also known as clubfoot, and is a condition in which the infant's foot looks as if it has been turned inward at the ankle, forcing a child of walking age to walk on the side of the foot or the ankle.

Q66.3   Other congenital varus deformities of feet

This includes a hallux varus birth defect in which the joint of the big toe is displaced and turns away from the rest of the toes.

Q66.5   Congenital pes planus

Congenital flat foot is a condition in which the arch of the foot never develops in childhood, which affects about one out of five people. Flat foot doesn't cause any complications as long as the feet remain supple and the Achilles tendon isn't tight; however this condition may present as a rigid flat foot, or even an everted flat foot with spastic muscles.

Q67.7   Pectus carinatum

Pectus carinatum is a birth deformity in which the chest is thrust outward and the sternum is prominent. This condition is also known as pigeon breast.

Q69   Polydactyly

Polydactyly is a deformity in which there are excess fingers or toes on a hand or foot. These extra digits are typically removed surgically.

Q70   Syndactyly

This condition occurs when flaps of excess skin, bone, or other tissue unite two or more digits, prohibiting them from functioning properly.

Q70.0   Fused fingers

Fused fingers is a complex form of syndactyly in which adjacent fingers are fused together by the union of bone or osseous material.

Q70.1   Webbed fingers

Webbing of the fingers appearing alone without other birth defects is an inherited condition in which adjacent fingers are joined partially or all the way to the fingertip by a flap of soft tissue. This results from a failure of the normal apoptosis enzymatic process to occur in the 16th week of gestation that dissolves the tissue between the longitudinal digits.

Q70.2   Fused toes

Fused toes is a complex form of syndactyly in which adjacent toes are fused together by the union of bone or osseous material.

Q70.3   Webbed toes

Webbing of the toes appearing alone without other birth defects is an inherited condition in which adjacent toes are joined partially or all the way to the tip by a flap of soft tissue. This results from a failure of the normal apoptosis enzymatic process to occur in the 16th week of gestation that dissolves the tissue between the longitudinal digits.

Q75.0   Craniosynostosis

Craniosynostosis is a birth defect condition that causes the fibrous sutures in the baby's head to close earlier than normal, disrupting the normal growth of the skull. The skull can no longer grow perpendicular to the suture line that is prematurely fused and grows in another direction, resulting in an abnormally shaped head. Different suture lines may be affected. Sagittal synostosis is the most common type, affecting the main suture on the very top of the head, which is seen more in boys than girls. The head then grows long and narrow. The frontal suture running from ear to ear on top of the head may also be affected, as well as a rare form affecting the suture close to the forehead, which results in a trigonocephalic-shaped head. Surgical treatment is done to ensure there is enough room in the cranial vault for the brain to grow and/or to relieve pressure on the brain.

Q75.2   Hypertelorism

Hypertelorism is an abnormally increased distance between two body parts, normally referring to the orbital sockets. The distance between the inner corners of the eyes and between pupils is greater than normal.

Q75.3   Macrocephaly

Macrocephaly, also called megalocephaly, is an abnormally large head and is diagnosed when the head circumference measures more than two standard deviations above the average for the child's age, sex, and race. Many conditions can cause macrocephaly, mainly megalencephaly, or an enlarged brain, and hydrocephalus, excessive cerebrospinal fluid in the brain. Many inborn metabolic diseases and chromosomal anomalies may also result in macrocephaly. Some cases may be benign, in which the only abnormality is an enlarged head that may be a familial trait.

Q76.0   Spina bifida occulta

Spina bifida occulta is a deformity in which there is a small hole in the spinal column, but it is too small to allow the protrusion of the spinal cord or the meninges.

Q76.1   Klippel-Feil syndrome

Klippel-Feil syndrome is diagnosed when two or more of the cervical vertebrae are fused together at birth. This condition greatly reduces the mobility of the upper spine, and the neck usually appears abnormally short. Other congenital deformities often appear with Klippel-Feil syndrome.

Q76.2   Congenital spondylolisthesis

Congenital spondylolisthesis is an inborn spinal condition in which a lumbar vertebra slips forward and downward over the adjacent vertebra below it.

Q76.41   Congenital kyphosis

The spine is normally straight from side-to-side, but has a gentle outward curve at the thoracic level of the spine and a gentle inward curve at the lumbar spine. Congenital kyphosis is a birth defect of the spine in which there is an abnormal degree of outward curvature in the vertebrae, giving the back a rounded or hunchback appearance.

Q76.42   Congenital lordosis

The spine is normally straight from side-to-side, but has a gentle outward curve at the thoracic level of the spine and a gentle inward curve at the lumbar spine. Congenital lordosis is a birth condition of the spine in which an abnormal inward curvature of the vertebrae in the lumbar area gives the back a swayback appearance.

Q77.6   Chondroectodermal dysplasia

Chondroectodermal dysplasia is a congenital condition affecting the cartilage of the growth plates in the long bones of the limbs. This usually results in dwarfism. Other associated symptoms are defects of the hair and teeth, as well as potentially fatal defects of the cardiac septum which divides the chambers of the heart.

Q78.0   Osteogenesis imperfecta

Osteogenesis imperfecta is a hereditary disease in which the bones are abnormally brittle and prone to fractures.

Q78.1   Polyostotic fibrous dysplasia

Polyostotic fibrous dysplasia is a genetic bone disorder that causes multiple areas of normal bone to be replaced by bands of abnormal, scar-like fibrous tissue. This causes pain, bony weakness, fractures, and deformity. It may affect only a single bone, or numerous bones. McCune-Albright syndrome is included, which is a genetic condition affecting the bones, skin, and hormone-producing endocrine glands. It addition to manifesting in the bones, brown cafe-au-lait spots with irregular borders appear on the skin, usually affecting one side of the body. Affected children have early onset puberty and other endocrine problems, such as thryroid enlargement with hyperthyroidism, and excessive growth hormone from the pituitary resulting in acromegaly.

Q78.2   Osteopetrosis

Osteopetrosis occurs as a result of a malfunction in the process by which old bone tissue is removed to be replaced by new bone cells, causing the bones to become abnormally dense.

Q78.3   Progressive diaphyseal dysplasia

Progressive diaphyseal dysplasia is a rare congenital bone condition that affects the growth plates of the long bones. Progressive bone formation occurs in the diaphyseal regions of the long bones--mainly affecting the femur and tibia, but the upper extremity long bones may be affected as well. Disease onset is usually in midchildhood, but the clinical presentations can vary widely from nearly asymptomatic to severely handicapped. Patients will typically suffer from muscular pain, wasting, and weakness, particularly around the pelvic area; abnormally short femurs; a wide-based waddling gait; flexion, varus, or valgus deformities of the knees; scoliosis and lumbar lordosis, and flat feet. The hands and fingers may also be unusually short, and patients may suffer from early onset arthritis in childhood. X-rays of the skull may show sclerosis or hyperostosis at the base of the skull. Complications of this condition include fractures of the long bones, optic nerve compression, raised intracranial pressure, and delayed puberty.

Note: This is also known as Camurati-Engelmann syndrome and osteopathic hyperostotica scleroticans multiplex infantalis.

Q78.8   Other specified osteochondrodysplasias

This includes osteopoikilosis, a condition which causes small, round areas of high bone density to appear on the ends of the long bones. This disease produces no symptoms, but is associated with other congenital conditions such as dwarfism, metabolic disorders, and cleft palate.

Q79.0   Congenital diaphragmatic hernia

Congenital diaphragmatic hernia is characterized by an abnormal opening in the diaphragm, the muscle that separates the abdominal cavity from the chest cavity, allowing abdominal organs such as the stomach, liver, spleen, kidney, and/or intestine to migrate upward into the chest. The lungs are not able to develop normally causing respiratory problems at birth. Bochdalek hernia is most common, occuring on the left side when the diaphragm fails to develop properly, or a section of intestine becomes trapped as the diaphragm is forming. Morgagni hernia is rare and occurs on the right side when a tendon in the center of the diaphragm fails to develop properly. There may be both genetic and environmental factors involved with this condition.

Q79.2   Exomphalos

This includes omphalocele, a distinct defect or weakness of the anterior abdominal wall around the umbilicus that failed to close completely. It is characterized by a membranous sac containing the fetal intestines and covered by the peritoneum that protrudes around the umbilical cord. Omphalocele often occurs in connection with other structural and chromosomal abnormalities. Half the incidences of omphalocele will also have additional abnormalities of other body parts or a third chromosome, as in trisomy. The condition occurs more often with mothers over 35 years of age.

Q79.3   Gastroschisis

Gastroschisis is a congenital defect of the anterior abdominal wall that lies adjacent, often to the right, of the umbilical cord insertion. The defect results when the developing abdominal wall fails to close completely. The fetal intestines then protrude through the defect without being protected by any membrane and suffer prolonged exposure to amniotic fluid. The intestines then become swollen and inflamed, increasing heat and fluid loss, and often becoming infected after birth. There are no syndromes associated with gastroschisis, but the incidence is higher in younger mothers and may be associated with other GI anomalies, such as atresia, stenosis, and malrotation.

Q79.4   Prune belly syndrome

Patients born with prune belly syndrome suffer from the absence of some or all of the abdominal muscles. The stomach will have a wrinkled, prune-like appearance, and the intestines will be visible protruding through the abdominal wall. The urinary system is also affected. The ureters are abnormally large or dilated, the bladder may be stretched, and other structures may be defective as well. This condition primarily affects males, in which the testicles will be undescended.

Q79.6   Ehlers-Danlos syndrome

Ehlers-Danlos syndrome (EDS) is a rare group of genetically inherited connective tissue disorders caused by defects in collagen synthesis. The condition can manifect in the musculoskeletal system with joint hyper-flexibility or instability and pain; in the skin with hyper-elasticity or fragility; and in the cardiovascular system with fragile blood vessels and valvular heart defects.

Q82.4   Ectodermal dysplasia (anhidrotic)

This code can be applied to any of the many disorders in which the ectoderm, or the outer layer of a developing baby, fails to develop properly. The teeth, hair, and skin are commonly affected, although other structures may also be abnormal. Hair may be sparse, the teeth may be misshapen, and the skin may be dry, reddish, or prone to rashes.

Q82.5   Congenital non-neoplastic nevus

Note: This includes birthmarks, port wine stains, strawberry nevus, and vascular nevus, or benign tumors of the blood vessels that resemble dark birthmarks.

Q83.8   Other congenital malformations of breast

Other congenital malformations of the breast includes ectopic breast tissue, hypoplasia of the areola, and congenitally inverted or invaginated nipples. Inverted nipples are those that actually sink or turn inward, appearing indented. They can occur in both men and women and are most often simply a normal anatomical variance seen in the population, although they can cause breast asymmetry and interfere with breastfeeding. Some cases of congenital nipple inversion may occur with Weaver syndrome, Fryns-Aftimos syndrome, chromosome 2q deletion, disorders of glycosylation types 1A or 1L, and Kennecknecht-Sorgo-Oberhoffer syndrome. Nipple inversion is usually classified as level I, II, or III based on how easily the nipple can be coaxed out, the degree of fibrosis, and the amount of milk duct damage or impairment. Level I is characterized by protraction induced with massage, cold exposure, or tactile stimulation. There is no milk duct compression, minimal or no fibrosis, and no soft tissue defects. Level II is characterized by protraction induced using strong suction with quick nipple retraction. Milk duct compression may be present and there is usually moderate fibrosis with mildly retracted lactiferous ducts. In Level III, the nipple rarely protracts, milk duct constriction is present along with marked or severe fibrosis, and severely retracted or shortened lactiferous ducts. Some classify truly congenitally inverted nipples as those that never protrude, even when stimulated due to connections to severely shortened milk ducts or other connective tissues, like ligaments, holding them permanently in place. Plastic surgery may be used to correct inverted nipples with complexity depending on the level of inversion. More severe cases usually require that the areola is incised and milk ducts and fibrous tissue are cut. Absorbable sutures are then placed behind the nipple to keep it protracted.

Q84.0   Congenital alopecia

Congenital alopecia is the absence of hair.

Q85.0   Neurofibromatosis (nonmalignant)

Neurofibromatosis is a set of genetic disorders which cause tumors to grow along various types of nerves and, in some cases, other tissues such as the bones or muscles.

Q85.01   Neurofibromatosis, type 1

Type 1 neurofibromatosis, also called von Recklinghausen's disease, presents with spots and/or nodules just beneath the skin. It can also cause enlargement and deformity of the bones as well as scoliosis.

Q85.02   Neurofibromatosis, type 2

Type 2 neurofibromatosis, also known as bilateral acoustic neurofibromatosis, is a much rarer form of the disease that presents with multiple tumors on the brain and/or cranial nerves. It often affects the auditory nerves so as to cause hearing loss, usually beginning in the teens or early 20s. Both forms are considered inherited genetic disorders. There is no cure for this disease, so treatment focuses on management and aiding the patient's quality of life rather than curing it.

Q85.03   Schwannomatosis

Schwannomatosis is a rare, but major type of neurofibromatosis (NF) that is distinct both clinically and genetically from type 1 and type 2 NF. About 15% of cases are linked to a genetic mutation. The disease causes multiple schwannomas to grow on cranial, spinal, and peripheral nerves, basically everywhere in the body--except on the eighth cranial (vestibular) nerve, as happens in neurofibromatosis type 2. Schwannomatosis does not cause development of neurofibromas. Schwannomas are tumors that develop on the nerve sheaths, or tissue coverings of nerves. The tumors may grow in a single part of the body, such as one arm, leg, or spinal segment, or tumors in multiple locations may be present. As the schwannoma enlarges, it causes intense pain as it compresses nerves or adjacent tissue, sometimes accompanied by numbness, tingling, or weakness in the fingers and toes. Most patients have significant or disabling pain that requires medication or surgery.

Q85.09   Other neurofibromatosis

This includes other cases of neurofibromatosis outside those specifically identified as type 1, type 2, or schwannomatosis, that are still encompassed within this set of distinct genetic disorders. Other neurofibromatoses cause neurofibroma tumors to grow anywhere on or in the body along various types of nerves, and even affect development of other types of tissue as well, such as bone and skin.

Q85.1   Tuberous sclerosis

Tuberous sclerosis is a condition in which benign tumors, called hamartoses, are found in the brain, retinas of the eyes, and other internal organs. These tumors arise from faulty development of the afflicted organs, and result in mental retardation and other problems.

Q87.1   Congenital malformation syndromes predominantly associated with short stature

This includes Prader-Willi syndrome, a condition caused by a defect of the 15th chromosome which results in short stature, mental retardation, obesity, and insufficient sex organs.

Q87.4   Marfan's syndrome

Marfan syndrome is caused by a defect to the FBN1 gene on the 15th chromosome. This condition results in a defect of the body's ability to manufacture fibrillin, which is used to make the elastic fibers comprising connective tissue. This results in elongated limbs, weak joints, heart conditions, and problems with vision.

Q89.3   Situs inversus

Situs inversus is a disorder in which the position of all major organs in the chest and abdomen are reversed horizontally and are located on the opposite side. The heart, for example, will be located on the right side of the chest. This condition usually presents with no adverse symptoms.

Q89.4   Conjoined twins

Conjoined twins are identical twins with a fused area of the body, most commonly the head, chest, or pelvis. This rare type of twin develops from a single fertilized egg cell with a common chorion, placenta, and amniotic sac. This conjoining can range in severity from a small membranous flap that can be easily separated to a connection at the head, abdomen, or chest, in which the fetuses share vital organs.

Q90   Down syndrome

Down's syndrome is a genetic disorder caused by the presence of 3 copies (trisomy) of chromosome number 21. The primary features of this condition are shortness of stature and mental retardation, as well as the characteristic slanted eyes and facial features. Patients with Down syndrome are also at increased risk of heart malformations and certain forms of leukemia, as well as various other malformations. There are three recognized variations of Trisomy 21: nonmosaicism, mosaicism, and Robertsonian translocation.

Q90.0   Trisomy 21, nonmosaicism (meiotic nondisjunction)

Down's syndrome is a genetic disorder caused by the presence of 3 copies (trisomy) of chromosome number 21. Nonmosaicism is most common, occurring in about 95% of cases, when either the male sperm or female egg has an extra copy of chromosome 21.

Q90.1   Trisomy 21, mosaicism (mitotic nondisjunction)

Down's syndrome is a genetic disorder caused by the presence of 3 copies (trisomy) of chromosome number 21. Mosaicism is uncommon, affecting 1-2 % of cases and results from a nondisjunction event that occurs on chromosome 21 during early cell division in a normal, 46 chromosome, fertilized egg causing some cells to have 47 chromosomes.

Q90.2   Trisomy 21, translocation

Robertsonian translocation, also known as Familial Down Sydrome, is uncommon and affects about 2-3 % of cases. This type of Down syndrome occurs when the long arm of chromosome 21 attaches to another chromosome, usually chromosome 14. The parent is phenotypically normal but a gamete can be formed that has an extra 21st chromosome.

Q91.3   Trisomy 18, unspecified

Edward's syndrome is diagnosed when the patient has three copies of the 18th chromosome. Infants born with this condition experience severe heart abnormalities, and most will die within the first year of life. Survivors must cope with severe mental retardation and other defects.

Q91.7   Trisomy 13, unspecified

Patau's syndrome occurs when the patient has three copies of the 13th chromosome. Due to heart defects caused by this disorder, an afflicted infant usually lives only a few days. Those who survive will have severe mental retardation, extra fingers, and facial deformities. Sensory perception problems are also common.

Q93.4   Deletion of short arm of chromosome 5

A condition in which a piece of chromosome five is missing is also called cri-du-chat syndrome. Symptoms include high-pitched crying due to underdevelopment of the larynx, an abnormally small head, mental retardation, and various other facial deformities.

Q93.81   Velo-cardio-facial syndrome

Velo-cardio-facial syndrome is a congenital condition in which a segment of the 22nd chromosome is missing. This condition results in a staggering array of abnormalities affecting nearly every bodily and mental process.

Q95.0   Balanced translocation and insertion in normal individual

In a balanced autosomal translocation and insertion in a normal individual, the patient has chromosomes which are out of sequence, yet has no adverse symptoms or conditions.

Q98.4   Klinefelter syndrome, unspecified

Klinefelter's syndrome is a chromosomal anomaly that occurs in males who have an extra X chromosome. Symptoms are enlarged breasts, sparse hair on the face and body, abnormally small testes, and the inability to produce sperm.

Q99.2   Fragile X chromosome

Fragile X syndrome is caused by a defect on the X sex chromosome and affects only males. It results in mental retardation, enlargement of the testes, and facial defects. It has also been linked to autism.

Malformations/Deformations/Abnormalities

Q93.4 – Q99.2

Symptoms, Signs and Abnormal Clinical and Laboratory Findings, Not Elsewhere Classified | R00-R99

R00.0 **Tachycardia, unspecified**
Tachycardia is an abnormally rapid heart beat.

R00.1 **Bradycardia, unspecified**
Bradycardia is an abnomally slow heart rate.

R00.2 **Palpitations**
Palpitations are the sensation of feeling the heart beat; an awareness of a slow, fast, or irregular heartbeat.

R04.0 **Epistaxis**
Epistaxis is bleeding from the nose.

R04.2 **Hemoptysis**
Hemoptysis is a cough with some type of pulmonary hemorrhage, or coughing up blood or bloody mucous.

R04.81 **Acute idiopathic pulmonary hemorrhage in infants**
Acute idiopathic pulmonary hemorrhage in infants is a very rare condition of bleeding in the lungs occurring in infants over 28 days old. Confirming the diagnosis follows proposed criteria set out by the CDC which include: pulmonary hemorrhage in a healthy infant over 32 weeks gestational age with no history of prior medical problems that could account for the bleeding; hemorrhage or blood in the airway that appears abruptly; a severe presentation leading to respiratory distress or failure that causes the patient to be hospitalized in pediatric intensive care with intubation and supportive mechanical respiration; diagnosis of von Willebrand's disease ruled out; bilateral diffuse pulmonary infiltrates seen on x-ray or CT scan.

Note: Use this code only for infants over 28 days old. Cases in newborns under 28 days old diagnosed with pulmonary hemorrhage are coded to P26.-.

R06.00 **Dyspnea, unspecified**
Dyspnea is discomfort or difficulty in breathing that occurs not as a normal breathlessness response of exertion, but as a sign of a more serious condition affecting the heart, lungs, or airways.

R06.01 **Orthopnea**
Orthopnea is difficulty breathing while sitting or lying down, often necessitating sleeping propped up in a chair.

R06.02 **Shortness of breath**
Shortness of breath is a condition in which a person is not able to inhale sufficient amounts of oxygen, causing the feeling of not getting enough air, or hungering for air. This may be a sign of some other heart or lung condition that affects the process of breathing.

R06.1 **Stridor**
Stridor is a condition in which an airway obstruction causes a harsh, shrill sound during breathing.

R06.2 **Wheezing**
Wheezing is reported when the patient struggles to breathe due to a narrowing of the airway.

R06.3 **Periodic breathing**
Periodic breathing, also known as Cheyne-Stokes breathing, is a type of abnormal breathing typically seen in comatose patients when they alternate between deep and shallow breathing.

R06.4 **Hyperventilation**
Hyperventilation is overbreathing, or breathing more rapidly or deeper than normal with a sense of anxiety or panic. Hyperventilation expells carbon dioxide from the body faster than it is produced, reducing the arterial concentration of CO2 in the blood, raising blood pH, and causing alkalosis. This begins a cascade effect of constricting blood vessels that supply the brain and transport oxygen that is necessary for proper functioning. Other symptoms of hyperventilation include numbness and tingling in the lips, hands, or feet; lightheadedness, dizziness, and nervous laughter; headache and chest pain; slurred speech; and even fainting.

R06.6 **Hiccough**
Hiccough is a spasm of the diaphragm that occurs as the glottis is closing, causing the familiar sharp sound of "hiccup" upon inhalation.

R06.81 **Apnea, not elsewhere classified**
Apnea is the temporary cessation of breathing.

R06.82 **Tachypnea, not elsewhere classified**
Tachypnea is an abnormally fast respiratory rate.

R07.2 **Precordial pain**
Precordial pain is a sudden, sharp chest pain in the area over the heart near the left nipple. The pain can be intense, but is temporary and short-lived, lasting for about 30 seconds up to 3 minutes. Precordial pain remains fairly localized without radiating and is most often experienced by children and young adults. It tends to worsen with movement, and cause temporary shallow breathing until the pain passes. Although the cause is not well understood, it is thought to be brought on by localized cramping of intercostal muscle fibers, particularly from nerve compression in the area, and has also been associated with stress and anxiety.

R09.01 **Asphyxia**
Asphyxia occurs when a person is unable to inhale or breathe normally for an extended period of time, such as during episodes of choking or smothering, with asthma attacks or laryngeal spasms, or when a foreign body is blocking the airway. This results in a severely deficient supply of oxygen reaching body tissues that can lead to unconsciousness and death very quickly.

R09.02 **Hypoxemia**
Hypoxemia refers to abnormally low levels of oxygen in the arterial bloodstream, commonly caused by various pulmonary conditions, the use of medications such as narcotics and anesthetics that depress respiratory function, and other types of airway blockages. Low levels of oxygen in the blood will cause symptoms of shortness of breath and can lead to hypoxia, in which the tissues and organs suffer from a lack of oxygen.

R09.1 **Pleurisy**
Pleurisy is a condition that occurs when the double membrane that surrounds each of the lungs and lines the chest wall, separating the two, becomes inflamed. The hallmark symptom of this condition is a sharp chest pain while inhaling or exhaling. Patients with pleurisy tend to take rapid shallow breaths. Other symptoms include chills, coughing, and fever. Coughing, sneezing, and moving worsens the pain. Normally, the two membranes glide smoothly against each other with inhalation and exhalation, but when they become inflamed, the two membranes rub against each other like sand paper. Any pleural effusion or accumulation of fluid in between may lessen the pain as it serves as a lubricant; however could rapidly become infected, causing empyema.

Note: When pleurisy is diagnosed as occurring with effusion, it is coded to J90.

R09.2   Respiratory arrest

Respiratory arrest is the cessation of breathing. This condition is a medical emergency as the patient stops breathing on his or her own. Cardiac arrest, unconsciousness, and death will soon follow if it is not reversed immediately. Many patients who suffer respiratory arrest are already experiencing cardiac arrest, and cardiorespiratory failure is included in respiratory arrest. Other causes may include airway blockage, or weakness or paralysis of the respiratory muscles.

R09.3   Abnormal sputum

Abnormal sputum may mean a copious amount of normal-appearing sputum, or the presence of an abnormal color, odor, or mucous in the sputum.

R09.82   Postnasal drip

The glands in the nose and throat continually produce mucus to keep the membranes healthy, trap and clear out foreign matter and infectious agents, and keep the air humidified. Postnasal drip is the sensation that this mucus is collecting in the back of the throat or dripping from the back of the nose. Postnasal drip is not only caused by an excessive production of thick secretion, but can also be a sign of disorders involving the throat muscles or the swallowing function.

R10.83   Colic

Colic usually affects newborns and infants between 3 and 12 weeks old, often peaking around 2 months and subsiding by 4 months. An otherwise healthy baby may cry loudly or scream frequently for extended periods of time without any discernible reason. Colic often begins suddenly, usually after a feeding. This can occur any time of the day or night, but typically in the late afternoon or early evening. The infant's belly may appear prominent or distended, the face red and flushed, the legs alternating between flexing and extending straight out, and fists clenched. Although this is very disconcerting, the condition is benign and there is no proven cause of colic.

R11.13   Vomiting of fecal matter

Vomiting of fecal matter, also called fecal emesis, copremesis, and stercoraceous vomiting is a medical emergency that requires immediate attention. Fecal matter has been drawn back up into the stomach from the intestines through gastric spasms and contractions of the muscles of the intestinal wall. This happens when there is an obstruction present, causing a blockage or back-up of partially-digested food or fecal matter. The underlying cause for the obstruction may be a tumor, twist, or torsion of the intestine.

R11.14   Bilious vomiting

Bile may be present in cases of severe vomiting when subsequent heaving causes contraction of the duodenum, forcing the bile to be regurgitated from the duodenum. In adults, bilious vomiting is usually an indication that the pyloric valve is open, and bile is flowing back into the stomach.

Note: Do not assign this code for newborns. This condition in newborns is an urgent condition that requires immediate attention and points to intestinal obstruction and is coded in the perinatal chapter to P92.01. In adults, intestinal obstruction causing a surgical condition is usually manifest by vomiting fecal matter, and not bile.

R12   Heartburn

Heartburn is the pain that occurs when stomach acid backflows into the esophagus.

R13.0   Aphagia

Aphagia is the inability to swallow.

R13.1   Dysphagia

Dysphagia is difficulty swallowing. This is a dynamic disorder that can manifest with problems related to any specific point in the pathway of food/liquid from the mouth to the stomach. Symptoms depend on the phase or phases in the swallowing function that are affected.

Note: Dysphagia resulting as a late effect of cerebrovascular disease is reported first with the appropriate code for sequelae of cerebrovascular disease from category I69, followed by a code from this subcategory to identify the type of dysphagia.

R14.0   Abdominal distension (gaseous)

Abdominal distension or bloating caused by excess gas in the digestive tract.

R14.2   Eructation

Eructation is burping or belching brought on by the escape of gas in the upper gastrointestinal tract through the esophagus. Belching most often results as a normal reaction to swallowing air when eating too rapidly, ingesting carbonated drinks, smoking, or chewing gum; but it may also be a sign of a more serious gastrointestinal condition, such as gastroesophageal reflux.

R15.0   Incomplete defecation

Incomplete defecation is also described as rectal tenesmus and is characterized by having the sensation of needing to pass stool that comes with pain, cramping, and straining, even involuntarily, while only little stool is passed and the bowel is not emptied. The inability or difficulty in completely evacuating the bowel results in a sensation of anal blockage. Patients often require digital manipulation in order to defecate completely.

R15.1   Fecal smearing

Fecal smearing or fecal soiling is the passage of bowel movements into clothing or other inappropriate place, often accompanying some form of fecal incontinence or functional fecal retention when liquid or watery stool leaks from the rectum while passing gas. Children may have non-retentive fecal soiling that may be caused by emotional disturbances triggered in relation to a certain person, place, or time of day. Fecal soiling may also occur when diarrhea or other conditions weaken the rectal sphincter muscles, which cannot hold back anymore.

R15.2   Fecal urgency

Fecal urgency is the sudden, irresistable or forceful need to have a bowel movement, making it very difficult to get to the bathroom in time. Fecal urgency is related to weak pelvic floor muscle strength.

R15.9   Full incontinence of feces

Full fecal incontinence is the complete loss of normal control over bowel movement. With the urge to defecate is the inability to hold it until reaching the bathroom. Fecal incontinence can affect people of all ages but is more common in older adults and women. It can be caused by damage to the anal sphincter; damage to the nerves that control the muscles of the sphincter or sense stool in the rectum; loss of storage capacity in the rectum from conditions that stiffen or scar the walls, making them less elastic; and dysfunction of pelvic floor muscles and nerves, most often from childbirth.

R16.0   Hepatomegaly, not elsewhere classified

Hepatomegaly is an abnormal enlargement of the liver.

R16.1   Splenomegaly, not elsewhere classified

Splenomegaly is an abnormal enlargement of the spleen.

R17   Unspecified jaundice

Jaundice is a yellowish tint to the skin and the whites of the eyes due to abnormal amounts of bile in the bloodstream.

R18.0   Malignant ascites

Malignant ascites is the abnormal accumulation of fluid containing cancer cells in the peritoneal cavity. This kind of ascites can be due to the metastatic spread of a malignancy into the peritoneal cavity, but it may also be due to a primary malignancy elsewhere, such as the ovary. This usually denotes a late stage of cancer. The most common symptoms are distended abdomen with pain, loss of appetite, shortness of breath, low blood pressure, weakness, and fatigue. Fluid is sampled by paracentesis and may be drained, or chemotherapeutic agents may be injected and diuretic medications given.

R18.8   Other ascites

Ascites is the abnormal or pathologic accumulation of fluid in the abdominal cavity, which is often a sign of cirrhosis of the liver.

R19.2   Visible peristalsis

Peristalsis is the rhythmic, one-way action of muscles encircling a tube-like organ contracting and relaxing, forcing the contents to move through the tube. Visible peristalsis is a condition in which the involuntary movements of the intestines increase, causing a rumbling or growling sound in the stomach, and wave-like movement in the abdomen that is discernible to the eye. Visible peristalsis may be a sign of an obstruction, pyloric stenosis, peptic ulcer, or other condition such as undiagnosed Crohn's or celiac disease; but it may also reflect normal perstaltic action in thin persons or those who are undernourished or have abdominal muscle atrophy.

R19.5   Other fecal abnormalities

This reports abnormal feces, in which the appearance, quantity, or consistency of the fecal matter is abnormal. The stool may contain fatty tissue, mucous, or other abnormal substances.

R23.0   Cyanosis

Cyanosis is a condition in which there is not enough oxygen in the bloodstream, causing a bluish tint to the skin.

R23.1   Pallor

Pallor is a lack of normal skin coloring; excessive paleness of the skin, especially of the face. This includes clammy skin, which is not only pale, but cool and moist instead of warm or dry. Pallor may be a sign of an impending emergency.

R23.2   Flushing

Flushing is a condition in which the skin appears with excessively blushing and takes on a reddish tint due to increased blood flow through the capillaries.

R23.3   Spontaneous ecchymoses

Spontaneous ecchymoses is a disorder in which blood from ruptured vessels near the skin forms a bluish discoloration of the skin surface. These spots resemble bruises or freckles, but occur without any kind of apparent skin trauma. This includes petechiae, minute red or purple spots appearing on the skin due to minor hemorrhaging from broken capillaries.

R26.0   Ataxic gait

An ataxic gait is a staggering gait that is distorted or impaired in some way from the normal voluntary movements of walking.

R26.1   Paralytic gait

A paralytic gait is an abnormal, spastic way of walking in which a person maintains the legs close together, dragging the feet or toes, and lacking flexibility in the ankles and knees. A person with a spastic gait typically has weak legs that are stiffer than normal. The person will walk without flexing and bending the legs normally. Long term contractions will cause the person to drag the feet or toes, usually on one side. This is a symptom usually associated with another condition such as cerebral palsy, multiple sclerosis, or a brain tumor, or it can be a sequelae of stroke or cerebral abscess.

R29.0   Tetany

Tetany is a medical sign marked by severe, involuntary spasming, twitching, or cramping of muscles, particularly of the extremities and the face, including carpopedal spasm or sharp flexion of the wrist and ankles. Tetany is most often due to low blood levels of calcium, causing hyperexcitability of nerves and muscles and may be a sign of vitamin D deficiency, parathyroid hypofunction, or alkalosis.

R29.1   Meningismus

Meningismus is an irritation of the meninges, the protective membranes around the brain and spinal cord, causing symptoms of meningitis, without an actual infection or inflammation present. The three typical signs are stiffness of the neck, photophobia, and headache. Meningismus often occurs in children at the onset of acute febrile illnesses.

R29.5   Transient paralysis

Transient paralysis of a limb is diagnosed when the paralysis comes and goes over time, rarely lasting more than a few hours at a time.

R29.891   Ocular torticollis

Ocular torticollis is a condition often seen in children, in which the head is tilted with a twisting of the neck in order to minimize the effect of some type of palsy or other abnormal action of an extraocular muscle (usually the superior oblique) in order to allow the person to see better.

R30.0   Dysuria

Dysuria is painful urination, often with a burning sensation, usually felt in the urethra or the perineal area. Dysuria is most often a sign of a urinary tract infection, although dysuria may also mean difficulty in urinating that may be a sign of another underlying condition.

R30.1   Vesical tenesmus

Vesical tenesmus is the feeling of incomplete voiding of the bladder and the desire to urinate after the bladder is empty.

R31.0   Gross hematuria

Gross hematuria is blood in the urine present in such high amounts that it is visible with the naked eye. It may be due to infections or stones within the urinary tract and is usually accompanied by pain.

R31.1   Benign essential microscopic hematuria

Blood present in the urine in such small amounts that it can only be detected with magnification under a microscope. Even a microscopic amount of blood in the urine is abnormal and requires investigation.

R31.9   Hematuria, unspecified

The presence of blood in the urine.

R32   Unspecified urinary incontinence

Urinary incontinence is the inability to control urination voluntarily.

R34   Anuria and oliguria

Oliguria occurs when the amount of urine expelled is inconsistently low with the amount of liquid that the patient consumes, and anuria is the absence of urination. These disorders often indicate renal or digestive problems.

R35.0   Frequency of micturition

Frequency of micturition is the need to urinate more often than is normal at shorter, frequent intervals. Frequent urination can be caused by increased urine formation, lower urinary tract infection, decreasing bladder capacity, and is often associated with incontinence.

R35.1   Nocturia

Nocturia is a condition in which the patient frequently wakes during sleep to urinate.

R35.8   Other polyuria

Polyuria is abnormally large amounts of urine.

R36.1   Hematospermia

Hematospermia occurs when blood is found in male ejaculate. This condition is usually due to infection or inflammation of one of the many organs that contribute to the composition of semen.

R39.0   Extravasation of urine

Extravasation of urine is the leaking or pooling of urine into other body cavities, such as the scrotum, usually caused by a break or rupture in the urethra and often associated with a calculus.

Symptoms/Signs/Abnormal Clinical/Lab

R18.8 – R39.0

R39.11 Hesitancy of micturition

Urinary hesitancy, also called delayed urination, is difficulty starting the urinary stream. This can affect all ages and both sexes, but urinary hesitancy is most often a problem for older men with enlarged prostates. The condition often comes on gradually and may lead to urinary retention with a distended and uncomfortable bladder before it is really noticed. Delayed urination is caused by prostatic hypertrophy, prostatitis, cystitis, urinary tract infection, anticholinergic drugs, neurologic disorders, and shy or bashful bladder syndrome in young people.

R39.12 Poor urinary stream

A weak urinary stream.

R39.13 Splitting of urinary stream

Splitting of urinary stream occurs when the the urine being voided leaves the body in two distinguishable streams of urine. A split stream is related to an obstruction in the lower urinary tract such as a urethral stricture, a swollen prostate gland, or a collection of some residual substance within the urethra causing an area of narrowing. The restriction can occur anywhere from the bladder neck to the urethral meatus. Many split streams require no treatment, but if the urine flow is restricted or there is urinary retention, treatment of the underlying cause may be necessary.

R39.15 Urgency of urination

Urinary urgency is an excessively strong urge to urinate, making delay feel intolerable.

R39.16 Straining to void

Straining on urination, or consciously pushing to force the urinary stream can be a sign of urinary tract infection, phimosis or a tight foreskin, an enlarged prostate, or other obstruction to the urinary stream. Continued straining that puts too much pressure on the abdominal muscles may contribute to the development of a hernia.

R39.2 Extrarenal uremia

Extrarenal or prerenal uremia is a condition in which urine and other nitrogen-containing wastes are found in the blood. This is associated with kidney failure and the use of non-steroidal anti-inflammatories NSAIDs. It is often seen in elderly given ibuprofen as a primary treatment for pain and inflammation. Symptoms include lethargy, edema, loss of appetite, and depression. Extrarenal uremia can lead to convulsions and coma.

R39.81 Functional urinary incontinence

Functional urinary incontinence is mostly seen in settings where care is provided for the elderly with dementia. Functional urinary incontinence is leaking urine due to an irreversible cognitive impairment, severe physical disability, or immobility that leads to an individual's inability to have volitional control over bladder function. The progression, treatment, and outcomes associated with this type of incontinence are unique. Management focuses on control of complications, like skin breakdown and urinary tract infections.

R40.1 Stupor

Unspecified catatonia is reported here as stupor. Catatonia is defined as a state of apparent unresponsiveness in someone who is apparently awake to experience external stimuli. Unspecified catatonia displays the catatonic group of symptoms, but has not been attributed to depression, schizophrenia, or another underlying medical condition. Catatonic patients display a group of symptoms related to motor behavior disturbances and behavioral responses to others. One group of symptoms includes slowed motor activity or immobility in which the same rigid body position is held for days, weeks, or even months. Catatonic patients also display a waxy flexibility in which they may hold a body position placed by someone else. Other signs and symptoms relate to behavioral responses to others and include elective mutism, negativistic halting against or going along with blindly; automatic obedience; echolalia in which the patient automatically repeats the vocalizations made by another; echokinesis, the involuntary imitation of another's actions; and the inappropriate repetition of stereotypical movements such as body rocking, tapping, abdomen patting, and moving the jaw, eyes, or mouth. There is also an alternative presentation of catatonia in an excited state with agitated, purposeless movements unrelated to the environment, possible combativeness, and autonomic instability. Catatonic disorder requires rapid evaluation and management in order to give the patient long-term cessation of symptoms. Lab tests, imaging, and EEGs are used to rule out causes. Pharmacological management and electroconvulsive shock therapy is used to treat the condition.

R40.20 Unspecified coma

Coma is a state of unconsciousness from which the patient cannot be roused.

R40.3 Persistent vegetative state

A persistent vegetative state occurs when the patient is unconscious and has no activity in the cerebral cortex. This is a more serious condition than a coma, as the patient has most likely suffered severe and irreparable brain damage.

R40.4 Transient alteration of awareness

Transient alteration of awareness is a nonconvulsive event in which the patient's state of awareness differs from that of a normal, conscious person. The altered state may occur with incomplete recall of an event while maintaining automatic behaviours such as walking, talking, and even driving, although the person's awareness of their own actions is diminished.

R41.4 Neurologic neglect syndrome

Neurologic neglect syndrome is known by many other terms, including hemispatial neglect, visuospatial neglect, unilateral neglect, unilateral visual inattention, hemi-inattention, hemi-akinesia, or left-sided neglect. This is a neuropsychological condition in which a person is unable to process or perceive stimuli occuring on or around one side of the body or its environment after damage to a hemisphere of the brain has been sustained. The lack of awareness of the space on one side is usually contralateral, but it is possible to have ipsilateral hemineglect on the same side as the damage occurred.

R41.81 Age-related cognitive decline

Age-related cognitive decline is unspecified type of senility, or senility without any mention of psychosis that occurs with advanced age and is not usually treated or considered as a disorder in and of itself.

R41.82 Altered mental status, unspecified

Altered mental status is actually a symptom of many other kinds of illness. Underlying factors for an altered mental status are many and include: infections, neoplasms, trauma, endocrine disorders, neurological disorders, psychiatric disorders, drugs, alcohol, and even renal disorders. Altered mental status can be judged by others with a knowledge of the patient's base line of mental function. Assessment includes looking at factors like orientation, mood, language, judgement, memory, perception, and abnormal thought content.

R41.840 Attention and concentration deficit

Attention or concentration deficit is the inability to sustain attention focused on certain tasks and becoming easily distracted. A concentration or attention deficit may also present as a failure to pay close attention to detail or instructions; making careless mistakes; not being able to follow through with instructions completely; feeling restless; losing things of importance; and being seemingly unable to stay on track without becoming distracted.

Note: Use this code to identify this as a cognitive symptom not identified as a specific disorder or due to a specified condition.

R41.841 Cognitive communication deficit

Cognitive communication deficit refers to a lack of understanding or comprehension related to communication efforts in one situation or another, such as a deficit of self expression through spoken or written language, or the inability to take in information from others' communication and make a meaningul response. This does not refer to developmental disability or mental retardation, but a sign or symptom of cognition problems with modes of communication.

R41.842 Visuospatial deficit

Visuospatial refers to the capability to perceive the spatial relationship between objects visually. A deficit in the ability to judge the spatial relationship among objects in the field of vision can lead to many different impairments in daily activities. Visuospatial skills are used many ways every day. Visuospatial ability allows us to recognize shapes, do a jigsaw puzzle, navigate through a city, or even go from one room in the house to the next. A visuospatial deficit can cause many problems with activities such as driving, shopping, typing or working on the computer, and even finding the way home from a walk.

R41.843 Psychomotor deficit

Psychomotor refers to the relationship between mental processes and the planning of muscular activity that results in an intended physical movement. A psychomotor deficit is any disturbance or lack of ability in coordinating voluntary movements with thought. A deficit may manifest in different or particular areas such as dexterity, coordination, balance, or stability of movement intended to produce a desired outcome.

R41.844 Frontal lobe and executive function deficit

Executive function refers to critical cognitive skills. The exact elements of executive function are not well defined. Deficits in this area often accompany attention deficit problems. Executive function has been described by leading researchers in the field as actions we perform ourselves that are directing ourselves to accomplish goals, maintain self-control, and maximize future outcomes. Frontal lobe or executive function deficits may appear as problems with getting starting or finishing projects; remembering to complete homework or other responsibilities; being able to take apart components of an issue and analyze or organize ideas for problem solving; an inability to deal with frustration or manipulate information; and even problems with thinking before directing actions or speaking.

R42 Dizziness and giddiness

Dizziness and giddiness is a sensation of being off balance, light-headed, or experiencing vertigo of an unspecified cause.

R43.0 Anosmia

Anosmia is the lack of a sense of smell; the inability to perceive odors. Temporary cases occur with inflammation or obstruction of the nasal passages, such as when a person has a cold or seasonal allergies. Permanent cases may occur with destruction of the mucous membranes lining the nose or receptors in the brain, such as with a brain tumor.

R43.1 Parosmia

Parosmia is a dysfunction of the olfactory center of the brain that results in the inability to recognize a substance's natural odor, which is often transmuted into an unpleasant or foul-smelling aroma, although in some instances, it may turn to a pleasant odor. There may be just one stimulating odor or group of odors, and degeneration of the olfactory senses may also be noticed in one nostril and not the other.

R43.2 Parageusia

Parageusia is a disorder of the sense of taste in which there is an abnormal change or perversion of the sense of taste. It typically manifests as a bad, metallic taste in the mouth.

R44.0 Auditory hallucinations

An auditory hallucination is a sensory disturbance in which a person hears a sound without any outside stimulus being present. This is also known as paracusia and can occur as elementary or complex perceptions of hearing an extended tone, a hissing or whistling noise, or voices and music in the absence of any real, causative stimulus.

R44.1 Visual hallucinations

A visual hallucination is a sensory disturbance in which a person sees things that are not there with the same vividness as a real perception.

R44.2 Other hallucinations

An hallucination is any sensory modality disturbance in which a person perceives a stimulus that isn't actually there with the same vivid qualities of real perception. Other types of specific hallucinations other than auditory or visual can include olfactory, gustatory, and tactile hallucinations in which a person smells, tastes, or feels something that is not in reality present at the time.

R44.3 Hallucinations, unspecified

An hallucination is any sensory modality disturbance in which a person perceives a stimulus that isn't actually there with the same vivid qualities of real perception.

R45.0 Nervousness

Nervousness is a hyperexcited state of the nervous system, usually manifested by restlessness, shaken mental poise, and an acute, but uncomfortable awareness of one's own self.

R45.3 Demoralization and apathy

Demoralization and apathy reflects impassiveness, or being devoid of emotion or feeling; an overriding indifference and lack of concern or interest, even for things that are appealing or of importance.

R45.4 Irritability and anger

Irritability is a state characterized by testiness and petulant behavior and/or demonstrating abnormal or excessive sensitivity to a stimulus.

R45.850 Homicidal ideations

Homicidal ideation is the term used for thoughts about committing homicide. These ideations are not considered a disease in itself, but a result of another illness, such as psychosis or delirium. Patients with homicidal thoughts pose a dangerous risk to society and need to be monitored when they are identified as having this kind of potential for violent behavior.

R45.86 Emotional lability

Emotional lability may also be referred to as emotional incontinence. This refers to a pathological expression of laughter, crying, or smiling, sometimes uncontrollably in episodes that are not mood congruent—for instance, laughing uncontrollably when one is actually angry or frustrated.

R45.87 Impulsiveness

Impulsive behavior is that which initiates actions without thought or consideration given to consequences, costs, or outcomes.

R47.01 Aphasia

Aphasia is a lack of ability to communicate due to the inability to speak, write, or understand spoken or written language.

R47.02 Dysphasia

Dysphasia is an impairment or partial loss of verbal communication skills due to damage to the brain's language center. Dysphasia manifests in different forms, but commonly falls into three syndromes: expressive, receptive, and global. The basic language functions affected include comprehension of spoken language, naming or identifying, repetition of words and phrases, and speech. Cognitive function is not necessarily affected. Thoughts and feelings may be clear, while expressing those thoughts and feelings is disrupted. Expressive dysphasia, also called motor dysphasia, produces conscious disruption of speech production recognized by an impairment of speech initiation and grammatical sequencing, and proper formation and articulation of words. Receptive dysphasia, also called sensory dysphasia, impairs comprehension and meaning of language. Global dysphasia is a disruption in all language skills from damage to both the anterior and posterior regions of the language-dominating hemisphere.

R47.1 Dysarthria and anarthria

Dysarthria is a motor speech disorder caused by neurological injury that results in the inability to control or coordinate the muscles used in speaking. The muscles of the mouth, face, or throat may not move, move only slowly, or become weak. Symptoms appear as slow, slurred speech; soft or whispering speech; rapid, mumbling speech; abnormal rhythm and intonation; limited tongue, jaw, and/or lip movement; drooling; and hoarseness, depending on the location and extent of neurological damage. Dysarthria also occurs in Parkinson's disease, amyotrophic lateral sclerosis, multiple sclerosis, neurological conditions leading to facial weakness and paralysis, or excessive use of alcohol, sedatives, or narcotics.

Note: Do not use this code to report dysarthria that occurs specifically as a late effect of cerebrovascular disease, such as hemorrhaging, occlusion, and stenosis.

R47.82   Fluency disorder in conditions classified elsewhere

Fluency disorder is stuttering, or a disruption in the flow of speech production, that occurs due to another underlying condition such as Parkinson's disease. The fluency disorder may be marked by sound and syllable repetitions, articulatory blocks that prevent the speaker from moving forward with speech, and incorrect prolongations of speech sounds.

Note: Fluency disorder in childhood, adult onset fluency disorder not caused by an underlying condition, or fluency disorders identified as due to the late effect of a cerebrovascular accident are not coded here.

R48.0   Dyslexia and alexia

Alexia occurs when the brain is unable to comprehend written language, and dyslexia is a condition in which some letters appear backwards or transposed, making reading difficult.

R49   Voice and resonance disorders

Voice disturbance disorders are those related to phonation, or the actual production of vocal sounds, and connected with disorders of the larynx. Resonance disorders are related to nasal air flow, and are connected with the structure of the oral cavity or nasal passages.

R49.0   Dysphonia

Dysphonia is a phonation disorder, or a problem with voice production causing hoarseness. This is much less severe than aphonia, which is a complete loss of voice. Dysphonia is a symptom manifested with laryngeal disorders that affect the structure and/or function of the larynx. Spasmodic dysphonia is a neurological voice disorder in which involuntary spasms of the vocal cords cause the voice to sound tight, strained, or strangulated.

R49.1   Aphonia

Aphonia is the complete loss of the ability to produce vocal sounds.

R49.21   Hypernasality

Hypernasality is a distinct manifestation of a resonance disorder. Resonance and air flow disorders are due to any kind of impairment that affects the structure and/or function of the oral cavity, the nasal passages, and/or the velopharyngeal port. Hypernasality results in a vocal quality that is excessively nasal.

R49.22   Hyponasality

Hyponasality is a distinct manifestation of a resonance disorder. Resonance and air flow disorders are due to any kind of impairment that affects the structure and/or function of the oral cavity, the nasal passages, and/or the velopharyngeal port. Hyponasality results in a vocal quality of diminished nasality.

R50.84   Febrile nonhemolytic transfusion reaction

Febrile nonhemolytic transfusion reaction (FNHTR) is the occurrence of fever, chills, and rigors without hemolysis within 4 hours of a transfusion. Febrile reactions are the most common type of transfusion reaction reported back to blood banks. FNHTR commonly occurs with the transfusion of platelets. Identified triggers include the immune-mediated reaction between anti-leukocyte antibodies in the recipient's plasma and the leukocytes in the transfused platelet product; however even when leukocyte reduction filters are used and the incidence drops, FNHTR is still known to occur even on the first platelet transfusion. Another trigger is inflammatory cytokines released from the leukocytes during storage. Patients are treated with antipyretics but still often complain of chills and discomfort after the fever is reduced.

R50.9   Fever, unspecified

Fever is a body temperature elevated above the normal point, also known as pyrexia, and includes fever with chills.

R52   Pain, unspecified

Unspecified pain is reported as a symptom that is acute or generalized, but not otherwise specified. Localized pain not specified as to type is coded to pain by site.

Note: Types of acute and chronic pain, central pain syndrome, chronic pain syndrome, and neoplasm related pain are coded under category G89.

R53   Malaise and fatigue

Malaise and fatigue are nonspecific conditions in which the patient experiences a state of persistent tiredness and low tolerance for exercise, often accompanied by weakness.

R53.2   Functional quadriplegia

Functional quadriplegia is the inability to move due to severe physical frailty, disability, or other non-neurological condition, such as severe spasticity, arthritis, or severe muscle contracture, that renders the patient like a quadriplegic.

R53.81   Other malaise

Other malaise includes states described as chronic or nervous debility, and generalized physical deterioration.

R53.82   Chronic fatigue, unspecified

Chronic fatigue syndrome is a disorder in which the patient has a combination of symptoms such as sore throat, swollen lymph nodes, joint pain, headache, muscle pain, impairment of short term memory, and fatigue and malaise not related to exertion. Typically, the patient must have the symptoms chronically for six months or longer for a diagnosis of chronic fatigue syndrome to be made.

R53.83   Other fatigue

Other fatigue includes unspecified persistent tiredness, lack of energy, or lethargy.

R55   Syncope and collapse

Syncope and collapse reports an episode(s) of fainting or blackout, with collapse caused by a lack of blood flow to the brain. This includes vasovagal syncope or attack, which is the most common type of fainting in which the body overreacts to a certain trigger, such as extreme emotional distress. Heart rate and blood pressure drop suddenly, reducing the flow of blood reaching the brain, and temporary, brief loss of consciousness occurs.

R56.0   Febrile convulsions

Convulsions brought on by a high fever, usually seen in small children, and characterized by loss of consciousness with stiffness and jerking of the limbs. The skin may become pale or turn blue. Once the jerking subsides, the child goes limp and then normal color and consciousness return.

R56.00   Simple febrile convulsions

Febrile convulsions should be reported when convulsions are brought on by a high fever (over 102 degrees F).

R56.01   Complex febrile convulsions

Febrile convulsions generally occur between the ages of six months and five years as a rule. The peak age for experiencing a febrile seizure is 18 22 months. Brain maturation has a clinical relationship to bringing on a febrile seizure, which is associated with a fever greater than 102 degrees Fahrenheit or 38.5 degrees Celsius. A complex or complicated febrile seizure is defined as focal, not generalized tonic-clonic, lasting more than 15 minutes, and occurring in a cluster of two or more within a 24-hour period. Febrile seizures are benign and the risk of developing epilepsy is very low.

R56.1   Post traumatic seizures

Post traumatic seizures are a recognized complication of traumatic brain injury (TBI) and are defined by early onset occurring within one week of head trauma. These early onset seizures are considered an acute symptomatic event with a low likelihood for recurrence, but they do require following the patient for clinical treatment and prognostic considerations.

Note: Seizures occurring later following TBI are considered to be post traumatic epilepsy with a much different prognosis contributing to survivor disability.

R57   Shock, not elsewhere classified

Shock occurs when the body cannot pump enough blood to meet the requirements of functioning tissue. Blood pressure typically drops, and the body quickly begins to shut down in order to supply oxygen to vital systems, such as the heart, brain, and kidneys.

R57.0   Cardiogenic shock

Cardiogenic shock is a state of medical emergency in which the heart is damaged or disabled enough to prevent it from supplying sufficient blood to the body. Failure of the heart to pump effectively can be caused by myocardial infarction, cardiomyopathy, arrhythmia, leaky valves, ventricular septal defects, and ventricular outflow obstruction such as aortic or pulmonary artery stenosis. Cardiogenic shock is defined by prolonged hypotension, with blood pressure dropping many points upon standing up, and hypoperfusion of tissue. This leads to symptoms such as a rapid but weak and thready pulse; rapid and deep breathing; cold, clammy, and mottled skin; lethargy, weakness, and fatigue; decreased mental alertness and confusion with restlessness and agitation; profuse sweating; distended jugular veins; and oliguria. Life-saving treatment must be undertaken immediately. Around 80% of cardiogenic shock cases are fatal even with treatment. Intravenous fluids, oxygen, and medications to treat arrhythmia and increase blood pressure are given. Intra-aortic balloon pumping may be done to reduce the heart's workload and increase coronary perfusion. Ventricular assist devices also help the heart to pump. Surgical repair of underlying causes is done when feasible.

R57.9   Shock, unspecified

Failure of peripheral blood circulation to maintain blood pressure and sustain adequate perfusion of tissue with oxygen and nutrients.

R59.0   Localized enlarged lymph nodes

Lymph nodes are small, oval clusters of highly organized immune cells grouped along the course of lymphatic vessels that filter microorganisms and abnormal cells from extracellular fluid. Localized lymphadenopathy involves enlargement of a single node or multiple contiguous nodes in one particular region. Since each group of lymph nodes drains lymph from a certain region of the body, determining the location and drainage pattern is useful in discovering the etiology as is assessing the clinical presentation of the swollen node(s). In most cases, locally enlarged lymph nodes are caused by a drainage response to an infection, but may also be caused by accumulation of inflammatory cells from infection within the node itself (lymphadenitis), neoplastic growth of lymphocytes in malignancy (lymphoma), or the accumulation of macrophages loaded with metabolites in storage diseases. Enlarged nodes that are red, tender, warm to the touch, and fluctuating usually denote infectious etiology. Nodes that are nonmoveable, firm, nontender, or fixed together suggest malignancy. The cervical region is the most common area of localized lymphadenopathy, especially in children. All cases require clinical investigation to determine the cause and appropriate treatment.

R59.1   Generalized enlarged lymph nodes

Lymph nodes are small, oval clusters of highly organized immune cells grouped along the course of lymphatic vessels that filter microorganisms and abnormal cells from extracellular fluid. Generalized lymphadenopathy is defined as the enlargement of more than 2 contiguous lymph node groups and is often a sign of a more serious underlying condition that may require a thorough work-up for diagnosis and treatment. Generalized lymphadenopathy is most often associated with systemic viral infections such as cytomegalovirus, infectious mononucleosis, varicella, and adenovirus. Some bacterial infections known to cause generalized lymphadenopathy include typhoid, syphilis, tuberculosis, and plague. Autoimmune diseases like rheumatoid arthritis and acute drug reactions may also cause enlarged lymph nodes in multiple groups. Generalized lymphadenopathy is also an important manifestation in lipid storage diseases such as Niemann- Pick and Gaucher disease, a presenting symptom for human immunodeficiency virus infection, and is also present in many cases of acute leukemias in children.

Note: Although human immunodeficiency virus will cause generalized lymphadenopathy, it is only coded as a presenting sign or symptom. Known HIV disease resulting in generalized lymphadenopathy is coded to B20.

R60.9   Edema, unspecified

Edema is a retained accumulation of fluid causing swelling of tissues or organs.

R61   Generalized hyperhidrosis

Generalized hyperhidrosis is defined as excessive sweating for no known reason and includes night sweats.

R62.0   Delayed milestone in childhood

Delayed attainment of expected physiological development stages of childhood, such as walking or talking, which the child begins to master later than is normal.

R62.51   Failure to thrive (child)

A condition in which a child fails to gain weight normally, and may be a sign of a related medical disorder, or some kind of abuse or neglect.

R62.52   Short stature (child)

Short stature is a lack of growth, causing physical retardation relative to the child's age.

R63.0   Anorexia

Anorexia is an unexplained loss of appetite.

Note: Do not use this code to report anorexia nervosa (F50.0-).

R63.1   Polydipsia

Polydipsia is excessive thirst.

R63.2   Polyphagia

Polyphagia is a disorder of excessive eating, in which the patient has an impulse to eat abnormally large amounts of food.

R63.3   Feeding difficulties

Problems feeding, or with the management of feeding, generally occurs in infants and the elderly, who may refuse to eat.

Note: Feeding difficulties with a newborn is reported with P92.-.

R64   Cachexia

Cachexia is a condition in which the patient suffers from muscle loss or wasting, weakness, weight loss, and decreased mental agility, usually due to another chronic disease or condition.

R65.1   Systemic inflammatory response syndrome (SIRS) of non-infectious origin

Non-infectious triggers of SIRS may include trauma, burns, pancreatitis, ischemia, hemorrhage, anaphylaxis, or several insults combined. SIRS is a self defense mechanism involving the inflammatory cascade with local release of cytokines for wound repair and subsequent cytokine migration to the circulatory system leading to systemic over reaction and organ dysfunction. Two (2) or more of the following symptoms must be present: Temperature <36°C (96.8°F) or >38°C (100.4°F), HR >90 bpm, RR >20 or PaCO2 <32 mmHg, WBC <4000 µL or >12,000 µL or >10% bands (immature neutrophils).

Note: SIRS of non-infectious origin is coded together with a code that first identifies the underlying condition, such as heatstroke, T67.0, or traumatic injury coded within Chapter 19. SIRS related to sepsis is excluded.

Symptoms/Signs/Abnormal Clinical/Lab

R57 – R65.1

R65.11 Systemic inflammatory response syndrome (SIRS) of non-infectious origin with acute organ dysfunction

Note: When non-infectious SIRS occurs with acute organ dysfunction, an additional code must be assigned to identify the specific organ failure, such as the type of acute kidney failure, N17.-.

R65.2 Severe sepsis

Severe sepsis with or without shock is considered a systemic inflammatory response syndrome (SIRS) due to an infectious process with acute (or multiple) organ dysfunction. SIRS is a self defense mechanism involving the inflammatory cascade with local release of cytokines for wound repair and subsequent cytokine migration to the circulatory system leading to systemic over reaction and organ dysfunction. Two (2) or more of the following symptoms must be present: Temperature <36°C (96.8°F) or >38°C (100.4°F), HR >90 bpm, RR >20 or PaCO2 <32 mmHg, WBC <4000 µL or >12,000 µL or >10% bands (immature neutrophils).

Note: The underlying infection is coded first, such as sepsis NOS A41.9, and an additional code is used to identify the specific organ dysfunction, such as hepatic failure, K72.0-.

R65.21 Severe sepsis with septic shock

Septic shock is a life-threatening state of emergency caused by the progression of a septic infection of the bloodstream to the point where blood pressure falls dangerously low (to a hypotensive state of SBP < 90 mm Hg) due to the toxins from the bacteria and the cytokines produced by the immune system to fight the infection. The systemic inflammatory response to this condition causes blood vessels to dilate dramatically, reducing blood flow to vital organs despite the body's compensating attempts to increase the heart rate and the volume of blood being pumped. The increased pumping action weakens the heart and causes decreased output with even less perfusion to vital organs leading to circulatory collapse. Blood vessels may begin to leak and the lungs become overloaded. As septic shock worsens, several organs begin to fail. Large amounts of intravenous fluid and high doses of antibiotics are given. Surgery may be done to remove any gangrenous or necrotic tissue.

R68.0 Hypothermia, not associated with low environmental temperature

Hypothermia not due to ambient temperature is a failure of the body to maintain normal temperature regulation, causing the internal core temperature to fall below 95 degrees Fahrenheit. Hypothermia not associated with low environmental temperatures may be caused by the use of substances such as marijuana or alcohol, which keep blood vessels dilated and restrict the shivering response. Conditions such as underactive thyroid, dehydration, severe arthritis, or nerve or blood vessel disorders that affect sensation, limit activity, or restrict normal blood flow can also lead to failure of the body's temperature regulation.

R68.12 Fussy infant (baby)

Fussy infant is an irritable baby with no apparent medical problems.

R68.13 Apparent life threatening event in infant (ALTE)

The National Institutes of Health Consensus Development Conference has defined an apparent life threatening event (ALTE) in an infant as "an episode that is frightening to the observer and that is characterized by some combination of apnea (central or occasionally obstructive), color change (usually cyanotic or pallid but occasionally erythematous or plethoric), marked change in muscle tone (usually marked limpness), choking, or gagging. In some cases, the observer fears that the infant has died." This can occur during sleep, wakefulness, or feeding, and generally in infants born at more than 37 weeks gestation. Cyanosis and apnea are the predominant symptoms, followed by pallor, stiffness or floppiness, choking, red face, limb jerking, vomiting, and difficulty breathing. Home monitoring is done for infants who have experienced an ALTE.

Note: Code first a confirmed diagnosis, when known and assign additional codes to report the associated signs and symptoms manifested with the ALTE, even those that are not routinely associated with the confirmed diagnosis, but may provide information as to the cause of the ATLE.

R68.81 Early satiety

Early satiety is a condition in which the patient feels full after eating a very small amount of food.

R68.84 Jaw pain

Jaw pain consists of pain in the maxilla or mandible occurring without any specified cause related to the jaw structure or temporomandibular joint itself. Jaw pain is considered a symptom of the head and neck and may reflect a serious underlying occurrence such as myocardial infarction or some other systemic disease.

R70.0 Elevated erythrocyte sedimentation rate

This test measures the distance that red blood cells in a test tube will fall in one hour. Erythrocytes, or red blood cells (RBCs), will gradually settle in the bottom of the tube, but the presence of inflammation produces proteins which cause these cells to clump together and form heavier clusters that settle much quicker than normal. Tests for sedimentation rate were done more frequently in the past than they are now with the development of more specific ways of measuring inflammatory activity in the body. An elevated sedimentation rate (ESR) may be done in suspected cases of autoimmune disorders such as rheumatoid arthritis and polymyalgia rheumatica. Very high ESRs are seen in cases of autoimmune disorders, with marked increase in immune globulins due to a severe infection, and with an increased amount of fibrinogen in the blood, causing the RBCs to clump together. This test alone does not confirm any diagnosis.

R71.0 Precipitous drop in hematocrit

A precipitous drop in hematocrit is a steep drop in the volume of red blood cells circulating in the bloodstream.

R73.01 Impaired fasting glucose

Impaired fasting glucose occurs when the level of glucose measured in the blood is elevated after not having eaten anything for the last 8 hours. This test is done to measure the risk of diabetes and check for prediabetes. The blood glucose level is normally increased after having eaten to induce the pancreas to produce insulin. Levels that remain high when not having eaten are a sign of prediabetes, or risk for developing full diabetes.

R73.02 Impaired glucose tolerance (oral)

Oral glucose tolerance tests are used to determine the risk of diabetes, or cases of prediabetes. The patient is given a sweet drink containing sugar, or glucose, and then a series of blood glucose measurements are taken after ingesting the liquid. Levels that remain elevated are a sign of prediabetes or diabetes. This type of oral testing is commonly done to assess gestational diabetes and is not often used to diagnose diabetes in those who are not pregnant.

R74.0 Nonspecific elevation of levels of transaminase and lactic acid dehydrogenase [LDH]

Nonspecific elevation of levels of transaminase and lactic acid dehydrogenase [LDH] can indicate the presence of a liver disorder or dysfunction, or pulmonary embolism.

R75 Inconclusive laboratory evidence of human immunodeficiency virus [HIV]

Inconclusive laboratory evidence of human immunodeficiency virus reports when a blood serum test produces results that would seem to indicate that the patient is infected with the HIV virus; but then a specific HIV test must then be performed to confirm a positive HIV status diagnosis.

R76.11 Nonspecific reaction to tuberculin skin test without active tuberculosis

Nonspecific reaction to tuberculin skin test (TST) without active tuberculosis diagnosis reports a nonspecific reading from a traditional tuberculin skin test exam in which the patient later returns to a health care provider after the test has been administered to obtain a reading. This type of skin test has been used worldwide for many decades to diagnose both latent and active tuberculosis. This code includes an abnormal result of Mantoux test, positive PPD, and positive or reactor TST.

R76.12 Nonspecific reaction to cell mediated immunity measurement of gamma interferon antigen response without active tuberculosis

Nonspecific reaction to cell mediated immunity measurement of gamma interferon antigen reports a nonspecific reaction or response from the more recently approved blood test for the detection of Mycobacterium tuberculosis without active TB. This type of test measures the amount of interferon gamma released from cells in response to antigens that equate as M. tuberculosis when introduced. These blood tests for tuberculosis are known as interferon gamma release assays (IGRA) and the first such test, QuantiFERON-TB (QFT), was FDA approved in 2001. Another IGRA, called the TSpot TB test, was approved in 2008.

R78.81 Bacteremia

Bacteremia is the presence of bacteria in the bloodstream. This is usually a temporary condition in which some bacteria have been able to enter the bloodstream though events such as toothbrushing, dental procedures, surgery, or catheterization. The body is usually able to clear out small numbers of bacteria quickly, especially as the blood passes through the liver, so temporary bacteremia rarely causes symptoms and is not usually serious. Bacteremia can become dangerous with higher concentrations of bacteria, particularly in people with a compromised immune system or heart valve disease. To prevent bacteremia, antibiotics are usually given before dental and surgical procedures.

Note: Bacteremia is not to be confused with sepsis or septicemia. Sepsis is an infection in the blood, or blood poisoning, almost always caused by the presence of bacteria and their toxins in the bloodstream. This is a very serious condition, causing symptoms such as shaking, fever, chills, weakness, confusion, nausea, and vomiting, and requires immediate treatment with antibiotics to increase life expectancy.

Note: When the causative bacteria are known, assign an additional code from the infectious disease chapter to identify the organism(s).

R79.81 Abnormal blood-gas level

Abnormal oxygen or carbon dioxide content in the arterial bloodstream.

R79.82 Elevated C-reactive protein (CRP)

C-reactive protein is is a protein produced in the liver that is normally undetectable in the blood, but levels rise in response to acute tissue injury, infection, or inflammation. Elevated levels of CRP can help detect cases of infection such as osteomyelitis, pelvic inflammtatory disease, and sepsis. Elevated CRP can also help detect flare-ups of inflammation from autoimmune diseases and other chronic conditions, such as lupus, inflammatory bowel disease, rheumatoid arthritis, and giant cell arteritis; and the test may also be done to check for infection after surgery. If CRP levels remain high 3 days after the procedure, an infection is likely present. Patients with elevated CRP levels are also at an increased risk for cardiovascular disease.

R82.0 Chyluria

Chyluria, or chylous urine, is excess chyle found in the urine, making it appear milky white. Chyle is an alkaline, odorless, pale yellow fluid comprised of lymph fluid and emulsified fats that is a byproduct of digestion. Chylous leaks are rare and can occur from a variety of reasons such as surgical trauma that damages or obstructs the lymphatic system or blocks the thoracic duct; rupture of the renal lymphatic system into the tubules; or the presence of a fistula between the lymphatic ducts and the urinary tract. Parasitic infestation of the lymphatics, such as filariasis, causes chronic infection and obstruction that can create an opening, or leak in the kidney, ureters, or bladder resulting in chyluria. Tumors or infections, such as tuberculosis, can block the lymphatic system as well.

R82.1 Myoglobinuria

The presence of myoglobin found in a urine sample, which is often a sign of the destruction of muscle tissue.

R82.2 Biliuria

Biliuria is a condition in which bile pigments from the liver are found in a urine sample.

R82.3 Hemoglobinuria

Hemoglobinuria is reported when hemoglobin is found in the urine. The urine will appear reddish in color. Hemoglobin is a protein attached to red blood cells that functions as a transport molecule, moving oxygen and carbon dioxide through the body. The presence of hemoglobin in urine is usually associated with some form of hemolytic anemia, in which the body's red blood cells are being detroyed.

R82.4 Acetonuria

The presence of excess acetone found in a urine sample. This condition is often indicative of diabetic acidosis.

R85.61 Abnormal cytologic smear of anus

Anal cytology smears are interpreted and reported exactly the same way as those done on the cervix. Anal tissue consists of the same type of cells that are present in the cervix uteri. Both carry the same risk for developing dysplasia or cancer. The correlation between anal smears and abnormal cytology predicts this risk just as it does for cervical or vaginal pap smears. Abnormal findings from a cytologic smear test from the anus indicate that there is some kind of atypical cellular changes taking place. Abnormal glandular changes, and high and low grade squamous intraepithelial lesions, are results of cytology studies from screening tests only. The actual extent of cellular changes could be more or less. Low and high grade lesions can indicate mild or moderate dysplasia, which is a more definitive result.

Note: Dysplasias must be histologically confirmed, and tissue samples are obtained from biopsies. Diagnoses of mild and moderate anal dysplasia and anal intraepithelial neoplasia [AIN] I and II are reported elsewhere. Severe dysplasia and AIN III are reported as carcinoma in situ.

Note: Having a high risk human papilloma virus is the cause of many anal cancers; its presence can also be tested for through DNA to help determine which patients should have careful monitoring. If it has been demonstrated that the patient is DNA positive for anal high or low risk human papilloma virus, it may be reported in addition to the abnormal finding code reported here, but it is not an inherent factor for these results.

R85.616 Satisfactory anal smear but lacking transformation zone

The transformational zone exists in both the anus and the cervix where the mucosa becomes squamous. A cytology sample will normally contain cells from this zone, but is not necessarily unsatisfactory without them. For instance, a menopausal woman may lack these endocervical cells in the transformational zone due to normal body changes, but the smear will still be satisfactory for the screening test. An anal smear may also lack cells in the transformation zone without being unsatisfactory for cytological testing purposes.

R87.61 Abnormal cytological findings in specimens from cervix uteri

Abnormal findings from a cytologic smear test from the cervix indicate that there is some kind of atypical cellular changes taking place. Abnormal glandular changes, and high and low grade squamous intraepithelial lesions, are results of cytology studies from screening tests only. The actual extent of cellular changes could be more or less. Low and high grade lesions can indicate mild or moderate dysplasia, which is a more definitive result.

Symptoms/Signs/Abnormal Clinical/Lab

R76.12 – R87.61

Note: Dysplasias must be histologically confirmed, and tissue samples are usually obtained from biopsies taken during colposcopy. Diagnoses of mild and moderate cervical dysplasia and cervical intraepithelial neoplasia [CIN] I and II are reported elsewhere. Severe dysplasia and CIN III are reported as carcinoma in situ.

Note: Having a high risk human papilloma virus is the cause of most cervical cancers; its presence can also be tested for through DNA to help determine which patients should have careful monitoring. If it has been demonstrated that the patient is DNA positive for cervical high or low risk human papilloma virus, it may be reported in addition to the abnormal finding code reported here, but it is not an inherent factor for these results.

R87.615 Unsatisfactory cytologic smear of cervix

This code is used to report an inadequate Pap smear sampling of cervical cells that cannot be used for testing purposes.

R87.616 Satisfactory cervical smear but lacking transformation zone

The transformational zone exists in both the anus and cervix where the mucosa becomes squamous. A cytology sample will normally contain cells from this zone, but is not necessarily unsatisfactory without them. For instance, a menopausal woman may lack these endocervical cells in the transformational zone due to normal body changes, but the smear will still be satisfactory for the screening test.

R87.62 Abnormal cytological findings in specimens from vagina

Abnormal findings from a cytologic smear test from the vagina indicate that there is some kind of atypical cellular changes taking place. Abnormal glandular changes, and high and low grade squamous intraepithelial lesions, are results of cytology studies from screening tests only. The actual extent of cellular changes could be more or less. Low and high grade lesions can indicate mild or moderate dysplasia, which is a more definitive result.

Note: Dysplasias must be histologically confirmed, and tissue samples are obtained from biopsies taken during colposcopy. Diagnoses of mild and moderate vaginal dysplasia and vaginal intraepithelial neoplasia [VAIN] I and II are reported elsewhere. Severe dysplasia and VAIN III are reported as carcinoma in situ.

Note: Having a high risk human papilloma virus is the cause of most vaginal cancers; its presence can also be tested for through DNA to help determine which patients should have careful monitoring. If it has been demonstrated that the patient is DNA positive for vaginal high or low risk human papilloma virus, it may be reported in addition to the abnormal finding code reported here, but it is not an inherent factor for these results.

R87.810 Cervical high risk human papillomavirus (HPV) DNA test positive

Human papillomavirus can cause genital warts and increase a woman's likelihood of developing cervical cancer.

R89.8 Other abnormal findings in specimens from other organs, systems and tissues

This includes abnormal findings of chromosomal analysis, which can detect damaged or aberrant chromosomes that may manifest as other disorders, or be a genetic risk when passed on to the next generation.

R90.81 Abnormal echoencephalogram

Abnormal results from an ultrasound examination of the brain.

R91.1 Solitary pulmonary nodule

A solitary pulmonary nodule (SPN), also known as a small peripheral lung lesion, or coin lesion, appears as a round or oval opaque spot up to 3 cm in diameter that is well-marginated and embedded deep within lung parenchymal tissue in a sub-segmental branch of the bronchial tree. It is not associated with atelectasis or adenopathy. Biopsy by wedge resection or lobectomy can determine if the SPN is benign, malignant, carcinoma in situ,

or stems from another disease process, such as tuberculosis or infectious granuloma. Patients with a SPN are usually asymptomatic. Many lesions are found incidental to another medical service. Although many are benign, malignancy that is discovered early as a SPN less than 3 cm may be the only chance for a cure, given the fact that lung cancer is the leading cause of cancer death in the U.S. The risk of malignancy increases with age, smoking, occupational risk, and travel to areas with a high risk of endemic mycosis or tuberculosis.

R91.8 Other nonspecific abnormal finding of lung field

Other nonspecific abnormal findings of the lung field includes any kind of pulmonary infiltrate not otherwise identified, or a 'shadow' on the lung, which is an area of abnormal lung tissue that is more dense than healthy lung tissue, but nonspecific enough to include a multitude of possible causes.

R92.0 Mammographic microcalcification found on diagnostic imaging of breast

Mammographic microcalcifications are calcium deposits in breast tissue that are not palpable, but are seen on mammographic images. In conventional mammographic examinations, microcalcification is of some biological significance as a feature related to a proportion of cancers, although it is a nonspecific indicator of breast cancer. Lymph node involvement tends to be higher in those with microcalcification, suggesting that the deposition of calcium may be related to tumor metastasis. Sometimes nonpalpable breast carcinomas may be identified by the microcalcifications confined within, contiguous with, or surrounding the tumor, which appear on the mammogram, together with prompt biopsy.

R92.2 Inconclusive mammogram

Sometimes a routine mammogram may be inconclusive due to dense breast tissue. Dense breasts are not considered an abnormal condition in themselves; however, in order to determine that no malignant condition exists, further testing is required, since it cannot be noted on a routine mammogram.

R93.9 Diagnostic imaging inconclusive due to excess body fat of patient

This code is reported when the results of an imaging exam do not yield any conclusive data because the target organs or tissues could not be visualized due to body habitus of the patient. When there is too much excess fat, the lipomatous tissue creates too great an impedance for the diagnostic technology to reach deeper, internal structures, and the image produced is not of sufficient quality to visualize any pathology that may be present.

R94.01 Abnormal electroencephalogram [EEG]

Abnormal results from a study that measures the electrical activity of the brain.

R94.110 Abnormal electro-oculogram [EOG]

Abnormal results from a test which measures electrical activity in the cells between the retina and the wall of the eye. This study is usually done to diagnose the reason a patient's vision is blurry.

R97 Abnormal tumor markers

Abnormal tumor markers are specific antigens, usually glycoproteins, that are present in the body in correlation with certain neoplasms and neoplastic-related disease conditions. The antigen's presence is an indicator of the body's immune response to the particular tumor or disease process within the body. Sometimes, the tumor marker is a substance secreted by the aggressive cancer cells themselves, and sometimes it is secreted by normal cells in increased amounts due to the effect of fighting the neoplastic disease.

R97.0   Elevated carcinoembryonic antigen [CEA]

Carcinoembryonic antigen [CEA] is a glycoprotein that is secreted into the surface of epithelial cells of the gastrointestinal tract. CEA does occur normally in stool and secretions of the pancreas and biliary tract, but also appears in blood plasma with a group of neoplastic and nonneoplastic conditions, mainly adenocarcinoma of the colon; pancreas, lung, and stomach cancer; alcoholic cirrhosis; inflammatory bowel diseases; pancreatitis; and rectal polyps. Carcinoembryonic antigen is primarily tracked in order to monitor the body's response to colorectal cancer treatment.

R97.1   Elevated cancer antigen 125 [CA 125]

Elevated serum levels of cancer antigen 125 [CA 125] is another glycoprotein antigen associated with epithelial ovarian carcinomas, and also seen with some other malignant and benign pelvic disorders.

R97.2   Elevated prostate specific antigen [PSA]

Elevated levels of prostate specific antigen (PSA) in the bloodstream can indicate prostate cancer, or precursor conditions that can develop into prostate cancer.

Injury, Poisoning and Certain Other Consequences of External Causes | S00-T88

S03.0 Dislocation of jaw

A dislocation is a separation injury of a joint where two or more bones come together in which the ends of the involved bones are forced further apart than their normal positions. This occurs as a result of a hard blow to the joint and most often results in immediate pain and immobilization, visual deformity, numbness, and swelling. Dislocation is also known as luxation. A dislocated jaw occurs when the mandibular condyle becomes displaced from the articular groove where it connects to the temporal bone, making it impossible to close the jaw.

S03.4 Sprain of jaw

A sprain is an injury to a ligament. Ligaments are tough, elastic tissues that connect bones and hold them together, supporting joints for movement and rotation or protecting against abnormal motion. A sprain occurs when the ligaments of a joint are stretched or torn, often by direct injury such as a hit or full contact blow, a fall, or traumatic twisting of the joint. Sprains are graded by severity. In a mild Grade 1 sprain, ligaments are stretched beyond their normal range with some microscopic damage to the collagen fibrils, but no tearing. In a moderate Grade 2 sprain, ligaments are partially torn with the tearing affecting some but not all of the collagen fibers. There may be some loss of function with abnormal laxity in the joint. In severe Grade 3 sprains, the elastic fibers are nearly completely torn or ruptured and gross instability can result. A sprain of the jaw involves stretching or tearing of the temporomandibular ligament.

S06.0 Concussion

A concussion is a traumatic brain injury that alters the way the brain functions, usually only for a brief period. Concussions are normally caused by a blow to the head, but can also occur when the head and upper part of the body are shaken violently, causing the brain to slide or bounce back and forth inside the walls of the skull from sudden acceleration or deceleration of the head. Concussions can cause loss of consciousness, although most do not. Bleeding in or around the brain can also occur right away or develop later, which is why all concussions need to be monitored. Signs and symptoms of concussion include severe headache, amnesia of the event, nausea, vomiting, lack of physical coordination, dizziness, ringing in the ears, visual changes, confusion, disorientation, fluid discharge from the nose or ears, slurred speech, concentration and memory deficits, sleep disturbance, irritability, sensitivity to light and noise, and behavioral changes.

S06.4 Epidural hemorrhage

Traumatic epidural (extradural) hemorrhage is bleeding that occurs between the dura mater--the tough, outer layer of the protective covering around the brain, and the skull. Extradural bleeding arises from blunt traumatic head injury such as occurs in a fall, an assault, or other accident. It can increase intracranial pressure, causing compression of brain tissue and leading to coma; but in most cases, it is easily treated with a good prognosis. This type of traumatic hemorrhage is not brought on by head motion, such as acceleration and deceleration, but by disruption of the blood vessels in the dura and skull associated with fractures, mainly laceration of the middle meningeal artery and the dural sinuses.

S06.5 Traumatic subdural hemorrhage

Traumatic subdural hemorrhage is bleeding that occurs between the dura mater--the very outer layer of the protective membrane covering the brain, and the arachnoid mater--the middle layer of the covering around the brain. The arachnoid mater is attached very closely to the inside of the dura mater and is much more delicate. Acute subdural hemorrhaging is usually caused by severe head trauma and has the highest mortality rate of all types of head injuries. Bleeding fills the brain rapidly and compresses the brain tissue, which can lead to death. In the elderly, chronic subdural hemorrhaging has been known to occur with very minor head injury and go unnoticed for days or weeks.

S06.6 Traumatic subarachnoid hemorrhage

Traumatic subarachnoid intracranial hemorrhage is bleeding that occurs between the middle (arachnoid) and inner (pial) layers of the protective membrane covering the brain. Hemorrhage into the subarachnoid space caused by head injury is the most frequent kind of traumatic hemorrhage and does not usually exert localized pressure as the bleeding is diffuse and diluted by the cerebrospinal fluid. The blood does not usually clot except in massive hemorrhaging cases. Large amounts of hemorrhaging will raise intracranial pressure and can lead to impaired perfusion of the brain and hypoxic ischemic encephalopathy unless treated.

S13.4 Sprain of ligaments of cervical spine

A sprain is an injury to a ligament. Ligaments are tough, elastic tissues that connect bones and hold them together, supporting joints for movement and rotation or protecting against abnormal motion. A sprain occurs when the ligaments of a joint are stretched or torn, often by direct injury such as a hit or full contact blow, a fall, or traumatic twisting of the joint. Sprains are graded by severity. In a mild Grade 1 sprain, ligaments are stretched beyond their normal range with some microscopic damage to the collagen fibrils, but no tearing. In a moderate Grade 2 sprain, ligaments are partially torn with the tearing affecting some but not all of the collagen fibers. There may be some loss of function with abnormal laxity in the joint. In severe Grade 3 sprains, the elastic fibers are nearly completely torn or ruptured and gross instability can result. A sprain of the cervical spine includes whiplash injuries of the neck in which the head is suddenly thrown backward and then forward, affecting the joints of the cervical vertebrae.

S14.1 Other and unspecified injuries of cervical spinal cord

Damage to the spinal cord is specified as to location using the vertebrae level closest to the injury. Codes for injury to the cervical spinal cord in the neck must be reported to the highest level of cord injury. Damage can take on many different forms and is reported as complete lesion, central cord syndrome, anterior cord syndrome, Brown-Sequard syndrome, and incomplete lesion of cerivcal spinal cord.

S14.11 Complete lesion of cervical spinal cord

A complete lesion of the spinal cord occurs when the spinal cord is completely severed, resulting in permanent, complete paralysis and loss of sensation below the level of the lesion.

S14.12 Central cord syndrome of cervical spinal cord

Central cord syndrome is an acute cervical spinal cord injury. It is the most common type of incomplete spinal cord injury that occurs when the spine in hyperextended with the head forced or flung backwards, usually from some kind of blow. The cord is then squeezed or compressed both anteriorly and posteriorly between the cervical body in front and the posterior intraspinal canal ligament in the back, called the ligamentum flavum. This results in edema, hemorrhage, or ischemia causing paraplegia, or severe loss of strength and mobility to the upper limbs in particular, with varying degree of sensitivity loss.

S14.13 Anterior cord syndrome of cervical spinal cord

Anterior cord syndrome is another common type of incomplete cord lesion, caused by infarction or vascular insufficiency when the blood supply to the anterior portion of the spinal cord is interrupted. This is usually as a result of the artery that runs along the front of the spinal cord being compressed, possibly from stray bone fragments, or large disc herniation. Patients usually display complete loss of muscle strength and sensitivity to pain and temperature, with greater motor loss in the legs than arms, while the sense of position, proprioception, and vibration remains intact.

S14.14 Brown-Séquard syndrome of cervical spinal cord

Brown-Séquard syndrome is a type of incomplete spinal cord injury occurring to either side of the cervical spinal cord and causing unilateral damage to the spinal tract that results in muscle paralysis on the same side as the injury with loss of pain and temperature sensation on the opposite side. It is usually caused by penetrating trauma to one side of the spinal cord, or vertebral facet fracture or dislocation on one side.

S14.15 Other incomplete lesions of cervical spinal cord

This includes posterior cord syndrome, a rare type of incomplete lesion caused by interruption of the posterior spinal artery. There are differences in the loss of sensory and motor function below the level of the injury. The posterior spinal cord carries sensory information from the periphery to the brain. Although motor function is most often preserved, or not as severe as with other cord lesions, and the general sense of pain and temperature also remain, sensitivity is lost regarding the position of the body and limbs, vibration, and fine touch. There is also the presence of other odd sensations such as burning, prickling, tingling, or insects crawling on the skin. Posterior spinal column damage also results in L'Hermitte's Sign, in which the patient experiences electric shock sensations running down the back and into the limbs.

S23.3 Sprain of ligaments of thoracic spine

A sprain is an injury to a ligament. Ligaments are tough, elastic tissues that connect bones and hold them together, supporting joints for movement and rotation or protecting against abnormal motion. A sprain occurs when the ligaments of a joint are stretched or torn, often by direct injury such as a hit or full contact blow, a fall, or traumatic twisting of the joint. Sprains are graded by severity. In a mild Grade 1 sprain, ligaments are stretched beyond their normal range with some microscopic damage to the collagen fibrils, but no tearing. In a moderate Grade 2 sprain, ligaments are partially torn with the tearing affecting some but not all of the collagen fibers. There may be some loss of function with abnormal laxity in the joint. In severe Grade 3 sprains, the elastic fibers are nearly completely torn or ruptured and gross instability can result.

S23.4 Sprain of ribs and sternum

A sprain is an injury to a ligament. Ligaments are tough, elastic tissues that connect bones and hold them together, supporting joints for movement and rotation or protecting against abnormal motion. A sprain occurs when the ligaments of a joint are stretched or torn, often by direct injury such as a hit or full contact blow, a fall, or traumatic twisting of the joint. Sprains are graded by severity. In a mild Grade 1 sprain, ligaments are stretched beyond their normal range with some microscopic damage to the collagen fibrils, but no tearing. In a moderate Grade 2 sprain, ligaments are partially torn with the tearing affecting some but not all of the collagen fibers. There may be some loss of function with abnormal laxity in the joint. In severe Grade 3 sprains, the elastic fibers are nearly or completely torn or ruptured and gross instability can result. A sprain of the ribs or sternum most commonly occurs with vehicular accidents, a direct blow in contact sports, or from falls.

S23.421 Sprain of chondrosternal joint

The chondrosternal joint is also called the sternocostal joint and is the point where the cartilage of each true rib (except the first) articulates with the sternum. The first rib cartilage is fused with the sternum, creating a synchondrosis. Each costosternal articulation of ribs 2-7 allows slight movement only and involves several ligaments - the interarticular sternocostal ligaments, the radiate sternocostal ligaments, and the costoxyphoid ligaments. Sprains may be mild, moderate, or severe.

S32.81 Multiple fractures of pelvis with disruption of pelvic ring

The pelvic circle is composed of the paired innominate, pubic, and ischial bones and the sacrum. The sacroiliac joints and ligaments join the ring in the back and the symphysis pubis joins the front. The pelvic ring transfers weight from the vertebrae to the acetabulum for standing and to the ischial tuberosities for sitting. High energy fractures cause severe injury

producing pelvic ring disruption, which is assessed for anterior, posterior, and rotational displacement. Associated pathology includes embolism and hemorrhaging from the fracture, or blood vessel tears which can cause hypovolemia and hypotension. Pelvic fractures with disruption of the circle must be treated to restore anatomic continuity, prevent deformity, and return mobility and function. Open reduction and rigid internal fixation is done with plates placed over fracture lines. Percutaneous fixation may be used for disruption of the sacroiliac joint or sacrum stabilization.

S32.82 Multiple fractures of pelvis without disruption of pelvic ring

The pelvic circle is composed of the paired innominate, pubic, and ischial bones and the sacrum. The sacroiliac joints and ligaments join the ring in the back and the symphysis pubis joins the front. The pelvic ring transfers weight from the vertebrae to the acetabulum for standing and to the ischial tuberosities for sitting. Low energy incidents generally result in isolated fractures to individual bones without pelvic ring disruption. Pelvic fractures that are stable or only minimally displaced and do not disrupt the pelvic circle are treated with gentle mobilization and protected weight bearing on the injured side.

S33.5 Sprain of ligaments of lumbar spine

A sprain is an injury to a ligament. Ligaments are tough, elastic tissues that connect bones and hold them together, supporting joints for movement and rotation or protecting against abnormal motion. A sprain occurs when the ligaments of a joint are stretched or torn, often by direct injury such as a hit or full contact blow, a fall, or traumatic twisting of the joint. Sprains are graded by severity. In a mild Grade 1 sprain, ligaments are stretched beyond their normal range with some microscopic damage to the collagen fibrils, but no tearing. In a moderate Grade 2 sprain, ligaments are partially torn with the tearing affecting some but not all of the collagen fibers. There may be some loss of function with abnormal laxity in the joint. In severe Grade 3 sprains, the elastic fibers are nearly completely torn or ruptured and gross instability can result.

S33.6 Sprain of sacroiliac joint

A sprain is an injury to a ligament. Ligaments are tough, elastic tissues that connect bones and hold them together, supporting joints for movement and rotation or protecting against abnormal motion. A sprain occurs when the ligaments of a joint are stretched or torn, often by direct injury such as a hit or full contact blow, a fall, or traumatic twisting of the joint. Sprains are graded by severity. In a mild Grade 1 sprain, ligaments are stretched beyond their normal range with some microscopic damage to the collagen fibrils, but no tearing. In a moderate Grade 2 sprain, ligaments are partially torn with the tearing affecting some but not all of the collagen fibers. There may be some loss of function with abnormal laxity in the joint. In severe Grade 3 sprains, the elastic fibers are nearly completely torn or ruptured and gross instability can result. A sprain of the sacroiliac joint is ligamentous disruption of the joint in the bony pelvis where the ilium, or the large 'wing' of the pelvis connects on either side to the sacrum, which supports the spine in the middle. The two, paired kidney bean-shaped sacroiliac joints are strong, weight-bearing joints that move together as a single unit.

S36.2 Injury of pancreas

The pancreas lies behind the stomach and connects to the duodenum of the small intestine through a duct shared with the liver and gallbladder. It secretes pancreatic juice, which aids in the digestion of protein, and also produces insulin. The organ is divided into three main sections: the head, the curved portion near the intestine; the main body; and the tail, which terminates at the spleen.

S42.2 Fracture of upper end of humerus

Fractures of the proximal or upper end of the humerus are classified using the Neer system. The proximal humerus is divided into four parts—the humeral head, greater tuberosity, lesser tuberosity, and the diaphysis or shaft. These four parts are separated by epiphyseal lines, also called growth plates when the bones are still growing during the developmental years. The surgical neck is the narrowest aspect of the humerus just below the tubercles. When the proximal humerus is fractured, it typically occurs at the surgical neck and along one or more of the three epiphyseal lines. The

2016 Plain English Descriptions for ICD-10-CM   Chapter 19 Injury, Poisoning and Certain Other Consequences of External Causes | S42.27 – S43.21

Injury/Poisoning/Other External Causes   S42.27 – S43.21

proximal humerus may fracture into 2, 3, or 4 parts at the surgical neck which is why surgical neck fractures are designated as 2-part, 3-part, or 4-part subcategories.

S42.27   Torus fracture of upper end of humerus

Torus fractures are also called buckle fractures and are most commonly found in children, due to the softness of their bones. This type of fracture occurs when increased weight loading is placed on the axis of a long bone, such as falling onto an outstretched arm. The soft bone is longitudinally compressed, resulting in an incomplete fracture of the diaphysis of the long bone, with buckling of the bone cortex on the opposite side, which appears as localized bulging. Torus fractures are most common in the radius, but do also commonly occur in the ulna, humerus, femur, tibia, and fibula. This subcategory reports a torus fracture of the upper end of the humerus.

S42.31   Greenstick fracture of shaft of humerus

Greenstick fractures are a common type of fracture injury in children. This type of fracture occurs in young, soft bones that are more pliable than adult bones. When force is applied, the bone bends, but does not completely break into separate pieces, leaving one side of the bone broken and the other side of the bone bent. This is analogous to breaking a young, green, fresh tree branch when the outer side snaps and the inner side bends. Some greenstick fractures may appear with typical deformity and significant swelling, while others may be confused with sprains as they do not always present with much pain and swelling. The child may even continue to use the limb, but casting will immobilize and protect from complete breakage.

S42.32   Transverse fracture of shaft of humerus

A transverse fracture is a complete break straight across a bone in which the fracture line runs at a right angle to the long axis of the bone. Transverse fractures are usually caused by a very sharp direct blow across the bone or sometimes through a stress fracture.

S42.33   Oblique fracture of shaft of humerus

An oblique fracture is a slanted break in a bone in which the fracture line is direct, but angled diagonally across the shaft of the bone. This is usually caused by a hard, angled blow to the bone, such as in sports or falling down stairs.

S42.34   Spiral fracture of shaft of humerus

A spiral fracture is a break in a bone similar to an oblique fracture, but caused by a twisting force that results in an oblique fracture line that spirals around and through the bone like a corkscrew. Spiral fractures are rare and are often misdiagnosed initially as oblique fractures, but can be seen on x-ray as a spiral break. These are generally caused by severe twisting force when one part of the limb is caught or trapped and the adjoining bone is torsed.

S42.35   Comminuted fracture of shaft of humerus

A comminuted fracture is any fracture in which the bone involved is broken into at least 3 separate pieces. This is also known as a multi-fragmentary fracture and is often the result of a tremendous traumatic force. Comminuted fractures also occur in people with weakened bones, such as the elderly, and those with cancer or other diseases like osteogenesis imperfecta.

S42.36   Segmental fracture of shaft of humerus

A segmental fracture is a break in a bone in which two distinct parts of the same bone are broken, creating a segment of the shaft of the bone that is isolated by a proximal and a distal fracture line. This is also known as a double fracture.

S42.42   Comminuted supracondylar fracture without intercondylar fracture of humerus

A comminuted fracture is any fracture in which the bone involved is broken into at least 3 separate pieces. This is also known as a multi-fragmentary fracture and is often the result of a tremendous traumatic force. Comminuted fractures also occur in people with weakened bones, such as the elderly, and those with cancer or other diseases like osteogenesis imperfecta. A comminuted supracondylar fracture of the humerus without

intercondylar fracture is a break in the lower portion of the upper arm bone just above the elbow resulting in multiple fragments, and in which no breaks reach into the rounded projections at the end of the humerus forming the articulation points for moving the elbow joint.

S42.48   Torus fracture of lower end of humerus

Torus fractures are also called buckle fractures and are most commonly found in children, due to the softness of their bones. This type of fracture occurs when increased weight loading is placed on the axis of a long bone, such as falling onto an outstretched arm. The soft bone is longitudinally compressed, resulting in an incomplete fracture of the diaphysis of the long bone, with buckling of the bone cortex on the opposite side, which appears as localized bulging. Torus fractures are most common in the radius, but do also commonly occur in the ulna, humerus, femur, tibia, and fibula. This subcategory reports a torus fracture of the lower end of the humerus.

S43.0   Subluxation and dislocation of shoulder joint

Subluxation is a partial dislocation of a joint in which the bones are misaligned, but the articular surfaces remain in some kind of contact with each other. This causes some loss of normal joint relationship and function. A dislocation is a separation injury of a joint (where two or more bones come together) in which the ends of the involved bones are forced further apart than their normal positions. This occurs as a result of a hard blow to the joint and most often results in immediate pain and immobilization, visual deformity, numbness, and swelling. Dislocation is also known as luxation. A dislocation or subluxation of the shoulder joint involves the point where the round, ball-shaped head of the humerus, the upper arm bone, connects to the socket-shaped glenoid cavity of the scapula, or shoulder blade.

S43.1   Subluxation and dislocation of acromioclavicular joint

Subluxation is a partial dislocation of a joint in which the bones are misaligned, but the articular surfaces remain in some kind of contact with each other. This causes some loss of normal joint relationship and function. A dislocation is a separation injury of a joint (where two or more bones come together) in which the ends of the involved bones are forced further apart than their normal positions. This occurs as a result of a hard blow to the joint and most often results in immediate pain and immobilization, visual deformity, numbness, and swelling. Dislocation is also known as luxation. A dislocation or subluxation of the acromioclavicular joint, also known as the AC joint, involves the joint on top of the shoulder where the highest point of the scapula, the acromion, connects with the collarbone.

S43.2   Subluxation and dislocation of sternoclavicular joint

Subluxation is a partial dislocation of a joint in which the bones are misaligned, but the articular surfaces remain in some kind of contact with each other. This causes some loss of normal joint relationship and function. A dislocation is a separation injury of a joint (where two or more bones come together) in which the ends of the involved bones are forced further apart than their normal positions. This occurs as a result of a hard blow to the joint and most often results in immediate pain and immobilization, visual deformity, numbness, and swelling. Dislocation is also known as luxation. A dislocation or subluxation of the sternoclavicular joint, also known as the SC joint, involves the point where the sternum, or breastbone, connects to the clavicle (collarbone).

S43.21   Anterior subluxation and dislocation of sternoclavicular joint

With an anterior subluxation and dislocation of the sternoclavicular joint, the collarbone becomes displaced in front of the sternum. The end of the displaced clavicle can usually be seen bulging out in front along with pain and swelling. Anterior subluxations or dislocations are usually the result of an injury when the outer front of the shoulder is hit with force.

S43.22 Posterior subluxation and dislocation of sternoclavicular joint

With a posterior subluxation or dislocation of the sternoclavicular joint, the collarbone becomes displaced behind the sternum. This kind of dislocation is much more worrisome than anterior dislocations or subluxations because of the major blood vessels and the windpipe located behind the protective sternum. If the displaced end of the clavicle punctures these structures, life-threatening problems can result. Posterior dislocations may appear only as a subtle bump or dimpling over the skin of the joint, and may occur with difficulty breathing, pain when swallowing, and an abnormal pulse that occurs with compression of the esophagus, trachea, or important blood vessels. This type of subluxation or dislocation is often caused by blunt force directly hitting the front of the chest.

S43.4 Sprain of shoulder joint

A sprain is an injury to a ligament. Ligaments are tough, elastic tissues that connect bones and hold them together, supporting joints for movement and rotation or protecting against abnormal motion. A sprain occurs when the ligaments of a joint are stretched or torn, often by direct injury such as a hit or full contact blow, a fall, or traumatic twisting of the joint. Sprains are graded by severity. In a mild Grade 1 sprain, ligaments are stretched beyond their normal range with some microscopic damage to the collagen fibrils, but no tearing. In a moderate Grade 2 sprain, ligaments are partially torn with the tearing affecting some but not all of the collagen fibers. There may be some loss of function with abnormal laxity in the joint. In severe Grade 3 sprains, the elastic fibers are nearly completely torn or ruptured and gross instability can result.

S43.5 Sprain of acromioclavicular joint

A sprain is an injury to a ligament. Ligaments are tough, elastic tissues that connect bones and hold them together, supporting joints for movement and rotation or protecting against abnormal motion. A sprain occurs when the ligaments of a joint are stretched or torn, often by direct injury such as a hit or full contact blow, a fall, or traumatic twisting of the joint. Sprains are graded by severity. In a mild Grade 1 sprain, ligaments are stretched beyond their normal range with some microscopic damage to the collagen fibrils, but no tearing. In a moderate Grade 2 sprain, ligaments are partially torn with the tearing affecting some but not all of the collagen fibers. There may be some loss of function with abnormal laxity in the joint. In severe Grade 3 sprains, the elastic fibers are nearly completely torn or ruptured and gross instability can result. A sprain of the acromioclavicular joint located at the top of the shoulder, involves the junction between the highest point of the shoulder, the acromion, and the clavicle, or collarbone. This joint allows the arm to be lifted above the head.

S43.6 Sprain of sternoclavicular joint

A sprain is an injury to a ligament. Ligaments are tough, elastic tissues that connect bones and hold them together, supporting joints for movement and rotation or protecting against abnormal motion. A sprain occurs when the ligaments of a joint are stretched or torn, often by direct injury such as a hit or full contact blow, a fall, or traumatic twisting of the joint. Sprains are graded by severity. In a mild Grade 1 sprain, ligaments are stretched beyond their normal range with some microscopic damage to the collagen fibrils, but no tearing. In a moderate Grade 2 sprain, ligaments are partially torn with the tearing affecting some but not all of the collagen fibers. There may be some loss of function with abnormal laxity in the joint. In severe Grade 3 sprains, the elastic fibers are nearly completely torn or ruptured and gross instability can result. A sprain of the sternoclavicular joint is involves the connection between the breastbone and the collarbone.

S49.0 Physeal fracture of upper end of humerus

Physeal fractures may also be referred to as Salter-Harris fractures or traumatic epiphyseal separations. These fractures occur along the physeal (growth) plates in bones that have not reached their full growth and in which the plates are still open and filled with cartilaginous tissue. Salter-Harris fractures are classified into 9 types. Types I-IV have specific codes for

fractures of the upper end of the humerus. Types V-IX are reported under other physeal fracture.

Note: The physis is the growth plate where the bone lengthens. The epiphysis is the rounded end of the bone that articulates with another bone. The metaphysis is the widened transitional zone between the diaphysis (the shaft of the bone), and the epiphysis, where the physeal plate is located.

S49.01 Salter-Harris Type I physeal fracture of upper end of humerus

A Salter-Harris Type I fracture is an epiphyseal separation with displacement of the epiphysis from the metaphysis at the physis.

S49.02 Salter-Harris Type II physeal fracture of upper end of humerus

A Salter-Harris Type II physeal fracture is a break through the physis and a portion of the metaphysis without fracture of the epiphysis.

S49.03 Salter-Harris Type III physeal fracture of upper end of humerus

A Salter-Harris Type III fracture is a break through the physis and epiphysis which damages the reproductive layer of the physis.

S49.04 Salter-Harris Type IV physeal fracture of upper end of humerus

A Salter-Harris Type IV fracture is a break through the metaphysis, physis, and epiphysis causing damage to the reproductive layer of the physis.

S49.09 Other physeal fracture of upper end of humerus

Other physeal fractures include types V-IX, which are less common types of physeal injuries and include crush or compression injuries involving the physis alone, injury involving perichondral structrures, an isolated injury of the epiphyseal plate or the metaphysis with potential endochondral ossification, and periosteum injury affecting growth of the membrane.

S49.1 Physeal fracture of lower end of humerus

Physeal fractures may also be referred to as Salter-Harris fractures or traumatic epiphyseal separations. These fractures occur along the physeal (growth) plates in bones that have not reached their full growth and in which the plates are still open and filled with cartilaginous tissue. Salter-Harris fractures are classified into 9 types. Types I-IV have specific codes for fractures of the lower end of the humerus. Types V-IX are reported under other physeal fracture.

Note: The physis is the growth plate where the bone lengthens. The epiphysis is the rounded end of the bone that articulates with another bone. The metaphysis is the widened transitional zone between the diaphysis (the shaft of the bone), and the epiphysis, where the physeal plate is located.

S49.11 Salter-Harris Type I physeal fracture of lower end of humerus

A Salter-Harris Type I fracture is an epiphyseal separation with displacement of the epiphysis from the metaphysis at the physis.

S49.12 Salter-Harris Type II physeal fracture of lower end of humerus

A Salter-Harris Type II physeal fracture is a break through the physis and a portion of the metaphysis without fracture of the epiphysis.

S49.13 Salter Harris Type III physeal fracture of lower end of humerus

A Salter-Harris Type III fracture is a break through the physis and epiphysis which damages the reproductive layer of the physis.

S49.14 Salter-Harris Type IV physeal fracture of lower end of humerus

A Salter-Harris Type IV fracture is a break through the metaphysis, physis, and epiphysis causing damage to the reproductive layer of the physis.

S49.19 Other physeal fracture of lower end of humerus

Other physeal fractures include types V-IX, which are less common types of physeal injuries and include crush or compression injuries involving the physis alone, injury involving perichondral structrures, an isolated injury of the epiphyseal plate or the metaphysis with potential endochondral ossification, and periosteum injury affecting growth of the membrane.

S52 Fracture of forearm

The Gustilo classification employed in 7th character extensions for fractures of some bones, such as the radius and ulna, applies to open fractures. The Gustilo open fracture classification groups fractures into three main categories designated as Type I, Type II, and Type III with Type III injuries being further divided into Type IIIA, Type IIIB, and Type IIIC subcategories. Each of these three main categories is defined by three major characteristics: mechanism of injury, extent of soft tissue damage, and degree of bone injury or involvement. The specific characteristics of each major type of open fracture determine the correct code placement.

Specific characteristics for **Type I** open fractures include a wound < 1 cm; minimal soft tissue damage; a clean wound bed; a typically low-energy type injury; and fracture types usually either simple transverse, short oblique, or minimally comminuted.

Specific characteristics for **Type II** open fractures include a wound > 1 cm; moderate soft tissue damage; minimal wound bed contamination; a typically low-energy type injury; and fracture types usually either simple transverse, short oblique, or minimally comminuted.

Specific characteristics for **Type III** open fractures include a wound > 1 cm; extensive soft tissue damage; a typically high-energy type injury; highly unstable fractures often with multiple bone fragments; and injury patterns usually resulting in open segmental or severely comminuted fractures. Traumatic involvement is seen as well, such as gun-shot wounds, neurovascular complications, severe contamination, traumatic amputations, and delayed treatment (over 8 hours). This last group of Type III fractures is further subdivided with the following specific characteristics: Type IIIA has adequate soft tissue coverage of the open wound with no local or distant flap coverage required, and the fracture may be open segmental or severely comminuted and still be subclassified as Type IIIA. Type IIIB has extensive soft tissue loss and local or distant flap coverage is required. Wound bed contamination requires serial irrigation and debridement to clean the open fracture site. Type IIIC has major arterial injury and extensive repair usually requires the skills of a vascular surgeon for limb salvage.

S52.01 Torus fracture of upper end of ulna

Torus fractures are also called buckle fractures and are most commonly found in children, due to the softness of their bones. This type of fracture occurs when increased weight loading is placed on the axis of a long bone, such as falling onto an outstretched arm. The soft bone is longitudinally compressed, resulting in an incomplete fracture of the diaphysis (shaft) of the long bone, with buckling of the bone cortex on the opposite side, which appears as localized bulging. Torus fractures are most common in the radius, but do also commonly occur in the ulna, humerus, femur, tibia, and fibula. This subcategory reports a torus fracture of the upper end of the ulna only, the bone on the inner, pinky finger side of the forearm.

S52.11 Torus fracture of upper end of radius

Torus fractures are also called buckle fractures and are most commonly found in children, due to the softness of their bones. This type of fracture occurs when increased weight loading is placed on the axis of a long bone, such as falling onto an outstretched arm. The soft bone is longitudinally compressed, resulting in an incomplete fracture of the diaphysis (shaft) of the long bone, with buckling of the bone cortex on the opposite side, which appears as localized bulging. This subcategory reports a torus fracture of the upper end of the radius only, but they do also commonly occur in the ulna,

humerus, femur, tibia, and fibula. Torus fractures are most common in the radius, the bone on the outer, thumb side of the forearm.

S52.21 Greenstick fracture of shaft of ulna

Greenstick fractures are a common type of fracture injury in children. This type of fracture occurs in young, soft bones that are more pliable than adult bones. When force is applied, the bone bends, but does not completely break into separate pieces, leaving one side of the bone broken and the other side of the bone bent. This is analogous to breaking a young, green, fresh tree branch when the outer side snaps and the inner side bends. Some greenstick fractures may appear with typical deformity and significant swelling, while others may be confused with sprains as they do not always present with much pain and swelling. The child may even continue to use the limb, but casting will immobilize and protect from complete breakage.

S52.22 Transverse fracture of shaft of ulna

A transverse fracture is a complete break straight across a bone in which the fracture line runs at a right angle to the long axis of the bone. Transverse fractures are usually caused by a very sharp direct blow across the bone or sometimes through a stress fracture.

S52.23 Oblique fracture of shaft of ulna

An oblique fracture is a slanted break in a bone in which the fracture line is direct, but angled diagonally across the shaft of the bone. This is usually caused by a hard, angled blow to the bone, such as in sports or falling down stairs.

S52.24 Spiral fracture of shaft of ulna

A spiral fracture is a break in a bone similar to an oblique fracture, but caused by a twisting force that results in an oblique fracture line that spirals around and through the bone like a corkscrew. Spiral fractures are rare and are often misdiagnosed initially as oblique fractures, but can be seen on x-ray as a spiral break. These are generally caused by severe twisting force when one part of the limb is caught or trapped and the adjoining bone is torsed.

S52.25 Comminuted fracture of shaft of ulna

A comminuted fracture is any fracture in which the bone involved is broken into at least 3 separate pieces. This is also known as a multi-fragmentary fracture and is often the result of a tremendous traumatic force. Comminuted fractures also occur in people with weakened bones, such as the elderly, and those with cancer or other diseases like osteogenesis imperfecta.

S52.26 Segmental fracture of shaft of ulna

A segmental fracture is a break in a bone in which two distinct parts of the same bone are broken, creating a segment of the shaft of the bone that is isolated by a proximal and a distal fracture line. This is also known as a double fracture.

S52.27 Monteggia's fracture of ulna

A Monteggia's fracture is a fracture of the upper (proximal third) shaft of the ulna with dislocation of the radial head. There are different types of Monteggia's fractures classified by the direction of the dislocation of the radial head and the angulation or point of ulnar fracture. Over half of Monteggia fractures are Type I, extension type fractures with anterior dislocation of the radial head and anterior angulated (usually proximal third) ulnar shaft fracture. Flexion type Monteggia's fractures (Type II) occur with posterior or posterolateral dislocation of the radial head and posterior angulation of the proximal ulnar fracture. Type III Monteggia fractures display lateral or anterolateral dislocation of the radial head and fracture of the ulnar metaphysis, or ulna fracture just distal to the coronoid process.

S52.31 Greenstick fracture of shaft of radius

Greenstick fractures are a common type of fracture injury in children. This type of fracture occurs in young, soft bones that are more pliable than adult bones. When force is applied, the bone bends, but does not completely break into separate pieces, leaving one side of the bone broken and the other side of the bone bent. This is analogous to breaking a young, green, fresh tree branch when the outer side snaps and the inner side bends. Some greenstick fractures may appear with typical deformity and significant swelling, while others may be confused with sprains as they do not always present with much pain and swelling. The child may even continue to use the limb, but casting will immobilize and protect from complete breakage.

S52.32   Transverse fracture of shaft of radius

A transverse fracture is a complete break straight across a bone in which the fracture line runs at a right angle to the long axis of the bone. Transverse fractures are usually caused by a very sharp direct blow across the bone or sometimes through a stress fracture.

S52.33   Oblique fracture of shaft of radius

An oblique fracture is a slanted break in a bone in which the fracture line is direct, but angled diagonally across the shaft of the bone. This is usually caused by a hard, angled blow to the bone, such as in sports or falling down stairs.

S52.34   Spiral fracture of shaft of radius

A spiral fracture is a break in a bone similar to an oblique fracture, but caused by a twisting force that results in an oblique fracture line that spirals around and through the bone like a corkscrew. Spiral fractures are rare and are often misdiagnosed initially as oblique fractures, but can be seen on x-ray as a spiral break. These are generally caused by severe twisting force when one part of the limb is caught or trapped and the adjoining bone is torsed.

S52.35   Comminuted fracture of shaft of radius

A comminuted fracture is any fracture in which the bone involved is broken into at least 3 separate pieces. This is also known as a multi-fragmentary fracture and is often the result of a tremendous traumatic force. Comminuted fractures also occur in people with weakened bones, such as the elderly, and those with cancer or other diseases like osteogenesis imperfecta.

S52.36   Segmental fracture of shaft of radius

A segmental fracture is a break in a bone in which two distinct parts of the same bone are broken, creating a segment of the shaft of the bone that is isolated by a proximal and a distal fracture line. This is also known as a double fracture.

S52.37   Galeazzi's fracture

A Galeazzi's fracture is a fracture of the lower shaft of the radius, occuring between the middle and distal thirds of the shaft, with dislocation of the distal radioulnar joint that usually occurs on the back side, but may be on the palmar side. In adults, the radioulnar joint injury tends to tear the ligaments or avulse the ulnar styloid with the triangular fibrocartilage complex in place, while in children there may be separation of the distal ulnar epiphysis. This type of fracture occurs as a result of direct blows or falls. In adults, Galeazzi fracture-dislocations are usually treated with open reduction and internal plate fixation, and K-wire fixation of unstable radioulnar dislocations. In young children, closed reduction may be possible.

S52.52   Torus fracture of lower end of radius

Torus fractures are also called buckle fractures and are most commonly found in children, due to the softness of their bones. This type of fracture occurs when increased weight loading is placed on the axis of a long bone, such as falling onto an outstretched arm. The soft bone is longitudinally compressed, resulting in an incomplete fracture of the diaphysis of the long bone, with buckling of the bone cortex on the opposite side, which appears as localized bulging. This code reports a torus fracture of the lower end of the radius only, but they do also commonly occur in the ulna, humerus, femur, tibia, and fibula. Torus fractures are most common in the radius, the bone on the outer, thumb side of the forearm.

S52.53   Colles' fracture

A Colles' fracture is a specific type of wrist fracture in which the distal end of the radius, the lower end of the bone in the forearm on the thumb side of the wrist, is broken with posterior (dorsal) displacement of the wrist. This type of fracture is very common and typically occurs with falling onto an outstretched arm and extended wrist, or getting hit on the ventral side of the lower forearm. Colles' fractures are seen in people playing contact sports, skiing, biking, and skating, and also in people with osteoporosis.

S52.54   Smith's fracture

A Smith's fracture is a certain type of broken wrist, often referred to as a reversed Colles' fracture, in which a fracture of the distal radius, the lower end of the bone in the forearm on the thumb side of the wrist, occurs with palmar side (volar) displacement of the wrist in front of its normal position. This type of fracture usually occurs after a fall onto the back side of the hand or flexed wrist, or a direct blow to the back of the lower forearm. Smith's fractures are much less common than Colles' types fractures.

S52.56   Barton's fracture

A Barton's fracture is an intra-articular fracture of the distal radius with dislocation of the radiocarpal joint. This is the most common type of fracture dislocation occuring in the wrist joint, usually caused by a fall onto an outstretched arm. The distal radial fracture may involve either the anterior or posterior bone cortex and the carpal dislocation may be either volarly or dorsally displaced. Volar Barton's fracture dislocations are more common. Dorsal Barton's fractures often occur with a fracture of the radial styloid. The carpal dislocation is the most obvious appearance on radiographs and thereby differs from either Colles or Smith fractures. Whether displaced in front of or in back of it's normal position, the rim of the distal radius is also seen displaced with the dislocated hand and wrist.

S52.62   Torus fracture of lower end of ulna

Torus fractures are also called buckle fractures and are most commonly found in children, due to the softness of their bones. This type of fracture occurs when increased weight loading is placed on the axis of a long bone, such as falling onto an outstretched arm. The soft bone is longitudinally compressed, resulting in an incomplete fracture of the diaphysis of the long bone, with buckling of the bone cortex on the opposite side, which appears as localized bulging. Torus fractures are most common in the radius, but do also commonly occur in the ulna, humerus, femur, tibia, and fibula. This code reports a torus fracture of the lower end of the ulna only, the bone on the inner, pinky finger side of the forearm.

S53.0   Subluxation and dislocation of radial head

Subluxation is a partial dislocation of a joint in which the bones are misaligned, but the articular surfaces remain in some kind of contact with each other. This causes some loss of normal joint relationship and function. A dislocation is a separation injury of a joint (where two or more bones come together) in which the ends of the involved bones are forced further apart than their normal positions. This occurs as a result of a hard blow to the joint and most often results in immediate pain and immobilization, visual deformity, numbness, and swelling. Dislocation is also known as luxation. Dislocation or subluxation of the radial head involves the point in the elbow where the bone on the thumb side of the forearm joins with the upper arm bone, called the radiohumeral joint.

S53.03   Nursemaid's elbow

Nursemaid's elbow is a subluxation of the radial head that is commonly seen in children under 5 years old. It is also known as a pulled elbow and derives its name from the causative action—a longitudinal yank to the arm, such as from a nursemaid, that forces the child's elbow into extension. The subluxation is reduced with firm supination at 90 degrees with extension. A sling or posterior splint is usually applied.

S53.1   Subluxation and dislocation of ulnohumeral joint

Subluxation is a partial dislocation of a joint in which the bones are misaligned, but the articular surfaces remain in some kind of contact with each other. This causes some loss of normal joint relationship and function. A dislocation is a separation injury of a joint (where two or more bones come together) in which the ends of the involved bones are forced further apart than their normal positions. This occurs as a result of a hard blow to the joint and most often results in immediate pain and immobilization, visual deformity, numbness, and swelling. Dislocation is also known as luxation. Dislocation or subluxation of the ulnohumeral joint involves the point in the elbow where the bone on the pinky side of the forearm joins with the upper arm bone.

S53.4   Sprain of elbow

A sprain is an injury to a ligament. Ligaments are tough, elastic tissues that connect bones and hold them together, supporting joints for movement and rotation. A sprain occurs when the ligaments of a joint are stretched or torn, often by direct injury such as falling or traumatic twisting of the joint. Sprains are graded by severity. In a mild Grade 1 sprain, ligaments are stretched beyond their normal range with some microscopic damage to the collagen fibrils, but no tearing. In a moderate Grade 2 sprain, ligaments are partially torn with the tearing affecting some but not all of the collagen fibers. There may be some loss of function with abnormal laxity in the joint. In severe Grade 3 sprains, the elastic fibers are nearly completely torn or ruptured and gross instability can result.

Note: Traumatic rupture of the collateral ligaments is coded in separate subcategories, S53.2 and S53.3.

S59.0   Physeal fracture of lower end of ulna

Physeal fractures may also be referred to as Salter-Harris fractures or traumatic epiphyseal separations. These fractures occur along the physeal (growth) plates in bones that have not reached their full growth and in which the plates are still open and filled with cartilaginous tissue. Salter-Harris fractures are classified into 9 types. Types I-IV have specific codes for fractures of the lower end of the ulna. Types V-IX are reported under other physeal fracture.

Note: The physis is the growth plate where the bone lengthens. The epiphysis is the rounded end of the bone that articulates with another bone. The metaphysis is the widened transitional zone between the diaphysis (the shaft of the bone), and the epiphysis, where the physeal plate is located.

S59.01   Salter-Harris Type I physeal fracture of lower end of ulna

A Salter-Harris Type I fracture is an epiphyseal separation with displacement of the epiphysis from the metaphysis at the physis.

S59.02   Salter-Harris Type II physeal fracture of lower end of ulna

A Salter-Harris Type II physeal fracture is a break through the physis and a portion of the metaphysis without fracture of the epiphysis.

S59.03   Salter-Harris Type III physeal fracture of lower end of ulna

A Salter-Harris Type III fracture is a break through the physis and epiphysis which damages the reproductive layer of the physis.

S59.04   Salter-Harris Type IV physeal fracture of lower end of ulna

A Salter-Harris Type IV fracture is a break through the metaphysis, physis, and epiphysis causing damage to the reproductive layer of the physis.

S59.09   Other physeal fracture of lower end of ulna

Other physeal fractures include types V-IX, which are less common types of physeal injuries and include crush or compression injuries involving the physis alone, injury involving perichondral structrures, an isolated injury of the epiphyseal plate or the metaphysis with potential endochondral ossification, and periosteum injury affecting growth of the membrane.

S59.1   Physeal fracture of upper end of radius

Physeal fractures may also be referred to as Salter-Harris fractures or traumatic epiphyseal separations. These fractures occur along the physeal (growth) plates in bones that have not reached their full growth and in which the plates are still open and filled with cartilaginous tissue. Salter-Harris fractures are classified into 9 types. Types I-IV have specific codes for

fractures of the upper end of the radius. Types V-IX are reported under other physeal fracture.

Note: The physis is the growth plate where the bone lengthens. The epiphysis is the rounded end of the bone that articulates with another bone. The metaphysis is the widened transitional zone between the diaphysis (the shaft of the bone), and the epiphysis, where the physeal plate is located.

S59.11   Salter-Harris Type I physeal fracture of upper end of radius

A Salter-Harris Type I fracture is an epiphyseal separation with displacement of the epiphysis from the metaphysis at the physis.

S59.12   Salter-Harris Type II physeal fracture of upper end of radius

A Salter-Harris Type II physeal fracture is a break through the physis and a portion of the metaphysis without fracture of the epiphysis.

S59.13   Salter-Harris Type III physeal fracture of upper end of radius

A Salter-Harris Type III fracture is a break through the physis and epiphysis which damages the reproductive layer of the physis.

S59.14   Salter-Harris Type IV physeal fracture of upper end of radius

A Salter-Harris Type IV fracture is a break through the metaphysis, physis, and epiphysis causing damage to the reproductive layer of the physis.

S59.19   Other physeal fracture of upper end of radius

Other physeal fractures include types V-IX, which are less common types of physeal injuries and include crush or compression injuries involving the physis alone, injury involving perichondral structrures, an isolated injury of the epiphyseal plate or the metaphysis with potential endochondral ossification, and periosteum injury affecting growth of the membrane.

S59.2   Physeal fracture of lower end of radius

Physeal fractures may also be referred to as Salter-Harris fractures or traumatic epiphyseal separations. These fractures occur along the physeal (growth) plates in bones that have not reached their full growth and in which the plates are still open and filled with cartilaginous tissue. Salter-Harris fractures are classified into 9 types. Types I-IV have specific codes for fractures of the lower end of the radius. Types V-IX are reported under other physeal fracture.

Note: The physis is the growth plate where the bone lengthens. The epiphysis is the rounded end of the bone that articulates with another bone. The metaphysis is the widened transitional zone between the diaphysis (the shaft of the bone), and the epiphysis, where the physeal plate is located.

S59.21   Salter-Harris Type I physeal fracture of lower end of radius

A Salter-Harris Type I fracture is an epiphyseal separation with displacement of the epiphysis from the metaphysis at the physis.

S59.22   Salter-Harris Type II physeal fracture of lower end of radius

A Salter-Harris Type II physeal fracture is a break through the physis and a portion of the metaphysis without fracture of the epiphysis.

S59.23   Salter-Harris Type III physeal fracture of lower end of radius

A Salter-Harris Type III fracture is a break through the physis and epiphysis which damages the reproductive layer of the physis.

S59.24 Salter-Harris Type IV physeal fracture of lower end of radius

A Salter-Harris Type IV fracture is a break through the metaphysis, physis, and epiphysis causing damage to the reproductive layer of the physis.

S59.29 Other physeal fracture of lower end of radius

Other physeal fractures include types V-IX, which are less common types of physeal injuries and include crush or compression injuries involving the physis alone, injury involving perichondral structrures, an isolated injury of the epiphyseal plate or the metaphysis with potential endochondral ossification, and periosteum injury affecting growth of the membrane.

S62.21 Bennett's fracture

A Bennett's fracture is a fracture dislocation of the base of the first metacarpal bone extending into the carpometacarpal joint. This intra-articular fracture of the base of the thumb affects the joint surface between the thumb and the trapezium and often involves significant displacement of the metacarpal bone. The fracture begins at the front ulnar side of the complex saddle joint and extends through the base of the metacarpal in an oblique fashion, leaving a triangular palmar fragment on the ulnar side of the base of the thumb attached to the trapezium by the strong stabilizing ligaments. The main, distal metacarpal fragment is then displaced dorsally and radially as well as rotated by the abductor pollicis longus and adductor pollicis. This highly unstable injury often occurs in football, rugby and other contact sports and requires prompt reduction and fixation to preserve function of this complex joint.

S62.22 Rolando's fracture

A Rolando's fracture is a comminuted, intra-articular fracture dislocation at the base of the first metacarpal. It affects the joint surface between the thumb and the trapezium as in a Bennett's fracture, but involves at least a three-part fracture, often in a Y or T shaped fragmentation. In addition to the fracture line that leaves a triangular palmar fragment on the ulnar side of the base of the thumb, there is also at least one other large dorsal fragment that continues to articulate with the trapezium, as well as the main distal metacarpal fragment that is then displaced. This complex injury is difficult to treat and has a less promising prognosis than a Bennett type fracture, usually requiring internal fixation by a specialized hand surgeon.

S63.0 Subluxation and dislocation of wrist and hand joints

Subluxation is a partial dislocation of a joint in which the bones are misaligned, but the articular surfaces remain in some kind of contact with each other. This causes some loss of normal joint relationship and function. A dislocation is a separation injury of a joint (where two or more bones come together) in which the ends of the involved bones are forced further apart than their normal positions. This occurs as a result of a hard blow to the joint and most often results in immediate pain and immobilization, visual deformity, numbness, and swelling. Dislocation is also known as luxation.

S63.5 Other and unspecified sprain of wrist

A sprain is an injury to a ligament. Ligaments are tough, elastic tissues that connect bones and hold them together, supporting joints for movement and rotation or protecting against abnormal motion. A sprain occurs when the ligaments of a joint are stretched or torn, often by direct injury such as a hit or full contact blow, a fall, or traumatic twisting of the joint. Sprains are graded by severity. In a mild Grade 1 sprain, ligaments are stretched beyond their normal range with some microscopic damage to the collagen fibrils, but no tearing. In a moderate Grade 2 sprain, ligaments are partially torn with the tearing affecting some but not all of the collagen fibers. There may be some loss of function with abnormal laxity in the joint. In severe Grade 3 sprains, the elastic fibers are nearly completely torn or ruptured and gross instability can result.

Note: A traumatic rupture of ligaments in the wrist is coded in subcategory S63.3 and not as a sprain.

S63.6 Other and unspecified sprain of finger(s)

A sprain is an injury to a ligament. Ligaments are tough, elastic tissues that connect bones and hold them together, supporting joints for movement and rotation or protecting against abnormal motion. A sprain occurs when the ligaments of a joint are stretched or torn, often by direct injury such as a hit or full contact blow, a fall, or traumatic twisting of the joint. Sprains are graded by severity. In a mild Grade 1 sprain, ligaments are stretched beyond their normal range with some microscopic damage to the collagen fibrils, but no tearing. In a moderate Grade 2 sprain, ligaments are partially torn with the tearing affecting some but not all of the collagen fibers. There may be some loss of function with abnormal laxity in the joint. In severe Grade 3 sprains, the elastic fibers are nearly completely torn or ruptured and gross instability can result.

Note: A traumatic rupture of ligaments of the fingers at the metacarpophalangeal and interphalangeal joints is coded in subcategory S63.4, and not as a sprain.

S72 Fracture of femur

The Gustilo classification employed in 7th character extensions for fractures of some long bones, such as the femur, applies to open fractures. The Gustilo open fracture classification groups fractures into three main categories designated as Type I, Type II, and Type III with Type III injuries being further divided into Type IIIA, Type IIIB, and Type IIIC subcategories. Each of these three main categories is defined by three major characteristics: mechanism of injury, extent of soft tissue damage, and degree of bone injury or involvement. The specific characteristics of each major type of open fracture determine the correct code placement.

Specific characteristics for **Type I** open fractures include a wound < 1 cm; minimal soft tissue damage; a clean wound bed; a typically low-energy type injury; and fracture types usually either simple transverse, short oblique, or minimally comminuted.

Specific characteristics for **Type II** open fractures include a wound > 1 cm; moderate soft tissue damage; minimal wound bed contamination; a typically low-energy type injury; and fracture types usually either simple transverse, short oblique, or minimally comminuted.

Specific characteristics for **Type III** open fractures include a wound > 1 cm; extensive soft tissue damage; a typically high-energy type injury; highly unstable fractures often with multiple bone fragments; and injury patterns usually resulting in open segmental or severely comminuted fractures. Traumatic involvement is seen as well, such as gun-shot wounds, neurovascular complications, severe contamination, traumatic amputations, and delayed treatment (over 8 hours). This last group of Type III fractures is further subdivided with the following specific characteristics: Type IIIA has adequate soft tissue coverage of the open wound with no local or distant flap coverage required, and the fracture may be open segmental or severely comminuted and still be subclassified as Type IIIA. Type IIIB has extensive soft tissue loss and local or distant flap coverage is required. Wound bed contamination requires serial irrigation and debridement to clean the open fracture site. Type IIIC has major arterial injury and extensive repair usually requires the skills of a vascular surgeon for limb salvage.

S72.32 Transverse fracture of shaft of femur

A transverse fracture is a complete break straight across a bone in which the fracture line runs at a right angle to the long axis of the bone. Transverse fractures are usually caused by a very sharp direct blow across the bone or sometimes through a stress fracture.

S72.33 Oblique fracture of shaft of femur

An oblique fracture is a slanted break in a bone in which the fracture line is direct, but angled diagonally across the shaft of the bone. This is usually caused by a hard, angled blow to the bone, such as in sports or falling down stairs.

S72.34 Spiral fracture of shaft of femur

A spiral fracture is a break in a bone similar to an oblique fracture, but caused by a twisting force that results in an oblique fracture line that spirals around and through the bone like a corkscrew. Spiral fractures are rare and are often misdiagnosed initially as oblique fractures, but can be seen on x-ray as a spiral break. These are generally caused by severe twisting force when one part of the limb is caught or trapped and the adjoining bone is torsed.

S72.35   Comminuted fracture of shaft of femur

A comminuted fracture is any fracture in which the bone involved is broken into at least 3 separate pieces. This is also known as a multi-fragmentary fracture and is often the result of a tremendous traumatic force. Comminuted fractures also occur in people with weakened bones, such as the elderly, and those with cancer or other diseases like osteogenesis imperfecta.

S72.36   Segmental fracture of shaft of femur

A segmental fracture is a break in a bone in which two distinct parts of the same bone are broken, creating a segment of the shaft of the bone that is isolated by a proximal and a distal fracture line. This is also known as a double fracture.

S72.47   Torus fracture of lower end of femur

Torus fractures are also called buckle fractures and are most commonly found in children, due to the softness of their bones. This type of fracture occurs when increased weight loading is placed on the axis of a long bone, such as falling onto an outstretched arm. The soft bone is longitudinally compressed, resulting in an incomplete fracture of the diaphysis of the long bone, with buckling of the bone cortex on the opposite side, which appears as localized bulging. Torus fractures are most common in the radius, but do also commonly occur in the ulna, humerus, femur, tibia, and fibula. This subcategory reports a torus fracture of the lower end of the femur.

S73.0   Subluxation and dislocation of hip

Subluxation is a partial dislocation of a joint in which the bones are misaligned, but the articular surfaces remain in some kind of contact with each other. This causes some loss of normal joint relationship and function. A dislocation is a separation injury of a joint (where two or more bones come together) in which the ends of the involved bones are forced further apart than their normal positions. This occurs as a result of a hard blow to the joint and most often results in immediate pain and immobilization, visual deformity, numbness, and swelling. Dislocation is also known as luxation. Subluxation and dislocation of the hip involves the ball-shaped head of the femur and the socket-shaped acetabulum of the pelvis. Traumatic dislocations of the hip are a medical emergency.

S73.01   Posterior subluxation and dislocation of hip

Posterior subluxations and dislocations of the hip are the most common type and account for nearly 90% of all cases. Posterior describes the position of the femoral head as being located behind the acetabulum. This occurs with force that is transmitted through the leg up and into a flexed hip joint.

S73.03   Other anterior dislocation of hip

An anterior dislocation of the hip describes the position of the femoral head being located in front of the acetabulum. This type of dislocation most commonly results from traumatic force causing hyperextension hitting against an abducted leg. The impact pops the femoral head out of its acetabular seat in an anterior direction. It may also be caused by a forward moving force hitting against the back of the femoral neck.

S73.04   Central dislocation of hip

A central dislocation of the hip is always accompanied by a fracture. The femoral head is positioned medially to a fractured acetabulum and occurs when a lateral force hits against an adducted femur.

S73.1   Sprain of hip

A sprain is an injury to a ligament. Ligaments are tough, elastic tissues that connect bones and hold them together, supporting joints for movement and rotation or protecting against abnormal motion. A sprain occurs when the ligaments of a joint are stretched or torn, often by direct injury such as a hit or full contact blow, a fall, or traumatic twisting of the joint. Sprains are graded by severity. In a mild Grade 1 sprain, ligaments are stretched beyond their normal range with some microscopic damage to the collagen fibrils, but no tearing. In a moderate Grade 2 sprain, ligaments are partially torn with the tearing affecting some but not all of the collagen fibers. There may be some loss of function with abnormal laxity in the joint. In severe Grade 3 sprains, the elastic fibers are nearly completely torn or ruptured and gross instability can result.

S79.0   Physeal fracture of upper end of femur

Physeal fractures may also be referred to as Salter-Harris fractures or traumatic epiphyseal separations. These fractures occur along the physeal (growth) plates in bones that have not reached their full growth and in which the plates are still open and filled with cartilaginous tissue. Salter-Harris fractures are classified into 9 types. Types I-IV generally have specific fracture codes while types V-IX are reported under other physeal fracture; however, for upper femoral physeal fractures, only type I for slipped or fractured capital femoral epiphysis is specifically coded, and all other upper physeal fractures of the femur are reported under 'other.'

Note: The physis is the growth plate where the bone lengthens. The epiphysis is the rounded end of the bone that articulates with another bone. The metaphysis is the widened transitional zone between the diaphysis (the shaft of the bone), and the epiphysis, where the physeal plate is located.

S79.01   Salter-Harris Type I physeal fracture of upper end of femur

A Salter-Harris Type I fracture is an epiphyseal separation with displacement of the epiphysis from the metaphysis at the physis.

S79.1   Physeal fracture of lower end of femur

Physeal fractures may also be referred to as Salter-Harris fractures or traumatic epiphyseal separations. These fractures occur along the physeal (growth) plates in bones that have not reached their full growth and in which the plates are still open and filled with cartilaginous tissue. Salter-Harris fractures are classified into 9 types. Types I-IV have specific codes for fractures of the lower end of the femur. Types V-IX are reported under other physeal fracture.

Note: The physis is the growth plate where the bone lengthens. The epiphysis is the rounded end of the bone that articulates with another bone. The metaphysis is the widened transitional zone between the diaphysis (the shaft of the bone), and the epiphysis, where the physeal plate is located.

S79.11   Salter-Harris Type I physeal fracture of lower end of femur

A Salter-Harris Type I fracture is an epiphyseal separation with displacement of the epiphysis from the metaphysis at the physis.

S79.12   Salter-Harris Type II physeal fracture of lower end of femur

A Salter-Harris Type II physeal fracture is a break through the physis and a portion of the metaphysis without fracture of the epiphysis.

S79.13   Salter-Harris Type III physeal fracture of lower end of femur

A Salter-Harris Type III fracture is a break through the physis and epiphysis which damages the reproductive layer of the physis.

S79.14   Salter-Harris Type IV physeal fracture of lower end of femur

A Salter-Harris Type IV fracture is a break through the metaphysis, physis, and epiphysis causing damage to the reproductive layer of the physis.

S79.19   Other physeal fracture of lower end of femur

Other physeal fractures include types V-IX, which are less common types of physeal injuries and include crush or compression injuries involving the physis alone, injury involving perichondral structrures, an isolated injury of the epiphyseal plate or the metaphysis with potential endochondral ossification, and periosteum injury affecting growth of the membrane.

S82   Fracture of lower leg, including ankle

The Gustilo classification employed in 7th character extensions for fractures of the bones of the lower leg applies to open fractures. The Gustilo open fracture classification groups fractures into three main categories designated as Type I, Type II, and Type III with Type III injuries being further divided into Type IIIA, Type IIIB, and Type IIIC subcategories. Each of these three main categories is defined by three major characteristics: mechanism of injury, extent of soft tissue damage, and degree of bone injury or involvement. The specific characteristics of each major type of open fracture determine the correct code placement.

Specific characteristics for **Type I** open fractures include a wound < 1 cm; minimal soft tissue damage; a clean wound bed; a typically low-energy type injury; and fracture types usually either simple transverse, short oblique, or minimally comminuted.

Specific characteristics for **Type II** open fractures include a wound > 1 cm; moderate soft tissue damage; minimal wound bed contamination; a typically low-energy type injury; and fracture types usually either simple transverse, short oblique, or minimally comminuted.

Specific characteristics for **Type III** open fractures include a wound > 1 cm; extensive soft tissue damage; a typically high-energy type injury; highly unstable fractures often with multiple bone fragments; and injury patterns usually resulting in open segmental or severely comminuted fractures. Traumatic involvement is seen as well, such as gun-shot wounds, neurovascular complications, severe contamination, traumatic amputations, and delayed treatment (over 8 hours). This last group of Type III fractures is further subdivided with the following specific characteristics: Type IIIA has adequate soft tissue coverage of the open wound with no local or distant flap coverage required, and the fracture may be open segmental or severely comminuted and still be subclassified as Type IIIA. Type IIIB has extensive soft tissue loss and local or distant flap coverage is required. Wound bed contamination requires serial irrigation and debridement to clean the open fracture site. Type IIIC has major arterial injury and extensive repair usually requires the skills of a vascular surgeon for limb salvage.

S82.01   Osteochondral fracture of patella

An osteochondral fracture of the patella is a break or tear in the articular cartilage of the kneecap along with a break in the bone. This leaves a fracture fragment of articular cartilage, and subchondral and supporting trabecular bone that may either remain stable and attached in place, or may displace and become a loose body in the joint. Nondisplaced osteochondral fractures usually just heal in time. Displaced fracture fragments require excision and sometimes stabilization with transosseous fixation screws.

S82.02   Longitudinal fracture of patella

A longitudinal fracture of the patella is a vertical break in the kneecap in which the fracture line runs in a superiorinferior direction. These types of fractures of the patella are rare.

S82.03   Transverse fracture of patella

A transverse fracture of the patella is a break in the kneecap in which the fracture line runs in a medial-lateral direction. Transverse fractures are seen most often in the central or distal third of the patella.

S82.04   Comminuted fracture of patella

A comminuted fracture is any fracture in which the bone involved is broken into at least 3 separate pieces. This is also known as a multi-fragmentary fracture and is often the result of a tremendous traumatic force. Comminuted fractures also occur in people with weakened bones, such as the elderly, and those with cancer or other diseases like osteogenesis imperfecta. The patella is a thick, flat, triangular-circular bone in front of the knee joint that covers and protects the interior structures, and articulates with the femur. The 'kneecap' bone is important to the mechanics of the knee joint and is often a site of orthopedic injury.

S82.16   Torus fracture of upper end of tibia

Torus fractures are also called buckle fractures and are most commonly found in children, due to the softness of their bones. This type of fracture occurs when increased weight loading is placed on the axis of a long bone, such as falling onto an outstretched arm. The soft bone is longitudinally compressed, resulting in an incomplete fracture of the diaphysis of the long bone, with buckling of the bone cortex on the opposite side, which appears as localized bulging. Torus fractures are most common in the radius, but do also commonly occur in the ulna, humerus, femur, tibia, and fibula. This subcategory reports a torus fracture of the upper end of the tibia.

S82.22   Transverse fracture of shaft of tibia

A transverse fracture is a complete break straight across a bone in which the fracture line runs at a right angle to the long axis of the bone. Transverse fractures are usually caused by a very sharp direct blow across the bone or sometimes through a stress fracture.

S82.23   Oblique fracture of shaft of tibia

An oblique fracture is a slanted break in a bone in which the fracture line is direct, but angled diagonally across the shaft of the bone. This is usually caused by a hard, angled blow to the bone, such as in sports or falling down stairs.

S82.24   Spiral fracture of shaft of tibia

A spiral fracture is a break in a bone similar to an oblique fracture, but caused by a twisting force that results in an oblique fracture line that spirals around and through the bone like a corkscrew. Spiral fractures are rare and are often misdiagnosed initially as oblique fractures, but can be seen on x-ray as a spiral break. These are generally caused by severe twisting force when one part of the limb is caught or trapped and the adjoining bone is torsed.

S82.25   Comminuted fracture of shaft of tibia

A comminuted fracture is any fracture in which the bone involved is broken into at least 3 separate pieces. This is also known as a multi-fragmentary fracture and is often the result of a tremendous traumatic force. Comminuted fractures also occur in people with weakened bones, such as the elderly, and those with cancer or other diseases like osteogenesis imperfecta.

S82.26   Segmental fracture of shaft of tibia

A segmental fracture is a break in a bone in which two distinct parts of the same bone are broken, creating a segment of the shaft of the bone that is isolated by a proximal and a distal fracture line. This is also known as a double fracture.

S82.31   Torus fracture of lower end of tibia

Torus fractures are also called buckle fractures and are most commonly found in children, due to the softness of their bones. This type of fracture occurs when increased weight loading is placed on the axis of a long bone, such as falling onto an outstretched arm. The soft bone is longitudinally compressed, resulting in an incomplete fracture of the diaphysis of the long bone, with buckling of the bone cortex on the opposite side, which appears as localized bulging. Torus fractures are most common in the radius, but do also commonly occur in the ulna, humerus, femur, tibia, and fibula. This subcategory reports a torus fracture of the lower end of the tibia.

S82.42   Transverse fracture of shaft of fibula

A transverse fracture is a complete break straight across a bone in which the fracture line runs at a right angle to the long axis of the bone. Transverse fractures are usually caused by a very sharp direct blow across the bone or sometimes through a stress fracture.

S82.43   Oblique fracture of shaft of fibula

An oblique fracture is a slanted break in a bone in which the fracture line is direct, but angled diagonally across the shaft of the bone. This is usually caused by a hard, angled blow to the bone, such as in sports or falling down stairs.

S82.44   Spiral fracture of shaft of fibula

A spiral fracture is a break in a bone similar to an oblique fracture, but caused by a twisting force that results in an oblique fracture line that spirals around and through the bone like a corkscrew. Spiral fractures are rare and are often misdiagnosed initially as oblique fractures, but can be seen on

2016 Plain English Descriptions for ICD-10-CM   Chapter 19 Injury, Poisoning and Certain Other Consequences of External Causes | S82.45 – S89.0

Injury/Poisoning/Other External Causes   S82.45 – S89.0

x-ray as a spiral break. These are generally caused by severe twisting force when one part of the limb is caught or trapped and the adjoining bone is torsed.

S82.45   Comminuted fracture of shaft of fibula

A comminuted fracture is any fracture in which the bone involved is broken into at least 3 separate pieces. This is also known as a multi-fragmentary fracture and is often the result of a tremendous traumatic force. Comminuted fractures also occur in people with weakened bones, such as the elderly, and those with cancer or other diseases like osteogenesis imperfecta.

S82.46   Segmental fracture of shaft of fibula

A segmental fracture is a break in a bone in which two distinct parts of the same bone are broken, creating a segment of the shaft of the bone that is isolated by a proximal and a distal fracture line. This is also known as a double fracture.

S82.81   Torus fracture of upper end of fibula

Torus fractures are also called buckle fractures and are most commonly found in children, due to the softness of their bones. This type of fracture occurs when increased weight loading is placed on the axis of a long bone, such as falling onto an outstretched arm. The soft bone is longitudinally compressed, resulting in an incomplete fracture of the diaphysis of the long bone, with buckling of the bone cortex on the opposite side, which appears as localized bulging. Torus fractures are most common in the radius, but do also commonly occur in the ulna, humerus, femur, tibia, and fibula. This subcategory reports a torus fracture of the upper end of the fibula.

S82.82   Torus fracture of lower end of fibula

Torus fractures are also called buckle fractures and are most commonly found in children, due to the softness of their bones. This type of fracture occurs when increased weight loading is placed on the axis of a long bone, such as falling onto an outstretched arm. The soft bone is longitudinally compressed, resulting in an incomplete fracture of the diaphysis of the long bone, with buckling of the bone cortex on the opposite side, which appears as localized bulging. Torus fractures are most common in the radius, but do also commonly occur in the ulna, humerus, femur, tibia, and fibula. This subcategory reports a torus fracture of the lower end of the fibula.

S83.0   Subluxation and dislocation of patella

Subluxation is a partial dislocation of a joint in which the bones are misaligned, but the articular surfaces remain in some kind of contact with each other. This causes some loss of normal joint relationship and function. A dislocation is a separation injury of a joint (where two or more bones come together) in which the ends of the involved bones are forced further apart than their normal positions. This occurs as a result of a hard blow to the joint and most often results in immediate pain and immobilization, visual deformity, numbness, and swelling. Dislocation is also known as luxation. The patella is a thick, flat, triangular-circular bone in front of the knee joint that covers and protects the interior structures, and articulates with the femur. A dislocation or subluxation of the patella involves the kneecap coming away from its normal position in the trochlear groove of the femoropatellar joint. This is a very common injury, especially in young people engaged in sports.

S83.01   Lateral subluxation and dislocation of patella

Most dislocations and subluxations of the patella coming out of its normal position in the trochlear groove of the femoropatellar joint occur laterally, or toward the outside, accompanied by significant pain and swelling. Since the kneecap will often spontaneously relocate or reduce itself back into its proper position when the knee is extended, many dislocation/subluxation injuries are inferred by signs and symptoms of concomitant problems, such as disruption or tearing of the supporting ligaments on the inside of the knee that allowed the kneecap to become displaced laterally, as well as small fragments of cartilage and bone that may be knocked off the kneecap or the lateral condyle of the femur.

S83.1   Subluxation and dislocation of knee

Subluxation is a partial dislocation of a joint in which the bones are misaligned, but the articular surfaces remain in some kind of contact with each other. This causes some loss of normal joint relationship and function. A dislocation is a separation injury of a joint (where two or more bones come together) in which the ends of the involved bones are forced further apart than their normal positions. This occurs as a result of a hard blow to the joint and most often results in immediate pain and immobilization, visual deformity, numbness, and swelling. Dislocation is also known as luxation.

S83.4   Sprain of collateral ligament of knee

A sprain is an injury to a ligament. Ligaments are tough, elastic tissues that connect bones and hold them together, supporting joints for movement and rotation or protecting against abnormal motion. A sprain occurs when the ligaments of a joint are stretched or torn, often by direct injury such as a hit or full contact blow, a fall, or traumatic twisting of the joint. Sprains are graded by severity. In a mild Grade 1 sprain, ligaments are stretched beyond their normal range with some microscopic damage to the collagen fibrils, but no tearing. In a moderate Grade 2 sprain, ligaments are partially torn with the tearing affecting some but not all of the collagen fibers. There may be some loss of function with abnormal laxity in the joint. In severe Grade 3 sprains, the elastic fibers are nearly completely torn or ruptured and gross instability can result. There are four major ligaments that stabilize the knee - the anterior and posterior cruciate ligaments (ACL, PCL) and the collateral ligaments. The medial collateral ligament (MCL) is located on the inner aspect of the knee and the lateral collateral ligament (LCL) is on the outer aspect. The MCL and LCL are less frequently sprained than the cruciate ligaments.

S83.5   Sprain of cruciate ligament of knee

A sprain is an injury to a ligament. Ligaments are tough, elastic tissues that connect bones and hold them together, supporting joints for movement and rotation or protecting against abnormal motion. A sprain occurs when the ligaments of a joint are stretched or torn, often by direct injury such as a hit or full contact blow, a fall, or traumatic twisting of the joint. Sprains are graded by severity. In a mild Grade 1 sprain, ligaments are stretched beyond their normal range with some microscopic damage to the collagen fibrils, but no tearing. In a moderate Grade 2 sprain, ligaments are partially torn with the tearing affecting some but not all of the collagen fibers. There may be some loss of function with abnormal laxity in the joint. In severe Grade 3 sprains, the elastic fibers are nearly completely torn or ruptured and gross instability can result. There are four major ligaments that stabilize the knee - the anterior and posterior cruciate ligaments and the collateral ligaments. The anterior cruciate ligament (ACL) is located in the center of the knee joint connecting the femur to the tibia. The posterior cruciate ligament (PCL) is located in the center of the knee behind the ACL and also connects the femur to the tibia. Both cruciate ligaments provide rotational stability in the knee. Injury to either ligament can cause the knee to buckle.

S83.6   Sprain of the superior tibiofibular joint and ligament

A sprain is an injury to a ligament. Ligaments are tough, elastic tissues that connect bones and hold them together, supporting joints for movement and rotation or protecting against abnormal motion. A sprain occurs when the ligaments of a joint are stretched or torn, often by direct injury such as a hit or full contact blow, a fall, or traumatic twisting of the joint. Sprains are graded by severity. In a mild Grade 1 sprain, ligaments are stretched beyond their normal range with some microscopic damage to the collagen fibrils, but no tearing. In a moderate Grade 2 sprain, ligaments are partially torn with the tearing affecting some but not all of the collagen fibers. There may be some loss of function with abnormal laxity in the joint. In severe Grade 3 sprains, the elastic fibers are nearly completely torn or ruptured and gross instability can result.

S89.0   Physeal fracture of upper end of tibia

Physeal fractures may also be referred to as Salter-Harris fractures or traumatic epiphyseal separations. These fractures occur along the physeal (growth) plates in bones that have not reached their full growth and in which the plates are still open and filled with cartilaginous tissue. Salter-Harris fractures are classified into 9 types. Types I-IV have specific codes for fractures of the upper end of the tibia. Types V-IX are reported under other physeal fracture.

Note: The physis is the growth plate where the bone lengthens. The epiphysis is the rounded end of the bone that articulates with another bone. The metaphysis is the widened transitional zone between the diaphysis (the shaft of the bone), and the epiphysis, where the physeal plate is located.

S89.01 Salter-Harris Type I physeal fracture of upper end of tibia

A Salter-Harris Type I fracture is an epiphyseal separation with displacement of the epiphysis from the metaphysis at the physis.

S89.02 Salter-Harris Type II physeal fracture of upper end of tibia

A Salter-Harris Type II physeal fracture is a break through the physis and a portion of the metaphysis without fracture of the epiphysis.

S89.03 Salter-Harris Type III physeal fracture of upper end of tibia

A Salter-Harris Type III fracture is a break through the physis and epiphysis which damages the reproductive layer of the physis.

S89.04 Salter-Harris Type IV physeal fracture of upper end of tibia

A Salter-Harris Type IV fracture is a break through the metaphysis, physis, and epiphysis causing damage to the reproductive layer of the physis.

S89.09 Other physeal fracture of upper end of tibia

Other physeal fractures include types V-IX, which are less common types of physeal injuries and include crush or compression injuries involving the physis alone, injury involving perichondral structrures, an isolated injury of the epiphyseal plate or the metaphysis with potential endochondral ossification, and periosteum injury affecting growth of the membrane.

S89.1 Physeal fracture of lower end of tibia

Physeal fractures may also be referred to as Salter-Harris fractures or traumatic epiphyseal separations. These fractures occur along the physeal (growth) plates in bones that have not reached their full growth and in which the plates are still open and filled with cartilaginous tissue. Salter-Harris fractures are classified into 9 types. Types I-IV have specific codes for fractures of the lower end of the tibia. Types V-IX are reported under other physeal fracture.

Note: The physis is the growth plate where the bone lengthens. The epiphysis is the rounded end of the bone that articulates with another bone. The metaphysis is the widened transitional zone between the diaphysis (the shaft of the bone), and the epiphysis, where the physeal plate is located.

S89.11 Salter-Harris Type I physeal fracture of lower end of tibia

A Salter-Harris Type I fracture is an epiphyseal separation with displacement of the epiphysis from the metaphysis at the physis.

S89.12 Salter-Harris Type II physeal fracture of lower end of tibia

A Salter-Harris Type II physeal fracture is a break through the physis and a portion of the metaphysis without fracture of the epiphysis.

S89.13 Salter-Harris Type III physeal fracture of lower end of tibia

A Salter-Harris Type III fracture is a break through the physis and epiphysis which damages the reproductive layer of the physis.

S89.14 Salter-Harris Type IV physeal fracture of lower end of tibia

A Salter-Harris Type IV fracture is a break through the metaphysis, physis, and epiphysis causing damage to the reproductive layer of the physis.

S89.19 Other physeal fracture of lower end of tibia

Other physeal fractures include types V-IX, which are less common types of physeal injuries and include crush or compression injuries involving the physis alone, injury involving perichondral structrures, an isolated injury of the epiphyseal plate or the metaphysis with potential endochondral ossification, and periosteum injury affecting growth of the membrane.

S89.2 Physeal fracture of upper end of fibula

Physeal fractures may also be referred to as Salter-Harris fractures or traumatic epiphyseal separations. These fractures occur along the physeal (growth) plates in bones that have not reached their full growth and in which the plates are still open and filled with cartilaginous tissue. Salter-Harris fractures are classified into 9 types. Types I-IV generally have specific fracture codes while types V-IX are reported under other physeal fracture; however, for upper fibular physeal fractures, only type I and II are specifically coded, and all others are reported under other physeal fractures.

Note: The physis is the growth plate where the bone lengthens. The epiphysis is the rounded end of the bone that articulates with another bone. The metaphysis is the widened transitional zone between the diaphysis (the shaft of the bone), and the epiphysis, where the physeal plate is located.

S89.21 Salter-Harris Type I physeal fracture of upper end of fibula

A Salter-Harris Type I fracture is an epiphyseal separation with displacement of the epiphysis from the metaphysis at the physis.

S89.22 Salter-Harris Type II physeal fracture of upper end of fibula

A Salter-Harris Type II physeal fracture is a break through the physis and a portion of the metaphysis without fracture of the epiphysis.

S89.29 Other physeal fracture of upper end of fibula

Other upper fibular physeal fractures include any other classified type that may include fractures through both the physis and epiphysis, or fractures through the metaphysis, physis, and epiphysis causing physeal damage as well as other less common types that may include isolated injuries to the physis, the epiphyseal plate, the metaphysis, or the periosteum alone.

S89.3 Physeal fracture of lower end of fibula

Physeal fractures may also be referred to as Salter-Harris fractures or traumatic epiphyseal separations. These fractures occur along the epiphyseal (growth) plates in bones that have not reached their full growth and in which the plates are still open and filled with cartilaginous tissue. Salter-Harris fractures are classified into 9 types. Types I-IV generally have specific fracture codes while types V-IX are reported under other physeal fracture; however, for lower fibular physeal fractures, only type I and II are specifically coded, and all others are reported under other physeal fracture.

Note: The physis is the growth plate where the bone lengthens. The epiphysis is the rounded end of the bone that articulates with another bone. The metaphysis is the widened transitional zone between the diaphysis (the shaft of the bone), and the epiphysis, where the physeal plate is located.

S89.31 Salter-Harris Type I physeal fracture of lower end of fibula

A Salter-Harris Type I fracture is an epiphyseal separation with displacement of the epiphysis from the metaphysis at the physis.

S89.32 Salter-Harris Type II physeal fracture of lower end of fibula

A Salter-Harris Type II physeal fracture is a break through the physis and a portion of the metaphysis without fracture of the epiphysis.

S89.39   Other physeal fracture of lower end of fibula

Other lower fibular physeal fractures include any other classified type that may include fractures through both the physis and epiphysis, or fractures through the metaphysis, physis, and epiphysis causing physeal damage as well as other less common types that may include isolated injuries to the physis, the epiphyseal plate, the metaphysis, or the periosteum alone.

S93.4   Sprain of ankle

A sprain is an injury to a ligament. Ligaments are tough, elastic tissues that connect bones and hold them together, supporting joints for movement and rotation or protecting against abnormal motion. A sprain occurs when the ligaments of a joint are stretched or torn, often by direct injury such as a hit or full contact blow, a fall, or traumatic twisting of the joint. Sprains are graded by severity. In a mild Grade 1 sprain, ligaments are stretched beyond their normal range with some microscopic damage to the collagen fibrils, but no tearing. In a moderate Grade 2 sprain, ligaments are partially torn with the tearing affecting some but not all of the collagen fibers. There may be some loss of function with abnormal laxity in the joint. In severe Grade 3 sprains, the elastic fibers are nearly completely torn or ruptured and gross instability can result.

S93.5   Sprain of toe

A sprain is an injury to a ligament. Ligaments are tough, elastic tissues that connect bones and hold them together, supporting joints for movement and rotation or protecting against abnormal motion. A sprain occurs when the ligaments of a joint are stretched or torn, often by direct injury such as a hit or full contact blow, a fall, or traumatic twisting of the joint. Sprains are graded by severity. In a mild Grade 1 sprain, ligaments are stretched beyond their normal range with some microscopic damage to the collagen fibrils, but no tearing. In a moderate Grade 2 sprain, ligaments are partially torn with the tearing affecting some but not all of the collagen fibers. There may be some loss of function with abnormal laxity in the joint. In severe Grade 3 sprains, the elastic fibers are nearly completely torn or ruptured and gross instability can result.

S93.6   Sprain of foot

A sprain is an injury to a ligament. Ligaments are tough, elastic tissues that connect bones and hold them together, supporting joints for movement and rotation or protecting against abnormal motion. A sprain occurs when the ligaments of a joint are stretched or torn, often by direct injury such as a hit or full contact blow, a fall, or traumatic twisting of the joint. Sprains are graded by severity. In a mild Grade 1 sprain, ligaments are stretched beyond their normal range with some microscopic damage to the collagen fibrils, but no tearing. In a moderate Grade 2 sprain, ligaments are partially torn with the tearing affecting some but not all of the collagen fibers. There may be some loss of function with abnormal laxity in the joint. In severe Grade 3 sprains, the elastic fibers are nearly completely torn or ruptured and gross instability can result.

T33   Superficial frostbite

A common complication of reduced temperature is frostbite, which occurs when prolonged exposure to extreme cold causes damage to the skin and other tissue. Exposed projections of the body are most at risk, such as the hands, feet, eyes, nose, and ears. Symptoms include discoloration of the skin, along with a painful itching or burning sensation. If the nerves or blood vessels under the skin become damaged, gangrene may set in, and the affected tissue must be amputated.

T34   Frostbite with tissue necrosis

A common complication of reduced temperature is frostbite, which occurs when prolonged exposure to extreme cold causes damage to the skin and other tissue. Exposed projections of the body are most at risk, such as the hands, feet, eyes, nose, and ears. Symptoms include discoloration of the skin, along with a painful itching or burning sensation. When the nerves and blood vessels under the skin become damaged, gangrene sets in, and the affected tissue becomes necrotic and dies.

T40.5X   Poisoning by, adverse effect of and underdosing of cocaine

Cocaine is an alkaloid extracted from the leaves of the coca plant. Besides abusive recreational use, it is also used in medicine as a topical anesthetic in ear, nose, and throat surgery. Cocaine acts on the central nervous system as a stimulant, causing euphoria, hyperactivity, increased blood pressure and heart rate, and may cause twitches, itching, hallucinations, and paranoid delusions. There is no antidote and it is rapidly metabolized by the body. Acute cases of poisoning are one of the most common causes of drug-related emergency department visits in the country. Poisoning causes tachydysrhythmias, stroke, subarachnoid hemorrhage, hyperthermia, and agitated delirium. Myocardial infarction can result from acute vasospasm and dysrhythmia. The cardiovascular effects from cocaine result from both its direct effects on the heart and its secondary effects of the central nervous system.

T67.0   Heatstroke and sunstroke

Heatstroke, also known as sunstroke, occurs when prolonged exposure to heat causes the body's ability to regulate body temperature to fail, resulting in cessation of sweating, accompanied by headache, nausea, dizziness, and possibly unconsciousness. Oral temperature will rapidly rise to over 103° F, and can go higher as the condition worsens. If treatment is not given immediately, death or permanent disability may occur.

T67.1   Heat syncope

Heat syncope occurs when prolonged heat exposure, most often with concomitant loss of body fluids and electrolytes, leads to low blood pressure, which causes the patient to collapse and become unconscious.

T67.2   Heat cramp

Heat cramps occur when excessive sweating from prolonged exposure to heat depletes the body's level of salts and other electrolytes, which leads to painful muscle cramping.

T67.3   Heat exhaustion, anhydrotic

Anhydrotic heat exhaustion is a common effect of excessive or prolonged exposure to heat. It causes dizziness, weakness, nausea, and prostration with lack of fluids in the patient's body, usually due to excessive sweating. This condition can be alleviated with rest, particularly out of the heat, and rehydration.

T67.4   Heat exhaustion due to salt depletion

Heat exhaustion due to salt depletion is a common effect of excessive or prolonged exposure to heat. It causes dizziness, weakness, nausea, and prostration with lack of salt and fluids in the patient's body, usually due to excessive sweating. This condition can be alleviated with rest, particularly out of the heat, and rehydration using salts and electrolytes.

T67.5   Heat exhaustion, unspecified

One of the most common effects of excessive heat exposure is heat exhaustion or heat prostration, which occurs when prolonged exposure to heat causes dizziness, weakness, and nausea. This condition requires rest, particularly in a cooler environment.

T67.6   Heat fatigue, transient

In transient heat fatigue, the patient experiences brief periods of discomfort, such as dizziness, weakness, and lack of energy when working outdoors in the heat. This condition is not serious and patients may need to rest frequently whenever they are outdoors in the heat and begin to feel uncomfortable.

T67.7   Heat edema

In heat edema, a part of the body swells with fluid due to excessive or prolonged exposure to heat. This condition typically occurs in the feet or hands.

T68   Hypothermia

Hypothermia is a condition in which the body temperature dips dangerously low as the result of low environmental temperature. Problems begin when body temperature dips below 95° F, producing symptoms such as shivering, drowsiness, cold dry skin, and reduced respiration and heart rate. The shivering will cease as the condition worsens. If core body temperature goes below 90° F, the person can become comatose and die.

T69   Other effects of reduced temperature

Other effects of reduced temperature on the body, often the result of exposure in low temperatures, or prolonged immersion in cold water.

T69.02   Immersion foot

Commonly known as trench foot, immersion foot occurs when the skin is immersed in water for a prolonged period of time. The feet will become numb and swollen, and will become red or blue as the problem progresses. Open sores and lesions may follow, which can result in fungal infections and/or gangrene.

T69.1   Chilblains

Chilblains is a condition that occurs when the small blood vessels below the skin become damaged by exposure to cold temperatures. A chilblain presents as an itchy, red, inflamed area on the skin surface. This condition occurs most often in the elderly and in females.

T70   Effects of air pressure and water pressure

Changes in air and water pressure from diving, flying, or otherwise traveling in high elevations can irritate or damage the ears and sinuses or cause diver's palsy or paralysis. Severe damage to body systems can be caused by pressure changes associated with explosions.

T70.0   Otitic barotrauma

Otitic barotrauma is damage to the middle ear, injured specifically by a pressure differential between the ear and the outside environment, often experienced during rapid descent during air travel. It can also occur in divers. Typical symptoms are pain, secretions into the middle ear chamber and, in severe cases, rupture or hemorrhage of the eardrum.

T70.1   Sinus barotrauma

Rapid changes in air pressure causing pain with a feeling of pressure in the sinuses.

T70.29   Other effects of high altitude

Altitude, alpine, or mountain sickness is another effect that can occur when at high altitudes. This condition is also known as 'the altitude bends' and hypobaropathy. This type of sickness is due to the decreased air pressure and lower oxygen levels present at high altitudes. The symptoms may range from mild to life-threatening and can affect the nervous system, respiratory system, heart, and muscles. Symptoms may depend on the rate at which the person ascends. Typical signs and sypmtoms present as headache, fatigue, dizziness, nosebleed, nausea and vomiting, rapid heart rate, and shortness of breath with exertion. Severe, acute altitude sickness presents with cyanosis, tightness in the chest, confusion, hemoptysis, shortness of breath at rest, and the inability to walk straight.

T70.3   Caisson disease [decompression sickness]

Caisson disease, also known as decompression sickness or "the bends" is a result of moving from a high pressure environment to a low pressure environment too rapidly. Although it can occur while flying in an unpressurized aircraft, the most common cause is diving. If a scuba diver surfaces too quickly after going deep underwater (100+ feet), nitrogen bubbles and other gases will enter the bloodstream, causing joint pain, chest pain, shortness of breath, muscle cramps, headache, and a variety of other symptoms. This condition can be fatal in severe cases.

T73.0   Starvation

Patients suffering from starvation, or the effects of hunger, will lose a good deal of fat and muscle mass, and the skin will appear pale and dry. Many other body systems will break down due to nutrient deficiencies. Lethargy, depression, and fatigue are usually pronounced, and heart failure can occur.

T73.1   Deprivation of water

Water deprivation, or dehydration, occurs when the body excretes more water than it takes in, usually around 2.5-3 liters a day in a temperate climate. Dehydrated patients will experience headache, irritability, and dizziness. Cases of total water deprivation are much more severe. After only a day or two without water, the patient will have dry, cracked lips and mucous membranes, intense headache, and a fever. Coma and death will follow in as little as 3-5 days.

T73.2   Exhaustion due to exposure

Exhaustion due to exposure typically occurs when a person is forced to spend a long period of time outdoors with no preparation, such as becoming lost in the woods or marooned at sea.

T74.12   Child physical abuse, confirmed

Physical abuse occurs whenever a child is subjected to intentional bodily injury. The child may be subjected to beatings, burns, lacerations, or any other acts of physical violence against the child which induce any type of physical injury or trauma.

T74.22   Child sexual abuse, confirmed

Child sexual abuse occur whenver a child is misused for the purpose of sexual gratification. This type of abuse ranges from allowing a child to view pornography to engaging in sexual intercourse with the child. Children subjected to physical sexual abuse often present with torn clothing, bleeding from the anus or genitalia, difficulty sitting or walking, and a host of psychological and behavioral problems. Other indicators are sexually transmitted diseases and pregnancy in young children.

T74.32   Child psychological abuse, confirmed

Psychological abuse of a child occurs when a parent or other significant adult in the child's life routinely rejects, ignores, terrorizes, isolates, or otherwise corrupts the child's healthy emotional, mental, and psychological state. The child may be told that they are unwanted or unloved, ignored, subjected to constant criticism and punishment, deprived of contact, or allowed to participate in or witness inappropriate activities. Note that in this type of abuse, the child is not deprived of food or harmed physically, although the result of this type of abuse can be just as damaging to the child. Emotional and/or psychological abuse is often the most difficult type of child abuse to diagnose.

T74.4   Shaken infant syndrome

Shaken baby syndrome occurs when an infant is injured due to violent shaking. This typically presents as head trauma or whiplash due to the head of the child moving back and forth. Physical symptoms may be hard to spot or absent, but one serious danger is bleeding inside the skull that can put pressure on the brain.

T75.0   Effects of lightning

Use this code to report the effects of a lightning strike, other than burns. In addition to burn injuries, lightning can also cause damage to the nervous system. Patients who are struck by lightning often have problems with concentration, memory, and complex mental tasks. Any or all aspects of the nervous system may be affected.

T75.1   Unspecified effects of drowning and nonfatal submersion

This code is used to report the nonspecific effects of immersion, or being submerged in water without dying.

Note: This codes excludes specified adverse effects caused by submersion, such as hypothermia and brain damage, which are coded to the specific effect.

T75.3   Motion sickness

Motion sickness occurs when the fluid of the inner ear becomes out of balance, causing confusion between real and perceived motion. This results in nausea, dizziness, and headache.

T78.0   Anaphylactic reaction due to food

Use a code from this subcategory to report anaphylactic reaction or shock due to an adverse reaction to food. Anaphylactic reactions are known as an immediate type I allergic hypersensitivity reaction that is elicited very

2016 Plain English Descriptions for ICD-10-CM   Chapter 19 Injury, Poisoning and Certain Other Consequences of External Causes | T78.2 – T80.21

Injury/Poisoning/Other External Causes   T78.2 – T80.21

rapidly after exposure to the causative antigen. It is mediated by antibodies in the blood that react to the initial introduction of an antigen and induce the synthesis of immunoglobulins, particularly IgE, which bind to specific receptors on the surface of circulating mast cells. The next time that same, specific antigen is introduced, it reacts with the IgE on the mast cells and induces them to release large amounts of histamine and other chemicals that cause the familiar reactions of bronchoconstriction, smooth muscle contraction, vasodilation, and increased vascular permeability. Not all anaphylactic reactions produce shock. Signs and symptoms include wheezing, hives, itching, nausea, vomiting, a weak pulse, rapid heartbeat, pallor, dizziness, and swelling in the throat and tongue that can interfere with breathing. Shock occurs when a sudden, severe drop in blood pressure occurs that can result in loss of consciousness and even death.

T78.2   Anaphylactic shock, unspecified

Use this code to report anaphylaxis--an anaphylactic reaction or allergic shock that is not otherwise specified. Anaphylactic reactions are induced by exposure to a specific antigen such as wasp or bee venom, a drug, a plant, or other substance. Anaphylactic reactions are known as an immediate type I allergic hypersensitivity reaction that is elicited very rapidly after exposure to the causative antigen. It is mediated by antibodies in the blood that react to the initial introduction of an antigen and induce the synthesis of immunoglobulins, particularly IgE, which bind to specific receptors on the surface of circulating mast cells. The next time that same, specific antigen is introduced, it reacts with the IgE on the mast cells and induces them to release large amounts of histamine and other chemicals that cause the familiar reactions of bronchoconstriction, smooth muscle contraction, vasodilation, and increased vascular permeability. Not all anaphylactic reactions produce shock. Signs and symptoms include wheezing, hives, itching, nausea, vomiting, a weak pulse, rapid heartbeat, pallor, dizziness, and swelling in the throat and tongue that can interfere with breathing. Shock occurs when a sudden, severe drop in blood pressure occurs that can result in loss of consciousness and even death.

Note: Anaphylaxis due to a correct medicine properly administered, an adverse reaction to food or serum, or the transfusion of blood products is reported elsewhere.

T78.41   Arthus phenomenon

Arthus phenomenon, also called arthus reaction, is an immediate hypersensitivity reaction that creates an inflammatory, indurated lesion, with redness, edema, hemorrhaging, and necrosis upon intradermal injection of an antigen into a person who has already been sensitized and has specific antibodies. The inflammation is an immune reaction precipitated by deposits of antigen-antibody complexes within tissue and blood vessels that in turn activate complement. Large numbers of phagocytic neutrophils then infiltrate the site and tissue destruction results by the neutrophil's release of lysosomal enzymes.

T79.2   Traumatic secondary and recurrent hemorrhage and seroma

A secondary traumatic, or post-traumatic seroma is a collection of fluid that develops in an area of soft tissue that has already been affected by previously suffering a large traumatic hematoma.

T79.A   Traumatic compartment syndrome

Compartment syndrome is an increase is tissue pressure within a fixed compartment bounded by muscle, fascia, and bone. This can occur from both traumatic and nontraumatic events. Traumatic events usually include direct tissue injury and burns. Compartment syndrome patients will have some kind of injury related to edema because edema and hemorrhage are the factors that quickly elevate compartment pressures high enough to cause ischemia in the muscles and nerves. When the pressure within the compartment exceeds the perfusion pressure of the arterioles, it causes muscle ischemia and tissue death. Symptoms of compartment syndrome include pain out of proportion with the injury that is not relieved by analgesics, edema, pain on flexion or extension, very painful passive motions, usually good capillary refill, paresthesia, weakness, and sometimes paralysis. Early recognition with fasciotomy often yields good results.

T79.A0   Compartment syndrome, unspecified

Note: Compartment syndrome that is unspecified as either a traumatic or nontraumatic event is coded by default under traumatic compartment syndrome.

T79.A1   Traumatic compartment syndrome of upper extremity

Traumatic compartment syndrome of the upper extremity is most commonly associated with fractures of the forearm, also with metacarpal-carpal dislocation, different kinds of soft tissue injury without fracture, and burns. Direct contusion injury or trauma to the extremity causes edema and hemorrhage within a fixed osteomyofascial compartment that quickly elevate compartment pressures high enough to cause ischemia in the muscles and nerves. Burns cause cellular damage associated with localized edema and cause compartment syndrome by three mechanisms: a) the formation of firm and inelastic eschars that encircle the limb and cause interstitial extravasation of fluids; b) burns caused by electrical conduction cause muscle and nerve damage in those compartments where the current traveled, leading to cell death; c) significant intravascular volume loss with systemic inflammation that requires careful volume replacement.

T79.A2   Traumatic compartment syndrome of lower extremity

Traumatic compartment syndrome of the lower extremity is most commonly associated with open or closed tibial fractures, significant soft tissue trauma without fracture, muscle rupture, and burns. Tissue trauma to the extremity causes edema and hemorrhage within a fixed osteomyofascial compartment that increases pressure high enough to cause ischemia in the muscles and nerves. Burns cause cellular damage associated with localized edema and cause compartment syndrome by three mechanisms: a) the formation of firm and inelastic eschars that encircle the limb and cause interstitial extravasation of fluids; b) burns caused by electrical conduction cause muscle and nerve damage in those compartments where the current traveled, leading to cell death; c) significant intravascular volume loss with systemic inflammation that requires careful volume replacement.

T79.A3   Traumatic compartment syndrome of abdomen

Traumatic compartment syndrome can occur in the abdomen, anywhere that soft tissue is affected within a fixed compartment bounded by muscle and fascia, when tissue injury results in hemorrhaging and subsequent swelling or edema enough to elevate intercompartmental pressures.

T80.21   Infection due to central venous catheter

Note: Types of catheters include PICC lines, triple-lumen catheters, umbilical venous catheters, Hickman catheters, and port-a-caths.

T80.211   Bloodstream infection due to central venous catheter

Bloodstream infections connected to central lines commonly occur in hospitals with about 250,000 cases a year. Bloodstream infections due to a central venous catheter are usually serious systemic infections that cause a prolonged hospital stay, increased use of resources and costs, and an increased risk of mortality. These are laboratory confirmed bloodstream infections due to a central line or umbilical catheter in place and not due to a secondary infection or community-acquired infection. There is no minimum of time that the central line must be in place for a bloodstream infection to be considered associated. A central line terminates at or near the heart in one of the great vessels such as the aorta, pulmonary artery, vena cavae, brachiocephalic veins, internal jugular, subclavian, common iliac, femoral, or external iliac veins, or the umbilical artery or vein in neonates.

T80.212   Local infection due to central venous catheter

A local infection due to a central venous catheter can occur in different places--at an exit site or insertion site, at the port or reservoir, or in the tunnel. Signs include pus or discharge, redness, pain, swelling, and tenderness at the site. Implantable venous access devices are associated with port or reservoir type infections in which discharge or purulent exudate may be present in the reservoir or its subcutaneous pocket. A tunnel type infection involves pain or inflammation in the area where the catheter runs under the skin.

T80.218 Other infection due to central venous catheter

This code reports any other specified type of central line or venous catheter-associated infection that is not further identified as either local or systemic.

T80.22 Acute infection following transfusion, infusion, or injection of blood and blood products

Acute infection following transfusion, infusion, or injection of blood and blood products reports infections caused by bacteria, viruses, parasites, or other infective micro-organisms transmitted through the receipt of whole blood, red blood cells, platelets, plasma, etc. This reports a diagnosis of acute cases, not chronic or longer term infections. These infections are monitored and treated as early as possible to avoid a more serious complication, such as sepsis.

T80.3 ABO incompatibility reaction due to transfusion of blood or blood products

ABO incompatibility is an immune reaction that occurs when two different, and incompatible, major blood groups are mixed together. There are three major blood types: A, B, and O. These groups are determined by very specific molecules present on the surface of the blood cells. These molecules, or antigens, act like immune system triggers against blood of a different group, i.e. A reacts against B, B reacts against A. Everyone has a combination of two of these surface antigens (Type A = AA or AO, Type B = BB or BO, Type AB). Type O lacks any surface antigens, and is known as the universal donor, because it will not trigger an immune response. However, type O can only receive type O, as it will react against the molecules on both type A and type B.

T80.30 ABO incompatibility reaction due to transfusion of blood or blood products, unspecified

An incompatibility reaction among differing blood groups causes clinical and laboratory signs of reaction and can present with back or flank pain, light-headedness, dyspnea, fever, chills, rigors, rash, and itching. Laboratory testing will show that the patient's and the donor's blood were not compatible.

Note: Use this code only when the type of ABO incompatibility transfusion reaction is not stated.

T80.310 ABO incompatibility with acute hemolytic transfusion reaction

An acute hemolytic transfusion reaction due to major blood group incompatibility causes rather immediate (within 24 hours) intravascular destruction of the transfused red blood cells by the patient's own immune system, which is producing antibodies to the transfused red blood cells. An acute hemolytic reaction produces abrupt onset of fever, chills, rigors, a feeling of heat in the vein being transfused, lumbar back pain, dyspnea, constricting pain in the chest, increased heart rate, hypotension, and hemoglobin in the blood and urine. A feeling of impending doom is often reported by the patient as an early sign of an acute hemolytic reaction. If the patient is unconscious or anesthetized, hypotension and uncontrolled bleeding from mucous membranes and incision sites from disseminated intravascular coagulation may be the only signs of an acute hemolytic transfusion reaction. The severity can be life-threatening and cause shock and acute renal failure. Treatment is aimed at maintaining blood pressure and renal blood flow with IV saline and furosemide.

T80.311 ABO incompatibility with delayed hemolytic transfusion reaction

A delayed hemolytic transfusion reaction due to major blood group incompatibility causes slowly accelerating extravascular destruction of transfused red blood cells by the patient's own immune system, which is producing antibodies against the transfused RBCs. A delayed reaction manifests any time after 1 day and up to 28 days following the transfusion, but most commonly within 4-8 days. Common signs are a dropping

hematocrit and a positive direct Coombs test. There may also be elevation of bilirubin and hemoglobin in the urine. Symptomatic patients will also have fever and appear to have an infection, demonstrating leukocytosis. Some cases may be so mild that they go undetected. Specific treatment is usually not necessary for delayed cases, although the patient may require supplemental transfusion of blood without the triggering antibody to replace the red blood cells that have been destroyed.

T80.319 ABO incompatibility with hemolytic transfusion reaction, unspecified

A hemolytic transfusion reaction due to major blood group incompatibility causes destruction of the transfused red blood cells by the patient's own immune system, which is producing antibodies to the transfused red blood cells. Hemolytic reactions can also produce fever, chills, rigor, low back or flank pain, and bloody urine. Lab tests demonstrate that the patient's and donor's blood were incompatible. Other tests may show high bilirubin counts, anemia, dropped hematocrit, and a positive direct Coomb's test.

Note: Use this code when the reaction is identified as hemolytic, due to major blood group incompatibility, but occurs at an unspecified time following the transfusion.

T80.39 Other ABO incompatibility reaction due to transfusion of blood or blood products

Use this code to report other types of transfusion reactions that are specifically identified as due to ABO, or major blood group incompatibility, such as delayed serologic transfusion reaction (DSTR). This is a positive posttransfusion finding on a direct antiglobulin test (DAT) and a newly developed alloantibody specificity, that occurs without clinical and/or laboratory evidence of hemolysis.

T80.4 Rh incompatibility reaction due to transfusion of blood or blood products

The presence of Rh antigens in the blood is another way to classify blood groups and is the second most important blood grouping system next to ABO. There are many defined Rh antigens; however only 5 are identified as the most important: D, C, c, E, and e. Rh factor refers to the strongest or most immunogenic of these antigens, D. Those without Rh factor present (Rh negative) do not have the D antigen on the surface of their red blood cells and will form antibodies against the Rh factor present in Rh positive blood if it is transfused. Most Rh incompatibility antigen-antibody response cases will be caused by the D antigen.

T80.40 Rh incompatibility reaction due to transfusion of blood or blood products, unspecified

This is an incompatibility reaction related to the patient's formation of antibodies against Rh antigens present in transfused blood. It causes clinical and laboratory signs of reaction and can present with back or flank pain, light-headedness, dyspnea, fever, chills, rigors, rash, and itching. Laboratory testing will show that the patient's and donor's blood were not compatible.

Note: Use this code only when the type of Rh incompatibility transfusion reaction is not stated.

T80.410 Rh incompatibility with acute hemolytic transfusion reaction

An acute hemolytic transfusion reaction due to Rh antigen incompatibility causes rather immediate (within 24 hours) intravascular destruction of the transfused red blood cells by the patient's own immune system, which is producing antibodies against the Rh antigen present in the transfused blood. An acute hemolytic reaction produces abrupt onset of fever, chills, rigors, a feeling of heat in the vein being transfused, lumbar back pain, dyspnea, constricting pain in the chest, increased heart rate, hypotension, and hemoglobin in the blood and urine. A feeling of impending doom is often reported by the patient as an early sign of an acute hemolytic reaction. If the patient is unconscious or anesthetized, hypotension and uncontrolled bleeding from mucous membranes and incision sites from disseminated intravascular coagulation may be the only signs of an acute hemolytic transfusion reaction. The severity can be life-threatening and cause shock and acute renal failure. Treatment is aimed at maintaining blood pressure and renal blood flow with IV saline and furosemide.

T80.411 Rh incompatibility with delayed hemolytic transfusion reaction

A delayed hemolytic transfusion reaction due to Rh antigen incompatibility causes slowly accelerating extravascular destruction of transfused red blood cells by the patient's own immune system, which is producing antibodies against the Rh antigen present on the transfused red blood cells. A delayed reaction manifests any time after 1 day and up to 28 days following the transfusion, but most commonly within 4-8 days. Common signs are a dropping hematocrit and a positive direct Coombs test. There may also be elevation of bilirubin and hemoglobin in the urine. Symptomatic patients will have fever and appear to have an infection, demonstrating leukocytosis. Some cases may be so mild that they go undetected. Specific treatment is usually not necessary for delayed cases, although the patient may require supplemental transfusion of blood without the triggering antibody to replace the red blood cells that have been destroyed.

T80.419 Rh incompatibility with hemolytic transfusion reaction, unspecified

A hemolytic transfusion reaction due to Rh antigen incompatibility causes destruction of the transfused red blood cells by the patient's own immune system, which developed antibodies against the Rh antigen present in the transfused blood. Hemolytic reactions can also produce fever, chills, rigor, low back or flank pain, and bloody urine. Lab tests demonstrate that the patient's and donor's blood were incompatible. Other tests may show high bilirubin counts, anemia, dropped hematocrit, and a positive direct Coomb's test.

Note: Use this code when the reaction is identified as hemolytic, due to Rh antigen incompatibility, but occurring at an unspecified time following the transfusion.

T80.49 Other Rh incompatibility reaction due to transfusion of blood or blood products

Use this code to report other types of transfusion reactions that are specifically identified as due to Rh antigen blood group incompatibility, such as delayed serologic transfusion reaction (DSTR). This is a positive posttransfusion finding on a direct antiglobulin test (DAT) and a newly developed alloantibody specificity, that occurs without clinical and/or laboratory evidence of hemolysis.

T80.5 Anaphylactic reaction due to serum

Codes in this subcategory report anaphylaxis, anaphylactic reaction, or allergic shock caused by an adverse reaction to a serum product, which may be a vaccination serum, blood serum, or other kind of serum. Anaphylactic reactions are known as a type I allergic hypersensitivity reaction. This is an immediate type hypersensitivity reaction that is elicited very rapidly after exposure to the causative antigen. It is mediated by antibodies in the blood that react to the initial introduction of an antigen and induce the synthesis of immunoglobulins, particularly IgE. The immunoglobulins bind to specific receptors on the surface of circulating mast cells. The next time that same, specific antigen is introduced, it reacts with the IgE on the mast cells and induces them to release large amounts of histamine and other chemicals that cause the familiar reactions of bronchoconstriction, smooth muscle contraction, vasodilation, and increased vascular permeability. Not all anaphylactic reactions produce shock. Signs and symptoms include wheezing, hives, itching, nausea, vomiting, a weak pulse, rapid heartbeat, pallor, dizziness, and swelling in the throat and tongue that can interfere with breathing. Shock occurs when a sudden, severe drop in blood pressure occurs that can result in loss of consciousness and even death.

Note: This group of codes has several exclusions: ABO incompatibility reactions and other types of serum reactions to the administration of blood or blood products, as well as anaphylactic reactions to drugs or chemicals.

T80.51 Anaphylactic reaction due to administration of blood and blood products

Most anaphylactic reactions to transfusions of blood and blood products occur in patients who have a hereditary immunoglobulin A (IgA) deficiency. They have developed complement-binding anti-IgA antibodies that react to donor IgA when exposed through transfusion. This causes anaphylaxis. Signs include the rapid development of chills, cramping, vomiting, diarrhea, and difficulty breathing. Anaphylactic reactions occur about 1 per every 20,000 transfused units.

T80.52 Anaphylactic reaction due to vaccination

Anaphylactic reactions to vaccines can be very serious and have the potential to be fatal when left without immediate treatment if anaphylactic or allergic shock occurs. Manifestations can be milder in less severe kinds of anaphylactoid reactions and produce allergy symptoms such as wheezing, hives, itching, and swelling. Severe anaphylactic reactions develop into a serious threat quickly after administration and include swelling of the tongue and throat impeding breathing, tightness in the chest, weak pulse, rapid heartbeat, cyanosis, dizziness, severe hives, swelling, itching, nausea, vomiting, abdominal cramping, and even a sudden drop in blood pressure (shock) and loss of consciousness. Since vaccines are complex and made of many different components, and anaphylactic reactions can also be triggered by many different substances, even from person to person, it is hard to pinpoint the cause.

T80.61 Other serum reaction due to administration of blood and blood products

Proteins in donor plasma are responsible for causing many other types of serum reactions besides anaphylactic reactions, such as protein sickness, serum rash, serum sickness, and serum urticaria. These less severe types of hypersensitivity reactions are seen more frequently in the transfusions of products that contain a large amount of plasma, such as whole blood, fresh frozen plasma, and pooled platelets. These reactions generally produce urticaria and may involve fever, joint pain, and swollen lymph nodes. Minor serum reactions to transfusions, along with nonhemolytic febrile reactions, are the most common and occur in 3-4% of transfusions.

T80.62 Other serum reaction due to vaccination

Vaccination can cause other serum reactions besides anaphylactic type, such as serum sickness, serum rash, and serum uticaria. These other kinds of reactions occur with injection of a vaccine, like an antitoxin, anti-infective, or antivenom produced in an animal. Serum sickness usually manifests after about 10 days, when the person's antibodies begin reacting against the vaccine serum, forming circulating antigen-antibody immune complexes that become deposited in tissues, causing further reaction and tissue damage. Symptoms may take up to three weeks to manifest and include itching, rash, fever, joint pain, and swollen lymph nodes.

T80.69 Other serum reaction due to other serum

Examples of other serum reactions include protein sickness or serum sickness, serum intoxication, serum rash, and urticaria due to serum. Serum sickness is a type III immune complex hypersensitivity reaction that involves IgG circulating antibodies that react with free antigens, forming circulating antigen-antibody immune complexes which become deposited in tissue. These deposits then cause further reaction with complement, and then tissue damage. This reaction develops with systematic exposure and manifests days or weeks later.

T80.81 Extravasation of vesicant agent

Extravasation means that a substance has leaked out of a blood vessel or organ where it is intended to be. This can occur with natural substances produced by the body, such as chyle, urine, or blood, or it can occur with an infused substance given intravenously. A vesicant is a substance that can cause tissue necrosis when it leaks from the infusion vessel. This can still occur despite great precautions taken to avoid it when catheters slip or become dislodged, separate, or break.

T80.810 Extravasation of vesicant antineoplastic chemotherapy

When a chemotherapy substance leaks from the vessel during infusion, the surrounding tissue can sustain significant damage. This is a very injurious event mainly occurring in an outpatient setting.

T80.89 Other complications following infusion, transfusion and therapeutic injection

Use this code to report other types of transfusion, infusion, or therapeutic injection reactions that are not specified as to the type of blood grouping incompatibility, such as delayed serologic transfusion reaction (DSTR). This is a positive posttransfusion finding on a direct antiglobulin test (DAT) and a newly developed alloantibody specificity, that occurs without clinical and/ or laboratory evidence of hemolysis.

T80.910 Acute hemolytic transfusion reaction, unspecified incompatibility

An acute hemolytic transfusion reaction due to an unspecified blood incompatibility causes rather immediate (within 24 hours) intravascular destruction of the transfused red blood cells by the patient's own immune system, which is producing antibodies against the antigen present in the transfused blood. An acute hemolytic reaction produces abrupt onset of fever, chills, rigors, a feeling of heat in the vein being transfused, lumbar back pain, dyspnea, constricting pain in the chest, increased heart rate, hypotension, and hemoglobin in the blood and urine. A feeling of impending doom is often reported by the patient as an early sign of an acute hemolytic reaction. If the patient is unconscious or anesthetized, hypotension and uncontrolled bleeding from mucous membranes and incision sites from disseminated intravascular coagulation may be the only signs of an acute hemolytic transfusion reaction. The severity can be life-threatening and cause shock and acute renal failure. Treatment is aimed at maintaining blood pressure and renal blood flow with IV saline and furosemide.

T80.911 Delayed hemolytic transfusion reaction, unspecified incompatibility

A delayed hemolytic transfusion reaction due to an unspecified blood incompatibility causes slowly accelerating extravascular destruction of transfused red blood cells by the patient's own immune system, which is producing antibodies against the antigen present on the transfused red blood cells. A delayed reaction manifests any time after 1 day and up to 28 days following the transfusion, but most commonly within 4-8 days. Common signs are a dropping hematocrit and a positive direct Coombs test. There may also be elevation of bilirubin and hemoglobin in the urine. Symptomatic patients will have fever and appear to have an infection, demonstrating leukocytosis. Some cases may be so mild that they go undetected. Specific treatment is usually not necessary for delayed cases, although the patient may require supplemental transfusion of blood without the triggering antibody to replace the red blood cells that have been destroyed.

T80.919 Hemolytic transfusion reaction, unspecified incompatibility, unspecified as acute or delayed

A hemolytic transfusion reaction due to blood incompatibility causes destruction of the transfused red blood cells by the patient's own immune system. Hemolytic reactions can also produce fever, chills, rigor, low back or flank pain, and bloody urine. Lab tests demonstrate that the patient's and donor's blood were incompatible. Other tests may show high bilirubin counts, anemia, dropped hematocrit, and a positive direct Coomb's test.

Note: Use this code when a transfusion reaction is identified as hemolytic due to an unspecified type of blood antigen incompatibility and not stated whether acute or delayed.

T80.92 Unspecified transfusion reaction

This code reports a blood group incompatibility infusion or transfusion reaction without any further information as to the type of reaction or the particular incompatibility that caused the reaction.

T80.A Non-ABO incompatibility reaction due to transfusion of blood or blood products

Incompatibility transfusion reactions can be caused by minor antigens also expressed on red blood cells, such as M, N, P, or S antigens, and Kell, Duffy, Lewis, Kidd, and Diego antigens. There are over 200 minor blood groups that can also cause problems with blood transfusions, and are known as rare blood types in addition to the major ABO designation. The Kell antigen is an example of one that can cause severe hemolytic disease when the tranfused person's immune system produces an anti-Kell response.

T80.A0 Non-ABO incompatibility reaction due to transfusion of blood or blood products, unspecified

This code reports an incompatibility reaction related to the patient's formation of antibodies against any minor blood grouping antigens present in transfused blood. The type of reaction is not further specified, but causes clinical and laboratory signs of reaction such as flushing, light-headedness, dyspnea, fever, chills, rigors, rash, and itching.

T80.A10 Non-ABO incompatibility with acute hemolytic transfusion reaction

Incompatibility transfusion reactions can be caused by minor antigens also expressed on red blood cells, such as M, N, P, or S antigens, and Kell, Duffy, Lewis, Kidd, and Diego antigens. There are over 200 minor, rare blood groups that can also cause problems with blood transfusions. The Kell antigen, for example, can cause severe hemolytic disease when the tranfused person's immune system produces an anti-Kell response. An acute hemolytic transfusion reaction causes rather immediate (within 24 hours) intravascular destruction of the transfused red blood cells by the patient's own immune system. The reaction produces abrupt onset of fever, chills, rigors, a feeling of heat in the vein being transfused, lumbar back pain, dyspnea, constricting pain in the chest, increased heart rate, hypotension, and hemoglobin in the blood and urine. A feeling of impending doom is often reported by the patient as an early sign of an acute hemolytic reaction. If the patient is unconscious or anesthetized, hypotension and uncontrolled bleeding from mucous membranes and incision sites from disseminated intravascular coagulation may be the only signs of an acute hemolytic transfusion reaction. The severity can be life-threatening and cause shock and acute renal failure. Treatment is aimed at maintaining blood pressure and renal blood flow with IV saline and furosemide.

T80.A11 Non-ABO incompatibility with delayed hemolytic transfusion reaction

A delayed hemolytic transfusion reaction due to a minor blood group antigen incompatibility causes slowly accelerating extravascular destruction of transfused red blood cells by the patient's own immune system. A delayed reaction manifests any time after 1 day up to 28 days following the transfusion, but most commonly within 4-8 days. Common signs are a dropping hematocrit and a positive direct Coombs test. There may also be elevation of bilirubin and hemoglobin in the urine. Symptomatic patients will have fever and appear to have an infection, demonstrating leukocytosis. Some cases may be so mild that they go undetected. Specific treatment is usually not necessary for delayed cases, although the patient may require supplemental transfusion of blood without the triggering antibody to replace the RBCs that have been destroyed.

T80.A19 Non-ABO incompatibility with hemolytic transfusion reaction, unspecified

Hemolytic incompatibility transfusion reactions can also produce fever, chills, rigor, low back or flank pain, and bloody urine. Lab tests demonstrate that the patient's and donor's blood were incompatible. Other tests may show high bilirubin counts, anemia, dropped hematocrit, and a positive direct Coomb's test.

Note: Use this code when the transfusion reaction is identified as hemolytic, due to any minor blood group antigen incompatibility, but occurring at an unspecified time following the transfusion.

T80.A9   Other non-ABO incompatibility reaction due to transfusion of blood or blood products

Minor antigens outside of the major ABO blood group and Rh antigens are also expressed on red blood cells, such as M, N, P, or S antigens, and Kell, Duffy, Lewis, Kidd, and Diego antigens. They can also cause other problems with blood transfusions, such as delayed serologic transfusion reaction (DSTR). This is a positive posttransfusion finding on a direct antiglobulin test (DAT) and a newly developed alloantibody specificity, that occurs without clinical and/or laboratory evidence of hemolysis.

T81.1   Postprocedural shock

Shock that occurs as a complication following major surgery is a physiological state marked by decreased perfusion of tissues with corresponding oxygen deprivation, the resulting effects of which are initially reversible but become dangerously irreversible very quickly. Symptoms of postprocederal shock include hypotension, rapid heart rate, cold, clammy skin, decreased kidney output, and altered mental state. Resulting end conditions from shock include organ injury or failure involving more than one system, and death. Different mechanisms occur in the body to produce different kinds of shock, all of which may occur postoperatively, and even concurrently. Codes in this subcategory report the different types of postoperative shock, such as cardiogenic and septic.

T81.10   Postprocedural shock unspecified

Unspecified postprocedural shock is used to report collapse, NOS either during or after a surgical procedure, and postoperative hypoperfusion or failure of peripheral circulation without any specification as to the mechanism or causative type of the perfusion/circulation failure.

T81.11   Postprocedural cardiogenic shock

Cardiogenic postprocedural shock is caused by failure of the heart's pumping ability resulting from postoperative myocardial infarction or systolic heart failure, causing global tissue hypoperfusion and both diastolic and systolic dysfunction. It is life threatening and treated as an emergency with inotropic agents, such as dopamine, dobutamine, epinephrine, norepinephrine, amrinone, and other medications to improve cardiac output and increase blood pressure.

T81.12   Postprocedural septic shock

Postprocedural septic shock originates from severe operative infections of the wound, lungs, blood, or vascular catheter that lead to septic shock, causing end-stage inflammatory response syndrome, organ ischemia, multisystem organ failure, procoagulant response with microvascular thrombosis, and death. Septic shock patients often have different components from the type of shock manifesting from other mechanisms, such as nonhemorrhagic hypovolemic shock from loss of fluids due to vomiting and diarrhea, or cardiogenic type from heart dysfunction. Septic shock is commonly seen with a distributive shock component due to inflammatory changes dilating systemic arterioles, decreasing vascular resistance, and affecting permeability. This emergency is treated with antibiotics, vasopressors to help manage persistent hypotension, and supportive measures necessary to restore fluid volume, reduce inflammation, inhibit thrombosis and promote fibrinolysis, and improve organ function.

T81.19   Other postprocedural shock

Other postprocedureal shock includes hypovolemic type shock that arises from a loss of intravascular volume, which can result from internal bleeding due to poor surgical technique or disseminated intravascular coagulation, and is treated with blood products. Hypovolemic postoperative shock may also occur with volume shifts, called "third spacing" that lead to a loss of fluid volume not caused by hemorrhaging. This type is treated with fluid resuscitation.

T83.711   Erosion of implanted vaginal mesh and other prosthetic materials to surrounding organ or tissue

Vaginal vault prolapse is treated surgically with abdominal sacral colpopexy in which a graft is used to suspend the sinking upper portion of the vagina to the anterior longitudinal ligament of the sacrum. Synthetic materials used for the implanted vaginal mesh can erode into surrounding organs or tissue, causing serious pelvic infections and requiring surgery to remove the mesh in addition to treating the infection. True erosions occur after healing due to the friction, compression, or tension caused by the implant. Erosion of organs besides the vagina include urethral, bladder, and rectal erosion, and even the erosion of more distant tissues.

T83.721   Exposure of implanted vaginal mesh and other prosthetic materials into vagina

Exposure of implanted vaginal mesh and other prosthetic materials into the vagina can occur when synthetic materials are placed in a colpopexy to suspend a prolapsing vagina. Vaginal exposure of the implant is not as serious as cases of mesh erosion into surrounding tissue. Exposure can be asymptomatic or cause leukorrhea, discharges, or slight spontaneous bleeding. This does not immediately mean infection, although it does carry a risk of infection. Exposed mesh is usually connected to a defect of vaginal healing and can sometimes be treated nonsurgically.

T84.01   Broken internal joint prosthesis

A prosthetic joint implant is not as strong or durable as the natural, normal, healthy joint and the patient cannot be guaranteed that a prosthetic implant will last for a lifetime. For instance, almost all prosthetic hips will need to be replaced or revised at some time. The longevity of a prosthesis varies from patient to patient with the type of implant, the joint being replaced, the amount of use, and other factors such as the patient's overall physical condition and level of activity, body weight, and the surgical technique used.

T84.05   Periprosthetic osteolysis of internal prosthetic joint

Periprosthetic osteolysis is the degeneration of bone tissue around an implanted prosthetic joint.

T85.44   Capsular contracture of breast implant

When a breast implant is placed, the body naturally begins to form a lining around it, called a capsule, or scar capsule, made of fibrous tissue. The body is programmed to shrink scar tissue somewhat and in some people, the capsule tightens and squeezes the implant, which makes it feel hard and look distortedly 'ball-like'.

T86   Complications of transplanted organs and tissue

Organ transplants are some of the most complicated medical procedures performed, and the risk of complication is extremely high. Transplanted organs are prone to infection and inflammation, and may be attacked by the body's immune system, causing rejection and the need for a new transplant organ. Blood clots can also develop around transplanted organs.

Note: Use additional codes to identify other specific complications, such as graft vs. host disease.

T86.5   Complications of stem cell transplant

Stem cells are found in the greatest concentration in bone marrow, but when bone marrow has been damaged from disease or treatment for neoplastic disease, hematopoietic stem cells can be transplanted to replace the dysfunctional marrow or even to destroy unhealthy marrow so the patient can produce healthy blood cells. In these cases, stem cells can be taken from the peripheral blood and from umbilical cord blood. Using peripheral stem cells collected from the bloodstream has a lower long-term relapse rate and provides a bigger graft in shorter time without surgical need for bone marrow donation. However, all stem cell transplantation poses many risks, including possibly fatal complications. The immune system may reject the stem cells and the graft may fail. The donor's stem cells may attack the recipient's body causing graft versus host disease. Organ damage or failure can occur, cataracts may appear, and secondary cancers can develop.

T88.3   Malignant hyperthermia due to anesthesia

This code is used to report malignant hyperthermia that occurs when the patient has a bad reaction to an anesthetic, usually halothane or succinylcholine. Symptoms of this condition are muscle rigidity, abnormally high metabolic rate, and abnormally high body temperature.

T88.52 Failed moderate sedation during procedure

When moderate conscious sedation is inadequate, the procedure is made much more difficult, dangerous, and unpleasant. Unsafe conditions result. Urgent intervention, particularly from someone trained to administer adequate moderate sedation, deep sedation, and/or anesthesia, becomes necessary. Failed moderate sedation includes times when the maximum amount of prudent and safe doses are given, but the patient remains inadequately sedated; the patient reacts idiosyncratically to the medication and becomes more deeply sedated than planned; the patient becomes unable to maintain a patent airway and has depressed respirations that compromise adequate air exchange; or other hemodynamic changes occur that pose potential risks.

T88.6 Anaphylactic reaction due to adverse effect of correct drug or medicament properly administered

Use this subcategory to report anaphylactic reaction or shock due to an adverse effect of a correct drug or medicament that was properly administered. Anaphylactic reactions are known as an immediate type I allergic hypersensitivity reaction that is elicited very rapidly after exposure to the causative antigen. It is mediated by antibodies in the blood that react to the initial introduction of an antigen and induce the synthesis of immunoglobulins, particularly IgE, which bind to specific receptors on the surface of circulating mast cells. The next time that same, specific antigen is introduced, it reacts with the IgE on the mast cells and induces them to release large amounts of histamine and other chemicals that cause the familiar reactions of bronchoconstriction, smooth muscle contraction, vasodilation, and increased vascular permeability. Not all anaphylactic reactions produce shock. Signs and symptoms include wheezing, hives, itching, nausea, vomiting, a weak pulse, rapid heartbeat, pallor, dizziness, and swelling in the throat and tongue that can interfere with breathing. Shock occurs when a sudden, severe drop in blood pressure occurs that can result in loss of consciousness and even death.

T88.7 Unspecified adverse effect of drug or medicament

A drug reaction or drug hypersensitivity, besides anaphylactic, without mention of any specified adverse effects.

Z00.11 Newborn health examination

Healthy supervision check-ups for newborns should be done following published recommendations from the American Academy of Pediatrics for post-hospital newborn care. The purpose of these follow-up visits is to weigh the infant; assess general health, hydration, and jaundice; observe feeding technique for adequate positioning, latch-on, and swallowing; review the newborn's elimination history; assess mother-infant interaction and bonding; review results of laboratory tests done before discharge; reinforce education in infant care; perform other screening tests; and set up a plan for continued health care maintenance and immunizations.

Z01.84 Encounter for antibody response examination

Pre-vaccination serologic antibody response testing is done to help ensure that persons who need a vaccine receive it and that those who are already adequately immunized are not overimmunized. When patients do not have adequate documentation, antibody response testing is indicated to determine the current immunity status as a precaution against unnecessary vaccinations. Pre-vaccination testing can also help reduce the cost of immunizing adult populations with a high prevalence for a given disease. Post-vaccination testing for antibody response is done to test for post-exposure prophylaxis and whether adequate immunity has been achieved. This can be particularly indicated for health care workers who have received a hepatitis B vaccine but are at ongoing risk from blood, patient contact, and injury from needle sticks.

Z11 Encounter for screening for infectious and parasitic diseases

The screening codes in this category are reported for testing that is done on asymptomatic patients to detect a disease or its precursor early enough that the right treatment can be provided for those who test positive.

Z11.51 Encounter for screening for human papillomavirus (HPV)

The human papillomavirus is a group of many viruses that can cause warts on the hands, feet, and genitals, and is known to contribute to the development of dysplasias and cancers of the anal canal and female reproductive organs.

Z11.59 Encounter for screening for other viral diseases

Other viral diseases inlcudes arthropod borne viruses, also called arboviruses, which are transmitted through a vector, such as a tick or mosquito. In cases such as West Nile Virus, St Louis encephalitis, and La Crosse encephalitis, the mosquito first becomes infected by feeding off an infected bird and then transmits the virus to the person being bitten. Dengue fever and dengue hemorrhagic fever are caused by four different serotypes of the Flavivirus and transmitted by the Aedes mosquito. Dengue is one of the most important mosquito-borne viral diseases affecting humans with a global distribution similar to malaria.

Note: Do not report Z11.59 for viral intestinal diseases, which are coded to Z11.0.

Z13 Encounter for screening for other diseases and disorders

Screening tests are done to detect the presence of a disease or disease precursors in those who are asymptomatic in order to provide early detection and treatment for those who are positive.

Z13.228 Encounter for screening for other metabolic disorders

This code reports a screening exam for inborn metabolic errors or other metabolic disorders besides lipoid disorders, such as cystic fibrosis, phenylketonuria, and galactosemia. Phenylketonuria [PKU] is a genetic disorder in which the body is unable to utilize phenylalanine, an essential amino acid and protein building block for the body. The enzyme that converts phenylalanine is completely or nearly deficient and so the blood levels rise. Infants born with PKU appear normal and may have fairer hair, skin, and eye color than other family members. If unscreened and untreated, symptoms appear as vomiting, irritability, eczema-type rash, mousy odor in the urine, and nervous system problems like increased muscle tone and hyperreactive tendon reflexes. Severe brain problems may occur later like retardation and seizures. Untreated children may also have microcephaly, protruding jaw and cheek bones, widely-spaced teeth, and poor teeth enamel. Galactosemia is a disorder in the body's ability to process the simple sugar, galactose, which is mainly a part of lactose and found in many foods, such as dairy products and baby formula. The different types of galactosemia are caused by a gene mutation that affects different enzymes responsible for breaking down galactose. Infants with the most severe, classic type will suffer life-threatening complications in a few days if not treated with a low-galactose diet. Symptoms include feeding difficulty, lethargy, lack of weight gain, jaundice, liver damage, bleeding, sepsis, and shock. Children may develop cataracts, speech difficulties, mental retardation, and ovarian failure.

Z13.5 Encounter for screening for eye and ear disorders

Ocular conditions that may be screened for in asymptomatic persons include cataract, glaucoma, congenital anomalies of the eye, and senile macular lesions. A cataract is a clouding in the normally clear lens of the eye, making it opaque and blocking vision. Some rare, congenital cataracts may be present or develop after birth, but most adult cataracts are associated with aging and develop slowly and painlessly, affecting vision, as the eye(s) get worse. Glaucoma is a disorder in which an increase in fluid pressure in the eye causes damage to the optic nerve, leading to vision loss and, if the disorder is not treated, permanent blindness. Glaucoma is caused when the outflow of ocular fluid, called the aqueous humor or aqueous fluid, is blocked. Glaucoma is painless and initially presents with no symptoms at all. However, as it progresses, the patient initially experiences loss of peripheral vision, while the center vision remains normal. As the disease continues, vision continues to narrow until blindness results. Senile macular lesions may be a hole, tear, or lesion in the foveal retina that may affect central vision and be only mildly apparent during driving or reading, or cause a scotoma, a blind spot in the central field of vision. Drusen is also an age-related macular lesion that appears as a round, yellowish lesion that evolves to macular degeneration. Choroidal neovascular lesions are abnormal blood vessels beneath the retinal pigment epithelium and are attributable to wet macular degeneration, a severe form leading to blindness.

Z13.71 Encounter for nonprocreative screening for genetic disease carrier status

This code reports special screening for a patient being evaluated to find out whether or not he or she is a carrier of a suspected hereditary disease that may be passed on to affected offspring, while the parent remains asymptomatic.

Note: This genetic screening code is for situations unrelated to procreation. When testing for a genetic disease carrier is done in relation to procreative management, use the appropriate male or female code for genetic disease carrier status testing.

Z13.820 Encounter for screening for osteoporosis

Osteoporosis is a bone disease in which bone mineral density is gradually reduced, making the bones porous, frail, and brittle, and leading to pathological fractures that occur almost spontaneously with very little stress. The bones most affected are those of the spine and hips. This disease most often affects females after menopause, but it also affects elderly men and anyone with particular hormonal disorders or chronic disease necessitating the long-term used of medications like corticosteroids.

Z13.850 Encounter for screening for traumatic brain injury

Traumatic brain injury occurs in many different ways--with intracranial injuries such as concussion, contusion, and subarachnoid hemorrhage; and with skull fracture, with or without open intracranial wound. Levels of loss of consciousness differ as do the neurological manifestations, and the late effects that develop over a longer time period. Each person's injury manifests in different ways.

Z13.89 Encounter for screening for other disorder

This code is reported for screenings done for congenital malformations or deformations, including a congenital hip dislocation. This is an abnormal musculoskeletal formation of the hip joint in which the femoral head is unstable within the socket, called the acetabulum. The ligaments may also be loose or stretched. The degree of instability varies. A baby born with this condition may have a loosely fitted ball in the hip socket, or it may be completely dislocated. If it is left untreated, it can cause the legs to be different lengths, with a duck-like walk, causing pain and early osteoarthritis. This condition is more commonly seen in girls than boys, in first-born children, those born breech, and usually affects the left hip more than the right. Usual treatment is to place the baby in a special harness with straps that let the baby move freely while holding the hip in place.

Z15 Genetic susceptibility to disease

Genetic susceptibility is the increased risk of developing a particular disease or illness due to the presence of one or more abnormal genes. The inherited genetic mutations predispose the individual to a higher chance of developing the disease than the average risk factors for the general population.

Z15.81 Genetic susceptibility to multiple endocrine neoplasia [MEN]

There are three distinct forms of multiple endocrine neoplasia [MEN] that are identified as inherited disorders and cause a syndrome of polyglandular malfunction. Type I, Werner's syndrome, is characterized by hyperplasia or tumors of the parathyroid, the pancreatic islet cells, and the pituitary gland. Type IIA, Sipple's syndrome, is characterized by a triad of medullary carcinoma of the thyroid, adrenal gland tumor, and hyperplasia of the parathyroid gland. Type IIB is similar to IIA but has mucosal neuromas without parathyroid involvement.

Z16 Resistance to antimicrobial drugs

Drug resistance is the ability of a micro-organism to withstand the effects of antibiotics, antimycotics, and other anti-infectives. Natural resistance evolves slowly over a long period of time through natural selection and resulting genetic mutations that endow subsequent generations of bacteria, viruses, etc, with the drug resistance. Once the resistant gene is generated, the micro-organism can even transfer the genetic information to other existing individual organisms by plasmid exchange. Due to the misuse of antibiotics and other anti-infectives, drug resistance is growing--brought on by overuse when the drugs are not necessary and by not completing the regimen as prescribed. This creation of 'superbugs' results in more dangerous infections that are harder to treat, and require more intensive care and even stronger medications.

Z16.2 Resistance to other antibiotics

Drug resistant microorganisms (DRMs) are common bacteria that have developed strains that cannot be controlled or killed with antibiotics. Some DRMs pose a serious public health problem and may include vancomycin resistant Enterococcus (VRE) and multiple drug resistant Mycobacterium tuberculosis (MDR-TB).

Z18.01 Retained depleted uranium fragments

Depleted uranium (DU) is a slightly radioactive heavy metal used in aircraft, armor, and ammunition. A person with a retained fragment of depleted uranium, such as veterans, are not radioactive, nor dangerous to others. When the fragment is left in place rather than taking the risk of damaging other tissue to dig it out, the amount of DU leaving the body in urine over time is monitored to determine if the kidneys must be watched closely, since exposure to large amounts of DU damages the kidneys.

Z18.11 Retained magnetic metal fragments

Any retained magnetic metal foreign body is a contraindication to an MRI exam, which uses a powerful magnetic field to systematically align the naturally occuring hydrogen atoms in the body. The magnetic field produced by the hydrogen nuclei is detected by the scanner to produce an image. The presence of an embedded magnetic foreign body interferes with the use of this imaging method.

Z18.2 Retained plastic fragments

Retained plastic fragments are not quite as common as embedded splinters of wood, glass, or metal, but are still a foreign material often encountered embedded in tissue. Unlike wood splinters or other embedded organic material, plastic fragments are relatively inert if the piece of plastic was uncontaminated. The retained fragment may cause only a mild reaction that presents as encapsulation. There are many chemicals used in the manufacturing of plastics that may leach out into tissue over time and present a carcinogenic risk factor later.

Note: Plastic foreign bodies include arcrylics, isocyanates, and diethylhexylphthalates.

Z18.31 Retained animal quills or spines

Animal quills or spines such as those of the porcupine have sharp, microscopic, backward-facing barbs that attach to skin and make them difficult to extract. If the quill becomes embedded, these barbs actually pull the quills deeper and deeper into the flesh in which it is embedded several millimeters per day just by the normal muscle movement of the victim. Animal quills or spines that remain embedded cause serious problems due to penetration and infection.

Z18.32 Retained tooth

A retained tooth, particularly a deciduous tooth, causes oral problems. No two teeth of the same kind should be present at the same time, occupying the same space. The retained tooth will force the permanent tooth into an abnormal position as it redirects the new tooth's growth, which then erupts through the gum at an improper angle. A retained deciduous tooth can cause damage to the oral soft tissues from sharp teeth protruding at wrong angles, excessive wear from malocclusion, pain, and increased, early onset of gum disease. A retained root that remains in the jaw after an extraction or tooth fracture causes mouth infections and pain, and may even act as a mobile foreign body. Roots encased in bone can remain buried in the jaw without causing problems for years.

Z18.33 Retained wood fragments

Splinters made of wood are one of the most commonly retained foreign bodies. Wood fragments are highly inflammatory and can cause severe reactions. Any wood splinter that is not removed completely causes complications like inflammation, infection, toxic or allergic reactions, and the formation of abnormal granulation tissue. Older injuries may not present with any kind of visible track leading to the foreign body but with symptoms such as swelling, pain associated with a mass, a draining sinus, tenderness, or infections such as cellulitis, abscess, bursitis, synovitis, osteomyelitis, and even sterile monoarticular arthritis. Deeper wood fragments can be difficult to detect by plain radiography and may require CT scanning or MRI for detection, especially when the splinters are lodged near bone.

Z18.39 Other retained organic fragments

Other retained organic fragments may include rose thorns, blackthorns, cactus spines, and other plant or vegetative material.

Z18.81   Retained glass fragments

Retained glass fragments are a common type of embedded foreign object along with wood and metallic splinters. Unlike wood splinters or other embedded organic material, glass fragments are relatively inert if the piece of glass was uncontaminated. The retained fragment may cause only a mild reaction that presents as encapsulation.

Z20   Contact with and (suspected) exposure to communicable diseases

These codes are used when the concern exists that a patient who does not currently display any symptoms or have a confirmed diagnosis may end up contracting a particular infectious disease through contact or exposure to it. Testing is done and may be positive for exposure, but this does not automatically mean the patient will contract the disease.

Z21   Asymptomatic human immunodeficiency virus [HIV] infection status

Note: This code is only to be used to identify a patient that has tested HIV positive and has no symptoms of the infection. It cannot be assigned if the patient has ever had any HIV-related illness

Z22   Carrier of infectious disease

An asymptomatic carrier of an infectious disease is an individual who acts as a host for the colonization of specific micro-organisms, but does not show any apparent signs of suffering from the illness themselves. The host harbors the disease-causing organisms in his or her own body, which can then be passed on and spread the disease-causing infection in others, but without the host manifesting any symptoms of the disease.

Both carriers and suspected carriers are capable of transmitting infectious diseases to others. A suspected carrier is someone who has come into contact with another known to have the disease, but does not currently display any signs or symptoms.

Z22.321   Carrier or suspected carrier of Methicillin susceptible Staphylococcus aureus

Staphylococcus aureus is a bacterium that commonly colonizes in the human respiratory tract and on the skin and may lead to acute infections. Methicillin susceptible Staphylococcus aureus (MSSA) is a strain of the bacterium sensitive to first line antibiotics including penicillins and cephalosporins.

Z22.322   Carrier or suspected carrier of Methicillin resistant Staphylococcus aureus

Staphylococcus aureus is a bacterium that commonly colonizes in the human respiratory tract and on the skin and may lead to acute infections. Methicillin resistant Staphylococcus aureus (MRSA) is a strain of the bacterium resistant to first line antibiotics including penicillins and cephalosporins. MRSA is not more virulent than other strains, but it is more difficult to treat.

Z23   Encounter for immunization

Vaccinations for immunization can be given orally or injected intramuscularly, subcutaneously, or intradermally, sometimes even given intranasally. A vaccine provides active, long-term immunity by exposing the recipient's immune system to altered versions of the bacteria or virus that will not actually cause the disease. Altered versions may be weakened, synthetic, purified, inactivated, or killed organisms that induce the immune system to produce its own antibodies against the invading micro-organism. The body then remembers how to make the specific antibodies when it is exposed to the antigen again.

Z28.3   Underimmunization status

A significant number of children are underimmunized, which means they may have received only some, or even none, of the recommended immunizations. Reasons for this include: immigration to the US, foreign adoptions, moving from the area of one's regular healthcare provider and failing to establish care with a new provider, and lack of healthcare insurance. Studies show that once immunizations fall behind, the catch-up rate is very poor. Underimmunized persons and those who are behind

schedule in their immunizations place themselves and others at risk for a given disease.

Z30   Encounter for contraceptive management

Category Z30 codes can be used as the first-listed diagnosis when the encounter is solely for purposes related to contraception, such as counseling or prescribing contraception; inserting, removing, and reimplanting an IUD device; and sterilizing or verifying sterilization. Different forms of contraceptives include dermal implants or patches with time-release medication, oral hormones taken daily, and physical barriers, or devices used internally, such as foams, diaphragms, or IUDs.

Z30.2   Encounter for sterilization

This is the principal diagnosis used when a patient comes in to have elective surgery for tubal ligation or vasectomy.

Z31   Encounter for procreative management

Procreative management is the opposite intent of contraceptive management. These codes relate to health care services for the purpose of creating offspring, or the ability to reproduce. The services described with these codes cover fertility testing, genetic testing and counseling, fertility preservation procedures, reversal of sterilization procedures, artificial insemination, and general counsel and advice for procreative management.

Z31.62   Encounter for fertility preservation counseling

Some types of cancer treatment affect the ability to conceive or maintain pregnancy. The infertility that results from treatments may be temporary or permanent and depends upon the kinds of drugs and dosage given, the method of delivery, the type of cancer, the body site being irradiated, and the patient's age and gender. If it may be possible to preserve fertility, patients are advised to talk with a specialist to review options such as different types of treatment; conceiving before treatment; banking tissue such as sperm, eggs, or embryos prior to treatment; or surgical modification to preserve the uterus.

Note: The use of this code is not limited to patients seeking fertility preservation advice prior to cancer treatment only. Assign this code for individuals seeking advice prior to other kinds of treatment that could also affect fertility, such as gonad removal.

Z31.84   Encounter for fertility preservation procedure

Assign this code when the purpose of the healthcare encounter is to perform a procedure, such as removing sperm or eggs for banking, in order to preserve fertility before a patient undergoes treatment (chemotherapy, removal of gonads) that may affect his or her ability to conceive or carry a pregnancy.

Z34   Encounter for supervision of normal pregnancy

A pregnancy can only be considered 'normal' when there is no problem or condition present that complicates the maternal state. When such a condition is present, the appropriate code(s) are reported from the pregnancy, childbirth, and puerperium chapter.

Note: Supervision codes for normal pregnancy are only used as the principal-listed code, generally in outpatient settings, when a visit is made for routine care or supervision during a first-time, or other normal pregnancy. These codes cannot be used or assigned in addition to any other pregnancy codes.

Z36   Encounter for antenatal screening of mother

Antenatal screening of the mother is done to help identify potential increased risks to the fetus' or mother's health prenatally. Alpha-fetoprotein (AFP) is a normal protein derived from the fetus that passes into the amniotic fluid, but can also be detected in maternal blood serum in concentrations much less than in the amniotic fluid. Raised levels of alpha-fetoprotein in maternal serum during the second trimester have been found to be a marker of placental dysfunction and an indicator of increased risk of unexplained stillbirth. Raised AFP levels are also a useful prenatal diagnosis tool for other fetal malformations, Down syndrome, open neural tube defects, spina bifida, anencephaly, and threatened abortion.

Antenatal screening of the mother may also help identify potential increased risks to the fetus' or mother's health from isoimmunization. This is incompatibility of blood groups and protein types between the mother and fetus. When a woman is Rh negative, she does not have a certain protein on the surface of her red blood cells (RBCs). An Rh positive fetus does have the protein and this creates a blood type incompatibility. The mother's immune system recognizes the baby's Rh positive RBCs as a foreign invader and begins producing antibodies against the baby's blood cells. This does not usually cause a problem in the first pregnancy, but will attack subsequent pregnancies and can result in jaundice, anemia, and retardation. In severe cases, hemolytic disease of the newborn develops and causes death in utero or shortly after birth.

Note: Isoimmunization that is currently affecting the management of the pregnant mother is reported in category O36.

Note: This code is used when the purpose of the visit is solely to conduct the screening test. Fetal conditions that are already suspected and looked for, but ruled out, are reported to subcategory Z03.7-.

Z37   Outcome of delivery

These codes are intended to be assigned on the mother's record for the delivery admission. Do not report Z37 codes on the newborn's record. These codes will show on the mother's chart whether the birth was single, twin, or multiple, and whether the birth(s) resulted in live or stillborn infant(s).

Z39   Encounter for maternal postpartum care and examination

The postpartum period begins immediately after birth and lasts for six weeks. These codes are used as a principal diagnosis, usually in an outpatient setting, when care or follow-up during the postpartum period is done for routine care or supervision in uncomplicated cases. If any postpartum complications are present, the appropriate codes from the pregnancy, childbirth, and puerperium chapter must be reported.

Z39.0   Encounter for care and examination of mother immediately after delivery

This code would be assigned when a woman has delivered outside of the hospital and is then admitted directly to a facility for care in an uncomplicated case.

Z43   Encounter for attention to artificial openings

Artificial openings are surgically created passageways from a site inside the body out to the skin surface. This includes stomas as well as an artificially created vagina. Stomas are created to provide an alternative site for certain key bodily functions, through a direct connection to an external surface, such as breathing through a tracheostomy or expelling fecal matter through a colostomy.

Note: Z43 codes are appropriate as the first-listed diagnosis when the encounter is for removing a catheter from the stoma; closing the stoma; checking patency, such as by passing a sound or bougie; or reforming or cleansing the stoma. Complications that need attention because of the stoma, or reporting the status only when no care is required are coded elsewhere.

Z44   Encounter for fitting and adjustment of external prosthetic device

A prosthetic device serves as a replacement for a missing body part. The need for such a device to be properly seated or fitted may require a health care visit, even if an adjustment to a previously fitted prosthetic is all that's necessary.

Z45.42   Encounter for adjustment and management of neuropacemaker (brain) (peripheral nerve) (spinal cord)

A neuropacemaker of the brain is an implanted electrode that may be placed in the basal ganglia of the brain to treat movement disorders such

as Parkinson's, dystonia, essential tremor, spasticity, Tourette's syndrome, myoclonus, and other disorders with deep brain stimulation. The electrode emits continuous, high-frequency electrical pulses and builds up a field of stimulation in the brain. A lead connects the electrode to the pacemaker battery under the skin near the collar bone. A neuropacemaker device may be placed in the spinal cord for neurostimulation therapy to manage chronic, intractable pain in the trunk, arms, or legs.

Z46.51   Encounter for fitting and adjustment of gastric lap band

A gastric lap band is a device used in bariatric surgery to treat obesity. The band is a restrictive device that functions as an inflatable silicone prosthesis placed around the top part of the stomach to reduce its size and restrict food intake without surgical removal of any part of the stomach. The temporary reduction in size and allowable food intake results in weight loss. A port is inserted to let the patient self-adjust the band. Occasionally, however, the device needs to be adjusted professionally to achieve optimal restriction of intake while still assuring the right nutrition, especially when the patient is pregnant. This kind of adjustment is best done in a physician office.

Z46.81   Encounter for fitting and adjustment of insulin pump

Insulin pumps are devices worn continuously outside the body with an implantable tube in the subcutaneous tissue. The device holds a reservoir of insulin, which is delivered before meals, and maintained throughout the day, as an alternative to daily injections.

Z47.3   Aftercare following explantation of joint prosthesis

Codes in this category are used for aftercare following the surgical removal of a joint prosthesis, including a staged procedure. This code also includes an encounter for joint prosthesis insertion following the prior surgical removal of the joint prosthesis.

Z49.31   Encounter for adequacy testing for hemodialysis

Hemodialysis is a mechanical means of removing waste products from the blood when the kidneys are not able to perform their function. The blood flows on a circuit outside the body through a special filter, or dialyzer, that contains a dialysate, or dialysis solution, in one section and blood flowing through the other section. The two sections are separated by a semipermeable membrane that allows excess water and waste, but not blood cells, to pass through it. The dialysate is a mixture of pure water, electrolytes, and salts, like bicarbonate and sodium that pulls toxins from the blood into the dialysate through diffusion. Since the concentration of toxins and wastes is much higher in the blood, they diffuse across the membrane into the dialysate seeking to equalize the concentration. The dialysate and waste is flushed away and clean blood is returned to the body. This code reports an encounter to test the adequacy of the procedure in clearing the blood.

Z49.32   Encounter for adequacy testing for peritoneal dialysis

Peritoneal dialysis is another method of removing waste products from the blood, used to treat end stage renal disease. It allows for the process to be done at home and uses the peritoneum that lines the patient's abdomen as the membrane for performing filtration. The dialysate is put into the patient's abdomen through a special peritoneal dialysis catheter. The cleansing solution pulls the waste and excess fluid from the blood into the peritoneal cavity. This solution remains in the abdomen for a certain dwell time before being drained and replaced with fresh solution to cleanse the blood. This code reports an encounter to test the adequacy of the procedure in clearing the blood, such as a peritoneal equilibration test that tests the transport function of the peritoneal membrane. Solute transport rates are assessed via the rates of equilibration between the blood in the capillaries of the peritoneum and the dialysate. The ratio of solute concentration in the dialysate vs the plasma at specific dwell times determines the equilibration ratio, which can be calculated for any solute, such as urea, phosphate, electrolyes, proteins, and creatinine, that is transported from the capillary blood into the dialysate.

Z51.11   Encounter for antineoplastic chemotherapy

Antineoplastic chemotherapy is the treatment of malignancy using chemicals introduced into the body that are toxic to cells, particularly the cancerous ones growing out of control.

Z51.12   Encounter for antineoplastic immunotherapy

Antineoplastic immunotherapy is a biological treatment to stimulate the body's own immune system to reject and attack those cells responsible for the cancer. The immune system is either trained to recognize the malignant cells as targets to be destroyed, or put into action to destroy tumor cells through therapeutic antibodies.

Z51.5   Encounter for palliative care

Palliative care is given to patients with a terminal condition and is intended to make the patient as comfortable as possible and not to treat the illness. This may be known as hospice care, end-of-life care, or terminal illness care.

Z51.81   Encounter for therapeutic drug level monitoring

Encounters for lab testing to monitor therapeutic drug levels in blood are necessary with the use of some drugs, particularly those with a small therapeutic window and those that present potential health hazards upon discontinuance.

Note: Use this code as the principal diagnosis in conjunction with a code(s) to identify any long term current use of the specific type of drug(s).

Z51.89   Encounter for other specified aftercare

An encounter for prophylactic or protective isolation may be necessary for two reasons. A patient may need to be removed from his or her own surroundings to protect the individual and provide a safe environment. A person may need to be separated from others to prevent the spread of a harmful and highly contagious disease after the individual has been exposed. Patients who are elderly, immunocompromised, already suffering an illness, or have had indwelling devices implanted are at higher risk for serious infection. In these cases, prophylactic isolation may also be necessary to protect the patient and others. An encounter for allergic desensitization is done by slowly exposing the patient to an allergen in incremental doses over a period of time to improve immunity and prevent dangerous, severe allergic reactions.

Z52   Donors of organs and tissues

These codes identify the type of tissue or organ that a donor is giving for transplantation into another patient, as well as the type of blood donor, and egg recipient. These codes are listed first in situations where the sole reason for the admission or encounter is to donate organ or tissue.

Note: An encounter to examine a potential donor is reported with Z00.5.

Z56   Problems related to employment and unemployment

This category is used to report when a person has problems or difficulties affecting his or her physical and/or mental health and well-being which are related to the work environment and work schedule. A person may be working in an unsuitable career, experiencing physical or mental strain at work, dealing with difficult conditions or a dangerous environment in the workplace, the stress of an odd or irregular schedule, or disharmonious or hostile interactions with the boss or colleagues.

Z59   Problems related to housing and economic circumstances

Housing and economic circumstances play a role in receiving or carrying out effective care. Reasons that may pose a problem for the patient include a lack of proper housing, not enough financial resources, or a lack of adequate food and safe drinking water.

Z65.5   Exposure to disaster, war and other hostilities

A soldier who has returned from active military duty may experience both physical and psychological problems related to the deployment. Medical issues which arise from this history need to be monitored for all individuals coping with the effects of their deployment, whether they are military personnel, federal civilian employee, or contract worker serving among the non-military in areas of armed conflict. Tracking this history will also help in learning whether there is any increase in diseases or conditions among those who served in military deployment arenas.

Note: This code does not pertain only to military personnel, but civilians who have also experienced war zones, war torn areas, natural disasters, or other cultural, ethnic, or racial hostilities.

Z66   Do not resuscitate

The care and services that a patient receives during a particular encounter may be different from the normal choices for care that would otherwise be the case when the patient has an order of 'do not resuscitate' in the chart.

Z68   Body mass index [BMI]

Body Mass Index (BMI) is a measurement of height and weight that is used to assess the total proportion of fat in the body. BMI is not however a direct measure of body fat. BMI is calculated by the following formula: (Weight in pounds x 703) divided by (height in inches squared); or (weight in kilograms) divided by (height in meters squared).

Z68.4   Body mass index (BMI) 40 or greater, adult

A BMI of 40 or greater is considered morbidly obese. BMI does not measure body fat directly but does correlate with direct measures that can be made of body fat, such as underwater weighing and bioelectrical impedance, among others. The CDC uses BMI 40 and over to assess morbid obesity in the population. Morbid obesity is the point where so much body fat has built up that it has an adverse effect on health leading to a reduced life expectancy, particularly from diseases such as diabetes, hypertension, heart disease, breathing failures during sleep, and cancer. Obesity is one of the most serious health problems of the 21st century and the leading cause of preventable death.

Z74.2   Need for assistance at home and no other household member able to render care

This circumstance includes when the home care-giver is temporarily away from the residence, or when the patient's only family member residing at home is too handicapped, ill, or otherwise incapable of providing the patient with care.

Z75.5   Holiday relief care

Holiday care reports institutional or facility care given to one who is usually cared for at home, when the caregiver takes a vacation.

Z76.2   Encounter for health supervision and care of other healthy infant and child

A healthy child or infant receiving care may include medical or nursing supervision in many different types of circumstances. For instance, an encounter for care of a healthy infant or child may be necessary when the mother is ill or has physical or psychiatric disabilities; when the conditions at home are adverse to maintaining proper care of the infant continually; or when there are too many children at home which prevents or interferes with normal care required by the infant.

Z77.011   Contact with and (suspected) exposure to lead

Lead is a metallic element that is purely toxic. Whereas other heavy metals, such as molybdenum, manganese, chromium, nickel, and selenium are actually required nutrients at low levels and become toxic at higher doses, lead is entirely toxic. No safe level of exposure to lead has been found. Even small doses lead to health problems. It particularly affects the central nervous system, the production of red blood cells, and vital organ functioning, such as of the liver and kidneys. Lead is transported by the bloodstream and is stored, even for decades, in the bones.

Factors Influencing Health Status

Z51.11 – Z77.011

Z77.012 Contact with and (suspected) exposure to uranium

Uranium occurs naturally in low levels on the earth within rock, soil, and water. Because uranium forms highly soluble complexes in an alkaline environment, it leads to increased leeching to groundwater and soil from the making, testing, or depletion of nuclear weapons, mining, ore processing, and phosphate fertilizer production. Humans are exposed mainly by inhaling dust or ingesting contaminated water and food. Insoluble uranium compounds ingested via the lungs or entering the bloodstream accumulate in tissue, such as bone due to its phosphate affinity, and remain for many years. The uranium compounds damage organs such as the kidneys, liver, heart, and brain, as well as the functioning of entire systems such as the reproductive and immune systems. Uranium itself is only weakly radioactive and alpha particles emitted are not absorbed by the skin but its radioactive decay products, such as radon, pose significant health threats.

Z77.090 Contact with and (suspected) exposure to asbestos

Asbestos is naturally occurring fiber-like minerals that can be separated and woven as very fine threads. It has been used for many years in products like cement, brake linings, roof shingles, and insulation. Asbestos is not dangerous until it is broken up and the tiny air-borne fibers are inhaled or swallowed. Exposure to asbestos causes side effects of shortness of breath, coughing, and permanent lung damage. Diseases caused by asbestos include asbestosis—chronic inflammation and scar tissue from the fibers inbedded in the lungs that cannot be expelled or destroyed by the body; lung cancer; mesothelioma—a rare cancer in the lining of the chest and abdomen; and other cancers of the throat, gastrointestinal tract, and kidneys.

Z77.121 Contact with and (suspected) exposure to harmful algae and algae toxins

Blue-green algae, also known as pond scum, are actually cyanobacteria--photosynthetic bacteria that live in lakes, ponds, and slow-moving streams that have warm water enriched with nutrients like phosphorus and nitrogen. Most species are buoyant and float on the top, forming scum layers, or mats, known as blue-green algae bloom. Certain species produce chemical compounds in their cells that are toxic. The toxins are released when the cells are broken open. Exposure to these neurotoxins produces stomach cramps, headache, fever, diarrhea, vomiting, muscle weakness, and difficulty breathing.

Note: This code identifies the possible contact with algae bloom for a person who has been in the vicinity but has not developed suspicious symptoms.

Z77.21 Contact with and (suspected) exposure to potentially hazardous body fluids

Potentially hazardous body fluids (blood, serum, cerebrospinal fluid, urine, semen, other exudates) are any that harbor an infectious disease such as hepatitis, human immunodeficiency virus, etc., that could potentially be transmitted to another and contracted through contact with the infected fluid.

Z79 Long term (current) drug therapy

Long-term current drug use codes note specific kinds of medications that a patient has been accustomed to taking for an extended period of time and is still currently using. The use of some medications may potentially present inherent health hazards that need to be carefully monitored, or create health hazards upon discontinuance.

Note: These codes include long term current drug use as a prophylactic approach.

Note: Encounters for lab tests to monitor therapeutic blood levels are necessary with the use of some drugs. Use these codes with Z51.81 Encounter for therapeutic drug level monitoring to note such cases.

Z79.81 Long term (current) use of agents affecting estrogen receptors and estrogen levels

When a tumor tests positive for estrogen receptors (ER+), the levels of estrogen in the body have a significant effect on the growth of the tumor. The hormone binds to its receptor protein on the tumor cells and stimulates growth. This type of cancer may stop growing when treated with a drug that blocks estrogen from binding, called selective estrogen receptor modulators (SERMS). Some drugs used to treat ER+ cancers do not act as blocking agents to prevent hormone binding to the receptors, but work to reduce estrogen levels present in the body, called aromatase inhibitors.

Note: These drugs are also used both to prevent a recurrence of a treated malignant neoplasm and to prevent the metastasis of a malignancy still currently under treatment.

Note: The agents reported here exclude hormone replacement therapies. The prophylactic use of these agents as a preventative measure before malignancy appears; following completed treatment for a malignancy; or with a current malignant neoplasm means Z79.81- codes are used in addition to a current malignant neoplasm diagnosis code, or they may be reported with additional codes to identify the family or personal history of cancer, or the genetic susceptibility to cancer. Additional Z17 codes are also appropriate for estrogen receptor positive status with current breast malignancy.

Z79.83 Long term (current) use of bisphosphonates

Long term use of bisphosphonates carries a significant risk of bone-related problems. Fractures of the subtrochanteric region or shaft of the femur are a common result. The fractures are pathological and/or stress related, such as occur with osteoporosis or altered mineral metabolism. These type of breaks are considered atypical and may be complete, extending across both cortices, or incomplete with only the lateral cortex involved. There are other distinctive features, such as transverse or short oblique orientation, minimal or no trauma, lack of comminution, and a few others. The long-term use of bisphosphonates is also related to osteonecrosis of the jaw following tooth extraction or minor trauma that exposes the bone. The jaw bone tissue fails to heal and begins to die, particularly in cancer patients who have received bisphosphonates for chemotherapy or osteoporosis patients who have taken oral bisphosphonates.

Z80 Family history of primary malignant neoplasm

A family history of malignant neoplasm makes one more prone through genetics to developing cancer. A known family history of cancer alerts health care providers to the need for vigilant or special screening, or prophylactic measures that should be considered, including surgery to remove the tissue at risk. This is particularly the case where the most common types of cancer are concerned, such as breast, colon, and prostate cancers.

Z82 Family history of certain disabilities and chronic diseases (leading to disablement)

This category includes a family history of stroke, sudden cardiac death, epilepsy and other neurological diseases, deafness, blindness, asthma, arthritis, osteopororsis, and polycystic kidney and other congenital malformations. Many of these diseases are hereditary. When a physician knows there is a family history of these, he or she can order special screening and diagnostic tests, and treat the particular signs, symptoms, or conditions quickly when they first appear.

Z82.41 Family history of sudden cardiac death

This code reports a family history of sudden cardiac death (SCD), also known as sudden cardiac arrest, which results from an unexpected and abrupt cessation of heart function and occurs within minutes of symptoms appearing. All known heart diseases can lead to sudden cardiac death, which usually occurs when the electrical impulses in the diseased heart become too rapid and chaotic. The most common cause is coronary artery disease. The American Heart Association estimates that 90 percent of adult victims of sudden cardiac death have two or more major coronary arteries narrowed by fatty plaque build-up. "Massive heart attack" is often incorrectly used in these cases; however, this refers to the death of heart muscle tissue, or myocardial infarction, from ischemic causes, not necessarily resulting in sudden cardiac arrest or death, although it is possible. Brain death begins in just under 6 minutes of sudden cardiac arrest, which is reversible in most patients if treated with CPR and/or electrical shock to the heart to restore normal rhythm within a few minutes.

Note: This code should not be reported for a family history of MI, myocardial infarction, or ischemic heart disease as this is not the same thing as sudden cardiac death, although it can possibly cause SCD.

Z83   Family history of other specific disorders

This category includes diabetes mellitus, glaucoma, colonic polyps, other endocrine and metabolic diseases such as MEN syndrome, HIV disease, and other blood and immune mechanism disorders. Many of these conditions are hereditary or may have a stronger tendency to occur within a family. When a physician knows there is a family history of these, he or she can order special screening and diagnostic tests, and treat the particular signs, symptoms, or conditions quickly when they first appear.

Z83.41   Family history of multiple endocrine neoplasia [MEN] syndrome

There are three distinct forms of MEN that are identified as inherited disorders and cause a syndrome of polyglandular malfunction. Type I, Werner's syndrome, is characterized by hyperplasia or tumors of the parathyroid, the pancreatic islet cells, and the pituitary gland. Type IIA, Sipple's syndrome, is characterized by a triad of medullary carcinoma of the thyroid, adrenal gland tumor, and hyperplasia of the parathyroid gland. Type IIB is similar to IIA but has mucosal neuromas without parathyroid involvement.

Z83.511   Family history of glaucoma

Glaucoma is known as the silent thief of sight as it causes gradual loss in vision that may not be detected until it's too late. Heredity plays a big role in this devastating disease. Although anyone is at risk, those with a family history of glaucoma have a greater chance of also developing the disease. There are several types of glaucoma. Open angle glaucoma is the most common with heredity being the most common factor. Pressure builds up in the eye and blocks the drainage canals that allow acqueous humor to flow out of the eye. This increased pressure damages the optic nerve and vision deteriorates, fades, and leads to blindness.

Z83.71   Family history of colonic polyps

Colonic polyps are overgrowths of mucosa that project out from the lining of the colon into the lumen of the bowel. Polyps are not immediately harmful but are considered a precursor to colon cancer. Polyps may occur in anyone, but those with a history are much more likely to develop them. Anyone with a personal or family history of colonic polyps should have regular exams. Sigmoidoscopy or colonoscopy is done with biopsies and polypectomy to remove them before they become cancerous.

Z84.3   Family history of consanguinity

Consanguinity means having the same blood or being of the same family lineage as another person. Reproduction with someone who has a close degree of consanguinity always elevates the risk of genetic defects and problems. Increased genetic diseases and anomalies occur with histories of inbreeding.

Z85   Personal history of malignant neoplasm

These codes are used as supplementary codes to identify specific malignancies with which a patient has been diagnosed in the past. The cancer has been previously treated or removed, and the disease is no longer evident, nor is the patient undergoing current treatment for it. Personal history of malignancy codes may indicate the need for adjunctive or prophylactic treatment, or special screening.

Z85.020   Personal history of malignant carcinoid tumor of stomach

Malignant carcinoid tumors are the most common form of malignant neuroendocrine tumors that arise from hormone-producing cells throughout the body and are grouped according to their embryonic site of origin in the fore-, mid-, or hindgut. The majority of these type of tumors occur in the appendix, small bowel, stomach, and duodenum. They are very slow-growing tumors that act benignly in the early stages, often with no symptoms, then turn malignant. Metastasis depends on the size of the primary tumor: those under 1 cm rarely metastasize, while those over 2 cm frequently metastasize to cause secondary tumors.

Z85.030   Personal history of malignant carcinoid tumor of large intestine

Malignant carcinoid tumors are the most common form of malignant neuroendocrine tumors that arise from hormone-producing cells throughout the body and are grouped according to their embryonic site of origin in the fore-, mid-, or hindgut. The majority of these type of tumors occur in the appendix, small bowel, stomach, and duodenum. They are very slow-growing tumors that act benignly in the early stages, often with no symptoms, then turn malignant. Metastasis depends on the size of the primary tumor: those under 1cm rarely metastasize, while those over 2 cm frequently metastasize to cause secondary tumors.

Z85.060   Personal history of malignant carcinoid tumor of small intestine

Malignant carcinoid tumors are the most common form of malignant neuroendocrine tumors that arise from hormone-producing cells throughout the body and are grouped according to their embryonic site of origin in the fore-, mid-, or hindgut. The majority of these type of tumors occur in the appendix, small bowel, stomach, and duodenum. They are very slow-growing tumors that act benignly in the early stages, often with no symptoms, then turn malignant. Metastasis depends on the size of the primary tumor: those under 1 cm rarely metastasize, while those over 2 cm frequently metastasize to cause secondary tumors.

Z85.821   Personal history of Merkel cell carcinoma

Merkel cell carcinoma is an aggressive and lethal neuroendocrine cancer of the skin with a mortality rate much higher than that of melanoma. Merkel cells tumors occur mainly in the elderly and do not have a distinctive appearance but grow rapidly as a painless, firm bump that may be flesh-colored, red, or bluish in appearance with overlying skin breaking down.

Z85.828   Personal history of other malignant neoplasm of skin

Personal history of other malignant neoplasms of the skin includes having previously had a basal cell carcinoma or a squamous cell carcinoma. Basal cell carcinomas (BCC) and squamous cell carcinomas (SCC) begin from the keratinocytes or keratin producing cells found in the outer layer of skin and arise most commonly in areas exposed to the sun. Rarely, BCC tumors may develop on nonexposed areas. Basal cell carcinomas begin in the lowest layer of the epidermis where the cells divide and mature into keratinocytes. This type is the most common skin cancer and accounts for about 8 out of 10 skin cancers. They rarely metastasize and are very slow growing, but can damage surrounding tissue, causing destruction or disfigurement when tumors are large or more aggressive. Squamous cell carcinomas (SCC) are the second most common type of skin cancer. Squamous cell carcinomas begin in the cells of the upper layer of the epidermis and in mucous membranes. SCC also arises most commonly from chronically sun-exposed areas but can occur on any area of the body, particularly from burns, scars, areas of chronic inflammation or open sores, and areas exposed to radiation or chemicals like petroleum by-products. These carcinomas typically look like a persistent, thick, rough, scaly patch, a wart-like growth, and a raised growth with central depression, that all occasionally bleed or crust.

Z86.32   Personal history of gestational diabetes

Gestational diabetes develops during pregnancy and affects how the cells utilize glucose for energy, causing high blood sugar that can affect the pregnancy and the health of the baby. For many women, this does not cause significant signs or symptoms, but may cause increased urination and thirst. Blood sugar usually returns to normal after the pregnancy, but those who have had gestational diabetes are at higher risk for developing type 2 diabetes later.

Z86.51 Personal history of combat and operational stress reaction

Army Behavioral Health defines combat and operational stress reaction (COSR) as "expected and predictable emotional, intellectual, physical, and/or behavioral reactions from exposure to stressful event(s)... not restricted to combat operations. These reactions may occur as the result of combat-like conditions that are present throughout the entire spectrum of military operations to include: training, all phases of the deployment cycle, peacekeeping missions, humanitarian missions, stability and reconstruction, and government support missions." This personal history code identifies persons who have once had COSR and are being treated for symptoms that have developed later due to this experience.

Z86.711 Personal history of pulmonary embolism

A pulmonary embolism is a blood clot or thromboembolus that blocks the pulmonary artery from the heart in the left or right branch or at the point where it divides into the left and right main pulmonary arteries, blocking both. The emboli originate in the lower extremity veins and travel through the venous system to the vena cava, through the right atrium and ventricle, into the pulmonary artery. The embolus becomes lodged where the larger vessel divides into smaller ones and there it occludes the pulmonary artery, preventing blood from entering the lungs. It can be life-threatening and result in irreversible effects from ischemia and lack of perfusion. A patient with a history of a pulmonary embolism may also be at risk for the development of future embolisms, particularly in the face of chronic conditions that cause the thrombi to form and then travel.

Z86.73 Personal history of transient ischemic attack (TIA), and cerebral infarction without residual deficits

This code should only be assigned when there are no residual effects from a previous TIA or stroke, or when there is a personal history of prolonged reversible ischemic neurological deficit.

Z86.74 Personal history of sudden cardiac arrest

This code reports a personal history of sudden cardiac arrest that was successfully resuscitated. Sudden cardiac arrest results from an unexpected and abrupt cessation of heart function and occurs within minutes of symptoms appearing. All known heart diseases can lead to sudden cardiac arrest, which usually occurs when the electrical impulses in the diseased heart become too rapid and chaotic. The most common cause is coronary artery disease. The American Heart Association estimates that 90 percent of adult victims of sudden cardiac arrest have two or more major coronary arteries narrowed by fatty plaque build-up. "Massive heart attack" is often incorrectly used in these cases; however, this refers to the death of heart muscle tissue from ischemic causes, not necessarily resulting in sudden cardiac arrest, although it is possible. Brain death begins in just under 6 minutes of cardiac arrest, which is reversible in most patients if treated with CPR and/or electrical shock to the heart to restore normal rhythm within a few minutes.

Z87.31 Personal history of (healed) nontraumatic fracture

Patients with osteoporosis or other bone conditions are very susceptible to pathological fractures. This subcategory identifies those patients who have had a pathologic or stress fracture in the past due to osteoporosis, some other form of bone disease, or repetitive bone stress and overuse, and not trauma. This puts them at risk for future fractures and affects their treatment.

Z87.410 Personal history of cervical dysplasia

Cervical dysplasia is an abnormality in the structure and growth of cells lining the surface of the uterine cervix and can range from a slight irregularity to a full-thickness abnormality. It is also referred to as cervical intraepithelial neoplasia (CIN) and is graded for severity. Some cases, particularly mild cases, may regress on their own and return to normal, but dysplasia is considered a precursor to cancer and can develop into malignancy over time if not properly treated. This code reports when a patient has a (now resolved) history of cervical dysplasia conditions.

Z87.411 Personal history of vaginal dysplasia

Vaginal dysplasia is a condition in which abnormal, dystrophic cell growth is found in the vagina. Although the dystrophic changes in the vaginal epithelium are not considered dangerous, the dysplasia is considered a precursor to cancer. This personal history code identifies persons who have once had vaginal dysplasia.

Z87.412 Personal history of vulvar dysplasia

Vulvar dysplasia is dystrophy of the external female genitalia with abnormal growth of cells on the surface of the skin, most often in the outer labia, considered to be a precancerous condition called vulvar intraepithelial neoplasia (VIN) I and II. VIN I is the first degree of dystrophic cells in the vulva, displaying mild dysplasia with only one third of the epithelial lining having changes. VIN II is moderate vulvar dysplasia with about half the thickness of epithelium affected, showing discolored raised skin lesions. This personal history code identifies persons who have once had VIN I or II.

Z87.7 Personal history of (corrected) congenital malformations

The codes in this subcategory report a personal history of a congenital anomaly that was previously repaired. Many congenital conditions are now being repaired with little or no residual effect, but the history of the anomaly should still be reported. The codes are organized to note anomalies by body system.

Z87.710 Personal history of (corrected) hypospadias

This code reports a personal history of previous hypospadias repair. Hypospadias occurs most commonly in males and manifests as an abnormally placed urethral opening on the bottom of the penis instead of at the tip of the glans.

Z87.718 Personal history of other specified (corrected) congenital malformations of genitourinary system

Congenital anatomic malformations of the genitourinary tract are more common than anomalies in other organ systems. Some of the most common congenital genitourinary malformations that may have a history of surgical correction include obstruction of the ureteropelvic and ureterovesicular junction, and malformed genitalia.

Z87.721 Personal history of (corrected) congenital malformations of ear

Corrected congenital malformations of the ear includes corrected absence of the external ear, microtia, and accessory auricle.

Z87.738 Personal history of other specified (corrected) congenital malformations of digestive system

Other specified corrected congenital malformations of the digestive system may include tracheo-esophageal fistula, omphalocele, hypertrophic pyloric stenosis, congenital hiatal hernia, esophageal stenosis or stricture, imperforate or webbed esophagus, and atresia and stenosis of intestines, rectum, or anal canal.

Z87.74 Personal history of (corrected) congenital malformations of heart and circulatory system

Corrected congenital malformations of the heart and circulatory system may include transposition of the great vessels, tetralogy of Fallot, atrial or ventricular septal defects, endocardial cushion defects, anomalous pulmonary venous connections, anomalies of the peripheral vascular system, and congenital aneurysms.

Z87.75 Personal history of (corrected) congenital malformations of respiratory system

Corrected congenital malformations of the respiratory system may include choanal atresia, and atresia and other anomalies of the larynx, trachea, or bronchus.

Z87.76   Personal history of (corrected) congenital malformations of integument, limbs and musculoskeletal system

Corrected congenital malformations of integument, limbs, and musculoskeletal system may include club foot, congenital dislocation of hip, syndactyly, and vascular hamartoses or port-wine stains.

Z87.790   Personal history of (corrected) congenital malformations of face and neck

Corrected congenital malformations of the face and neck includes corrected absence of the external nose, an accessory nose, nasal deformities, webbing of the neck, and branchial cleft sinus or fistula.

Z87.820   Personal history of traumatic brain injury

Traumatic brain injury occurs in many different ways - with intracranial injuries such as concussion, contusion, and subarachnoid hemorrhage, or with skull fractures occurring with or without open intracranial wound. Neurological manifestations can develop later at different time periods as late effects. Each person's injury manifests in different ways. When a person has a history of traumatic brain injury, late effect manifestations, or sequelae, may remain for years or not even appear until years later.

Z87.821   Personal history of retained foreign body fully removed

Any embedded foreign object carries a potential for infection, not only due to the presence of the fragment itself, but also due to any bacteria that were present on the object when it entered the body. Some may pose longer-term health risks or toxic hazards, such as lead or certain metal alloys, like tungsten. This code is to be used as a status code that identifies potential health hazards associated with having had an embedded foreign body that is now completely removed.

Z87.892   Personal history of anaphylaxis

Anaphylactic reactions are an immediate type I hypersensitivity reaction elicited very rapidly after exposure to the causative antigen. Antibodies in the blood react to the initial introduction of an antigen and induce the synthesis of immunoglobulins that bind to specific receptors on the surface of circulating mast cells. The next time that same, specific antigen is introduced, it reacts with the immunoglobulins on the mast cells and induces them to release large amounts of histamine and other chemicals that cause the familiar reactions of bronchoconstriction, smooth muscle contraction, and vasodilation with wheezing, hives, itching, nausea, vomiting, a weak pulse, rapid heartbeat, pallor, dizziness, and swelling in the throat and tongue that can interfere with breathing and can become life-threatening. A patient with a history of a previous anaphylactic reaction is at risk for another each time contact is made with the original causative antigen.

Z88   Allergy status to drugs, medicaments and biological substances

An allergy is a disorder of the immune system manifesting with a hypersensitivity reaction after the body is exposed to substances called allergens. Symptoms of an allergic reaction include rashes, welts, or hives on the skin; itching; wheezing or difficulty breathing; swelling, particularly of the lips, face, and tongue; and a rapid pulse. Allergic reactions to drugs or medicinal agents can be dangerous or life threatening. An allergic reaction may not happen the first time a person is exposed to a particular drug, but as the body builds antibodies against the allergen, a subsequent exposure will cause a reaction. When a patient is known to have a particular drug allergy status, measures can be taken to avoid exposure and reduce the risk of dangerous reactions. Once a person has had an allergic reaction to a medicinal agent, he or she is always considered allergic to that substance.

Z89.23   Acquired absence of shoulder

Codes in this subcategory are used to denote the status of a patient who has had a shoulder joint prosthesis surgically removed, with or without placement of an antibiotic-impregnated cement spacer. These status codes reflect the reason for the absent joint as specifically due to previous prosthetic joint removal as opposed to other clinical reasons, such as

trauma, neoplasm, or infection that may cause the acquired destruction of a joint.

Z89.52   Acquired absence of knee

Codes in this subcategory are used to denote the status of a patient who has had a knee joint prosthesis surgically removed, with or without placement of an antibiotic-impregnated cement spacer. These status codes reflect the reason for the absent knee as specifically due to previous prosthetic joint removal as opposed to other clinical reasons, such as trauma, neoplasm, or infection that may cause the acquired destruction of a joint.

Z89.62   Acquired absence of hip

Codes in this subcategory are used to denote the status of a patient who has had a hip joint prosthesis surgically removed, with or without placement of an antibiotic-impregnated cement spacer. These status codes reflect the reason for the absent joint as specifically due to previous prosthetic joint removal or disarticulation that has occurred at the hip level as opposed to other clinical reasons, such as trauma, neoplasm, or infection that may cause the acquired destruction of a joint.

Z90.410   Acquired total absence of pancreas

Completely removing the pancreas is used as treatment for cancers, chronic pancreatitis, extensive neuroendocrine tumors, and for those with a family history of pancreatic cancer and premalignant lesions. Total absence of the pancreas requires special management, such as autologous islet cell transplantation, and glucagon-rescue therapy with dependence on long-acting insulin formulations to counter life-threatening risks from the lack of pancreatic hormones, particularly insulin.

Z90.411   Acquired partial absence of pancreas

Endocrine cells make up about 5% of pancreatic mass and are found scattered throughout the pancreas in clusters called 'islets.' Specialized cells within the islets produce their specific pancreatic hormone. Because of the small mass and distribution of these islets of specialized cells, diabetes does not usually ensue until after the pancreas has been removed at more than 60%, sometimes up to 90%. Once the pancreas fails to produce sufficient amounts of its endocrine hormones, the resulting deficiencies in insulin and glucagon production cause problems with blood sugar regulation, fluid and salt balance, and digestion. Replacement therapy is then necessary.

Z91.041   Radiographic dye allergy status

Reporting when a patient has an allergy to contrast media used in diagnostic radiography is important not only for alerting care givers that exposure to this allergen should be avoided for the patient's health and safety, but also serves to justify the need medically for using a different contrast, such as low osmolar contrast, which may be more expensive.

Z91.15   Patient's noncompliance with renal dialysis

When a person requires renal dialysis to filter and clean the blood as a mechanical replacement for kidney function and the person is noncompliant with scheduled treatments, the risk of fluid overload and chronic kidney disease complications increases dramatically.

Z91.83   Wandering in diseases classified elsewhere

Most patients with dementia will have behavioral disturbances at some point, which includes wandering off, hoarding, aggressiveness, sexual disinhibitions, screaming or incessant vocalizations, perseveration on bathroom activities, attention seeking, and combative or violent behavior that puts patients and others in danger. Wandering off is a common behavioral problem that refers to the urge to walk about and leave home. This may be unpredictable or a warning sign that the patient needs stimulation, exercise, mobility, and more social contact. Wandering often occurs when a person walks about their own familiar environment but then cannot find their way back, or if a person feels confused, threatened, or over-stimulated in their environment. Persons also wander off who are bored, in pain, have excess energy, or were used to going for walks habitually. Wandering poses a challenge for the dementia patient's safety and wellbeing and is reported separately in addition to the code for dementia with behavioral disturbances.

Factors Influencing Health Status

Z87.76 – Z91.83

Z92.23 Personal history of estrogen therapy

Estrogen therapy is used to treat certain conditions like delayed onset of puberty, menopausal symptoms, vaginal atrophy, irregular menstrual cycles, and reproductive and endocrine disorders. The risks of hormone therapy depend upon the woman's age or the years since menopause. The effects of having estrogen therapy include the potential for dangerous blood clots, high blood pressure, and blood sugar abnormalities. Other harmful side effects include the worsening of estrogen-dependent conditions like uterine fibroids and endometriosis as well as estrogen receptive breast cancers and endometrial (uterine) cancer.

Z92.240 Personal history of inhaled steroid therapy

Inhaled steroid therapy is used to treat asthma and COPD. Treatment with topical, inhaled, steroid administration can cause a condition referred to as steroid inhaler laryngitis, a chemical-induced laryngopharyngitis. The laryngitis manifests with dysphonia and other laryngeal findings that range from mucosal edema, leukoplakia, and granulation, to laryngopharyngeal reflux and infectious disease processes like candidiasis.

Z92.241 Personal history of systemic steroid therapy

Systemic steroids are those taken by mouth or given by injection and are prescribed for a large number of serious diseases. Excessive use can cause Cushing's syndrome. The skin also becomes prone to many adverse reactions from prolonged use, such as bacterial and fungal infections, purpura (easy bruising), stretch marks, and subcutaneous atrophy, or a loss of fat under the skin. Other adverse side effects from prolonged use of more than a month include: reduction of natural cortisol production, causing lack of response to stress, trauma, or infection; osteoporosis; muscle weakness; increased circulation of triglycerides; diabetes mellitus; salt retention; shaking and tremors; glaucoma; headaches and raised intracranial pressure; and even psychological effects.

Note: A history of systemic steroid therapy includes the use of prednisone, prednisolone, methylprednisolone, betamethasone, dexamethasone, triamcinolone, and hydrocortisone.

Z92.25 Personal history of immunosupression therapy

Immunosuppressive drugs inhibit or prevent the normal activity and functioning of the immune system. They are used to treat against rejection of transplanted organs and for autoimmune diseases like rheumatoid arthritis, multiple sclerosis, systemic lupus erythematosus, pemphigus, and ulcerative colitis. Side effects of using immunosuppression drugs include hypertension, hyperglycemia, peptic ulcers, dyslipidemia, and liver and kidney injury besides the lack of ability to fight off infection or the spread of malignant cells.

Z92.82 Status post administration of tPA (rtPA) in a different facility within the last 24 hours prior to admission to current facility

Tissue plasminogen activator is approved as a treatment for acute stroke and myocardial infarction victims when started as soon as possible, within the first three hours. Giving tPA immediately maximizes its benefits. Small suburban or rural hospitals that do not have a system capable of handling the complications that may arise with lytic therapy for stroke cases will transfer patients from the emergency department to another facility after initiating IV tPA therapy. The status reported with this code is a critical factor in assessing the resources used in the US health care system for acute stroke.

Z92.83 Personal history of failed moderate sedation

When moderate conscious sedation is inadequate, the procedure is made much more difficult and unpleasant. Unsafe conditions result. Urgent intervention, particularly from someone trained to administer adequate moderate sedation, deep sedation, and/or anesthesia, becomes necessary. Failed moderate sedation includes times when the maximum amount of prudent and safe doses are given, but the patient remains inadequately sedated; the patient reacts idiosyncratically to the medication and becomes more deeply sedated than planned; the patient becomes unable to maintain a patent airway and has depressed respirations that compromise adequate air exchange; or other hemodynamic changes occur that pose potential risks. When failed sedation has occurred in a previous procedure as is reported with this code, it is necessary to make planned interventions for subsequent procedures.

Z98.85 Transplanted organ removal status

An existing transplant may develop many kinds of complications, including failure, rejection, and infection. In some cases, it becomes necessary to remove the transplanted organ. Patients may now receive more than one transplant in a lifetime. When an existing transplant needs to be removed, it may be some time before a new transplant becomes available. This code is used to mark the status of a patient who has had a previous transplant now removed.

Note: When the patient encounter is specifically for the surgical removal of the transplanted organ, code the complication of the transplant.

Z99.2 Dependence on renal dialysis

Use this code to denote when a patient requires any kind of renal dialysis, whether peritoneal or hemodialysis, even if intermittently required. This status code also reports that a patient has an arteriovenous shunt in place for the purpose of renal dialysis.

Z99.3 Dependence on wheelchair

People bound to a wheelchair have an increased risk of acquiring a variety of medical problems such as infections and pressure ulcers.

Note: The causative condition that results in wheelchair dependence, such as morbid obesity or muscular dystrophy, should be coded first.